**Here's what they're saying about
Jesse and the book:**

"George Foreman gave me great advice. When I told him my husband ran 100 miles nonstop he said, 'Sara, don't try to understand a man like that. Just love him.'"

—Sara Blakely, founder of Spanx, and Jesse's wife

"Most of us go through life on autopilot. New day...same routine. This guy beamed a 'live action hero' into his living room for 31 days to shake up his life. Sometimes you have to have the guts to do something radical to get results."

—Dolvett Quince, health and fitness trainer,
The Biggest Loser

"The relationship between these guys is outrageous...But with all the insanity there are strong life messages, hysterical moments, and great lessons to be learned. Like Jesse, this book is a HIT!"

—Jake Steinfeld, chairman and founder
of Body by Jake

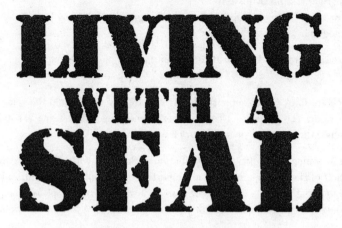

LIVING
WITH A
SEAL

31 DAYS TRAINING WITH THE
TOUGHEST MAN ON THE PLANET

JESSE ITZLER

CENTER STREET

New York Boston Nashville

Center Street
Hachette Book Group
1290 Avenue of the Americas, New York, NY 10104
centerstreet.com
twitter.com/centerstreet

Originally published in hardcover and ebook by Center Street in November
2015
First trade paperback edition: November 2016

Center Street is a division of Hachette Book Group, Inc. The Center Street
name and logo are trademarks of Hachette Book Group, Inc.

The publisher is not responsible for websites (or their content) that are not
owned by the publisher.

The Hachette Speakers Bureau provides a wide range of authors for speaking
events. To find out more, go to www.HachetteSpeakersBureau.com or call
(866) 376-6591.

LCCN: 2015028519

ISBN: 978-1-4555-3468-5 (trade pbk.)

Printed in the United States of America

LSC-C

10 9

This book is dedicated to my mom and dad, who have been at every game, every event, and every BIG moment in my life. Also, to my wife, who continues to teach me about unwavering support and love. Plus, she has the patience to put up with me.

Disclaimer

The events of this book have been re-created from memory and in some cases have been compressed to convey the substance of what occurred or was said. I tried to keep the time sequence of my experiences in order, but it's possible that events occurred either earlier or later in reality than they do in this story. Although every workout written is true and happened, it's important to note, I'm not recommending you do or try any of the workouts in this book. First off, I don't want anyone to get hurt. Second, who wants to get sued?

Like any activity involving speed, equipment, endurance, and environmental factors, the workouts described in *Living with a SEAL* pose some very serious risks. All readers should take full responsibility for their safety and know their limits. As a trainer, SEAL knew his stuff, and he factored into every single one of his workouts my level of experience, aptitude, training—and how much I could handle.

I kept a detailed diary during my time living with SEAL, which instantly became a blog. It was primarily for friends and family, but as the insanity of my workouts grew, so did my audience. The result is this book.

You will notice in the following pages that the person with whom I trained is referred to only as "SEAL." He asked that I not disclose his name. And he didn't say please.

Contents

Introduction

People ask me why I hired SEAL. One answer is this: When it comes to physical fitness, I tend to be a creature of habit. I guess compared to most people my age, I was in excellent shape and in a great place in my personal life. At the time I was married (still am) to a fantastic woman, and we had our first beautiful eighteen-month-old son (two more since). I began running in 1992, just after I graduated from college. I've missed maybe a handful of days since. I've run eighteen New York City marathons in a row, and it's been the same drill every year. Training schedule—the same. Running route—the same. The store I buy bananas from the day before the race—the same. The Patsy's pizza I order the night before each race—the same.

I like routine.

And routine can be good, especially when it comes to working out. But routine can also be a rut.

Many of us live our lives on autopilot. We do the same thing every day; wake up, go to work, come home, have dinner. Repeat. I found myself drifting in that direction. It was as if my cruise control settings had been set and I wasn't improving. I wanted to get off it; I wanted to shake things up in a big way. My Central Park West life and SEAL's nomadic take-no-prisoners life merging (or I should say, colliding) for a period of time was what I needed. It was unexpected, it was unique. It was insane (okay, I admit it), but research shows that stepping out of our routine in life is great for the body and spirit...the brain too. Mix it up! Do the outrageous; think out of the box. Life is short, why not? As SEAL says, "This ain't a dress rehearsal, bitch."

While this is a story about our month together, it's just as much a story about two people that had to step outside of their comfort zones. SEAL and me. He was as uncomfortable with doormen, chefs, and drivers as I was with sleeping in a chair and intentionally waking up in the middle of the night to run in the worst possible conditions. His no rhyme or reason approach to our workout schedule actually brought a lot of clarity into my life.

SEAL had something I wanted, but I just wasn't sure what it was. And I wanted to find out. Do you remember Mr. Miyagi from *The Karate Kid*? He had a very unorthodox approach to training. Daniel LaRusso, played by Ralph Macchio, wants to learn martial arts, but Mr. Miyagi starts him off with menial chores to help him. And Daniel unknowingly develops the defensive blocks through muscle memory, but what he eventually learns is a lot more than martial arts. That's kind of what I was looking for when I asked SEAL to move in and train me. I wanted to train my body, but also my mind and spirit. The difference was I wasn't training for protection or a trophy. And I had already gotten the girl. I just wanted to get better.

I've also always had an unorthodox approach to business and life in general. It's served me well. I don't believe in résumés in the traditional sense, I believe in life résumés. Do more. Create memories. Only when looking back on my successes and failures am I able to connect the dots. I could have never predicted or planned to go from being a rapper on MTV in the 1990s to eventually owning and operating my own private jet company. My normal has always been abnormal.

I don't know if I was thinking about my mortality, or fretting over how many more peak years I had left, or anything like that. I just felt that now was as good a time as any to shake things up. You know, to break up that *same* routine.

I believe the best ideas are the ones you don't spend too much time thinking through. My time with SEAL was no different and I got a lot more than I bargained for. Most of my successes in life have come from learning how to be comfortable with being uncomfortable. Like I said, I just want to get better.

Every day do something that makes you uncomfortable.

—SEAL

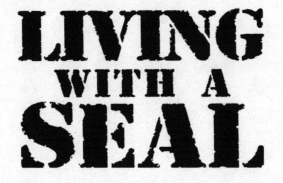

PROLOGUE

SEAL moved into my home to train me in December 2010. That winter went on to be one of the snowiest on record. Airports closed. Trains were delayed. A nor'easter dropped more than twenty inches of snow on New York City in one day. The winds were so strong they pushed the falling snow into drifts that measured up to four feet. City bus drivers abandoned their vehicles in the middle of the streets. So did regular drivers. Plows couldn't remove the snow for days. I was sure my mission with SEAL would be compromised. But that was before I knew him.

DAY 1

The Arrival

I'm trained to disappear.
—SEAL

New York City
14°
0638

I pour oatmeal into a bowl, fill the pot with water, light the stove, and set the timer. I click play on the remote and position Lazer, my eighteen-month-old son, so he can see his *Baby Einstein* video. I peek into the guest room to make sure the bed is made. My son is giggling, which comforts me. I check on my wife, Sara, who's still sleeping, and then recheck the guest room to make sure it's shipshape, or whatever the heck they say in the Navy. I hear the timer go off. I cut up some bananas and pour honey on them. I look at the clock on the microwave: 6:38 a.m.

ETA: twenty-two minutes.

I'm filled with nervous energy.

I sit with my son, feed him breakfast, and watch the rest of *Baby Einstein*. The bananas are still in my bowl. I'm not hungry. I go into the bathroom and look at myself in the mirror. I push my hair back with my hands. I grin at my reflection to check my teeth. They're clean.

I go back to the living room.

I do as many push-ups as I can: twenty-two.

I look at the clock: 6:44 a.m.

What if he has trouble getting a cab? Does a guy like him even take a cab? Maybe he's going to run to my house. The plane might be delayed? He could've changed his mind? Maybe I should call. What am I talking about? The guy's probably parachuted into foreign countries; he has to know how to get to my house on time. Right?

But he *NEVER* asked for my address, *NEVER* inquired what to bring. He *wouldn't* give me his flight information and *didn't* request a car service. *NOTHING*. In fact, the only thing the man said was:

"I arrive at oh seven hundred." That's military time for 7:00 a.m.

* * *

I first saw "SEAL" at a twenty-four-hour relay race in San Diego. After several marathons, this was my first "ultra." I was on a team of six ultra-marathoners who would each take turns running twenty-minute legs. The objective: Run more miles than every other team in twenty-four hours.

There were teams registered from all over the country.

You know, friends coming together to test themselves physically and mentally. SEAL, however, didn't have a team. He didn't have friends. He was running the entire race... himself.

The event was low budget, really low budget. The entire course was set around a one-mile loop in an unlit parking lot near the San Diego Zoo. It was unsupported, meaning you bring your own supplies. Whatever you needed, you were responsible for.

My team and I flew in the night before to get ready. When we got there we walked the course and mapped out our strategy. Before we went to sleep, we laid out our race gear and supplies so we were ready to go when we woke up. Water. Gatorade. Bananas. PowerBars. Band-Aids. We were ready.

Before the race, we stretched in a small circle on the grass. I was nervous and excited, but I couldn't help notice the guy ten feet away. To say he stood out would be an understatement. For starters, he was the only African-American in the race. Secondly, he weighed over 260 pounds whereas most of the other runners weighed between 140 and 165 pounds. Third, whereas everyone else was talkative and friendly, this guy seemed pissed. I mean he looked very angry.

He just sat there all by himself in a folding chair with his arms crossed waiting for the race to start. No stretching, no prep, no fancy shoes, and no teammates. No smiling. He just sat quietly with a don't-fuck-with-me expression on his face. His supplies for twenty-four hours: one box of crackers and water. That's it. He laid them out next to his chair.

The guy was a cross between a gladiator and the G.I. Joe action hero my son has, but life size. He looked indestructible. Battle tested. Dangerous. Alone. Determined.

Even the way he spit was scary. If he hit you with it, it likely would leave a scar. He was intimidating. Physically, the man looked like someone sprayed muscle paint all over his body. Ripped. Flawless.

Once the race started, in between our individual legs of running, we stretched and stayed hydrated to avoid injury, and applied plenty of Vaseline. As a friend of mine likes to say: "Brother, ultras are chafey." But as the race continued and I cheered on my teammates, I couldn't help but keep tabs on the guy who was running alone. Who *was* this guy?

There was magnetism to his fury. Underneath his scowl I sensed something I couldn't quite put my finger on. Maybe it was a sense of honor or integrity. Or purpose. Yeah, that's it. He ran with a sense of purpose that I couldn't quite comprehend. He ran as though lives depended on it, like he was running into a burning house to save someone, a kitten or an old woman. With each stride he took it seemed like he was creating mini-earthquakes beneath his feet, but at all times his form was perfect, his eyes locked in a stare, a focus that was diamond-tip PRECISE. He just ran...checked his splits on his watch...and ran for a hundred miles straight.

When the twenty-four-hour race was over, I was cooked. My thighs were so tight I could barely walk a yard. As my teammates and I slowly gathered our extra sneakers, lawn chairs, and personal belongings, I noticed him again, this massive, two-hundred-plus-pound block of carbon steel, being helped to the parking lot by a woman (whom I would later find out was his wife), looking like he just survived a plane crash.

I concluded two things:

1. I had never seen anyone like this.
2. I had to meet him.

Back home, after some investigating and some Googling, I was able to ascertain a few pertinent things about him, including the fact that he was a Navy SEAL, a highly decorated Navy SEAL at that. Then I tracked down a contact number and called him cold. He was on the West Coast.

This is a habit I have. When I see or read about someone interesting, I call them up and basically ask them to be my friend. My wife says it reminds her of middle school when you hand someone a note and ask, "Do you want to be my friend? Check yes or no." Well, I guess I never outgrew that phase.

"Yeah?" he answered.

"Is this SEAL?"

"That depends on who's asking," he said.

I hadn't experienced these kind of nerves since I called Sue my senior year in high school to ask her to the prom. I started talking about the race and babbling on, until halfway through my rap I realized that I sounded like someone I would've hung up on. In fact, I wasn't completely sure he hadn't hung up—there was dead silence coming from his end of the phone.

This was way worse than the call to Sue.

"Hello?" I asked.

"Yeah."

"Just give me fifteen minutes to propose something to you in person," I said finally. "I'm in New York City but can fly out tomorrow."

Silence.

"Hello?"

Silence.

"SEAL?"

Silence.

Finally: "You wanna come out…it's on you," he said.

Twenty-four hours later I was in California.

We met in a local restaurant in San Diego. After some small talk, which consisted of me talking and him saying nothing in response, I asked him to move into my house to train me.

He stared at me with cold, flat eyes. I couldn't tell if he thought I was nuts or if he was figuring out if I was worth his time. He was sizing me up.

One minute passed. Then another.

"Okay, I'll do it with one condition," he said in a tone that was slightly motivational in a psychopathic drill sergeant way. "You do everything I say."

"Yes."

"And that means EVERYTHING."

"Okay."

"I can wake you at any time; I can push you to any extreme."

"Ummm."

"NOTHING is off limits. NOTHING."

"Well..."

"By the time we're done you'll be able to do a thousand push-ups in a day."

"A thousand?"

This wasn't going to be anything like the prom, I thought.

* * *

At exactly 7:00 a.m. there's a knock on my door.

He has *NO luggage. NO suitcases. NO expression.* In spite of the fact that it's December and it's *freezing* out, he's wearing *NO coat. NO hat. NO gloves.* And there's NO greeting.

He simply says, "You ready?"

That's it? No warm-up pitch? No "nice to see you again"? No "it's cold out, huh?" Maybe something nice and easy, right down the middle? Instead, I get a Mariano Rivera cut fastball.

"I'm so glad you're here," I say. "Anything you need, please feel free to help yourself. Make yourself at home. Our home is your home."

"Nah, bro! Not at all, this is *your* home. I don't have a home."

I laugh.

SEAL doesn't laugh.

"It was only an expression," I answer. "Make yourself at home, that's an expression."

"I don't operate in expressions, dude. I operate in actions. That needs to be clear immediately," he says. "Understand?"

"Okay."

"Huh?"

"Yes . . . sir?"

"I'm trained to disappear. You won't EVER even know when I'm here."

"Okay."

"Ah'ite. Let's get into this shit. Meet me here in nine minutes. And don't bring your cowfuck expressions."

Cowfuck?

I change into my standard cold-weather workout gear, which consists of two sweatshirts, two hats, and gloves. I walk back out to the front door, where SEAL is already standing, looking at his watch. It's fourteen degrees out and nippy. He's wearing shorts, a T-shirt, and a knit hat. Nothing else.

"Man, I may need to borrow some gloves," says SEAL.

"You *may* need gloves?"

"Yeah, or some kinda mittens or some shit like that."

"That's it. Only gloves?"

"That's it."

"It's fourteen degrees outside," I say.

"To you it's fourteen degrees 'cause you're telling yourself it's fourteen degrees!"

"No. It really is. It's fourteen degrees. Like that's the real actual temperature outside. It says so on my computer."

SEAL pauses for a moment like I may have disappointed him. "On your computer, huh?"

He begins to laugh, but it's a haunting laugh, like the Count on *Sesame Street*.

"The temperature is what you think it is, bro, not what your computer thinks it is. If you think it's fourteen degrees, then it's fourteen degrees. Personally, I'm looking at it like it's in the mid-fifties."

Rather than argue—after all, we're still just getting to know each other—I just say: "Got it."

"You ever spent any time in freezing water, Jesse?" SEAL asks.

I'm thinking to myself, Like on purpose? But I respond with a "no."

"Well, is it freezing? OR is your *mind* just saying it's freezing? Which is it?" He laughs again. "Control your *mind*, Jesse."

"Got it." (I'm going to have to put that on the to-do list: *Control mind.*)

"Exactly. Enjoy this shit. If you want it to be seventy and sunny...it's seventy and sunny. Just run. The elements are in your mind. I don't ever check the temperature when I run. Who gives a fuck what the temperature on the computer says? The computer isn't out there running, is it?"

He's got me there, but instead of saying "got it" again, I try to keep the banter going.

"Does that work the same way in heat? I mean, if it's ninety-five degrees outside, can you make it snow in your mind?"

"Nah, man, it's a one-way system, bro. Cold to hot only. When it's hot outside...it's just fucking hot!"

If one of my friends tried to give me the same logic, I'd laugh, but coming from SEAL's mouth, I almost believe him.

However, I can feel the draft coming from our windows and I don't care what SEAL says—it really is fourteen degrees outside.

"Well, then, what's the strategy in the heat?"

"In extreme heat, it's a totally different mind-set, bro. You have to get medieval. Embrace it! Grind it out. Think about how others are suffering. Enjoy the pain."

"Yours or theirs?" I ask.

SEAL levels me with his stare.

"Both," he says. Then SEAL nods at me, the signal that it's "go" time.

We head to Central Park and run six miles at a 9:20-mile pace. I think SEAL wants to feel me out. Although I am an experienced marathoner, I was never a fast runner. I can run at a seven-minute pace, but I prefer not to. I like to take my time running; my pace is more the you-should-be-able-to-talk-to-a-friend-while-running pace. It's more enjoyable. I'm way more of an endurance guy than a sprint guy. I find that endurance running is more of a mental challenge than a physical challenge, and I'm pretty good at blocking out the pain and boredom of long runs.

This pace suits me well. I think to myself, I can do this.

An hour later…

After a warm shower and quickly returning some work emails, I give SEAL a quick tour of our apartment. We live at 15 Central Park West on the Upper West Side of Manhattan.

The building has been written and blogged about as a famous New York City building and also been featured for its amazing views, architecture, and residents. Many of the world's top CEOs, athletes, and entertainers live in the building.

I convinced Sara two years ago we should move in because the building had a pool. "We can swim every day, honey." Well, here we are two years later. We bought the apartment but we have not been in the pool once.

Although my wife and I don't consider ourselves to be "fancy," the building sure is. In fact, when we first moved in, the elevator concierge (not the elevator operator; the elevator *concierge*) told me to get off of the elevator because the elevators are "only for residents." I guess I didn't look the part of resident in my ski hat and shorts.

I start the tour by showing SEAL how to use the remotes for the television. I figure that is something a guest who is staying with us for over a month will want to know, right?

"This is how you turn it on," I say, pointing to the power button.

"We won't be watching much TV," he says, interrupting me.

"Okay then... Moving on," I say.

I set the remote down and then lead him over to the kitchen. If we aren't going to be watching television, then we certainly will be eating, I assume. I pull out the first drawer.

"So this is where all the forks, spoons, and knives are," I say.

"I won't be using your utensils," he says.

Huh? I close the drawer.

Maybe I'll have more luck in the laundry room.

As I am about to show him how to use the washer and dryer, he interrupts me again and says, "Yo, man, you can skip all this tour shit. Just tell me how to get to the gym."

Okay. The tour is officially over and we head to the gym.

For the first time I can see SEAL's front teeth as a smile starts to form. He is ecstatic; I can see the change in his expression just from walking inside of the gym. It's almost like watching *The Wizard of Oz* for the first time when you see the screen go from black and white to color. It's a whole new world. He walks over to the pull-up bar, jumps up, grabs the bar, and hangs. He starts to swing and swing some more and swing until he finally jumps off. I guess he approves because his smile has grown.

"This is perfect. You ready?" he asks.

"For what?"

"Your pulls."

"You mean like right now?"

"Give me ten. All the way down and all the way up. Let's see where your pull-up game is at."

I jump up and grab the bar and pull my two hundred pounds of body weight up until my chin is over the bar. "One."

I go down. When I get to number eight, I start kicking my legs around frantically to try to get some momentum. I need to get my chin over this damn bar, but I can't. I drop to the floor. SEAL tells me to take a forty-five-second break and do it again.

Forty-five seconds later I jump back up and grab the bar. I've never been good at doing pull-ups. In fact, I hate doing them. Somehow I manage to squeak out six more before I drop back to the ground. This time I think for good. SEAL tells me to take another forty-five seconds and then do it again.

Another forty-five seconds go by and this time I'm able to get three solid pull-ups in before I drop to the ground. Each time I'm dropping, my legs give out a little more. That's seventeen pull-ups. I'm *done*. I'm literally maxed out. I don't think I have ever done seventeen pull-ups so fast, or *ever*, for that matter. I grab my left bicep with my right hand and my right bicep with my left hand and squeeze. It feels like there are nails in my biceps.

"Seventeen! Cool, that's my max number. I didn't think I could even do that. Amazing! Let's head back upstairs."

As I start to look up, SEAL is staring at me with a blank expression...deadpan. "We're going to stay here until you do a hundred."

WHAT?

"I can't do a hundred. That's impossible," I say.

"You better find a way," he says to me like a father might tell his son to clean his bedroom. "You got a shitty-ass attitude."

I do one and drop to the floor.

I walk around the gym trying to delay the inevitable. My arms sag at my sides and SEAL watches me. I can't procrastinate any longer. I return to the pull-up bar. I do another one and drop to the ground. I take another lap around the gym

and I'm back to the pull-up bar. I drop. Lap...Pull-up...
Drop...Lap...Pull-up...Drop...

Ninety minutes later I'm on ninety-seven.

Training is definitely under way.

> **Workout totals: 6 miles and 100 pull-ups**

No Novocain

I like to sit back and enjoy the pain. I earned it.
—SEAL

I grew up on Long Island in Roslyn, New York, with two older sisters and a brother. I was the youngest by five years. As suburban as you can get, Roslyn has developments of houses that all are pretty much the same with connected backyards that were patrolled by an army of kids my age. My mom owned a cowbell. I could be six or seven houses away and I'd hear my mom's bell calling me home. I was trained like a cow; it was slightly embarrassing. The rule was: Do your homework and you can go outside, but when you hear the bell, you'd better come home and you'd better be home in five minutes. My mom was the most unconditionally loving mom, but my mom was a hard-ass. Nobody messed with her. I've never heard her curse, but she has this look that she'd give you: her go-to move. Silence. It got me every time.

My mom was also something of a dichotomy when it came to traditional child healthcare. On one hand, she'd let me eat cheeseburgers, bacon, ice cream, and Oreo cookies, whatever I wanted, and all at once; but she was freaked out by X-ray machines, fluoride, and Novocain. She didn't think there had been enough research and testing done on certain things in the 1970s, and she didn't want me to be the lab rat. I got my first X-ray only after they invented that big lead vest they put on you, and she thought fluoride was just the most toxic thing. Not having X-rays and fluoride in my life was easy to take. What was hard was no Novocain.

My dentist's name was Henry Schmitzer, and his office was about a forty-five-minute drive from our house. I guess he was the only dentist my mom could find who would drill a kid's mouth without an anesthetic. Henry might have been Laurence Olivier's inspiration for the character he played in *Marathon Man.*

So while all of my friends were getting gassed-up, pain-free, and lollipoped visits to their dentists around the corner, I'd be sitting in the back of the car for forty-five minutes, staring out the window, sweating, thinking...we are actually driving out of our way for this shit. That sound, and smell, like burning bone, of the drill. The anticipation was grueling, to say the least. It was a full-on event for me. The walk from the parking lot to the office always sparked thoughts and temptations to just run away as fast as I could. But my mother would give me a sympathetic smile as she held the door for me to go inside—she really believed she was doing the best for me.

Inside, Schmitzer the motherfucker, would start drilling my mouth. (I'm literally holding my mouth as I'm writing this.) The taste of that fire, the sound, the excruciating pain, and my mouth would be sore forever. It was crazy. You'd think that would have been motivation to brush better, but it always seemed like I had at least one cavity every checkup.

My dad was basically the complete opposite from Mom, in a go-with-the-flow type of way. He owned a plumbing supply store in Mineola and worked six days a week (a half day on Saturday). Even with all the time he invested at work, he was a hands-on dad. He showed up for every game, every event, and made it a point to be home for family dinner every night.

At home he was like a mad scientist—he had a workshop in his basement, and that was his spot. He wasn't into watching sports or hanging out with friends, he liked to invent. When the movie *Back to the Future* came out and "Doc" created the Flux Capacitor...I was like, *"That's my dad!!"*

I remember one time in elementary school when I had to make a diorama. The assignment was simple: Take a shoebox and create a replica of your own house. Well, by the time my dad "helped out," my diorama had running water and electricity. I kid you not. You could also push a button and the little garage door on the diorama would open.

I definitely think I got my creativity from my dad. And as far as I know he's pro-Novocain, but unfortunately he wasn't the one driving me to the dentist.

The part of me that would grow up to hire a Navy SEAL, that came from Mom.

DAY 2

Nature's Gatorade

I'm the surprise-or. Not the surprise-ee.
—SEAL

New York City to Boston
20° to 16°
0700

I had a hard time sleeping last night. It's a combination of nerves and excitement mixed in with the fact that my biceps are jacked up from the pull-ups. They are sore to the touch. I don't think they moved once from the ninety-degree flexed position they were stuck in all night.

As far as nerves go, I am unusually nervous right now. It's not the typical type of nerves someone might get from having to go on a job interview or something like that, but it's nervousness in the sense that I don't want to disappoint SEAL by not being able to do the workouts. This anxiety started to build before he ever arrived. And the thought of not wanting to get hurt is playing like background music in my head. It's a little like the nerves I feel before a marathon. There's a level of uncertainty of what will and might happen. Plus, the way SEAL expected me to do a hundred pull-ups yesterday was borderline certifiable. And he refused to leave the gym until they were all done.

It freaked me out.

·Anyway, before we went to bed last night, SEAL told me to set my alarm clock for 0630 (6:30 a.m.) in preparation for a run at 0700 (7:00 a.m.)...SHARP.

Well, there was no alarm clock needed because at 6:00 a.m. I hear someone walking around the foyer of the apartment. Not tiptoeing, but making what feels like intentional noise to wake me up. I hear an excessive loud fake coughing...the slamming of the front door...and music being turned up extra loud.

What an asshole.

I grab two sweatshirts, two hats, and gloves. SEAL is in the same summer attire as yesterday with the addition of some old gloves I lent him. We head out.

As we walk by the front desk, I can tell the doormen are curious as to who SEAL is. I thought I overheard one of them asking the other if he was Jerry Rice, the football great.

"Nah, this guy is way bigger than Jerry Rice," the other said.

We run the same loop of Central Park as we did yesterday at the same nine-minute-mile pace. There is *no* talking. There is *no* joking. There is *no* communication. I'm not so sure this guy wants to be my friend...and I'm not so sure I now want to be his.

My arms hurt like hell from the pull-ups, but I don't say anything. I just keep stride. I have run long distances in my life, but when I'm not training on a daily basis, a six-mile run is a pain in the ass. It's *long* and definitely can be boring. No matter how you slice it, six miles is going to take me fifty to sixty minutes. That's a long time to be running.

Any runner will tell you that some days a run can fly by and be enjoyable. And sometimes that same exact run on the same exact path feels like torture and is excruciatingly slow. Today the clock seems to be ticking particularly slowly. Maybe it's the awkwardness of running with a stranger. It's very odd running with someone you don't know and who doesn't speak. The silence is very uncomfortable. It's like running with someone who speaks a language you don't understand...except this someone is very intimidating and will be living with you for another thirty days. Whatever it is, this run feels twice as long as it did the last time I ran it.

When we get home I make a quick shake, shower, and head to work.

Three hours later...

I haven't told SEAL that today I have to fly to Boston for a business meeting around noon. But I have good reason for the trip. I recently started a company called the 100 Mile Group. I'm fairly good at identifying trends and predicting the next big thing. The 100 Mile Group is set up to take advantage of that. If I find a product or service that I know customers will want and I have authentic passion for it, then our company will invest, market, or launch it.

Our first product is a new brand called Zico Coconut Water. As a runner I am well aware of the amazing hydrating qualities of coconut water and am convinced the category is going to take off. I had also noticed that every four years or so, a new, natural health drink would hit the market and explode off the shelves. Pomegranate juice had just stormed the castle—everywhere you looked there was an ad for the stuff. I believed coconut water was next.

Initially I looked into importing coconut water from overseas and having a go at it myself. After trips to Jamaica and Brazil, I quickly realized I would be much better off partnering with an existing brand and helping them grow their business.

I was introduced to Mark Rampolla, the founder of Zico Coconut Water, that summer. Zico was a small company at the time with about $5 million in sales, but my Spidey senses told me they were onto something, plus I really liked Mark. I ended up partnering with the company and simultaneously brokered a deal with Coca-Cola where they came in as a minority partner.

Coca-Cola had recently established a division called VEB, Venturing & Emerging Brands. This is the branch of Coke that looks for the next billion-dollar brand and partners with them during their early growth period. They were responsible for acquiring Honest Tea, Illy Coffee, and other hot brands. My friend Lance Collins had founded Fuze and just sold it to Coke. He introduced me to the president of the division, and after several trips to Atlanta we formed a three-way partnership: Zico, the 100 Mile Group, and Coca-Cola. Coke retained an option to acquire the whole company based on certain sales triggers. Zico is starting to take off, so this is a big meeting for me.

I eventually tell SEAL we have to go to Boston for the

meeting. I totally forgot to give him the heads-up, but I'm sure he'll understand—it's business.

"This is some bullshit, Jesse. I'm gonna do it, but this is some pure cow BULLSHIT. No more motherfuckin' surprises, Jesse. I'm the surprise-or, not the surprise-ee. I'm not playin'. NO MORE FUCKING SURPRISES. We can't deviate." He is livid.

"I promise we'll be back by seven p.m. tonight to train," I say, hoping to smooth over his disappointment. He agrees, but in my mind I'm thinking, What real choice does he have? I have to work, right?

It's noon. We go straight to the airport from my office. There's no need to stop by my apartment and pack because I'm positive we'll be back in time for our evening workout. I have an extra pair of shorts and a T-shirt under my desk at work so I grab them...just in case.

The fact that I'm going to be meeting with Boston Celtic and basketball legend Kevin Garnett does very little to impress SEAL. This is my first time meeting Garnett and I'm looking forward to it. I've been good friends with his sports agent for a while, and I'd heard Garnett was a fan of Zico, even though he's officially an endorser of Gatorade. And Garnett is a fitness freak.

In the off season Garnett lives in Malibu. But Garnett does not technically have an off season because as soon as the season ends, he gets right to training. He prides himself on working out early and often. "I like my feet to be the first footprints in the sand," he's said many times. I love the guy's intensity and focus on wellness. I think he'll be a perfect fit as an investor and endorser for Zico. Plus, it would be huge for us to lure him away from Gatorade, and I believe his contract with them is coming up for renewal. Needless to say, I'm excited for this meeting.

On the jet, I buckle my seat belt as tight as I can and point the air valve directly at me. Then I pull the shade down over the window. I've never been the greatest flyer (which is ironic because I started a private jet company). As part of my superstition, I go through a kind of preflight checklist every time I get on a plane. I say a prayer, put on Carole King, and click my heels three times. And this time I'm glad I do. To say the takeoff is bumpy doesn't capture the experience. It's a nauseating roller coaster. The plane is being tossed around like a pinball from side to side.

In between the free falls, I glance over at SEAL. He's still in the same running shorts and T-shirt he ran in this a.m., and he's reading *Sports Illustrated*. I'm not sure SEAL realizes we even took off yet as he casually flips the pages of his magazine. He's unfazed.

Twenty minutes into the flight a beeping noise chimes indicating a warning and the buckle-your-seat-belt sign illuminates. The pilot instructs the flight attendants to "return to their seats and stop service" as the turbulence is so severe. I'm flipped out and have convinced myself we are going down. Beads of sweat are pouring down my forehead and my palms are drenched. But SEAL, he doesn't so much as flinch. He's just reading. Casually flipping the pages and yawning.

Finally we are wheels down in Boston. I'm ecstatic that we are on the ground in one piece.

SEAL couldn't give two shits. He turns to me and says, "Great flight."

1600

We walk into the conference room of the Boston Celtics' practice facility and there's Kevin Garnett, his agent, and one of his financial guys. Kevin is much taller than I anticipated, and he is super ripped. The guy looks way more muscular and intimidating in person. He had just finished a three-hour practice and was showered up and ready to discuss business.

We're led to a large room that overlooks the court where the team's executives sit when they watch practice. I'm feeling pretty good. I enjoy putting people and products that I believe in together and am quite at ease in this kind of meeting, so going in my confidence level is on high.

"Hey, Kevin, man, Jesse Itzler..." I go to shake Garnett's hand, which is the size of a Hamburger Helper hand, but I realize he's not looking at me. He's looking at SEAL.

"And this is SEAL," I say.

SEAL nods, then Garnett does. It's like a silent standoff—two gunslingers in the Wild West evaluating each other.

"I hired a Navy SEAL to live with me for a month or so," I say to explain. "You know, to train me. To shake some shit up in my life."

Garnett's eyebrows arch as if I'm the first person to bring a Navy SEAL to a business meeting with him.

"Is it okay if he joins us for the meeting?"

I hand Garnett a Zico Coconut Water, smile, and jump right into my pitch: "If Mother Nature went into the sports drink business, Zico would be her Gatorade..."

"How many miles you run a day?" Garnett asks SEAL, finally breaking the silence that has been building between them.

"Depends," SEAL says with a shrug.

"Do weights or resistance training?"

"Yes and no," SEAL says.

"Anaerobic threshold?"

"Body composition?"

"Maximum heart rate?"

"Your VO2?"

Garnett fires the questions and SEAL parries them back. It's not a gunfight, it's more like Garnett is in the quarter-finals at the U.S. Open in Flushing, Queens, and SEAL is playing badminton at a cookout.

Hours pass. Not once do we talk about Zico. I'm just sitting there. We talk about workouts. Or rather *they* talk about workouts. I can tell that SEAL is digging Garnett. There is some kind of mutual warrior vibe going on that they are connecting with. I'm picking it up too, but I'm not on the same warrior vibe radio station as them.

Weather starts to roll in. The meeting goes on, and on, *and on*!

"Ah'ite," Garnett finally says, signaling the meeting's over.

What about Zico? I'm wondering.

Garnett and SEAL turn and look at me like I've just magically reappeared. They give each other a bear hug and we say our good-byes.

Finally Garnett turns to me. "It's as simple as this, yo. Whatever you motherfuckers do," Garnett says, "I want in."

2000

I give SEAL a high fist bump as we walk out of the building. The euphoria quickly turns into fear as we walk out into a full-fledged snow squall. This isn't good, I think to myself. This is what SEAL might refer to as a surprise, but this one's on Mother Nature—not me. We don't even attempt to go to the airport, and I find us a hotel near the Boston Garden. It's getting late as we check into our rooms. I'm tired and need to rest. Maybe I'll rent a movie and order room service. Just as I lie down on the bed I hear a knock.

"Let's go," the voice says through the door. "Meet in the lobby in ten minutes."

"But it's freezing and snowing."

"Ten minutes."

"But we ran already this morning."

"Ten minutes."

"But I don't have anything warm?"

Eight minutes later I get off the elevator in the lobby. SEAL is ready. He's waiting at the front desk. He looks at me like I'm late when in actuality I'm two minutes early. It's our second run of the day, and the temperature keeps dropping. I'm in shorts, a T-shirt, a hat, and the sweatshirt I wore to the meeting. That's it. It's eighteen degrees outside and we run along the Boston waterfront. It's bitter cold, windy with a misty snow. I really *don't* want to be out here, but I have no choice. I'm freezing my ass off. I want to be in my hotel room ordering room service and watching the snow from behind

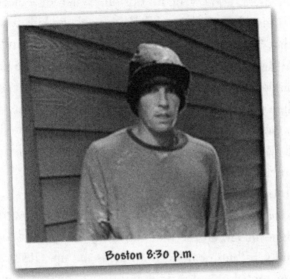

Boston 8:30 p.m.

my window. Plus, all I really want to do is think about the next steps with Zico and Garnett while it's fresh on my mind.

I try to break down the Garnett meeting with SEAL and discuss the win.

"That meeting was awesome," I say.

No response.

"You think his financial guy dug it?"

No response.

"What did you think of his financial guy anyway?"

No response. About one minute later SEAL finally says, "Motherfucker, it's KG's show." I'll leave it at that.

I'm not sure exactly what body of water we are running next to this evening, but I assume it's the Charles River. I have *nothing* to base that off of other than the fact that it's the only river I know of in Boston. Whether I'm right or wrong, I visualize the river filled with college kids rowing on a hot day. I'm not sure SEAL is visualizing anything. He is just staring straight ahead as if he is anticipating an ambush. But no enemies appear.

When we get back to the hotel, my fingertips are frozen. I go to Google "frostbite" on my laptop, but I can't work the keypad. We just logged six more miles. That's twelve for the day and eighteen so far.

I throw my wet clothes in the bathtub, lay my sweatshirt out on the heater in the room to dry, and call Sara to check in. Whenever I'm on the road, it's tough being away from my wife and son (but a call always warms me up). It's 9:30 p.m. real time and she's not picking up. It just keeps ringing.

Sara likes to go to bed early. It's been like that since the day I met her in 2006 at a poker tournament in Las Vegas.

Sara was a customer of mine at Marquis Jet, the private jet company I co-founded in 2001. Our partner, NetJets, was hosting a poker tournament, and we were allocated only forty seats at the tables. We had three thousand–plus customers at that point, and picking forty was hard to do. Every sales rep got to submit a list of four or five clients they thought were worthy of being invited, and then my partner Kenny and I would choose one person from each region to invite.

My Georgia sales rep called me and said she had a young businesswoman who she thought should get a ticket. The rep then emailed me a photo of her. The picture was a headshot of a pretty blonde with an apple on her head. *What?* I was intrigued. She was a cutie! So I told the rep not to send any other applications my way and to go ahead and invite her, the girl with the apple on her head.

The night of the tournament, about fifteen of us went out to dinner, and the woman with the apple on her head was in the group. Then, thirty minutes into the dinner, she said it was past her bedtime and was going back to her room. I looked at my phone. It was 9:30 p.m. Who goes to bed at 9:30 at night in Vegas? What an odd bird, I thought. Two years later I was married to that odd bird.

My call goes into voicemail and I leave a message. Since it's past 9:00 p.m., Sara must be sound asleep, and it's time for me to call it a night. With all of the weather delays, I assume the airport will be backed up and I want to get there early in the morning.

Workout totals: 12 miles in freezing rain

DAY 3

My Nuts

You need to feel the pace.
—SEAL

Boston
28°
0500

The hotel phone is ringing. What time is it? I didn't request
a wake-up call. Obviously it's SEAL, so I roll over in bed and
pick it up.

"It's go time" is the first thing I hear.

Yesterday, SEAL told me he wanted me to run six miles
in the morning and three miles at night for the first three
days he's here to build my "base."

Three days to build a base? That sounds ridiculous.
Doesn't it take months to build a base?

Anyway, I wasn't expecting to be in Boston overnight, so
I have no extra clothes to change into, plus my clothing from
last night is still soaking wet and cold from the snow and

sweat. Before we head down I meet SEAL in the hallway between our rooms to discuss a little issue I have.

"SEAL, I have a problem," I say to him. "I didn't bring any extra underwear."

"So what?"

"I can't run without underwear."

"Nah, bro, you can't run without legs. It's on."

So I throw on my freezing wet clothes from last night. I'm cold and miserable before I even head out. My underwear is so wet that I can't put it on, so I go "commando" style.

We meet in the lobby.

Today's pace is faster than last night's, like a minute per mile faster. And somebody forgot to give the sun a wake-up call because it's still pitch black out. We dart in and out of the headlights of incoming traffic like inmates fleeing the yard in a prison break. We zig, horns beep, and we zag, horns blast. I'm just trying to keep pace.

Apparently SEAL prefers to run on the street facing traffic and as close to the moving cars as possible. Like why not run on the sidewalk? Why are we on the street? The answer is I'm not really sure why. Maybe he likes the adrenaline rush. I don't. I prefer to run on a quiet street where there's no exhaust and cars aren't coming within an inch of killing me! Whatever the reason, he insists on running that way.

There's a sidewalk two feet from us that we can easily jump on. It may even be *for* runners. It's clean, empty, safe, and appealing. SEAL ignores it. We stay on the street narrowly avoiding cars and jumping over potholes. It's driving me crazy. WHY CAN'T HE GO ON THE SIDEWALK?

After twenty minutes or so, SEAL has only said two words to me.

"Stay close."

At about three miles into our six-mile run, it's time to turn around to run back to the hotel, so we do. The sun begins to peek through. It's 5:30 a.m. I'm getting better at dodging traffic, but I still don't like it.

It's on the route home when I begin to realize something isn't quite right. It's my nuts. They're starting to rub against the fabric of my shorts because I'm running without underwear. It's not a pleasurable feeling.

Without breaking stride I put my right hand on my balls, pull my fingers out of my shorts, and look...Blood! Confirmed. It's my nuts. My balls are bleeding from the friction. Jesus!

"SEAL, my nuts are bleeding."

"Who gives a fuck about your tiny nuts?" he says.

We keep pace.

About a mile later I realize I don't recognize anything. The buildings...the trees...nothing on the way back to the hotel looks familiar. This is not the way we came.

"Sorry, man, but nothing looks familiar. I assume it's impossible that you could get lost?" I manage to ask in between gasps. "Not with your training?"

He glares at me. "Ranger school, bro...No chance."

After forty-eight minutes of running, his watch beeps for the sixth time indicating we've hit the six-mile mark, but no hotel in sight. I'm thinking three miles out, three miles back...Run should be over, right? Come on, man. My nuts are fucking bloody.

At 8.3 miles, we finally find the hotel.

I'm pissed off about the extra mileage. SEAL is satisfied. It's like he thinks he got extra credit or something. The second we get inside, SEAL pulls out his training log and jots down a recap of the workout. Date. Time. Pace. Mileage, etc. He writes so small he has the details of his whole year of workouts on two pages. I walk bow-legged across the lobby. It hurts. I wonder if the concierge can help with bleeding nuts.

"Ranger school, bro."

Three hours later...

I call SEAL's room and tell him we'd better get to the airport.

"Roger that," he says.

It's 9:00 a.m. We're stuck for hours at Logan. Nothing's flying. I make some calls. I'm happy thinking over the way the Garnett meeting went down. I read some magazines. I walk around. I make some more calls. SEAL just sits there, staring straight ahead. He doesn't move off the chair. He doesn't go to the bathroom. I'm not even sure he blinks. He's just staring.

I look over in the direction of what he's staring at to identify it. I follow his eyes to a blank brick wall. There is nothing there. I look back at him to double check I'm lining up his sight line correctly. And again, it takes me to the brick wall. He is just staring. Like the stone lion in front of the New York Public Library.

SEAL has two gears: idle and full out. But his idle isn't like normal idle at all; it's more like the moment between ignition and blastoff. I get the feeling around him that things could get hairy quickly. And yet I also have a feeling of absolute safety around him. I don't mean my own personal safety, though there's that too. I mean like national defense safety.

For three more hours I pace, eat, shop, and read. SEAL just stares. We finally board our flight.

Still Day 3. That night.

Thankfully, the flight is much smoother than the ride to Boston. I am able to close my eyes for the fifty minutes to New York, and it feels like I am in a full REM cycle. I'm out cold. We land at LaGuardia and jump in a cab back to the city. It's a short thirty-minute ride to the West Side. It's almost 8:00 p.m. by the time we get back to my apartment.

SEAL throws a banana at me and says, "Fuel up." I have only eaten airport food all day and I'm starving. I'd love to order in Josie's, the local health food restaurant, but that's not on SEAL's menu. His specials tonight are tossed bananas and running miles.

"Let's knock these three little miles out," he says. "Six in the a.m. and three miles at night," he repeats. "We need to build this foundation."

Maybe I'm calculating wrong but we did 8.3 miles this a.m. If we round up, we are done for the day.

I'm not 100 percent sure why SEAL agreed to come "work" with me. As eager as I was to shake up my life, I bet in some way he was equally curious to see how I lived. To learn. To get some ideas about business, travel, family, and life after the military. I'm not really sure. It's too early in our relationship, but I make a mental note to ask him down the road.

Winter in NYC can be very cold, and tonight the big CNN video screen that's displayed across from my apartment says seventeen degrees. SEAL puts on the same outfit he has had on for the past five runs. I mean the exact same outfit. How did all his shit dry?

I go into my room and layer up in long-sleeve running shirts. I also grab two hats and throw them on. It's a universally accepted fact that you lose a lot of warmth through your head. If you keep your head warm in the severe cold, you will have won half the battle of keeping your body warm. I usually always prefer to run in shorts (regardless of the temperature), but tonight I choose to put on a thin thermal legging because it's so damn cold.

During the ride down the thirty-seven flights on the elevator, SEAL doesn't even look at me. It's like he's infuriated with me. Actually, he looks like he is mad at something way bigger than just me. Is he mad at the world?

"Let's get the fuck out of here," he says as the elevator opens. "Fuck it. Let's do six," SEAL says as we leave. I don't even question it 'cause he looks so mad.

We run six miles in Central Park. Usually I run the loop of Central Park in a clockwise direction, but tonight he wants to run it in the opposite direction. He tells me we hit way more hills going this way. Not sure I really get that. To me it sounds like a word problem I had in eighth-grade math, but there's no time to discuss. Off we go.

SEAL does not look at his watch once during the run,

and when we finish he hits the stop button on his GPS. I hear it beep indicating the run is done and logged. "We did those in nines," he says. He then looks down at his watch...exactly fifty-four minutes. It's like he is a human GPS.

"SEAL, how the *fuck* did you know we were running nines without checking your watch?"

"Instincts. You need to feel the pace."

This guy is like the Obi-Wan Kenobi of running!

Twenty minutes later...

It's about 10:00 p.m. and I'm starting to think about sleep. I'm usually not hungry after I work out and tonight is no different. I guzzle a glass of water and wash up. Sara is reading *People* magazine in the living room.

Ten minutes later...

I walk to SEAL's room to say good night and see if he needs anything. Our relationship is still in the infancy stages, and I want to make sure he feels welcome. I lightly knock on his door three times and then peek my head in. He's sitting upright in his bed like he knew I was going to come in.

"Hey, man," I say. "You cool?"

"You know what, Jesse?" SEAL says. "No, I'm not cool. I'm sick of this shit." SEAL pounds his fist on the bed. "You're too pretty, man. Too cute. Fuck you."

What?

"Go grab a chair. The most uncomfortable chair you can find."

I have no idea what he's talking about, but I go and get a wooden chair, one with no armrests, out of my home office and return to his room.

"This?"

"This is perfect!" SEAL says. "Sit down."

I sit in the chair.

"Now go grab a fucking blanket," he says.

"Wait. What?"

He doesn't really think I'm going to sleep in A CHAIR?

"You got to get out of your comfort zone, Jesse," he says. "Enough of this comfy shit. Fuck this Park Avenue bullshit." He repeats himself under his breath: "Fucking Park Avenue bullshit."

But we live on Central Park West...

So I grab a blanket and try to get comfortable sitting in the chair. Every time I try to stretch out to get into more of a reclined/bed position, I slide down off the chair. Then Sara walks in.

"Hey, honey! Umm...what are you doing?"

"Sweetie, SEAL says I need to get out of my comfort zone. He wants me to sleep in this chair. It must be a mental thing." I'm trying to spin this as positively as I can. It's almost like I'm trying to convince myself that this is a great idea.

"Jess, you're a forty-two-year-old father. Please go and get into your bed."

My wife knows what I signed up for, but she slightly rolls her eyes, a judgmental expression that's somewhat neutralized by her smile. Sara also knows I'm going to make every

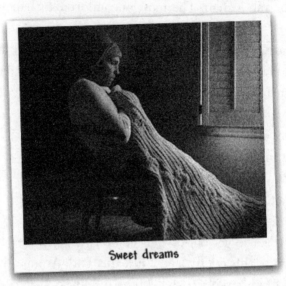
Sweet dreams

attempt to complete any and all of SEAL's challenges. But she didn't think I'd be told to sleep in a chair.

The blanket isn't helping, and the chair squeaks every time I shift positions. My wife shakes her head, turns, and walks back to the bedroom to our comfy bazillion-thread-count-sheet bed (my wife likes nice sheets).

It's midnight. Lights out.

Workout totals: 14.3 miles (8.3 miles in the morning and 6 miles at night)

Sara's First Sighting

I don't do shit for applauses. I don't do shit for
fanfare. I do shit for me.
—SEAL

The first time Sara saw SEAL was before he moved in with
us, but after I flew to the West Coast to offer my invitation.
I'd told my wife I wanted to run the Badwater race—it's
a grueling 135-mile ultra-marathon through the Mojave
Desert's Death Valley in 130-degree heat (and that's in the
shade). Sara thought that was the dumbest thing she ever
heard and insisted I first go watch the race to see what it was
all about before I entered it myself. And like a good husband,
I agreed. And because of the extreme nature of the race and
inherent danger, she decided that she ought to come too. You
know, for a second opinion.

I'd always wanted to complete the Badwater race. It is
considered the toughest footrace on Earth, and rightfully so.
135 miles. 130-degree heat. Plus, the last thirteen miles of
the race are a straight ascent up Mount Whitney. I also knew
SEAL was running in it.

I just felt like this race was *the* race to do for my life
résumé. It was the ultimate physical and mental challenge,
and I wanted to take the test. I guess I also wanted to be able
to look other runners in the face and say, "I completed Badwater." Like I said earlier, I want to get better.

So that summer for our family "vacation," we flew across

the country in July to watch the race. Since there are no direct flights (or any flights, for that matter) into Death Valley, we had to fly into Las Vegas, rent a car, and drive a few hours to the desert. The ride to Death Valley is long and boring, straight through the desert. Not a great way to spend your vacation if you're Sara (but I was psyched to watch the race). We got there just after the final wave of runners started the race. We drove out about twenty miles past the start to cheer on the competitors.

Any description I could offer here wouldn't do justice to how hot it was. As we arrived, the thermometer in the car showed the outside temp to be 128 degrees. It was so hot that at first Sara wouldn't even get out of the car. We parked at the thirty-mile mark and watched the racers pass with the air conditioner inside blasting.

Now, I'm not sure if you have ever seen an ultra-marathon before, but the competitors are an interesting breed of humans. As Sara said, "It's like they put ninety people from an insane asylum onto a Greyhound bus, drove them out to the desert, blew a whistle, and said run for two days." She wasn't far off. Most of the runners looked like a cross between scrawny science teachers and confused goat herders. As we cheered on the runners, they enjoyed our support by thanking us and giving us high-fives. Some even engaged in light conversation. Sara could not believe the group. She anticipated super-fit athletes, not folks who looked like mad scientists in running shorts.

But then, over the horizon, she saw what she thought was a mirage coming toward us. It was like the music from *Chariots of Fire* started playing in Death Valley as he approached.

The guy was a machine. He stared straight ahead like there was nothing in his path and ran. His muscles were like a locomotive train. As he passed us, Sara jumped up and down and yelled, "GO! GO! GO!" Although there wasn't another human within a mile of us or him, he didn't even react. No "thank you"...no smile...no anything.

"Holy shit," she exclaimed. "What the hell was that?"

Several months later "that" moved into our house.

DAY 4

Fitness Test

I don't think about yesterday. I think about today
and getting better.
—SEAL

New York City
25°
0530

I've been in and out of sleep all night but officially wake up
in the chair at 5:30 a.m. I've never been more happy to be
up at 5:30 a.m. in my life. My neck is *KILLING* me. I have
an L-shaped back and my knees are locked. I think I got
two hours of sleep...MAX. SEAL meets me in the den at
0545. He looks like he's already showered, had coffee, and
read the morning paper. Maybe he has. He doesn't say a
word about the chair. Nothing.

Now that we are three days into his stay and have "built
a foundation," SEAL decides he wants to test where I'm at...

physically. We "agreed" last night to an 0600 start time for our "fit test." Agreed means he told me when we're waking up.

Before SEAL got here, I had no idea how to convert military time into regular human time (the time the rest of the world operates on). But now I'm completely fluent in the conversion. So, at 0545 we head down to the gym for our test.

Before we get started, SEAL takes his shirt off. He looks at himself in the gym mirror. It's almost like he is doing it in slow motion. Checking to see if he added more definition to his Hulk-like body overnight. I apologize and explain that he has to keep his clothing on in the building gym, that those are the rules…that other residents will be coming down soon.

He acts like I'm taking a toy away from him and telling him to brush his teeth, like it's my rule. Like I'm the stuffy one.

"That's the dumbest shit ever," he says. "This is a gym. Gyms have mirrors."

"I know but that's the rules."

"Well, whoever made that rule is an asshole."

He reluctantly keeps his shirt on, and we walk over to the pull-up bar for what he has coined "nickels and dimes." We do five pull-ups (nickels) and then ten push-ups (dimes) "every minute on the minute."

We start every time the second hand is on the 12. If we finish in forty seconds, we then have twenty seconds of rest. We do this for ten minutes (fifty pull-ups and a hundred push-ups). However, by the time we get to four minutes, I have to drop my pull-up count to three. I can't keep up. I'm a runner, but this is a totally different skill set. I assume most forty-three-year-old men aren't doing eight pull-ups, let alone fifty.

SEAL doesn't say anything. He just pulls out his tiny journal and scribbles in it.

I'm already incredibly sore and struggling. Pull-ups are not my thing. Plus I'm still sore from the pull-ups three days ago.

SEAL says, "Okay, now we get started."

"What?"

We head over to the treadmill. SEAL hands me two twenty-pound dumbbells and sets the controls. Incline: 8. Speed: 4.0. He pushes the start button. I do this for eight minutes. It's like a brisk walk up a moderate-size hill carrying a couple of suitcases. Then, every minute thereafter, SEAL increases the incline by 1. By incline 10 it feels like I'm walking up a steep hill carrying two camp trucks; by 15, I'm climbing the side of a *mountain* holding two minivans! When I'm done, my shoulder blades feel like they're on fire. My thighs are jacked up. My lungs are so expanded it feels like they're going to burst my rib cage.

SEAL pulls out his tiny journal and marks it as such.

In fact, I tell him to jot it down in bold: MISERABLE.

We head over to the box jump. It's twenty-four inches high. He times me on how long it takes me to do fifty: 1 minute, 57 seconds.

SEAL pulls out his tiny journal and marks it as such.

Then we go outside and run six miles. It takes me an hour. I'm miserable. *Miserable.*

SEAL pulls out his tiny journal and marks it as such.

What's amazing is that SEAL not only does almost every

single workout with me, *but* he also does his own personal workouts on top of this. It was like the workouts we're doing that are knocking me out are not nearly enough for him. My workouts are like his jumping jacks for a warm-up.

We have only been together for a few days and I never really see SEAL lifting weights, but the guy is always doing push-ups. It's like push-ups are his hobby or more like it's his job. Or better yet, it's his hobby *and* his job. Anytime I go into the kitchen I see him doing push-ups in his room or in the hallway. He'll be in position, pushing up and down. And completely out of nowhere the guy will just drop and give himself twenty—at work, in the lobby, in the restroom. Any-where and everywhere. It's not normal.

Today, for example, when the doorman came to the apartment to drop off some packages that were delivered, SEAL answered the door and welcomed him in. As the door-man was placing the package by the wall, he tried to engage SEAL in conversation.

"You good?" the doorman asks.

Rather than answer and continue a normal conversation, SEAL drops to the floor and starts doing rapid-fire push-ups.

"Hey, man, just leave that shit by the wall. Appreciate it," he says as he goes up and down…up and down…up and down.

Workout totals: 6 miles, 15-minute treadmill test, 50 box jumps, 36 pull-ups, and 100 push-ups

DAY 5

Escape Vehicle

It doesn't have to be fun. It has to be effective.
—SEAL

New York City
20°
0800

I'm on the couch reading the *New York Post*. The door to the apartment opens. It's SEAL. He's back from doing an errand.

"This is fucking amazing."

SEAL is holding a fifty-pound camouflage backpack and four oars.

"What's that for?" I set down the paper and sit up a little straighter on the couch.

"It's your escape vehicle out of Manhattan," he says. "In this backpack is an inflatable raft that carries a maximum load of 450 pounds. Pull this cord and it inflates instantly." He shows me the cord. "You, Sara, and Lazer can all fit in it comfortably and paddle to Jersey."

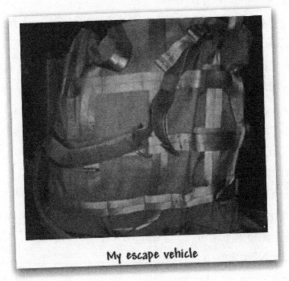

My escape vehicle

"Brilliant!" I say.

"Man, this shit is so badass," he says. "It's low to the water and impossible to see at night. It has an attachable motor. If you time your escape right, you can get out of Dodge undetected. POOF!"

This is the most animated I've seen SEAL since he got here.

"But why would we want to escape?" I ask.

"In case some 9/11 shit happens again. There's only one way out—the river. The city shuts down all bridges and tunnels and access points. How the fuck else do you plan to get out? What's the plan?"

"Plan? I don't have a plan."

"Well you do now. You're gonna row row row your boat the fuck out of here."

Makes sense to me.

As SEAL and I are admiring the fifty-pound backpack and the four oars, Sara walks in the front door.

My wife looks down at the backpack and then up at us. She is a bit confused.

"Sweetie, SEAL got us a backpack that turns into an inflatable raft in case we need to get out of the city," I say.

"An inflatable raft? We live on the thirty-seventh floor in an apartment in Manhattan."

"Yeah, SEAL said the bridges and tunnels get shut down during an emergency. It's protocol. A raft is the only way out. We just bring it to the Hudson River and inflate it. Then we paddle to New Jersey."

"Okay, love." She sets the mail down on the kitchen counter.

"That's it? Just 'okay, love'? Any thoughts?"

"Well, just so I understand. I'm supposed to grab my son, strap a fifty-pound pack on my shoulders, carry four oars, walk a mile to the river, inflate this survival raft, and then paddle to New Jersey...in the middle of a national emergency?"

There is dead silence in the room.

Then...more dead silence.

Sara chimes in and says, "I'm not even sure I could lift this thing."

"Nah, you'll be fine," SEAL says as he grabs the backpack and puts it on Sara's back.

She falls straight over backward.

I think to myself, she has a point.

Finally SEAL interjects. I can tell he is about to lose it and has been holding in his words. But now he can't hold them in any longer. "Sara, don't EVER underestimate the power of adrenaline," he says.

So we put the backpack behind the bar.

Four hours later...

"Come on, we're going to do the one hundred workout."

SEAL explains the routine, and I realize that he needs help with his math...it's really the *five hundred* workout.

We jump on the elevator and head down to the gym. There are already three other people working out when we get there. While the gym is fully operational and is loaded with equipment, it's rare that more than a handful of residents are ever there working out at the same time.

There's a guy with blond hair doing what looks like a serious core workout.

SEAL looks at the guy and then back at me.

"What the fuck is Billy Idol doing here?" SEAL asks.

"That's Sting," I whisper. "He lives in the building."

We do a hundred dumbbell bench presses (2X), no rest, and I start with thirty-pound weights but end with twenty-pounders. Total: 200.

100 lateral pull-downs (2X). 75 pounds. Total: 200
100 shoulder presses (seated). Total: 100

Like I said, that's five hundred, not one hundred.

Extra credit: 2X light triceps pull-downs and 2X curls

It's time to leave. We make our way out of the gym.

"Well, that didn't look fun," Sting says.

7:00 p.m.

It's Saturday night and most of the people I know are watching college football. Not us, because apparently SEAL does have a friend—someone he met in my gym yesterday. They must have become close because the guy lets SEAL borrow his fifty-pound weight vest. SEAL hands it to me.

"Put it on."

I grab it and put one arm in at a time. I throw the vest over my shoulders and strap it on. My immediate reaction is *This is heavy*. Like really heavy. It's like having a big suitcase on your back.

We do fifteen sets of ten push-ups, with thirty seconds of rest between sets.

Total: 150.

It takes me twenty-two minutes.

It takes SEAL fifteen minutes.

"This is no punk," SEAL says.

And it's not. It's so hard that even SEAL can't go straight to ten without dropping to his knees after the sixth set. Yet all he keeps saying is: "This is great."

This is not great. This is brutally hard.

I found out SEAL once entered a race where you could either run for twenty-four or forty-eight hours. Shocker: SEAL signed up for the forty-eight-hour one. At around the twenty-three-hour mark, he'd run approximately 130 miles, but he'd also torn his quad. He asked the race officials if they could just clock him out at twenty-four hours. When he was told they couldn't do that, he said, "ROGER THAT," asked for a roll of tape, and wrapped his quad. He walked (limped) on a torn quad for the last twenty-four hours to finish the race and complete the entire forty-eight hours.

"When you think you're done, you're only at forty percent of what your body is capable of doing. That's just the limit that we put on ourselves."

> Workout totals: 500 workout (bench presses, lat pull-downs, shoulder presses) and 150 push-ups

Señoras de la Limieza

I don't need new friends. I like to keep my
shit lean and tight.
—SEAL

We have two cleaning ladies who come to the apartment twice a week. They don't speak a lick of English, and I don't speak a lick of Spanish. So I have to use props and diagrams to communicate. If I want them to vacuum, I go get a magazine and show them a picture of a vacuum. If I want them to clean the windows, I show them a photo of Windex and point to the glass.

I keep a stash of *Us Weekly* around just for communication purposes. I'm always pointing to stuff and showing them a picture of what I need them to do. It's kind of like a combination of American Sign Language and charades. It can get challenging.

But when SEAL came into their world, there was no way I could explain him to them. I mean, what do I do? Show them a picture of Russell Crowe in *Gladiator*? Or Stallone's *Rambo*? But as I've come to learn, some things don't need to be communicated. These women were immediately obsessed with him. I mean, SEAL is a nice-looking man. Have I mentioned that? And he walks around without a shirt a lot. *A lot!* In fact, I'm starting to notice that Sara's friends are coming over lately for no reason. I guess they want to just look at SEAL.

Since he's moved in, the cleaning gals seem to be spending an extra hour or two cleaning. They also seem to be spending a lot time in his room despite the fact the guy is spotless. His room doesn't need cleaning—*ever*! Military corners, you could bounce a quarter off the bed after he makes it, all his gear is stowed. I mean, the bedroom looks like it's right out of a boot camp. But the ladies are always in there when SEAL's around, talking to each other in Spanish and giggling.

In the other direction, SEAL doesn't even acknowledge them. He's not exactly rude to them, it's more like a silent assessment—and he doesn't trust them.

Yesterday he ordered something that was FedExed to the apartment and one of the cleaning ladies accepted the package, he freaked out—not to them, but to me.

"It's a breach of security," he said.

Breach of security?

"The integrity of the delivery was compromised."

He went on to lecture me about my naiveté when it comes to insubordination of the people who work for me. The only thing he ever said about anyone was they should be fired. SEAL didn't think anyone who worked for the Itzlers cared enough or did their job like they should. He was really mad or suspicious of everyone he came into contact with except for Sara, Lazer, and me. According to SEAL, if my driver, Smith, was a minute late, it was because he didn't study the routes correctly. If there was traffic, Smith should have anticipated the accident.

In looking back on it now, I'm not sure SEAL was wrong. He was taught that if you have a job to do, you do it with 120 percent effort. I have been operating under the assumption that if someone that works for me does something 80 percent of the way I would do it, that's enough. SEAL is teaching me that we can all do so much more.

DAY 6

That Damn Finger

It's really not that complicated.
—SEAL

New York City
29°
0400

It's 4:00 a.m. I hear some banging and mumbling in the living room. Banging...mumbling...banging...mumbling. Although I am half asleep, I decide to check it out.

When I get to the living room, SEAL is on the couch holding the remote control. Well, holding is not really an appropriate description. He is slamming the remote control against the armrest of the couch as if that may turn the TV on.

"This motherfucker," he mumbles, "is too complicated. Too many buttons. It's making me fucking nuts."

SEAL looks like he may implode. His eyebrows are arched and he looks like he could attack...anything. Right now, he is attacking the remote but since I'm the closest human, I'm alarmed.

So, I immediately grab the remote and hit POWER then switch the command to CABLE 1. I put on ESPN and hand SEAL the remote.

"Just use the channel and volume controls for now. No need to even shut it off. I will shut off the TV in the morning."

SEAL's eyebrows contort back to normal as he watches some football highlights.

I go back to bed.

0600.

I hear my bedroom door slowly open. There's no nice way to put this, but it's a bit unnerving because my wife is in bed next to me and I can sense someone else in the room with us. I feel a tap.

I half open my eyes and imagine I see a long black finger on my shoulder. I roll over. My wife is sound asleep. Plus, the finger I'm imagining doesn't look anything like her finger.

I ignore the finger. I must be dreaming.

Ten seconds later, I feel another tap on my shoulder. I'm hoping it's my wife, but this finger does not belong to her. The finger keeps tapping me. In the other hand, is a remote.

I ignore it again.

Twenty seconds later, I feel hot breath whispering into my ear in a monotone voice. I guess the loud-intentional-noises-in-the-hallway trick wasn't working for him.

"Get up, motherfucker," SEAL says.

I get up. Fast. Sara remains motionless and oblivious next to me.

SEAL tells me we'll run another six miles in Central Park this a.m. That this is our last "primer." Then we start.

Start? I thought we started days ago.

I go into the living room and shut the TV off.

Central Park is where most of our training occurs. Park Drive is a 6.1-mile loop in the heart of Manhattan. Back in the 1970s, before they routed the race through the five boroughs, the New York City Marathon was held in Central Park. The marathoners ran around the loop four times plus. I've run the course hundreds of times since I moved to Manhattan, as it serves as a perfect training ground with its rolling hills, few cars at this time of the morning (which probably disappoints SEAL), and other runners and bikers to interact with.

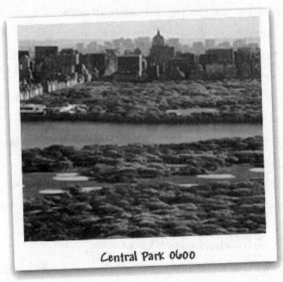

Central Park 0600

It's chilly today with the wind, but only until we start running. Our breath comes out in puffs of white. That's all that comes out of SEAL. He doesn't make a sound. He runs like a submarine. Silent. Deadly. The thought reminds me of a fart joke I heard in the fifth grade.

We do the first three miles at a ten-minute pace. Then the next two at an eight-minute pace. And the final mile is seven minutes. When we get home my son is still asleep. So is my wife. She doesn't even know there was a finger tapping me in bed earlier.

The past two days when we came home from our morning runs I have been drenched in sweat. *Soaked.* My routine has been simple: I shower, grab a bowl of fruit and some bananas, then go to work.

I eat only fruit until noon. That's been my thing since I read *Fit for Life* by Harvey Diamond in 1992. For over twenty-five years, just fruit till noon.

Harvey is another of the "interesting people" that I cold-called to be my friend. His story is fascinating. Harvey was exposed to Agent Orange, perhaps the most toxic molecule ever synthesized by man, during the Vietnam War. Agent Orange has been linked to various cancers, lymphomas, and multiple chronic diseases.

As far as I know, Harvey is the only American soldier who was exposed to the deadly chemical and is still alive. He credits it to a philosophy and lifestyle called "natural hygiene," and he lays out the road map in *Fit for Life*. I read the book three times, and it completely changed my life.

So one day I decided to call Harvey and introduce

myself. No different from SEAL. I tracked down his number, picked up the phone, and got him on the line. He checked the "yes" box to being my friend and we have been great friends since.

He's another character in my life that my wife tolerates. Every time we talk, he ends the call with "Fruit till noon, brother." One of the main underlying philosophies in his book is that we use more energy for digestion than all other bodily functions combined. That's why we are usually tired after a big meal. That said, the average American will eat seventy tons of food in their lifetime. Imagine how hard the body has to work to process and break down all of that food. The more efficiently we can digest all this food and the less stress we put on the digestive process, the more energy we will have for everything else.

According to *Fit for Life*, fruit is the perfect food because on top of being sweet and delicious, it's super-easy to digest. In fact, it is the only food that bypasses the stomach and is digested in the small intestines. It unleashes all its nutrients and goodness without using much, if any, energy, which frees up your energy for other things. As long as you eat fruit on an empty stomach, you can reap amazing benefits.

According to Diamond, you don't have to look beyond the animal kingdom to see evidence of this. The strongest animals in the world thrive on a fruit- and plant-based diet. Silverback gorillas, for example, are thirty times as strong as man and three times our size. Their DNA is 99 percent similar to that of humans, and they are our closest living relatives next to chimps. How are they so strong? Oh yeah, their diet is made up mostly of fruit and leaves. The silverback gorilla doesn't eat turkey sandwiches, chips, and McDonald's. Makes sense to me.

After reading the book in 1992, I decided to try the concept out for myself. I religiously stuck to a fruit-only diet until noon every day for ten days. After noon I generally kept it pretty clean—no fried foods, no dairy, no meats, but I didn't waver from the fruit *only* in the a.m. I had an enormous amount of energy during that span and very "efficient" digestion. I felt so good that the ten-day trial period turned into twenty-plus years of following this routine. It doesn't matter if I'm running a full marathon in the morning; I still stick to this program. Fruit till noon!

1:00 p.m.

Forty-five minutes after I get to the office this morning, SEAL arrives.

I'm back sitting in front of my computer when he gets there. I ordered in a salmon platter and some veggie dumplings from Josie's. I ate them like a wrestler right after his weigh-in. It's been about an hour since I had lunch. Zico's marketing team has presented some new packaging, and we are reviewing the options. SEAL sits in a chair in my office, motionless. That is, until he jumps out of the chair, unprompted.

"Burpee test, motherfucker," he barks.

"I'm sorry, what?"

"Burpee test, motherfucker. Why do I have to keep repeating myself?"

"I just didn't know what you meant."

"Dude, you know what a fucking burpee is, right?" He's not really asking but telling me.

"Yeah, I know what a burpee is."

"And you know what a motherfuckin' test is, right?"

"Yes. I know what a test is."

"Well then, motherfucker, this is a burpee test."

SEAL tells me he wants to time how long it takes me to do a hundred burpees. "It's a fitness test," he says, and makes sure to emphasize these are burpees with push-ups. He explains that anything under ten minutes is solid, under eleven minutes is acceptable, and he finds over thirteen minutes is unacceptable.

"In fact, if you don't go under thirteen minutes, we are doing them again," he says.

Well, I'm not really good at burpees, and I find doing one set of fifteen to be a friggin' pain.

SEAL takes off his watch and presses the start button.

BEEP!

"Wait, I have to change into something."

"Clock's already started, bitch."

I immediately drop to the floor in a plank position, do a push-up, kick my knees to my chest, and jump up into a jumping jack. One.

I get to ten in fifty-five seconds. I'm on pace. Problem is, I'm already starting to sweat, and I'm in my work clothes. I'm in my work clothes *because*...I'm at work. Plus, I need to look presentable for my meetings today. I don't want to get them all sweaty.

So, I use or waste, however you want to look at it, the next ten precious seconds taking my shirt off and then my shoes and socks. And finally my pants. I'm now in my boxers in my office. Eleven, twelve, thirteen...I keep going.

The clock is ticking and I'm at fifty at 5:30. I'm slowing down, but I'm still on pace for "acceptable." I can feel sweat on my face and rolling down the center of my back.

The door opens.

But I only see the back of her head before the blond hair quickly exits.

It's Jennifer Kish, my right-hand person at the office. She's gone before I can explain. I want to yell "burpee test, motherfucker" but the door is already closed behind her. I wonder what she's thinking.

I keep going.

When I get to sixty, I start breaking down the remaining forty burpees into sets of ten. Ten burpees and then a ten- to fifteen-second rest.

Eleven minutes, forty-five seconds. Done.

I grab an old T-shirt I happen to have lying around and wipe myself off. I'm soaked. It takes about twenty minutes for me to stop sweating, and my thighs feel like they are *broken*. I throw the soaking-wet T-shirt into the garbage can by my desk and put on my work clothes.

Soon enough I'm back at my computer looking at the color options on the packaging. My legs tremble and shake under my desk. Work resumes and a slight smile comes over my face as I think, *Burpee test, bitch!*

I work for nine hours straight.

2200

I walk home from work at 10:00 p.m. with SEAL. It's been a long day. We've been working on Zico all day with the design people, and I'm wiped out. While we were able to be additive with the new packaging, a big part of our role is generating sizzle for the brand. Every day we ask ourselves: How do we generate buzz and excitement around our products? But generating the buzz today took a lot out of me. I just want to turn on the television. Maybe watch the fourth quarter of the Knicks game and veg out. I lie down on the couch and look for the remote. SEAL has been with me all day at the office, and he's seen how intense it's been. The only real time I was alone today was when I went to the bathroom. It might have been the best five minutes of my day. I'm beat, so I'm not going to say anything about working out if he doesn't, plus we have already run six miles and done one hundred burpees. I grab the remote and flip on the television.

SEAL doesn't watch much TV. I feel like he just watches me watch TV. It's very uncomfortable. And it makes me not want to watch TV.

"You a Knicks fan?" he asks.

"All my life," I say.

"You ever go to the games?"

"I do," I say. I've had season tickets for years. "I even wrote their theme song back in the day."

"A song?"

"Rap song, theme song sort of like an anthem," I say, then

sing a little: "*Go New York, Go New York, Go*...You ever hear of it?"

"That's it?"

"That's what?"

"That's the whole song?"

"No. That's only the chorus, there's a whole verse and then you repeat the chorus, you know?"

"Doesn't seem that complicated."

"I'm not sure if it's complicated or if it's simple, but I do know that it worked," I respond.

I was a twenty-three-year-old recording artist signed to a small independent record label called Delicious Vinyl when I wrote "Go New York Go" in 1993. I somehow convinced the Knicks brass they needed a new theme song and that we could get Spike Lee and other celebs in a video around the song if we did it correctly. They gave me a shot. "Go New York Go" became the Knicks' anthem and the number-one most requested song on New York radio during the 1993–1994 NBA playoffs. The lyrics were licensed by Budweiser, Foot Locker, and other major brands. I felt like I had finally *arrived*. I was *big time*.

Well, not really big time. The Knicks paid me $4,000 to write the song. After I paid the studio, engineer, producer, and musicians, I think I netted about $300, and a net worth of $300 isn't really big time. But to me it was. Any success I have ever had in my life usually occurred when I was *not* chasing the money but was doing things out of passion. And as far as music, I was never in it for the money.

But it's not like I just woke up one day and said I want to write and record a hip-hop theme song for the New York Knicks. It started much earlier than that.

After graduation from American University, my plan A was to get a record deal and to be on MTV. That's it. There was no plan B. There was no financial goal. I just wanted to be on MTV.

Getting a record deal is one of the hardest things you can ever do. The odds of even getting a meeting with the right person are very low, and the odds of getting signed—well, those are virtually astronomical. If you don't have a powerful lawyer or know someone, then the astronomical odds become...ridiculously astronomical. I didn't have either.

In 1988, a show on MTV called *Yo! MTV Raps* debuted. The program was like the Jackie Robinson of rap TV—it broke all sorts of barriers and injected rap into mainstream culture. Still, by 1990, you could count the number of white hip-hop artists who were receiving any kind of acceptance in the larger community on one of Ice Cube's hands. The Beastie Boys were at the top of the list along with 3rd Bass. Maybe it was naiveté or pure determination—probably both—but despite the enormous odds facing me, I knew what I was going to do. I was going to be on *Yo! MTV Raps*.

A few weeks after "Pomp and Circumstance" played at my graduation ceremony, I got a phone call from a fraternity brother who had moved to LA to be a production assistant on a movie called *The Bonfire of the Vanities*. As he got settled in California, he invited me out to LA to check out the movie set (uh-hemm...and the girls).

I had never been to Cali, so I hopped on a plane and headed west.

At the time, there was a hot new independent label called Delicious Vinyl located off Sunset Boulevard. Delicious was an ultra-hip recording outfit with two of the hottest artists on pop radio: Tone-Loc and Young MC. Loc's song "Wild Thing" was the number-one-selling single in the country, and Young's "Bust a Move" was blowing up the charts. If I could write my own script, this would be the perfect label for me. Fun. Irreverent. Successful. Different. I had to meet the owners.

The guy who was the head of Delicious was named Mike Ross. In the music business, creating and distributing a song usually works like this: There's the artist who is signed by a label. Once that deal is done, either the artist has a particular producer they always work with to create and record the songs (Michael Jackson, for example, was always produced by Quincy Jones), or the label hires a producer to work with the artist. That is, of course, unless the artist does it all himself. Mike Ross was one of those rare label owners who also produced the music his label released. Along with his partner, Matt Dike, Ross was one of the most dynamic rap producers in the business.

I had read that Mike was a big fan of a Brooklyn-born rapper named Dana Dane. A big fan. As it turns out, Dana Dane recorded at Hurby "Luv Bug" Azor's studio (the same studio I recorded at), and one night while I was at the studio, I saw an advance copy of Dana's album lying on the mix board. I decided to "borrow" it while nobody was looking. Couldn't hurt. It was his second album and highly anticipated in the music community. I brought the cassette with me to LA. Nobody outside of Dana's inner clique had even heard it yet.

After only two days in LA, I decided to cold-call Mike Ross at Delicious Vinyl. "Why not?" I thought. If I was going to take a shot, I might as well take one from outside the arc. I literally got his office number out of the phone book and called the main line. I didn't have a game plan other than try to get a meeting with Mike:

"Delicious Vinyl, may I help you?" the receptionist said.

"Mike Ross, please."

"Sure, please hold."

Forty-five seconds later...

"This is Dina, Mike Ross's assistant. Can I help you?"

"Mike, please."

"Mike's not in. Who's calling?"

"Jesse."

"Jesse who?"

"Jesse. I'm a friend of Dana Dane's. Dana wanted me to drop off his new cassette for Mike while I'm in town. I'm leaving tomorrow. He said it's urgent. Mike knows about it."

"Please hold."

I covered the receiver with my hand and whispered to my friend Jon. "I'm on hold."

Maybe it was my thick Long Island accent disconnecting with her Cali vibe or maybe it was the universe wanting me to get in that door, but thirty seconds later she comes back:

"So you're Dana Dane?".

Obviously I don't look like Dana (he's African American and I'm white...he has a gold front tooth and I don't...etc.). I guess I could have cleared up the misunderstanding right then and there, *but*...when your foot is half in the door, you don't pull it out. So, without pausing, I say...

"Yes! I'm Dana."

"Okay, hold on."

One minute later...

"Dana, Mike is excited to meet you. Can you come in today around 2:00 p.m.?"

"Yes, ma'am. I'll be there."

Game on, motherfucker!

At precisely two o'clock I show up at the Delicious Vinyl offices. I'm twenty-one years old. I walk up the stairs to the second floor, where the buzzer to announce yourself is located. I push the button for entry. A very sexy receptionist voice chimes in through the speaker box:

"Who is it?"

"Oh, it's Dana Dane here to see Mike Ross please," I respond.

Ten seconds later...

BUZZZZZZ.

I'm in!

Mike Ross's assistant leads me to his office and sits me down right on the chair across from Mike's big-ass executive desk. "Mike will be back in five minutes, Dana," she tells me, right before she offers me some water.

She closes the door behind her and there I am. Just me...sitting in Mike's big, cool, unlit office. There are gold records hanging on the walls, different album covers, photos, and really cool graffiti. A patchouli candle is burning on his desk. The office is amazing. I start to read the credits on Tone-Loc's platinum album hanging on the wall and check out some of the awards on Mike's desk. Then the door opens and Mike Ross appeared. He is baffled.

"Who are you?" he said.

"What's up, Mike? I'm Jesse. I work with Dana. He's running a little late."

"Late?

"Yeah, he's maybe like twenty minutes behind."

"How do you know Dana?"

(I'd never met Dana.)

"I record with him at the same studio. My producer is part of his production crew called Idolmakers, and I did a few songs for him too."

"You sing?"

"No. I actually rap."

"You rap? With Dana?"

I figured I would continue to confuse him as it has worked thus far...

"Yeah. Well, not with him directly, but I'm part of a group signed to Virgin. But Dana thinks I should do a solo thing."

"Virgin? Do you have any songs with you?"

"Yeah! I do. Can I pop this cassette in while we wait?"

"Sure."

I handed Mike a copy of my three-song demo, and "College Girls" comes on first.

Anywhere I go a fly girl will please me
East to west college girls are easy.

He listens for thirty seconds and stops the tape.

"This is fucking amazing."

"Man, thanks, brother. I think it's a hit!"

"Who is your lawyer?"

"Excuse me?"

"Who is your lawyer?" he asks again.

And just like that—just like that!!!—after two years of getting doors slammed in my face, he hit me with the four magic words every artist shopping a demo tape wants to hear: "*Who is your lawyer?*" In fact, he asked me twice!

Since I didn't have a lawyer and I didn't even know any lawyers, I told him: "Oh, my dad is."

"Your dad is an entertainment lawyer?"

At the time my dad owned a plumbing supply company, but it was the first answer that popped into my head (I'm a "get your foot in the door, figure it out later guy") so I responded with a firm "Yes." "Yep…my dad does all my stuff."

"I'm gonna have my attorney contact your dad. I want to buy this song for Loc."

"That's incredible, if Loc did this song…" Then I paused. Loc? I realized that this song was *my* ticket to a deal. Sure,

I could have sold it to Tone-Loc. "Wild Thing" had sold over 3 million units at the time, but this was the lead song on my demo. So I responded, "Actually, I really think this song is a big hit. I gotta keep this one for me. It's going on *my* album."

"That makes sense. Well, would you be willing to write for Loc then?"

And that was the *official* start of my music career.

Mike gave me the instrumentals for four songs he wanted me to write for Tone-Loc and sent me back to my friend's apartment. Two hours later, I called him on his Nokia with lyrics for all of the songs. He was at a Dodgers game and could barely hear me over the din of the stadium. But he heard enough to meet me back at his office when the game was over. There I not only signed a deal to write songs for Tone-Loc, but he signed me on the spot for my own album. (Dana later became a great friend and we still laugh about it.) Thanks, Dana!

Maybe the best part about my music career was the fact that I didn't sell that many records. As my wife likes to say, "Failure is just life's way of nudging you and letting you know you're off course." Yes, I was on MTV and got to tour the country, but the hockey-stick-curve sales trajectory wasn't there. So, I decided to "call an audible" and look for other opportunities in music. Writing theme songs for sports teams seemed like a great niche. I loved music. Loved sports. And *nobody* else was doing it. The result was "Go New York Go." I started a niche...sports music.

There must be an echo in here because I keep hearing SEAL say "Doesn't seem that complicated." SEAL is a lot of things, but he is not a music critic. Rather than debate this, out of my mouth comes:

"You're right. It's really not that complicated. Pretty simple actually."

"Yeah, it's simple," he says.

I start flipping the channels. I don't even find the Knicks game on the tube before SEAL suggests we take the conversation outside and get in another workout. It's 10:45 p.m. The upside is this is the first time he's actually asking questions about me. Not that I want him to, but it makes it easier to get to know someone when there's a back-and-forth. As my wife likes to remind me, "When I talk to you...please play tennis with me and hit the ball back. It's called 'communication,' and it's important to a marriage." And although I'm not looking to get married to SEAL, my wife has a valid point.

Our workout is basically the same routine as the morning, a loop around Central Park, except tonight comes with a bonus: Every half mile we do twenty-five push-ups. The other difference is that SEAL wants the pace to escalate, meaning every mile has to be slightly faster than the previous mile.

We start out at a nine-minute pace and at 4:30 into the run, we drop and do twenty-five push-ups, then we increase to an 8:50-mile pace and 4:25 into the run, we drop and do twenty-five push-ups. This continues all the way down to an 8:10 pace for the last mile.

Every time we drop to do the push-ups, blood rushes to my head and I get slightly faint. I'm breathing so hard when we do the push-ups (plus it's friggin' *brick cold* outside) that I'm slightly hyperventilating. SEAL is knocking out the push-ups like a programmed robot. Up. Down. Up. Down. Up. Down. I'm at around nine by the time he is done with his twenty-five and already standing to start running again. Every time.

> **Workout totals: 12 miles (6 miles "escalation" pace), 300 push-ups, and 100 burpees**

DAY 7

Mix Up Your Runs

If it doesn't suck, we don't do it.
—SEAL

New York City to Atlanta
36° to 75°
0530

"Your runs are too predictable," SEAL says as he stares at me stone-faced.

"Predictable?"

"Yeah, motherfucker...predictable. It's like your legs know what's coming next. It's making shit too comfy. Your body is used to your bullshit jogging routine. Gear up and meet me in five; we're doing intervals."

I throw on my gear and grab a brand-new pair of New Balance running shoes. I have been wearing New Balance for twenty years. They are the only things I run in. Once the bottoms get fairly worn out (but not all the way worn out), I replace them with a new pair. I read that having the proper cushion on your sneakers minimizes the impact on your legs when running and therefore reduces the chance of injury. I don't know if that is true or if that was created by a sneaker company, but I bought into it hook, line, and sneaker. Regardless, New Balance are part of my routine.

Five minutes later, we're on our way to Central Park for a seven-mile run. We do the first mile at a ten-minute pace to warm up, then every quarter mile after that we runasfastaswecan. After sprinting a quarter mile we slow down to a ten-minute pace again.

SEAL pushes me so hard on the quarter miles I can feel my pulse pounding in my neck. I can literally take my pulse by just counting the thumps exploding through my neck.

At the end of the run I'm gasping for air. But it's not my heart or lungs I'm worried about.

"Man, my legs are really messed up. It feels like a knife is in my calf," I complain. "Like I can cramp any second." I grab my leg and walk stiff-legged, keeping my legs totally straight like Herman Munster from *The Munsters*.

"Perfect," SEAL says. "There's only one rule in training: If it doesn't suck, we don't do it."

I probably should have broken in my new sneakers because I feel a blister forming on my right big toe. It hurts, but that pain is trumped by the pain in my calf. The blister is more like the middle child at the dinner table—not even part of the conversation. It's like I don't even pay it any mind, but I know it's there. It's like SEAL has made blisters that previously would have been big deals almost seem insignificant.

As a reward for my pain, I get to do 275 push-ups when we get home. To make matters worse, SEAL tells me we are doing them wet.

"Wet?"

"Wet!"

"What does wet mean in push-up land?"

He tells me that we don't change out of our wet, sweaty-ass clothing. We do the push-ups wet.

"Why are we doing wet push-ups?"

"'Cause that's the way I ordered them up today. That's why. I don't give a fuck how you give them to me, but I want all two seventy-five."

This guy is out of his mind.

I drop down and do my first set of ten. My body heat is dropping fast as I cool off from the run. I'm starting to get very cold. Like shivering cold. Every time my shirt touches my skin, it feels like a wet ice pack. I look at SEAL and he is warm. Lukewarm. He is just going down, up, down, up, down, up. Fifty. Down, up, down, up...sixty...Who is this motherfucker, and where did he come from?

I don't know much about SEAL's childhood, but I do know that he always wanted to be in the Special Forces. The other day while we were sitting around he mentioned that he used to play Rambo as a kid. *Not* the way I would play Rambo (with a Toys "R" Us Rambo doll), but like real Rambo.

When SEAL was fifteen or sixteen, he would go out into the deep woods alone around 11:00 p.m. and pretend he was picking off the enemy. He said he would stay out there for hours at a time training. I found the story to be very interesting and scary.

I don't know when it dawned on me, but at some point during that story I realized I had a Navy SEAL living in my house now—for every second of the day. This guy is using my toilet, he's in my fridge, he's answering my door, and he's sleeping in the room next to my kid's. He's everywhere. I mean, I knew I had a Navy SEAL living with me in *theory* because I invited him, but in practice it was slightly disconcerting.

In fact, I'm starting to realize I know very little about SEAL. Actually, I don't really know *anything* about him. It's sorta like inviting your taxi driver home to live with you and your family and having him drive you everywhere, but you know nothing about the taxi driver.

So now I'm wondering: What if I say something he doesn't like politically? What if I say something that pisses him off? What if I accidentally offend him and he gets even angrier than he already is? I mean, I did a full background check before I hired my first assistant, and she came from a nice family I already knew. SEAL is trained to eliminate the enemy if ordered and is now living with me . . . and I have done nothing.

Luckily, I keep these thoughts in my head.

I know I'm being a little crazy and there's probably nothing to worry about. I mean, really. But, honestly, what the fuck was I thinking? I don't even like strangers being in my house for a couple of minutes. I hate it when the cable guy comes. And yet I now have a trained hunting machine in my midst—not only my midst, but my wife's and my son's midst. He's right in the middle of our midst.

I wish there was someone I could talk to about this. I'd tell my wife, but I can't because it'll scare her. And then she'd be like, "You have to get rid of him." And I know there's no way I can get rid of him. How can you get rid of someone like him? "Oh, excuse me, Mr. SEAL, this isn't working out, so get your gear and beat it." Right?!

So instead I do the exact opposite and say stuff to my wife like, "You know, SEAL's the nicest guy..." Or "It's really amazing how someone who looks so indestructible and scary can be so cool." I have to oversell him. But I think Sara is starting to see through my ruse. Thank God, SEAL is the perfect houseguest. He's quiet, clean, and well mannered. And thank God he and Sara are getting along well.

Seven hours later....

We show up at Teterboro Airport in New Jersey at 1:30 p.m. for our flight to Atlanta, where Spanx, my wife's company, is headquartered. Today we are flying on a Marquis Jet Citation X. I love the Citation X because it is superfast but also quite roomy. It can knock off significant travel time on a flight like this.

In the late 1990s my partner at the time, Kenny Dichter, and I were guests on a private plane. From the minute we stepped on board we were in love with the convenience of flying private; comfort and ease at its very best. When we got home from the trip, we never wanted to get back on a commercial plane again. We assumed if we wanted to fly this way, there must be a heck of a lot of others who would want to as well. There has to be a market for this, we thought.

At the time, there were only three ways to fly private: One was to buy your own plane, which was impossible unless you were Mark Cuban or the Sultan of Brunei; two, buy a fraction of a jet, which comes with a very expensive five-year commitment; or, three, charter a plane, a process that has a lot of moving parts and inconsistencies. None of those options was very appealing to us, nor would they be appealing to any potential clients if we tried to start a company, which we had begun to think about.

We wanted to create something more realistic for a much larger demographic—people who wanted to fly privately a few times a year. So we came up with this idea: What if you could buy twenty-five hours a year of private flight time? It would be almost like a Starbucks card, or a prepaid gift card, to fly.

At the time NetJets was the 800-pound gorilla of fractional jet ownership. Warren Buffett owned the company. The CEO was a guy named Richard Santulli, and the president was a guy named Jim Jacobs. When we got the idea for Marquis Jet, we knew the first call we should make was to Jacobs.

A couple of years before, during the time I was still in music and connected to a lot of artists, I'd gotten a call from a friend who wanted a favor. I don't really remember why, maybe he was doing a business deal or maybe he just wanted to do something nice for someone, but he asked me if I could get tickets to a Christina Aguilera concert in Connecticut for a friend's daughter. My friend knew that I had a relationship with Christina's manager. So I called up the manager and not only did I get the guy and his daughter great seats, but I worked out having his daughter onstage as a backup singer if she wanted to (they would shut her mic off). I mean, for a teenager, this was a life-altering moment.

The next day the guy who went to the concert with his daughter called me up and said, "I don't know who you are, but I want to let you know that I owe you one in a big way. If there's anything I can ever do..."

That guy was Jim Jacobs.

So now it's a year later, and there *is* something Jim Jacobs can do for me. I call him. I think it took him five minutes just to figure out who I was: "Who is this again?" Jim asked.

"Jesse. Christina Aguilera. Not only backstage but *on*stage," I said. "Genie in a Bottle Itzler? You said if I ever needed anything to call you." It was the same shit as when I got my record deal, I confused him. Just throwing words at him. It was Harry Truman who said, "If you can't convince them, confuse them." It's a tactic I still use instinctively. It buys time.

"Oh, yeah," he said.

"Can I steal thirty minutes of your time?" I said.

We set up a meeting with Jim Jacobs and Rich Santulli a week later. Kenny and I drove to their Woodbury, New

Jersey, headquarters with our PowerPoint deck and presentation ready to start our new private jet timeshare company. We weren't exactly sure at the time what the company was, but we knew we had a great idea. We walked into the meeting and Jim and Rich were already seated in their conference room. They were suited up, and I mean Italy suited up. About twenty minutes into the meeting, Rich Santulli said, "No way am I letting two twenty-nine-year-olds use my fleet of five hundred planes. Good to meet you, guys." Then he threw us out of his office.

"I guess we need a new idea," I said to Kenny after we walked out of there. And that's when my phone rang. It was Jim.

When I started apologizing to him for wasting his time, he cut me off.

"That was amazing! Great meeting," he said.

"Great meeting?"

"Yeah, Rich doesn't give twenty minutes to anyone. I think it went great. The idea is brilliant! I think there's something here. Why don't you tweak your presentation a little bit and come back? Let me see if I can get you another meeting."

By this time, I knew a lot of athletes and entertainers and Kenny knew a lot of Wall Street guys we both felt would be interested in buying twenty-five hours of private jet time if it was available. We realized we needed a different pitch. We needed to show Santulli and Jacobs, not tell them. So we put together our own focus group.

A week later, we were back in Santulli's office with Carl

Banks from the New York Giants, the guys from Run-DMC, a top sports agent for NBA players, and a successful Wall Street guy who ran his own firm and wanted to use jets occasionally for entertaining. One by one our focus group participants explained to Rich how they would never buy a NetJets fraction, but they *would* spend 100K or 200K on a jet card every year. They discussed how they needed the flexibility of being able to choose their flights year by year. And they talked about why they or their clients would buy a card. And how if things went well, they would eventually graduate into the fractional program NetJets already offered.

Although Santulli didn't take the bait right away, we could tell he was nibbling. It would take three or four more meetings to set the hook, but eventually Santulli told us if we were willing to put up our own money to try this idea we were calling "Marquis Jet," then he'd give us a shot at it. We did and it worked. BIG TIME.

Sara and SEAL don't really say much to each other on the plane—it's only been seven days since he moved in and they haven't had much quality time with each other—but there is a mutual respect and friendship forming.

Sara acts 100 percent normal around SEAL, as if it's not strange at all having a Navy SEAL shadow me 24/7 all of a sudden. But her disposition being normal is not abnormal to me, as sometimes my wife is in her own world. I mean, she is *brilliant* but also has her blond moments. I like to say she is 50 percent Lucille Ball and 50 percent Einstein. For example, she built a highly successful global brand with just $5,000 of savings but asks me what day of the week it is often, and means it. That said, as long as she gets seven hours of sleep and has her Starbucks in hand when the sun comes up, life is good.

My wife's name is Sara Blakely, and she's the founder and inventor of Spanx. If you're a woman, you probably know what Spanx are. If you're a guy, Sara is like the Michael Jordan of women's underwear.

When I first started dating her, I didn't get it. But now, after witnessing the love for her brand firsthand, I totally do. Women go crazy for her products. Strangers are always hugging Sara and flashing her their undergarments in public. It's wild.

What I love most about Sara's story is that, growing up, she always wanted to be a lawyer, but she failed the LSATs... twice. So instead of heading to law school after college, she decided to go to Disney World and try out to be Goofy... naturally. When she arrived, she was too short for the job (minimum height is 5'8" and Sara is 5'6") so they asked her to be a chipmunk instead.

After a short stint at Disney, Sara accepted a job with an office supply company called Danka and sold fax machines door to door... for seven years. One night before heading out for a party, she didn't like the way her own butt looked in white pants. She took a pair of scissors and cut off the feet of her pantyhose to avoid panty lines and have a smoother look under her clothes. Voilà, her invention was born.

Over the course of the next two years, Sara worked on

developing her new idea after work, at night, and on the weekends. She took $5,000 she had set aside in savings to start the company. Since she had never taken a business course in her life, she operated on instinct and guts.

Instead of using her entire budget on legal fees to patent her product, Sara bought a book on patents and wrote her own patent. She used bold colors on her packaging to make her products pop off the shelves. She spent twelve hours a day in department stores promoting her products. It worked!

The name Spanks came to Sara while sitting in traffic in Atlanta. She knew that Kodak and Coca-Cola were two of the most recognized brand names in the world and that both names shared a strong "k" sound. She figured it must be good luck. She changed the "ks" to an "x" at the last minute because she had read that made-up words are easier to trademark than real words.

Sara trademarked the company online for $150 at www .uspto.com. Today Spanx has over 150 products, hundreds of employees, and is sold worldwide.

Our newly SEAL-infused family touches down in Atlanta and we start to gather our things. Needless to say, we spend a lot of time in Atlanta because Spanx is headquartered here, but I'm not ready to give up on New York just yet. The amount of time we're spending here is also increasing, so we're renovating a new house. It's exactly two miles from our current house in Atlanta. Sara wants to check on the progress of construction.

SEAL tells me we'll run there and back as we pull into the driveway. Sara teases she will drive there and she will drive back. We quickly change and head out on our run to the house to meet Sara.

It's a nice leisurely run along shaded streets lined with beautiful homes and huge trees. We're not really pounding it and I'm thinking about how pleasant everything is today. Then, just about a mile into our run, I hear something that sounds like the crack of a huge thunderbolt. I can't pinpoint where the sound is coming from or what it is, but it sounds dangerous and close. In that instant, I turn to look at SEAL. But his arms are stretched out and he's heading toward me. He looks like an eagle. There's a woman who happens to be walking her dog on the sidewalk about five feet away. Now SEAL has both of us in his wingspan and is practically lifting us off the ground as he pushes us. It's then I see a huge branch fall twenty-five feet from a tree directly above us. It hits the ground with a massive *thud* and explodes. The thing is about eighteen inches in diameter and bursts into small pieces when it hits the cement. It would have killed us.

"Let's go. Keep pace," SEAL says, and continues on.

The entire rest of the run I'm in complete awe. It was almost as if he knew the branch would fall. How did he identify what was going on so quickly, and how did he know where the branch was coming from? This was not the type of shit you learn in a manual.

When we get to the new home, I'm still half in shock.

"How was your run?" Sara asks.

I look at SEAL expecting him to say something about the branch. Instead, he says: "Good. Your husband is improving."

Good?

He doesn't mention the branch. It was like branches falling and almost hitting him in the head is a regular thing. No biggie. Not worth a mention.

2045

Sara's watching *Oprah* repeats and I'm in my go-to-sleep clothes. SEAL appears in my room to check up on me.

"How ya legs feel?" he asks.

"Terrible. They're sore and tight."

"Cool. Put your shorts and sneakers on."

"No," I say.

"Oh, yes indeed."

It's our third run of the day. I've previously done some two-a-days while training for long races or to try to get in fast shape, but three-a-days is new territory, especially at this intensity. And especially at my age. And really especially at 8:45 p.m. at night.

One and a half miles into our six-mile run, SEAL talks for the first time.

"You okay?"

"No. I don't feel well," I say as I keep pace.

"Fuck, yeah," he celebrates. "Now you're seeing what it's like to train, Jesse. I hope you enjoy this shit." He begins to laugh, which soon becomes an all-out cackle. "You look like a pile of spilt fuck," he says.

When we return, Sara is still watching *Oprah*. It's like we never even left.

> **Workout totals: 17 miles and 275 push-ups in the morning**

DAY 8

No Peeing Allowed

This isn't piss time. It's run time.
—SEAL

Atlanta to New York City

34° to 18°

0800

After a super-early flight from Atlanta, we land back in Teterboro. The flight time to Teterboro is only about one hour and forty minutes. Since we live relatively close to the airport in Atlanta, the door-to-door travel time is close to two hours. Not a bad commute.

Thirty minutes later...

SEAL and I put on our gear to run six miles outside. Maybe it's from the flight or maybe I'm just not drinking enough, but I feel a little dehydrated before the run. This is confirmed by the fact my urine is almost brown. So, before heading out, I drink two full glasses of water. Then we're off.

About one mile into the run, I have to pee so bad it hurts. If I could cross my legs, I would. I ask SEAL if we can pull over.

"SEAL, man, I gotta pee...BAD."

"NOW? In the middle of the fucking run? On my time? Why didn't you plan your piss BEFORE the run? What the fuck do you think you're doing pissing now when this is run time? This isn't piss time."

SEAL is genuinely mad. I offended him by having to urinate on our run. So, after his thirty-second rant on the subject, I decide that I no longer have to piss anymore. I hold it in. For the next five miles of the run, all I'm thinking about is *not* peeing.

When we complete the run, I ask SEAL politely if I can urinate. "It's your time now. Do whatever the fuck you want."

One hour later...

We're at the breakfast table, one big happy family. Sara feeds Lazer applesauce, I'm reading the sports section of the *New York Post* devouring some more bananas, and a morning TV show is on in the background. SEAL slides a box of fancy granola off to the side. SEAL isn't big on rations from Whole Foods. He shakes his head when Sara offers him a bowlful. I noticed yesterday I haven't seen SEAL eating at all. I mean...as in *nothing* since he's been here. That's seven days and three meals a day and I haven't seen him eat a single bite.

But it's Sara who asks, "SEAL, are you on a diet?"

"Nah, I just like to go to sleep hungry...so I wake up hungry. Life is all about staying out of your comfort zone."

"And what's the reasoning behind that?"

My wife is very inquisitive, but not in a pushy way. She loves to learn and hear every detail when she's curious about something, and I can say with confidence that she likes to talk. Her favorite thing is having a long meal and talking about the meaning of life. SEAL is polite, but you couldn't build a dinner party around him. He looks like he's going to pull a muscle trying to converse. After about twenty questions from Sara ranging from his upbringing to what should she make for dinner tonight, I decide to cut SEAL a break and change the topic by making a suggestion.

"So what do you guys think about heading up to Connecticut to the lake house for the Christmas holiday?"

"Sounds good," SEAL says. "I want to check your security up there anyway."

"Security?" Sara says. "We don't need security; it's a private community."

"A private community? So is the White House," he answers.

The house is on Candlewood Lake in Danbury, Connecticut. Candlewood is the largest lake in Connecticut, and it's a great vacation spot. We mostly go up there as a summer retreat, but we also like to do a trip around Christmas as well. The house is in a gated community of a hundred homes.

Lawns are perfectly manicured, houses are superbly well kept, and if there is one piece of litter on the streets, it would be considered dirty. Needless to say, crime is not an issue.

"Who checked it last?" SEAL asks.

My wife looks at me and shrugs.

"That's it," SEAL says, tossing his cloth napkin on the table. "I'm going to take a look."

SEAL has a mission. He finds a clipboard I didn't even know we owned and grabs a pen.

I have a few meetings in the office, so I can't go along. I call Smith, my driver, and ask if he minds taking SEAL up to Connecticut for the night. We're scheduled to have a plumber come to the lake house the next day, so it's perfect.

"What time?" Smith asks.

SEAL is standing there with the clipboard looking at me. "I think he's ready to go now," I say.

"Tell him I'll be there in three minutes," Smith says.

I met Smith through Jam Master Jay of Run-DMC. I knew Jay from the mid-1990s. After I wrote "Go New York Go" for the Knicks, I cofounded a company called Alphabet City. Alphabet City was a vehicle for me to sell more theme songs to teams. I was at a trade show and I saw Jay across the way from our booth. I decided to go over and introduce myself. Jay was my Ringo Starr: not the front guy of the band, but the guy that held it together. He was the guy I looked up to in the music business. We hit it off from minute one.

A month after meeting, Jay called me up. He had been working out of an office at Def Jam Records and wanted to relocate. We had created one big "war room" at Alphabet

City, and I told him he could have the desk next to mine. At that time he had just started JMJ Records and was producing a number of artists including Onyx of "Slam" fame.

Jam Master Jay had one secretary/manager and two interns who also worked out of our office. One of the interns was a young rapper from Queens named Kaeson, and the other was a rapper/boxer from Queens named Curtis. I *loved* Kaeson's music and signed him to my own private label. I didn't see the same star power in Curtis, but he helped me with a bunch of sports songs. Well, shortly after interning for us, Curtis Jackson, calling himself 50 Cent, went on his own and signed with Eminem. 50 Cent became one of the top-selling artists of the decade. BIG miss on my part.

Smith was Jay's friend, and that's how I got to know him—Smith was always at Jay's office and ultimately ended up working for Jay. Smith isn't a tough-looking guy, but you can tell he's tough. He's someone you'd let win an argument because you're afraid he'd fight you. But his exterior belies his interior. He's a gentle soul at heart.

One of the first things you learn about Smith is that he's one of those guys who always just missed. If Smith bought a Mega Millions lottery ticket today, his numbers would come in tomorrow. He's always one inch away from greatness. Smith was like the fourth member of Run-DMC no one knew about. In the early 1980s the group wanted him to be the original DJ, but he was dating a girl in Texas and didn't want to commit to the group. So instead of the meteoric fame his friends enjoyed, he ended up doing sound checks and what-ever else the group needed. Plus, he broke up with the girl.

To find out how long Smith has been just missing, you

have to go all the way back to his days in junior high. His full name is Darnell Smith, which apparently didn't single him out because there was another Darnell Smith in his class. On the playground one day in eighth grade, the two Darnell Smiths decided to play rock, paper, scissors to see who would be called "Darnell" and who would be called "Smith." And Smith just barely missed with a throw of rock only trumped by paper. He's been known as Smith ever since.

Through Jay, Smith became a close friend. After a while, our friendship felt like any of the friendships I had with the guys I grew up with except that Smith was much tougher than the guys I grew up with. After Jay was murdered by an unknown assailant at his music studio in Queens in 2002, Smith needed a job. I ran into him a couple of months after the funeral and asked him if he had a driver's license. He held up a MetroCard.

"Does this count?" he said. He was only kidding. He had a license, so I asked him if he wanted to drive for me.

"What would it entail?" he asked.

"Mostly it entails driving for me."

He's been working for me for ten years now, but he's much more than an employee—he's part of my family. He's someone I can trust and count on.

Smith drives SEAL up to the house in Connecticut. They're both going to spend the night and meet with the plumber the next morning. The plumber is going to give me an estimate on replacing some damaged tile in the steam room. I call them before I go to bed just to make sure everything is okay.

"All cool," says Smith.

But apparently it doesn't stay all cool. In the middle of the night Smith decides he's hungry and tiptoes downstairs to the kitchen because he doesn't want to wake SEAL, who's in one of the bedrooms. Smith doesn't even want to turn on the lights, so he makes his way from the bottom of the staircase to the kitchen using his cell phone for light until he manages to find the handle of the refrigerator, which he pulls open to give more light. He walks over to the counter and grabs a bag of cookies. What Smith didn't know was that we have a motion detector we turn on when we're not using the house. It goes on automatically at night. Maybe this scored some points with SEAL when he inspected the house's security. So when Smith pops the first cookie into his mouth, the alarm is triggered and sends off this earsplitting sound.

Now, Smith knows there's no intruder in the house because he triggered the alarm, but Smith also knows that SEAL doesn't know what Smith knows. Smith might have a bit of intruder experience in his repertoire, but he has absolutely none when it comes to dealing with a pissed-off Navy SEAL who might think he's an intruder.

Smith drops to the ground and crawls over underneath the kitchen table and begins to scream, "SEEEEEEEEEEEE EEEEEEEEEEEEEEEEEEEEEEEAL, IT'S MEEEEEEEE, IT'S SMIIIIIIIIIIIIIIIIIIITH, IT'S ME, SMITH!"

When the alarm company notified me, I called SEAL. He told me he found Smith trembling underneath the kitchen table, kneeling in a pool of spilled milk, cookie crumbs all over his face.

The next day SEAL drives back to New York and sits me down in our conference room with a report of his inspection.

He looks even more serious than when he is about to tell me what workout or run we are going to do. He's prepared.

"Man, this is fucked up. You guys are FUCKED up there."

I'm trying not to laugh. "We're on a beautiful, tranquil lake. Even the deer feel safe up there."

"The northeast windows are warped. The perimeter is exposed...too many entry points...too much glass."

I try to take a look at his report.

"This is a fucking disaster zone," he says.

"For real?"

"Man, I couldn't live in this place. NO FUCKING WAY. I can't even comprehend how you and Sara live there."

This may be the most animated I've ever seen SEAL.

"Wow...Well, what do you suggest we do?"

"We need to swap out all the doors IMMEDIATELY. Lock down all the nonprimary windows. AND bulletproof the glass."

"Bulletproof the glass?"

"Yep, bulletproof the glass."

"Is that really necessary? It's a lake house...in the middle of nowhere."

"CRITICAL...I'm going to contact my boy and price that sucker out."

That evening, SEAL is waiting inside the doorway when I get home. He's holding a file in his right hand. His muscles are tense. His expression is so stern it's like his face is cut from rock. He doesn't say hello. He gets right into it.

"We have two options as I see it," he says in a deadly whisper.

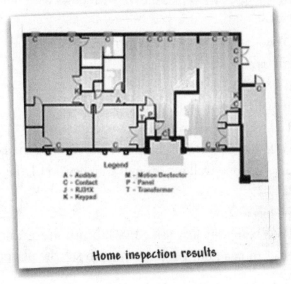

Home inspection results

"Okay."

"We can replace all the lower and midlevel windows for $450,000, or...we can say *Fuck it* and do the whole house for $785,000, which personally I think is a no-brainer."

"Seven hundred eighty-five thousand dollars?"

"Yep, but man, look. Rambo can be standing outside with an M16...and you can stick your middle finger up at him and say, '*FUCK YOU, RAMBO*'... And he won't be able to get in. This is military-grade shit. *It works.* Unless Rambo brings a bazooka, you can sleep knowing your shit is on lockdown."

Sara comes home, and I sit her down to discuss our options.

"Sweetie, SEAL gave me a quote on the security system for the lake house."

"Great, honey," she says as Lazer runs into her arms.

"He suggests we replace all our windows with bulletproof glass."

"Okay, love." She smiles while combing her fingers through our son's hair.

"It's $785,000."

My wife says nothing.

"Thoughts?" I ask with a manufactured smile.

"Well, let me ask you this, sweetie. When is the last time you saw someone walking around Candlewood Lake with an M16?"

She has a point.

"Love, can you just ask SEAL to put fire extinguishers in all the rooms and teach me how to set the alarm?" Sara smiles.

Workout totals: 6 miles

Google Me, Motherfucker

I don't like motherfuckin' freeloaders. You
better work hard for your shit or we aren't gonna
get along very well.
—SEAL

Next day...

I get a call from the plumber who went in to check the steam room tiles at the Connecticut house. The conversation went something like this:

"Hello, Mr. Itzler?"

"Yes."

"Please tell that man I did not Google you and that I would have quoted the same price if you lived in the South Bronx."

"Excuse me?"

"I don't want any trouble. But I do want you to know I've contacted my lawyer."

"What?"

"I'll take thirty percent off."

"I don't know what you're talking about."

"Okay, forty percent, damn it! Do you mind if I make a living? I have a family too!"

"Uhhh?" was all I could manage before he hung up.

It turns out SEAL had taken exception to the price the plumber quoted for the work and accused the man of going on the Internet, determining our net worth and the location of our primary residence at 15 CPW, and then trying to gouge us based on that information. The way SEAL expressed his displeasure at the plumber was to pound his fist on the tile until it began to crack while yelling: "You Googled them! You Googled them! Well, Google me, motherfucker!"

"I don't want any trouble," the plumber said on the phone. "Please. I beg you."

DAY 9

Oxygen Deprivation

Train for the unexpected.
—SEAL

New York City
23°
0600

It's only been a little over a week...nine days to be exact...
but it feels like SEAL has been living with me for fifteen
years. It's not like we're exchanging friendship bracelets,
though I do feel I understand him a bit better. He's still
spending a lot of time in his room at night, but he feels a
little more integrated into our daily lives.

Today I wake up *sore*. Or maybe stiff is the more accurate
description. I've never been one for stretching out. And I can
honestly say I've never formally stretched in all my years of
running. Not pre-run. Not post-run. It's not that I'm against
it; it's just not my thing. But today I'm going to need to figure
something out. I'm in this stiff-like locked mode and my body

can't function normally. I reach for the beeping alarm clock, and my arm can't move from a ninety-degree angle. It's stuck in an imaginary sling.

To get up, I have to clasp my hands under my legs and hurl them both out of bed. I basically have to generate enough momentum to swing my legs over the side of the bed and onto the floor. They are that stiff.

H E L P !

As I get to an upright position, I bend down and try to touch my hands to the floor. I barely get past my knees. It makes me realize that SEAL does not do any stretching either. When we do our workouts, we just start. There is no "pregame" before the runs and there are no cooldowns after. Eventually I make it out of my bedroom and see SEAL in the living room writing something down in his tiny workout log.

"SEAL, are we going to do any stretching during this whole ordeal?" I ask.

First his eyebrows arch. Then instantly his expression turns to a scowl. SEAL takes two steps closer to me and gets in real close. I can feel and hear his nostrils breathing. I think I insulted his expertise.

"What do you want, a fucking leotard? Man, we start, and then, motherfucker, we finish. That's what we do up here," he says.

Okay then.

So at 0600 today we head out to Central Park for *another* run.

No stretching.

No preparation.

My warm-up is putting on my warm clothing.

I get it.

It takes me a solid three miles to get going, but surprisingly, once we find our pace and break a sweat, my legs really loosen up. In fact, I go from feeling like a stick figure to someone performing in Cirque du Soleil—okay, maybe that's a bit of an exaggeration, but I feel good—real good. Odd. I mention it to SEAL as we run and he just replies, "Jesse, I really don't give a fuck."

As we come close to the end of the run, SEAL finds a tree with a long branch hanging straight out. We stop. SEAL jumps up and knocks out twenty-five pull-ups. No kipping. No using his legs for momentum. Just twenty-five perfect all-American pull-ups. He instructs me to do ten.

"Even if you have to stop. Do all ten."

I'm soaking wet in sweat after our six-mile run. I do six nonstop pull-ups and then drop to the ground. Back up for the last four. We return home.

I make a hot bath in my bathroom. As the warm water fills the tub I dump an entire box of Epsom salts into the water and mix it around with my hand. I have no idea if this product works, but it has been said to help muscle pain. The box says to add two scoops for every so and so gallon of water, but I'm so stiff again now that there will be no measuring. I pour the entire box in. I strip down and climb in slowly to get used to the heat. I grab a magazine, kick my feet up on top of the tub, and relax!

It feels good to be working out so hard, but I'm also starting to feel and see hints of my body breaking down. It's much harder to get out of bed in the morning, although I do appreciate my bed more, especially when I see that wooden chair. But I know I can do this.

Four hours later...

I have a meeting in my conference room. We have an idea for a new business we are calling "Sheets," and we are going through some early-stage strategy. "Sheets" are small dissolvable strips that you place on your tongue (think Listerine strip) that are loaded with caffeine, B-12, and other vitamins and nutrients. The hope is that this product could one day compete with or even replace 5-hour Energy or other on-the-go energy products. The product has unique benefits in its fast delivery system of caffeine and its portable packaging.

SEAL is in the meeting. Well...SEAL is sitting in the meeting, but I wouldn't say he is active. He is listening, but I can tell something is bothering him. He is looking at me like he is pissed off. When the group decides to take a ten-minute break to "check emails," SEAL asks if he can chat with me for a second.

Thirty seconds later we are alone in my office.

"This morning was incomplete. I got shortchanged," he says.

"Excuse me?"

"We ran. We did push-ups. We did pull-ups. But we didn't get our sit-ups in. It was an incomplete session."

"But I did everything you asked me to do," I say.

"Well, now I'm telling you that our shit was incomplete and it's fucking me up. So we are going to do them NOW."

"Now? I'm in the middle of a big meeting."

"No you're not. You're in the middle of a break."

SEAL tells me to sit my ass on the floor and then he steps on my feet.

"Lie all the way down," he says.

Then he tells me to sit up and touch his knees. I do that a hundred times. After about thirty-five I have to lie flat on the floor after every five sit-ups to get my energy and strength to do the next five. When we are done I am sweating profusely. At that exact moment, Kish comes into my office and tells me we are resuming the meeting.

SEAL and I head back to the conference room. Everyone is staring at me as sweat pours off my forehead like a faucet that has been left on. SEAL looks at the group and can clearly sense the tension.

"Jesse had some unfinished work," SEAL says. "He is ready now."

The meeting resumes.

1800 (6:00 p.m.)

Dinner.

2000 (8:00 p.m.)

Shower.

2200 (10:00 p.m.)

I hear a noise coming from SEAL's room like he's landing a helicopter in there. I knock gently on the door. Nothing. I knock a little louder. Nothing.

I'm POUNDING on the door.

"WHAT?" SEAL yells.

He opens the door and there's a camp tent on the floor. Not folded or packed away, but set up like he's going to build a campfire and roast marshmallows in the middle of my Manhattan apartment. The tent is hooked up to some type of generator with a hose. The generator is pumping full tilt. It's loud.

"Whatcha doing?" I ask casually.

"Huh?"

"WHAT ARE YOU DOING?"

"Getting ready for bed," he says.

"Ah, okay. What's that?"

"What?"

I point at the tent.

"That's a tent."

"OHHHH! It's a tent," I say.

"Yep!"

"I know it's a fucking tent, but why?"

"'Cause I'm gonna sleep in it tonight."

"You're gonna sleep in a tent? In a bedroom? On Central Park West?"

"Yes."

"Can I ask why?"

"Oxygen deprivation."

"Huh?"

"This tent deprives you of oxygen."

SEAL zips himself in and says, "I'm training too, dude. Kill the lights."

I later learn it's called an altitude-simulation tent, and

when the generator is hooked up it sucks the O2 out of the tent and helps the body produce more red blood cells. It makes your cardio system work like you're sleeping on top of Mount Everest.

I'd have to bet I'm the only guy on the Upper West Side of NYC with an inflatable raft, an oxygen deprivation tank, a tent, and a SEAL in his apartment. I get into my bed and open the window in our room. I suck in the cold NY air coming into my apartment off Central Park. It feels great. As I fall asleep I think about the lack of oxygen in SEAL's tent and again think to myself…I'm such a pussy.

Workout totals: 6 miles, 10 pull-ups, 100 sit-ups

DAY 10

The Honor Code

If you want to be pushed to your limits, you have
to train to your limits.
—SEAL

New York City
21°
0500

Sara is sound asleep. My son Lazer is asleep. Most of the
continental United States is asleep.

SEAL is *not* asleep.

SEAL is in the den.

SEAL is dressed.

Same T-shirt.

Same shorts.

He looks like he's been up for hours. Fresh. Unfazed.
Wide awake and giddy.

Me? I look like I just got off the red-eye. Tired. Worn
and pissed that I'm up.

SEAL looks like he has nothing else to do but this. Me? I have a ton of shit on my mind with Zico and making sure Coke is happy with our work to date. I'm concerned about the new Sheets product. I'm preoccupied. He is not occupied.

"You ready?" SEAL says.

"Go fuck yourself," I reply.

It's 5:00 a.m. It's way too early. I hate this.

There's generally a moment in every endeavor I undertake, be it business, love, or fitness, when I say to myself: *What the hell was I thinking?*

I'm just now experiencing that moment. Sleeping in a chair, bleeding nuts, and almost getting sued by a plumber was not what I was expecting. Sure, I pictured grueling workouts, sweat pouring off my face, and challenging my limits when I hired SEAL, but all this?

I know my friends think I'm insane right now, and they've seen me do some crazy stuff before. But this has to be at the top of the list. My whole path has been nontraditional. Any time when you live a little outside of the norm people look at you: (a) with some admiration and (b) like you're crazy. I never cared about that and I still don't. I have a complete stranger living in my apartment; I'm getting up super early and running every day when it's freezing. I think some people wished they could do it but they never would. The will to keep doing this and the will to put myself through this is what people think is crazy, and I'm paying for this, literally and metaphorically. Maybe I *am* crazy.

I know it's normal to have second thoughts about some of my decisions, but what about third, fourth, and fifth thoughts? It's pitch dark and twenty-one degrees out, for

God's sake! Maybe I'll just wrap it up, I think. Pay him for the month, and wish him happy trails.

Then I remember the one condition I agreed to when I hired him: Do anything he asks. SEAL built his career around honor. At a minimum I have to honor my commitment to him.

I go change into my workout clothes.

0515

This is our push-up routine: Do one push-up then stand up and wait fifteen seconds, then go down and do two push-ups and wait fifteen seconds and so on, until we get up to ten push-ups, and then we start taking thirty-second breaks. For push-ups sixteen, seventeen, and eighteen, SEAL allows us to take forty-five seconds between sets. What a guy! I do sets of push-ups one to eighteen for a total of 171. Followed by thirty pull-ups. (No time limit. As long as it takes to knock out thirty even if I drop from the bar.) Then we go and run quarter-mile intervals. We run the quarter miles at a fast pace. Then we walk one minute. We repeat this for two miles. Quarter-mile sprint...one-minute walk.

SEAL says he wants to get me up to a hundred miles of running a week.

What? Even when I trained for marathons, my highest weekly mileage per week was forty miles. One hundred miles of running a week sounds like that can be dangerous. That feels like shin-splint territory.

Meanwhile, I'm so sore from all of the push-ups I can't even wash my hair.

SEAL doesn't care, nor is he very concerned.

"If you want to be pushed to your limits, you have to train to your limits. If you get hurt, you will recover. What the fuck is the problem?"

Three hours later...

SEAL calls me into his room for a sidebar. He tells me he has to "go away" for three days. I guess he really is the "surprise-or." He's doing a seventy-five-mile race and traveling for business. I don't ask any questions.

Sometimes at night he makes calls, but I have no idea to whom or for what. I occasionally hear him talking on the phone in his room behind a closed door in a low whisper. It's not like I'm spying on him or anything, but I have to walk by his room to get to Lazer's room. I've never overheard anything he said on the phone. But it does make me wonder.

"Keep up the program while I'm gone," he says. "Do six-mile runs in the mornings and three at night. And don't forget to hit the push-ups. Make sure you get two hundred in every day. I'm going off the grid. Do this shit on the honor code."

Roger that.

I can't help but speculate where SEAL is going. Yes, he runs races. Yes, he does Ironmans. So he might be doing something like that.

But he also could be going on a secret mission. Who knows? My mind is racing with ideas.

> **Workout totals: 2-mile interval run, 171 push-ups, 30 pull-ups**

Date Night?

*I'm not into sit-down dinners and fancy shit like
that. I'm into fueling up and being on my way.*
—SEAL

With SEAL gone for three days, Sara plans a lovely dinner
for just the two of us. I mean, I have some input too, but
Sara wants to cook—and she's terrific. It's to be a time for
us to catch up on any topic we see fit, nothing is off limits,
and share some "quality alone time," as my wife calls it. I'm
all in. I'd taken for granted the sacrifice Sara had made. She
agreed to let someone who was basically a stranger live with
us. And although she grew fond of SEAL, we had zero alone
time.

At 3:00 p.m. she calls me at work to tell me she's leaving
for Whole Foods with a list of items for our date. She's making homemade veggie burgers, pasta, a salad, steamed spinach, and baked potatoes. My favorites!

"Six thirty sharp!!!! Be home at six thirty *sharp!*" she
says. Sara has a tendency to repeat words in sentences if they
are *really* important.

So, I leave my office at 6:00 p.m. My apartment is only a
twenty-minute walk from my office. I make it with six minutes to spare.

I peek into the kitchen: Flour. Boiling water. Veggies.
Game on!

"This looks great, honey. Can I help?"

"Please set the table and get water for us both," she says with a smile. "Dinner will be ready in four minutes." Sara pauses for a moment. "Four minutes."

In the dining room, I grab forks, spoons, knives, and two plates. I place the silverware on the side of the plates in no special order. I can't find napkins and I don't want to bother Sara. There's a powder room right off of the dining room. I unroll about three feet of toilet paper, tear it in two, and fold each section. Now we have napkins! I pull out another three feet in case we need extra. I put two of the "napkins" under the silverware and the rest in the middle of the table.

"Table is set," I yell.

"Great," she responds. "COME AND GET IT!!!!"

I walk into the kitchen with both of our plates. "This looks fantastic," I say, admiring the wonderful meal my wife has cooked. I kiss her on the forehead.

"Please, honey, you first," I say, handing her a plate.

Sara carefully constructs her meal with salad, a veggie burger, and some steamed spinach. Her plate looks like it's from a photo spread in *Bon Appétit* magazine.

"Honey, I'll meet you in the dining room," she says as she heads out of the kitchen. "I'm so excited," she adds.

As she leaves, I start filling up my plate...nibbling away during the process. One scoop of veggies on the plate...one scoop directly into my mouth.

I'm eager to sit down and eat, but food for me is fuel. I inhale...I don't eat. I think sitting through a long dinner is an inefficient use of time. I like to stand when I eat. Why not...take in the calories fast...and be on our way? With that mentality baked in my DNA, I start ingesting the food on my plate as I walk into the dining room. First a fingerful. Then a handful. Then a full-on attack. I'm starving from all the working out.

I get to the dining room table.

"Sweetie, where's your food?" Sara asks.

I look down at my empty plate.

"Did you eat all your food already????"

I shake my head no. I can't say no, because my mouth is filled with veggie burger.

Now I don't know what to do. I'm done. To me, we had a great date, no? So I sit and watch my wife eat. There's not a lot of no-limits discussion at the table. In fact, it's pretty quiet. The thought that I might have put a slight damper on our date creeps into my consciousness.

After Sara finishes eating, she wipes her mouth with the toilet-paper napkins.

"Sweetie," she says, holding the flatware between her thumb and index finger. "This is a *fork*! A F-O-R-K. Fork! A fork is an eating utensil. It's used to get food off of your plate and bring it into your mouth without getting it all over you. A fork is what *adults* use to eat."

She places the fork on the table and then holds her hand up and wiggles her fingers. "And these are called *fingers*. Fingers are used to hold the fork. They are *not* used to scoop up pasta...squeeze it into a ball...and eat it like an apple. Repeat after me: *fingers*."

"Fingers," I say.

"Are *not*," she says.

"Are *not*," I repeat.
"Used."
"Used."
"To pick up food."
"To pick up food."
Great date!

Three Years Earlier: First Date

I imagine I'm a hard guy to have a relationship with.
—SEAL

The first time I met Sara, I overheard her saying she was hosting a charity event to raise money for college scholarships for underprivileged women in Africa.

When I got back to New York, I looked the charity up. It was called the Sara Blakely Foundation, and the event was called the Give a Damn Party. The money raised was to help women in Africa attend university. I bought a table of ten on the condition it was right next to the host's table. Then I called Sara and commented on how amazing it was we were both so passionate about sending underprivileged African women to school. What a coincidence!

The night of the event, my table was indeed right next to Sara's, but I couldn't convince anyone other than one of my high school friends to fly down to Atlanta with me—there were going to be only two of us at a table for ten. So, the day of the event, I called Sara's office and they filled the table with people I didn't know. I didn't care, I was there for one reason (with all due respect to the underprivileged African women). As it turned out, I didn't get a whole lot of Sara's time that night. As the host, she didn't have a lot of time to give. But she knew I came, of course, and that was the whole point.

I must admit, while Sara intrigued me before the party, I was more interested by the time the night ended. She was even more beautiful than the first time I saw her, and she performed her duties as host with an elegant self-assuredness that was incredibly attractive. She had organized quite a night: Sir Richard Branson was there, Jewel and Collective Soul performed, but to be honest, I paid very little attention to what was going on around me. I couldn't take my eyes off Sara.

Not too long after the charity dinner, I found out, and I really don't remember how I did, that Sara had broken up with her boyfriend. I immediately emailed and invited her to go with me to the Final Four basketball championship, which was being held in Atlanta that year. She didn't know anything about basketball, but you really don't have to know anything about basketball to have fun at the NCAA Men's Finals, and she did.

Two weeks later she came up to New York for business, and I asked her out on our first official date. I told her I made reservations at a day spa and a sushi place for dinner.

"Terrific," she said.

Now, describing where we were going as a day spa was stretching it a bit. "Illegal Russian bath" was perhaps a more apt representation. I love hot saunas, and this place had a sauna so hot they made us wear felt hats so we didn't burn the roots of our hair. Sara showed up having just had her hair done that afternoon and thinking she was going to get a pedicure and a foot massage. Instead, she was led into a changing room where a Russian woman with calves the size of fire hydrants gave her a paper bottom to wear. Just the bottom.

Sara came out with her arms wrapped around her boobs to cover them up. Remember, this is our first real date.

The sauna was set for 185 degrees. Ivan the Russian therapist then comes in and performs a platza treatment on us where he beats us both with wet oak leaves to generate more body heat and takes our body temperatures to unbearable highs. Then, when he feels we can't take any more heat, he takes us to a room where he pours glacially cold water all over us. Then back to 185 degrees.

It was so romantic...

Then we went to dinner.

As I look across the dinner table in a fancy New York sushi restaurant, Sara's hair is still soaking wet and she has some mascara running down her face. The poor woman looks like she'd been boiled. However, she never once complains and we have a great time.

Sara and Jesse... Game on!

DAYS 11–12

(not counting the days I was on my own)

Enjoy the Pain

I earned it. Now I'm going to enjoy it.
—SEAL

New York City
38°
0800

I was on my own for the past two days while SEAL disappeared, and I honestly stuck with the program—Honor Code. I did six-mile runs in the morning and three-mile runs at night. And two hundred push-ups in the middle like an Oreo cookie. It was actually a bit lonely doing the workouts on my own. Not that I miss the guy, but maybe a little?

Today is no different. I did a six-mile run this morning. At 11:00 a.m. my cell phone rings and it's SEAL. He tells me he's on his way back to NYC and that he just completed the seventy-five-mile race.

"How was it?"

"Hard," he says.

"Really? Seventy-five miles was hard?"

"It had a climb," he says. "The terrain was tough."

I know SEAL well enough by now to know that if he says a race was "hard," had a "climb," and the terrain was "tough"...then it was TOUGH!

"And...I broke all the metatarsals in both feet."

Huh? Check that. Tough times twenty.

"But I finished strong," he says.

He *finished*?!

"What are you going to do?" I ask.

"What do you mean?"

"You going to go get them looked at?"

"Get what looked at?"

"Your feet."

"Why would I get them looked at?"

"'Cause they're broken!"

"Come on, man. The doctor will only tell me they're busted up. But I already know they're busted up. Why would I waste my fucking time driving to the doctor and then pay a man to tell me my feet are fucked up when I already know that? I gotta go. Call you back."

He has a point, I guess.

One hour later...

I'm in my home office when I get an email SEAL sends while he's in the car on the way to the airport:

From: SEAL
To: Jesse Itzler
Subject: On my way

Training will go on.

The guy breaks every bone in both his feet but can still run? Training will go on?

11:00 p.m.

The front door of the apartment swings open. It's SEAL. He has a key, but since he's been living with us, we hardly ever lock the door during the day. What's the purpose? Today is no different, and he opens the door.

As he makes his way in, SEAL is walking like he's stepping on broken glass. He's limping and in obvious pain. He's not wearing any shoes, and his toes are really messed up. SEAL is missing the toenail on his right big toe, and he has a few blisters that look like his toes swallowed giant red grapes. OUCH.

"Man…that looks bad. You gotta do something for it," I say.

"Nah, I'm just gonna sit on the couch and enjoy the pain," he says. "I earned it. Now I'm going to enjoy it." He starts to laugh to himself.

At first I thought that maybe he wanted to impress me and create this crazy persona. Like overplay some of this stuff for effect. But now as I look at his battered feet, I realize that there is no overplaying this kind of thing. There is no effect. He really means it. He really wants to enjoy the pain.

Next day

I'm at my office getting caught up on work when I get a call from Mark Rampolla, the CEO of Zico. He gets right into it.

"A lot of people in the Zico office are reading your blog about SEAL," he says.

"Awesome," I say. "Thanks for sharing."

"Yeah, they can't believe you are doing this. You're nuts. You must be getting in great shape, and you must be exhausted."

"Yes...and definitely YES!"

"Well, anyway, we want to know if SEAL would endorse Zico. You know, use it at races and talk about the product, et cetera?" he asks as his words hang in the air like a puff of white smoke.

I feel like telling Rampolla that SEAL doesn't really talk, but I say "great idea" and I will ask. "Call ya back," I say.

I hang up and tell SEAL about the conversation.

"You are blogging about this?"

"Yeah, at first I just sent it to a few friends who love to work out, but now it is catching on. And it's kind of spread a little bit, but just a little bit," I say.

"Okay, cool, but I don't want any part of that shit. None."

"Any interest in endorsing Zico?"

"I race for me. I don't race for products, Jesse. I race for me."

We leave it at that.

Dinner
1730

I hear the *Rocky* theme playing in SEAL's bedroom. It plays once and then I hear it again. Then again. And again. Then the song repeats approximately thirty times. What the fuck is he doing in there?

I choose not to knock on the door but can tell there's something serious going on in that room. I can almost feel heat coming out of the door. I'm curious.

Finally, after the thirty-first time of the song repeating, SEAL walks out. He is soaking wet and leaving puddles of sweat all over the floor.

"You okay?" I ask.

"Twenty-five hundred push-ups, motherfucker. Yes, I am okay."

Sara walks into the room as she too is curious. However, I can tell her curiosity suddenly changes to concern. Something is bothering her. Really bothering her. I can see it on her face she's trying to tell me what's on her mind...without talking. She's sending me some kind of husband-wife telepathy through her eyebrows and expression, but I'm not getting the message clearly. I wonder if I get points for at least knowing she's trying to send me subliminal Morse code?

Then her eyes slowly shift from my eyes to the floor. They go there in slow motion, taking my eyes with them. It is there that I see a puddle of sweat growing larger by the second on our silk Oriental rug. It's the same rug that has been passed down from generation to generation and was given to Sara by her grandmother. With every passing second the puddle spreads out like it's raining all in one spot… dead smack in the middle of the family rug. As SEAL sits on our couch, sweat pours off his nose and lands on the rug in a steady flow.

I immediately go to the bathroom and get two towels, one for SEAL and one to place on the rug. I'm in trouble.

Sara calls me into our bedroom.

"Don't ever let that happen again," Sara says to me. "I'm dead serious." She says it in a tone that is way scarier than anything SEAL has said or done to me to date. It even rivals my mother's silent treatment. "Never," she repeats.

Thirty minutes later…

It's 8:30 p.m. and we are on our first workout of the day (well, at least I am). We do a series of push-up sets one to eighteen, for a total of 171. Then we head downstairs to the gym. Residents have 24/7 access. It's pitch dark when we get down there but I immediately flip on the gym lights.

I never ran on a treadmill until I met SEAL. I'm an old-fashioned, lace-on-the-kicks-and-run-out-the-front-door kind of runner. SEAL thinks a treadmill is a good training tool because it's controlled. Yeah. Like Chinese water torture.

He has me walk for five minutes at a 12.5 incline at a

fifteen-minute pace. Then, he reduces me to a 3.0 incline, but makes me do:

1/4 mile: 9:30 pace
1/4 mile: 6:50 pace
1/4 mile: 9:20 pace
1/4 mile: 6:40 pace
1/4 mile: 9:20 pace
1/4 mile: 6:30 pace
1/4 mile: 9:00 pace
1/4 mile: 6:20 pace

Approximately three hours later (11:30 p.m.)

SEAL tells me it's time for some sit-ups. It's like we are cramming for a test trying to get our daily double workout in before midnight.

He always makes sure I have proper form. As in all the way up and all the way down, as fast as you can do them, or they don't count:

44 unassisted ("Unassisted" means no help with lots of yelling.)
1 minute rest
44 unassisted
1 minute rest
44 unassisted
1 minute rest
Total: 132

Push-ups:

15X @ 7 sets (on the minute): 105 total
Rest 1:30
12X @ 9 sets (on 50-second mark): 108 total
Rest 1:30
10x @ 10 sets (on the 45-second mark): 100 total
Total: 313

I'm wiped out. But I'm so wired from endorphins I can't fall asleep. Never in my life have I worked out late at night. I'm used to knocking it out first thing in the morning.

SEAL comes in and tells me to set my alarm for 0730. We are starting at 0800 sharp tomorrow, so I set my alarm for 0745. I want those extra fifteen minutes of sleep. It dawns on me that SEAL doesn't have an alarm clock. Yet he never oversleeps; he's always up when I get up. In fact, now that I think about it, I've never actually seen him asleep. I've never seen him yawn, never even seen him stretch or even seen him close his eyes for any length of time. This dude is a robot.

> **Workout totals: 5-minute walk on a steep incline, 8 miles (2 miles of which were intervals), 132 sit-ups, 484 push-ups**

DAY 13

Sick Fuck Friday

Every day is a challenge, otherwise it's not a
regular day.
—SEAL

New York City
21°
0800

It's been less than eight hours since I did my 484 push-ups.
Five hours since I fell asleep. When I get up, SEAL is already
up. I mean, *wide awake* up. He tells me he has been outside
surveying our running route, checking the terrain, feeling it
out.

"The terrain?"

"It's not a regular day in Central Park," he says.

"No?"

"Nope. Nobody's smiling. There are only a few stragglers
out running. One guy is walking a dog. Saw one delivery guy."

"Okay."

"Nah, man, it's not okay," he says. "Only the loonies are out there today, bro. Only the demented...It's sick fuck Friday."

I'm not sure what he means.

I walk out the front door as SEAL limps.

We set out to run five miles at an eight-minute pace, but SEAL wants the run to be mostly hills. He settles on running the small back part of Central Park by 110th Street. So we run uptown and when we get there, we do the small loop of the 110th Street hill. The hill is only about a quarter of a mile up, but it's steep. To hold an eight-minute pace is *very* challenging.

As we ascend, my shoulders kill from the 484 push-ups yesterday. I mean *they are killing me.*

My arms dangle from my sides as I run to ease the sharp pain in my shoulders. They're not sore. I'm beyond being sore. I'm trying any technique to ease the pain. *Nothing works.* At the end of our run, I bend over huffing and puffing. My arms hang like they're dead. I need to give them a day off.

"How are your shoulders feeling, bitch?" he asks.

I don't even respond.

"Tonight more push-ups. I'm gonna test your shoulders," SEAL says, limping past me. "Be ready."

1:00 p.m.

I decided to work from home today, so SEAL is in his room "chilling out" and I'm in my room making calls. I can't lift anything (even my cell phone) because my shoulders hurt so much, and I'm not exaggerating. SEAL walks into my room.

"I'm going down to the gym to get a quick workout in."

"Okay," I respond.

Two hours later

SEAL returns to the apartment holding his hands up to show me his palms. They look like he fell off his bike and braced his fall with his hands. They're battered.

"What happened?"

"I knocked out my pull-ups."

"How many you get?"

"I did five pull-ups on the minute for two hours."

"You just did six hundred pull-ups? Just now? Just like that?"

"Roger that. So go fuck your bullshit shoulders," he says. "Whatever you got going on, someone else has more pain. You gotta learn how to fight through it. No matter what it is...Think about someone else and take a suck-shit pill."

I think he means a suck-it-up pill, but I don't question him. "Suck-shit pill" sounds good to me!

2200

SEAL has been in his room the entire afternoon and evening. I have no idea what he's doing but he has not once come out and looked for me. Is he mad? I didn't dare to bother him;

who wants to wake up a sleeping giant? As the night creeps in, I realize I'm exhausted. Plus, I need to let my shoulders recover. I crawl into bed with my clothes on and fall sound asleep at 10:00 p.m. I'm zonked out.

At 12:30 a.m. my alarm goes off. Now, I know I didn't set my alarm. I know my wife didn't set the alarm. And I'm damn sure Lazer didn't set the alarm.

"Trick or treat," SEAL says.

He's sitting in my room on a chair four feet from my bed in his running gear. I think he's eating a banana. I rub my eyes to make sure I'm not dreaming, and, sadly, I'm not. I'm more freaked out than the first time I saw *Silence of the Lambs*. The only way this could be worse is if he told me to put the lotion in the basket.

He walks over to my side of the bed, bends down so his mouth is basically inside my right ear, and starts quietly whispering the lyrics to the Geto Boys hit song, "At night I can't sleep, I toss and I turn..."

I pretend like I'm sleeping, but he repeats that line over and over...louder and LOUDER...until I finally get up.

We head outside. It's the middle of the night. Well, actually, it's the start of the middle of the night. Actually, it's one hour past midnight.

It's about twenty degrees but feels like minus-five degrees with the wind. We do a three-mile run around the lower loop of Central Park, forty jumping jacks, then ten push-ups, and repeat. We do twenty sets of the jacks and push-ups in fifteen minutes. That's eight hundred jumping jacks and two hundred push-ups in *fifteen minutes*!

There was not a living thing stirring in Central Park while

we trained. Not a civilian. Not a police officer. Not even a squirrel. I'm bruised and battered. The only way I could feel worse is if SEAL made me carry him home.

I don't give him any ideas. I just want to be warm. Who trains at 1:00 a.m. outside in the middle of winter?

When we get inside, I take off all my clothing and throw on some dry boxer shorts and an old short-sleeve tee. Then I grab my winter jacket from the foyer closet and put it on. I was so damn cold from the run my jacket is the only thing that is appealing to me. I zipper it up to my chin and climb into bed. I know I'm at 15 Central Park West, but it feels like I'm on a mission in Serbia in the winter. I look at Sara; she's in the fetal position in the middle of the bed spooning with her pillow. I throw the hood of the jacket over my head and pull it up until it covers my eyes. Lights out.

Workout totals: 8 miles, 800 jumping jacks, 200 push-ups

Lady in the Honda

Everyone is a potential threat.
—SEAL

SEAL and I head up to my lake house in Connecticut. I need to make sure the pipes didn't freeze and take care of some odds and ends. After we check everything off the list, we get ready to head back to New York. I ask SEAL if he'd mind doing the driving so I can get some work done.

"Roger that."

"How are your driving skills?"

"I'm well trained."

We start driving back to the city. SEAL apparently is a defensive driver. I note that he even uses the turn signal to pull out of the driveway. I nod left to confirm which way to the interstate. I grab my phone to check emails and then give him a nod when we need to take a right at the fork. I snatch a pen from the glove compartment to take a few notes. Eventually we get on the main road.

SEAL points his index finger at the first car we pass. Then he does it again to the next car. Like his hand is off the wheel pointing. Again he does it. Plus, he's talking to himself in a low melodic voice mumbling.

"Mblamblamblam," he mumbles and points.

"The pointing thing, is that some kind of—?"

"Yeah, it's a driving technique. You need to point at the target. Every target," SEAL says, pointing at an eighteen-wheeler.

"But these are just commuters. Guys coming home from work."

"That's what they are to you. To me, they're targets."

I check out the next car we pass. It's a mom with two kids in the back watching videos. SEAL points at her.

"You have no idea what the lady in that Honda can do," he says. "You have no clue what her reaction time is. You have no inkling to what that lady is thinking. Honestly, you don't know shit."

We sit in silence for a minute.

"Man, you wanna drive?" SEAL asks, sensing my discomfort.

"No, not at all. I've just never seen a technique like that. Where you point at every approaching car."

"You're too trusting, man. It just takes ONE pissed off mom. BAM. It happens that fast. A fucking nanosecond. Reach for your phone and KA-POW, you're blasted. You need to think prevention and stop singing that Elton John SHIT, Jesse!"

"Elton John?"

I have no idea what he's talking about.

"All cylinders, baby," he says. "This is no joke. This shit is like a video game behind this wheel. You can get gobbled up real quick. You need to have your shit tight on the roads out here."

DAY 14

Fireman's Carry

If you can't do the basics, you can't do shit.
—SEAL

New York City
22°
0945

SEAL has about ten pills in his hand, and he throws them all back in his mouth in one giant handful. He then takes a swig of water and opens his mouth.

"AHH," he says, and they are gone.

I'm not sure what SEAL is taking. Vitamins? Medicine? Anti-radiation tablets in the event of an attack? Who knows? All I know is he is taking horse-size pills in large quantities at odd hours.

"Let's stay inside for forty-five minutes," SEAL says.

"Why?"

"You'll see." SEAL chuckles.

We take the elevator down to the basement where there's

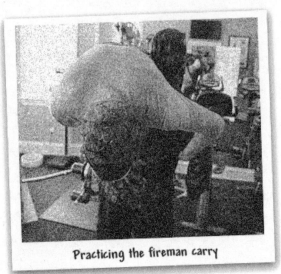

Practicing the fireman carry

a hallway that's about thirty yards long. SEAL says we're going to do fireman carries.

"It's a basic military workout," he says.

I have to throw SEAL over my shoulder and run thirty yards in the hallway of the basement, drop SEAL, do thirty-five reps (four count) of flutter kicks, flip to my knees and do twenty push-ups, then we switch and he carries me. We are to repeat this fourteen times.

By the twelfth repetition, I'm messed up. Like really screwed. This is up there with the worst I've ever felt in my life.

Carrying SEAL was brutal, but being carried by him was way worse. Imagine all the blood rushing to your head from being carried upside down. Plus, SEAL's shoulder is digging into my torso.

During one of the reps, the elevator opens and a resident

steps out of the elevator and into our hallway. I recognize
her, but I don't know her name. I've seen her on TV and I
think she's a real estate mogul or something, but at this hour,
who cares? I realize the people in my building must think
I'm crazy. They must be wondering what's going on. This is
a building with fancy handbags with poodles living in those
bags. We do not fit in. They must want to know why Rambo
is living in their building.

Anyway, she can sense the insanity, and she looks at
both of us, scared and yet curious. She walks unusually fast
toward the gym. It's almost like when you see someone on
the street and they suddenly realize they aren't where they
want to be and quickly change pace.

"This looks a bit intense," she says as she walks by me
and into the gym.

A little intense? I'm thinking. How about crazy intense?

3:00 p.m.

I walk into my office and SEAL is sitting by my desk on the
phone. He rocks back and forth in my comfy swivel chair.

"It's Garnett," SEAL says to me.

"Yeah, man, be cool," he says as he hangs up the phone.

Apparently SEAL and Garnett have stayed in touch. I
have no clue how either of them got each other's contact info,
nor do I know what those guys are possibly talking about, but
it makes me smile that they are connected.

SEAL gets up and I sit at my desk and power up my
computer.

"No need for that now," he says.

"What do you mean?"

"We are going to check in on your burpee progress. Same drill."

"Come on, man, I got shit to do today."

"So do I. Take your shit off and get started."

I strip down to my boxers.

One...two...three...ninety-nine...one hundred!

Ten minutes and twenty-seven seconds! I feel myself smile.

2218

I get home late from a New York Knicks game. I walked the twenty blocks to the Garden directly from work. Today I had multiple meetings, multiple conference calls, and had to put out multiple fires at work, plus the fireman workout killed me this morning. Then the burpees. And then the walk to the Garden.

I'm somewhere between the front door and comatose when I hear "Let's run eight."

"C'mon, man...It's over. Let's just do early tomorrow."

"Okay, if that's what you want," SEAL says, looking at me like I'm a pussy.

When SEAL wanted to become a SEAL, he weighed 290 pounds. You can't be 290 pounds and be a SEAL, he was told. So he lost 105 pounds in less than two months. I know it sounds impossible, but he lived on fresh fruit and water and worked out like a madman (naturally!).

In SEAL training, you're subjected to something called

"Hell Week." Over a five-and-a-half-day period he was allowed only two hours of sleep. His class had just finished exercises in freezing water when their instructor ordered them back in. A SEAL in training standing next to him stared vacantly. There was no expression in his classmate's eyes. They were hollow. SEAL called it "the Look." The classmate turned and walked away. He quit.

SEAL looks at me like I have the Look.

I man up. We get our shit on. It's twenty-two degrees outside. I'm mad as hell that I'm doing this. When we walk out of the front door, I turn to SEAL and say, "FUCK YOU."

"Let's go," he says.

11:00 p.m.

We start running to the Hudson River.

Before he pushes the button on his watch to start the run, I plead to do only four miles. He says eight. Miraculously we settle on six. We start.

I can honestly say there's *not one single person* other than us running at 11:25 p.m. on the West Side Highway. *Not one.*

As we run I notice my shoulders are in extreme pain from this morning's workout. I run with my arms dangling by my sides. That lasts for a half mile because this type of running style kills your thighs. (Try running fast for a half mile with your arms like this if you don't believe me.)

Now I have a choice: severe shoulder pain or running like an asshole with my arms dangling. I opt for the running-like-an-asshole look partly because there's not a soul on the streets to see me.

During the fifty-three-minute run, SEAL and I don't say one single sentence to each other. Not a peep. It's like *Night of the Living Dead*. He only says two words the entire run:

"Turn around" at the halfway mark.

Three miles back in silence. It's midnight when we finish.

"Tomorrow starts at oh six hundred," he says as we walk into my building. "Get some sleep."

> **Workout totals: 6 miles, 100 burpees, and 14 fireman carries**

DAY 15

It's All About the Push-ups

If you're gonna do 'em, do 'em right.

—SEAL

New York City to Atlanta
28° to 49°
0600

I walk into the kitchen and SEAL has a look on his face that I have never seen. It's a cross between furious and confused. It's scary. He's having a heated debate...with himself.

"Let's add some extra mileage today," SEAL says. "Nah, let's knock out a slow eight," he says back to himself. "Nah, fuck that. Let's knock out a slow six and then do two AFAWC."

When he says it, it sounds like "AFLAC" from the commercial with the duck, but it's not. It's AFAWC: as fast as we can.

"Yeah, motherfucker, we're gonna do six miles and then do two AFAWC."

It's about twenty-eight degrees outside today. However, today I decide to dress more like SEAL does and only wear shorts and two T-shirts, but double up on the hat and gloves. Without the extra layers, I'm feeling light and we fly on the run.

The first six miles are at an 8:06 pace, then SEAL takes the pace to 7:29 for the last two miles. As soon as we hit the six-mile mark, he says to me "sub seven thirty" and speeds up. He doesn't even look at his watch; he just programs his pace like someone would program a car to a certain speed on cruise control.

When we get home, I peel two bananas and dip them in honey. I one-bite them and am done in about ten seconds. I grab a Zico and hit the shower. We just flew through that run, and I'm feeling great...not just about the run, but how much I'm improving. How I have been able to hang in there.

The funny thing is, SEAL has not complimented me once, which is fine. It's not like I need his validation, but it would be encouraging. That said, I'm genuinely proud of myself. It's like this experience is a personal test of will... it's the ultimate "can I make it?"...and so far I think I'm winning.

I note it as such.

Five hours later...

We head to LaGuardia for a Delta flight to Atlanta. Sara wants to check in at Spanx HQ tomorrow, and we decided yesterday that we would all go. Although we have access to Marquis Jet, we often fly Delta. SEAL doesn't seem to mind either way, and he is totally indifferent about where we train just as long as there are NO FUCKING SURPRISES. I give him at least a twenty-four-hour heads-up before any travel now. I'm looking forward to the flight as it represents two to three hours where I can just read and listen to music. SEAL just sits and stares on a commercial flight. I can't even guess what he's thinking about. Truthfully I don't even want to know. So I'm usually not factored into the equation. I get comfortable in my seat and wonder what I should read first.

But today's flight is different. SEAL wants to talk.

"So tell me your shit," SEAL says.

"My shit?"

"Yeah, your shit."

"Okay," I say, reclining my seat back as far as it can go. "What story do you want to hear: (a) The Big Red Chicken; (b) Don't Let Them Boo You; (c) Larry the Coconut Guy; or (d) 1-800-PLAYMATE?"

"Who the fuck wants to hear a story about a big red chicken?"

"Well, it's not really about a chicken," I say.

"Keep your fucking chicken stories to yourself," he says. "I go with D, motherfucker...D."

"Well, I moved from LA back to New York in the summer of 1992. After I realized there would be no second album," I say.

I came up with an idea to start my own record label so I could sign my own artists. I partnered up with my friend Spit and we called it Riot Records. To be honest, that sounds a lot more impressive than it was. First of all, I didn't have enough money to rent an apartment so I was sleeping on friends' couches. Second, the first deal I made didn't exactly go according to plan.

The artist we lined up was a woman named "Crystal," who was confirmed to be a centerfold in an upcoming magazine issue. Mike Ross had suggested her to me. Maybe I should have known better since he turned her down. When I first talked to Crystal on the phone, I asked her to sing "Happy Birthday" to me as a kind of audition. The sound that came out of the phone was like someone with bronchitis trying to sing "Old McDonald Had a Farm"…while being strangled. But that centerfold thing…

So…I agreed to do it! Again, get that foot in the door… figure it out later!

Crystal already had some good marketing ideas in place. She'd worked out a deal with the magazine to publicize a contest where if you bought the record, you were given the chance to win a date with her. This promotion was going as an insert in the magazine that would be distributed to hundreds of thousands of people. I thought the idea guaranteed strong sales just to pimply-faced teenage boys alone.

One weekend we took Crystal out to the Hamptons summer share house where we were staying. She definitely didn't get the memo because she walked around the whole time topless. I'm not even sure she packed a top. Now, she's like a fifteen out of a possible ten. None of my college friends had ever been exposed to anything like her. She was like the hot chick they invented in the movie *Weird Science*. All of the pent-up sexual energy in the house made me think this was going to be a great idea.

My friend Spit's parents had a place in the mountains, and I moved all of my recording equipment into their house. The idea was we would block off a solid week and record her album with her at the house. One night after recording, we joined Spit's parents for dinner at their dining room table.

Everything went along just fine: the usual small talk and niceties. Then Spit's father brings up the Miss America Pageant that was on TV the night before.

"They asked some tough questions of the finalists," he said. "One was who they thought the most influential woman in the last century was."

"That's easy," Spit's mom said. "Eleanor Roosevelt."

Crystal didn't say a word. She was the perfect guest, albeit one with thirty-eight-inch perfectly shaped breasts that stretched the limits of the white Nirvana T-shirt she wore, but was quiet at dinner. Then, right on the heels of the name Eleanor Roosevelt coming out of Spit's mom's mouth, she decides to weigh in.

"ELEANOR ROOSEVELT???? I would *not* say she was that influential," she said.

"Why's that?" Spit's mom asks.

"Well, all she did was fuck a president," Crystal responded.

I thought Spit was going to choke on the Eli's baguette he was chomping on. Mrs. Spit looked like someone had just taken a crap on the dinner table in front of her; but Mr. Spit,

God bless him, sort of cocked his head and let his glance drop ever so slightly down on Kurt Cobain's face.

"She's got a point," he said.

We eventually made Crystal's record. While she waited for the magazine to come out, she decided to make some extra money dancing at a famous Manhattan strip club. One night she bumps (literally) into Baba Booey from *The Howard Stern Show*, who falls headfirst for her. Between dances, he tells her he wants her to come on Howard's show. She gives him my number. When he calls me, he tells me there is one condition: She has to come on the show completely naked. "From the second she gets off the elevator, she has to be nude." After consulting with Crystal, we booked the appearance.

I figured I'd milk this appearance for everything I could, so I got a 1-800 number that had the ability to take three hundred orders a minute. We'd charge $9.99 for the CD, which we'd split. Crystal would promote the record on the Stern show, give out the 800 number, and I was going to sit back and watch the orders roll in. Boo-ya!!!

The day Crystal went on the show I was home listening on the radio. Spit took Crystal to the studio. When Howard saw her walk in naked he went crazy—he said he'd never seen anyone so hot…EVER! It couldn't have gone any better—Howard's fully engaged, really funny, the interview even goes past the allotted time. By the time they played her song, I'd already started counting the money in my head. Then Howard asks her to tell his listeners how they can order the record.

We must have rehearsed what she was going to say the

night before twenty thousand times. Twenty thousand times. I did everything but tattoo the 800 number on her...well, her palm. But from the radio all I heard was the disturbing sound of nothing.

Howard Stern: "Is there a number they can call, Crystal? Crystal? Crystal?"

Silence.

I was screaming the number at the radio. Finally, Crystal begins to speak. But my relief quickly turns into utter disbelief. To a national audience on the highest-rated show on radio, she gives out *not* the 800 number that we practiced but my personal *home* phone number to call and order her record, which started to ring immediately.

Oh, my God. I thought.

Although I tried, any attempt to keep up with the demand was futile. In the few calls I did answer, the comments ranged from junior high stupid, to sexual offender stuff. I just stopped answering.

My phone rang without pause for three solid hours. Then, just when it seemed to slow down, the show aired on the West Coast. The onslaught happened all over again. We didn't sell a single CD, I had to change my phone number, and we ended up not releasing her album.

SEAL has a hint of a smile on his face. I think he likes the story.

"All the profit I made from my own album, which was about $50,000, I'd lost in a matter of months with Riot Records," I say.

"Poof," SEAL says. "Are you still friends with Crystal?"

1800

We land and head to baggage claim in Atlanta. A friend of mine, Lisa, comes over and says hello. She didn't realize we were on the same flight; neither did I. I do a quick introduction to her with SEAL.

"I know who you are," she says.

"That so," SEAL says.

"I read Jesse's blog," Lisa says, and she gives us a coy smile. SEAL still isn't smiling. He just looks at me and gives me a silent grunt and then looks back at Lisa.

She extends her hand and he shakes it.

"I know who you are too. You were sitting in seat fourteen C," SEAL says. "The guy next to you was dark-skinned and reading *Reader's Digest*. I'm aware."

Lisa looks at me with a "holy shit...what the fuck" face.

2200

After we get settled into the house in Atlanta, SEAL summons me to the living room.

SEAL believes push-ups are the single best exercise for strength. He also believes proper form is the key. You get more out of ten push-ups the right way than thirty done improperly.

Proper form: back straight, ass up slightly, neck straight (don't drop your neck). Go down and break ninety degrees with elbows, and make sure your chest hits the floor. Go all the way up (until arm is fully extended).

We begin doing our one to eighteen push-ups and then eighteen to one. So our first set has one push-up with a fifteen-second rest; then we do two push-ups with a fifteen-second rest. All the way to eighteen and then back down to one. In case you're counting, that's 342 total. So SEAL has me do eight more for good luck. That's 350 push-ups.

We finish around midnight.

Workout totals: 8 miles (2 AFAWC) and 350 push-ups

Perfect Position

I'm on alert. High alert. Even when you don't
think I'm on alert, I'm on alert. Even right now,
I'm on alert.
—SEAL

Sara and I have plans tonight for dinner. Friends of ours own a popular restaurant in Atlanta called 10 Degrees South, and we have a 7:00 p.m. reservation. The restaurant has a South African safari motif and cuisine. It's refined—no paper napkins, no bare feet—but it's not pretentious. We ask SEAL if he wants to join us.

"Roger that."

We drive to the restaurant.

I'm in jeans and a button-down. Sara wears a dress. SEAL is in a black T-shirt.

He takes the seat on the far side of the table so his back is against the wall. From there he can see the entire landscape of the restaurant and notifies us that he has the exits staked out.

"I'm in perfect position," he says.

Our table is fairly close to the kitchen door, which is heavy. It makes a small boom every time it closes, which makes SEAL clench and bounce up.

"Yo, you okay, man?" I whisper. "That jumping thing…"

"Yeah, I'm cool. Just them loud noises, man," SEAL says.

"The door?"

"Yeah, the door. It's freaking me out."

"It is?"

"It sounds like a fucking explosion or something. It's loud. It's unpredictable," he says.

"Should I have them leave the door open?"

"No. I'll block out the sound."

"You can do that?"

"Of course. You could explode the fucking Goodyear Blimp in here and if you're zoned in, you can block that shit out."

Sara and I look at each other but don't say anything.

A waiter comes over and hands us menus. He points to the specials on the board and takes our drink order. I've never seen SEAL drink anything other than water in a restaurant. At home he likes to drink special, "military-grade" shakes "that you can't get online." It's a combination of protein and carbs and comes in chocolate and vanilla. That's his "meal." You order it through a special website.

SEAL glares at the waiter as he takes our order.

"SEAL, what's up?"

He whispers, "Man, this motherfucker right here. I don't trust that dude."

"Our waiter?"

"Yeah, whatever he says he is," he says.

"I'm pretty sure he's just our waiter."

"Nah. I've seen this movie before, man. I don't trust that motherfucker at all."

"What makes you feel like that?"

"Well, for one, his whole pretty-boy act: his smile, his gear, his walk, his silly-ass laugh, the grin, that bullshit attire."

"I think that is his waiter's outfit."

"Fuck that," SEAL whispers. "Guy's a threat."

"Wow. I don't see that at all."

"Really?" SEAL's eyes go wide. "You don't? Man, he knows what time the cash comes in and out. He knows when this place opens and when it closes down. He has ties to all the delivery guys. You trust the fucking delivery guys here, Jesse?"

"I haven't given it a lot of thought."

"Oh, you haven't, huh?" SEAL is now livid. "You see who brings the shit into this place? The delivery guys. They know all the patterns. MAN! Just keep your eyes on that dude. That's all I'm saying, Jesse. Keep your eyes on that dude."

I look over at our waiter. Come to think of it, he does look a little sneaky.

"Everyone in this place is capable of something. Remember that, Jesse... EVERYONE."

Our waiter returns with our food. I keep one eye on him as he sets down the butterflied prawns. Sara is now looking at our waiter like she doesn't trust him now either.

DAY 16

Stay Lite

You can get through any workout because
everything ends.
—SEAL

Atlanta
55°
0700

As Sara heads out to the Spanx headquarters, SEAL and I
head out for a run in Atlanta. The route is simple: three miles
down Peachtree Road, turn around, and come home. It's a
beautiful day in Atlanta, fifty-five degrees and sunny, and it's
warming up fast as the sun starts to climb. SEAL takes his
shirt off and we take off.

Peachtree is a main road in Atlanta. There are like ten
different Peachtrees and I'm not sure which one is which, but
this is the main one. I'm still not familiar with the streets here,
so no matter where I have to go, I just take this version of
Peachtree. I know eventually it will get me where I need to go.

It's almost rush hour here and the street is starting to get crowded. Cars are backed up at red lights and traffic is slow moving. The sidewalk we're running on is roughly two feet from the oncoming traffic. If I look into the window of the cars we pass on the run, I can see the blemishes on the faces of the drivers. We are that close.

I can feel the eyes of the drivers in traffic looking at us. It's making me uncomfortable and also making me run faster. SEAL, well, he couldn't give two shits. He is so locked in on the run I don't think he notices one single car. But he has to. He has to know that he stands out like a sore thumb, right? He is a V-shaped mountain of African-American muscle running up Peachtree. Everyone is looking at him.

When Sara gets to Spanx, she hears rumblings throughout the office about the specimen running down Peachtree. Sara's office has about two hundred women, half of whom just passed SEAL on their morning commute to work. So you can imagine how quickly word spread throughout the office.

Buckhead, where Spanx is headquartered, has a pretty typical cast of characters. Men wear suits, basically all have the same haircut, and drive the same three cars—Mercedes, Range Rover, or BMW. So seeing SEAL wearing only short flimsy running shorts looking like every inch of his body was meticulously carved out of stone…seemed a little out of place to say the least…and caused quite a stir.

My phone rings…It's Sara. She says in a whisper, "Honey, everyone here is talking about SEAL, wondering who he is and where he came from. What do I do? Do I mention the 'specimen' is living with us?"

1430

After a late-morning flight, we arrive back in NYC and head home.

SEAL greets the FedEx guy at the door. It appears Christmas has come early for him, or maybe for me. He ordered me my very own fifty-pound metal-plated weight vest for push-ups and to "increase the level of difficulty" of my runs. You've got to love SEAL. I didn't even know my runs needed a higher degree of difficulty.

"It's on, motherfuckers!" he yells, jumping up and down as he opens the package. "It's on!"

I don't think I've seen SEAL this excited—ever. He takes the vest from the box and puts it on. It fits perfectly. The thing looks like a suicide bomber's vest. If he walked into a bank wearing it, people would dive under their desks and give him the combination to the vault without him even asking for it.

"Today we test it out." SEAL grins.

We have one vest and have to share it, so I go first.

We do a three-mile run with the extra fifty pounds strapped onto my body. The vest is uneven, so the weight shifts from one shoulder to the other. It's brutal and makes it hard as hell to run.

It's so painful the three miles take thirty-three minutes. Each step is torture.

SEAL asks for the vest. We switch off and I'm free. He's so happy you'd think he's putting on the Masters' green jacket.

We run three more miles. It takes him/us 22:30.

Total run: 55:30.

I come home and fall asleep on the couch. I literally can't move.

Sixty minutes later...

"Grab the vest," SEAL says.

"You're joking," I say.

"Actually, I'm not," he says. "Grab the vest, fucker."

I clutch the vest.

"I can't," I say. "I need to watch Lazer." Sara has a work function tonight, so my parenting duties are doubled.

"Bring him," SEAL says. "All three of us are training today."

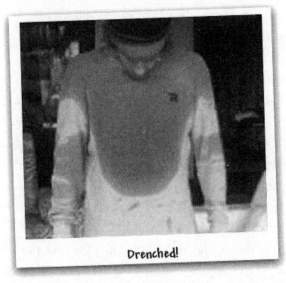

Drenched!

"But he's eighteen months old," I say. "And it's only twenty degrees outside."

"Bring him," SEAL says firmly.

I bundle up Lazer and we start running.

I'm wearing the vest. It weighs as much as a safe. SEAL pushes my son in the stroller next to us.

I go two and a half miles wearing the vest. It takes thirty-one minutes.

I've been on a thousand runs in my day. I've run eighteen New York City marathons in a row. I've done ultra-marathons of a hundred miles. This is one of the most brutal runs of my life. No question.

I pull over every hundred yards and drop to my knees and adjust the vest. I try to shift the weight to save my shoulders. The heft kills me. I shift again. It doesn't help. People in the park are starting to stare. They want to know what the fuck is wrong with me. They also want to know what the fuck two grown men in weight vests are doing pushing a baby stroller in twenty degrees.

I wish I knew…I wish I knew…

At this point I'm out of options; the shifting provides no temporary relief anymore. I'm done.

"What the hell are we doing? This is ridiculous. Can't you see this is killing me?"

"Relax, Jesse, you need to know that everything ends. Just do this shit and it will end."

We switch. SEAL puts on the vest.

We run another two and a half miles.

FAST.

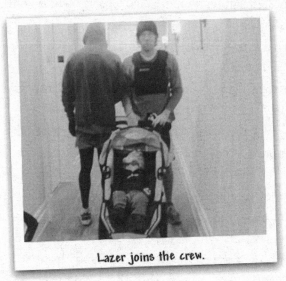

Lazer joins the crew.

8:00 p.m.

I'm starving. I feel like I need at least ten thousand calories. Maybe that is because I burned ten thousand calories today.

"SEAL, I'm ordering in some food. What'dya want?'

"I'm good."

"Come on, you gotta be starving."

"Nah, man, I'm good. I'm staying light."

I order in dinner for three and start to eat and I'm still hungry as I'm shoveling food in as fast as I can. SEAL grabs a banana and some almonds on his way to his room.

"See ya in the a.m.," he says.

With a mouthful of food I try to enunciate "See ya," and food flies out of my mouth as I do.

A few minutes later, Sara calls to check in. She asks to talk to Lazer who babbles "mama" into the phone. I pull the phone away and am so grateful Lazer hasn't learned the words "help me!"

"All is good here, honey...we've got it under control."

> **Workout totals: 17 miles (5.5 miles in 50-pound vest)**

DAY 17

Suicide Bombers

If a motherfucker looks crazy, usually the
motherfucker is crazy.
—SEAL

New York City
18°
0500

Sting is not in the gym when we walk in, but Bob Costas is.
He's on the treadmill watching the news on the tiny screen.
I see Costas a lot in the gym and love chatting sports in
between sets.

SEAL starts setting up the gym like a wedding planner
would set up a reception. He lays out the bench press bench
in one section, then grabs the curling bar and moves it to
another section. After a quick assessment, he spreads out a
rubber mat for sit-ups in another location. Before you know
it, we have a variety of circuits perfectly laid out.

He tells me the routine and we start:

Dumbbell bench press: 15 reps at 35 pounds, 12 reps at 40 pounds, 10 reps at 45 pounds, 8 reps at 50 pounds, and then 6 reps at 55 pounds.

Then, we do seated rows: 15–12–10–8–6 (medium weight). 51 reps.

Then, we do military press: 4 sets of 10 (medium weight). 40 reps.

Then, we do triceps pull-down: 15–12–10 (light weigh). 37 reps.

Curls: 15–12–10 (25 pound dumbbells). 37 reps.

Sit-ups: 50 . . . one minute rest . . . then 50 flutter kicks: 50 four-count flutter kicks (basically do a flutter kick for 4 seconds . . . that equals 1).

Costas is now ignoring the television and is focused on us. I fly through the workouts with *zero* talking. The workouts are starting to have a definite precision to them; meaning . . . SEAL is really focused on my form, and I'm finally getting comfortable with my technique. I think Costas has noticed the improvement. At least he has in my head. I grab my towel and we leave the gym.

SEAL pats me on the back and says, "Nice work."

My first real compliment!

0650

I have to be at work at 7:00 a.m. for a breakfast meeting (well, the guy I'm meeting will have breakfast, I will be having fruit), and SEAL makes me wear the weight vest to the office today. He wears the one he borrowed from the guy at the gym. Mine's under my jacket. SEAL just wears his vest over a T-shirt. We walk around Columbus Circle over toward my office on Park Avenue. It's not a bad walk, but today we stand out. I think we look like suicide bombers from a J.J. Abrams movie. Shoulder to shoulder, black guy, white guy, down Park Avenue looking like we're going to blow some shit up just for the sake of blowing some shit up. We are walking with some purpose down the street.

"We'll do this from now on," SEAL says.

I'm a bit freaked out. Not because of the weight of the vest, but because I'm thinking we are going to get stopped by the police. September 11 is still on people's minds, and we don't look at all sane. I'm worried that we will get asked to freeze and instructed to put our hands up and someone I know will see me. We keep walking.

We walk to work every day we're in New York, and something curious happens during these walks. Most of the time I spend with SEAL is either working out, getting ready to workout, recovering from working out, or talking about working out. Little of it is enjoyable. It isn't all misery (although much of it is), but there isn't a whole lot of human interaction.

However, during the walks to work that changes a little. Just a little.

Today he asks me what I do with my money. Meaning, do I invest it? In real estate? Stocks? He had saved some money from being in the military and is curious as to what to do with it. I thought that was very "human" of him!

Rather than go into detail about my portfolio, I give him a quote that my wife says about money. "Money is fun to make, fun to spend, and fun to give away. That sums it all up." He *loves* it! He looks at me like Sara had written the Gettysburg Address and I was reciting it. "Fuck yeah, Sara," he says.

So, I give him more. "Sara also likes to think of money as a big magnifying glass. If you are a good person before you had money…then money makes you an even better person. If you were a charitable person before you had money… then money makes you even *more* charitable. But if you were an asshole before you had money…well then, money makes you an even *bigger* asshole."

"That's some fucking real poetic shit right there," SEAL says. "Sara doesn't play."

We keep pace.

As the small talk disseminates, it becomes obvious to me that SEAL is very suspicious of some of the pedestrians on the street. Out of nowhere he says, "Cross the street" and then "I don't like the way things are looking on Fifty-first today."

I'm like, *really*?

One day on the walk to work, SEAL made us go all the way over to the West Side Highway, down to 57th Street, and then back up around to my office. This added an extra twenty minutes to the walk.

"Let's stay away from Trump Tower today," he said. "Trump been in the news too much lately."

We also talked some sports on our walks, and he put up with the ten thousand questions I asked him every day. I'd ask him ten thousand and he'd ask me none. He couldn't relate to my business accomplishments, and there's nothing I could do physically that would impress him because he's already done it longer, faster, and harder. So there was really nothing he could ask me.

When SEAL asks about money, it seems a little strange. I can tell it's purely out of curiosity. It's not like he's angling for anything. He just doesn't understand how I live the way I live. Can you imagine what it would be like if we switched places for a week? Like one of those Disney movies where we somehow magically switched bodies. I don't think either of us could function right away, but I'm sure by the end of the second act we would both learn valuable lessons from each other.

SEAL would laugh at how simple his life was and how complicated mine was. I would have a call list for the day, a schedule, my bag, appointments, calendars, and such, and he would literally grab his military card and $50, and that was all he needed for the day. That was his whole existence. He didn't have a car, a house, or anything to tie him down. If I fly someplace for a weekend, I always have to check my bag. He showed up at my house with a backpack. For thirty-plus days. One backpack. We have closets full of shit we never use, millions of pictures we took that we never look at, stacks of files that collect dust. He's a master at keeping it simple, and I have to say his simplicity looks attractive to me. I sort of want what he has, but I still want what I have.

SEAL has me thinking a lot about my own life as well as his. Mine seems ultra-calculating these days. It gets really complicated. You get pulled in a lot of directions. I know it sounds cliché, but the journey really is more important than the destination. Once you get where you're going, most of the magic drains out. I could really see myself as a minimalist, just taking life wherever it leads me.

I like my walks with SEAL in the morning.

2:00 p.m.

I throw two MorningStar veggie burgers in the microwave and cut up some raw carrots as a side for lunch. SEAL is in his room on the phone. I'm not sure who he is talking to, but he is being intentionally quiet. Before he can hang up, I have already inhaled both the veggie burgers. I throw two more into the microwave.

"You're done," SEAL says. "Time."

We head down to the gym and start our second workout of the day with an interval run on the treadmill. I grab a towel and leave it on the handrail of the treadmill because I know I'm going to need it:

Walk 5:00 at 12 incline (3.5 speed)
2:30 at 6.2 speed
2:30 at 8.7 speed
2:30 at 6.3 speed
2:30 at 8.8 speed

I grab the towel and wipe off my forehead. I'm starting to drip. My sweat is landing on the treadmill and making each stride super-slippery. I'm convinced I'm going to fly off like George Jetson did when I start sprinting.

2:30 at 6.4 speed
2:30 at 8.9 speed
2:30 at 6.5 speed
2:30 at 9.0 speed
5:00 walk/cooldown
1–30 push-ups (Time: 41 minutes)

Halfway through the run I start to feel like my Morning-Stars may come up. I'm cramping a bit but figure I can run through it. As the cramp moves from the side of my stomach to the center, I think it may be gas. I push. It is gas. I push a bit harder and a loud "fahhhhh" blasts out of my ass. It's like a thundercloud has burst out of me.

SEAL looks and me and says, "Fahhhhh," in the same exact pitch as my fart. I keep running but start laughing hysterically on the treadmill. SEAL is standing there just staring at my pace on the electronic dashboard of the machine. No smile. No laugh.

Ninety minutes later...around 3:00 p.m.

I want to pick up some gifts at Barneys, a fancy department store on Madison Avenue, for Sara and Lazer as the holidays are coming up soon. SEAL comes with me because SEAL comes everywhere with me. SEAL suggests we run there, but I tell him I don't want to be sweating while we're shopping.

"Well, we can run home then," he says.

"But we'll have all of the shopping bags and stuff," I say.

"Fuck it. Let's run there," he says.

So we run crosstown to Barneys. Since I know we are going to be holiday shopping on the Upper East Side of New York, I want to look somewhat respectable. So, I'm running in the nicest running outfit I have. I'm holding my credit card in my hand and a $20 bill in case we need to cab it back. By the time we get into the store, I've got a nice sweat going. SEAL looks like he took a cab there. He is unblemished.

I say to SEAL, "Let's make this fast, let's just go to the jewelry section." My wife certainly doesn't need anything, but she definitely needs to see the effort. If there is one thing I've learned about marriage, it's not the gift that counts, it's the effort. That's kind of like SEAL, I guess.

As we look at the jewelry in the glass case, I ask SEAL what he likes. "Man, this shit doesn't make any sense to me. Who would want a gold snake on their wrist for a few weeks' salary?" He has another point.

"I mean you work one hundred twenty hours and you go buy a bracelet? Shit is crazy to me."

And another point.

I pick up a few items (effort!), and ask the salesclerk to wrap them and throw the gifts in a bag. I have the $20 in my hand, but obviously we run home. Straight crosstown with a Barneys bag hanging from one arm. Bonus miles. Again, crazy. Two grown men running through Manhattan holding a Barneys bag.

> Workout totals: 3 miles (25 minutes of intervals on treadmill), 465 push-ups, 50 sit-ups, 50 flutter kicks, and SEAL circuit: dumbbell bench presses, seated rows, military press, tri pull-downs, curls

DAY 18

The Difference Five Minutes Can Make

Don't get too comfortable. Ever.
—SEAL

New York City
21°
0700

Miracle of miracles. We take the morning off.

"Hey, Lazer," I say to him in his highchair. "What do you think if Daddy stays home from work this morning to play?"

Lazer's smile lights up the room. First we start with his action figures and then we get into some serious block building. I haven't thought about anything other than how to build a higher tower in hours.

"Should we knock it down?" I ask Lazer.

And before the grin on his face is fully formed, the tower of blocks comes crashing down.

"Let's build it again," I say.

1145

SEAL walks in. He reminds me that it's almost noon and I have a 12:30 p.m. meeting today with the Zico sales team. I kiss my son on the forehead with a big smooch and head out the door with SEAL.

I've got on a winter coat and my Knicks knit hat. SEAL has a T-shirt and jeans on. His shoulders are angled up into his neck as we walk to work and his hands are in his pockets. He must be cold. This is unusual for him, I've never seen his body look like this before.

We are on a direct walking path to my office today, which is also unusual. Sara convinced SEAL the weighted vests were a bad idea so we look like civilians today. I guess SEAL doesn't think there are any imminent issues en route. Or maybe he feels the urge to change our pattern so we are less likely to be detected. Whatever the case, it's a normal person's commute—a direct shot.

As we hit the corner of 57th and Broadway, we wait for the WALK sign. "You ever worry about all these meetings you take? Like what if the direction isn't going the way you want it to go?"

"Never let them boo you," I say.

One of SEAL's eyebrows arches.

"No matter what, you can never let them 'boo' you. You have to control the situation."

His shoulders immediately drop down into a normal position and he asks, "What do you mean?"

"Can I tell you a story?" I ask. The WALK sign illuminates.

"Sure. Just as long as it's not about a big red chicken," he says.

"Okay, well after my video debuted on *Yo! MTV Raps*, I went on tour to support my CD. My first single, 'Shake It Like a White Girl,' was starting to get national radio play. While I was on the road, I got a call from Mike Ross. A promoter had reached out and asked if I would perform at the Increase the Peace charity benefit in Atlanta. Apparently, the promoter was getting African American artists and Caucasian artists to come together and play one big benefit show. Some of the biggest acts were confirmed. I guess Vanilla Ice was booked that day, 'cause they called me as the 'Caucasian' representative.

"The show was at the Georgia Dome in downtown Atlanta and they bused in about twenty-five thousand kids from all over Atlanta to attend. I'd known the crowd was going to be tough, but they were worse than I'd anticipated. The kids were unruly. There were fights in the stands. They were throwing shit at the stage. They had to keep putting the house lights on to control the audience. And...they booed everyone...I mean, EVERYONE. It was *insane*.

"Shortly before I was supposed to go onstage, LL Cool J was on. They had to move up his start time because he had another gig later that night and he had to fly out. The fans in Atlanta...they booed LL. I was like, 'If this crowd is booing LL, I'm in *big* trouble. Real big trouble. They are booing L and I'm supposed to go up and sing my song, "Shake It Like a

White Girl"?' I couldn't figure out how I was going to get out of this thing. I did not want to go on. I was physically sick.

"When the MC of the event introduced me, it was even worse.

"'Ladies and gentleman...all the way from Los Angeles, Californ-I-A...give it up for my MAIN MAN...JESSE JAYYYMEEES.'

"Silence.

"Radio silence.

"I could see the whites of the eyes of the fans in the first row. They were pissed. I don't know at what, but they were pissed. Before the crowd could even get the 'B' in 'Boo' out of their mouths, I came up with a crazy idea. My label had given me some free T-shirts to give away. I grabbed the cordless mic from the soundman backstage but also grabbed a pile of a hundred or so T-shirts and took them out with me onstage.

"'Atlanta, Georgia, do you want some FREE SHIIIIIT?' I yelled to the crowd.

"'YEAH!' they screamed back.

"'You all want some T-shirts up in the back section?'

"'Yeah!'

"'To my left?'

"'Yeah!'

"I kept throwing out T-shirts until they were all gone.

"Then, before anyone could even react, I said 'Good night, Atlanta. Love you guys and enjoy the show. Color Me Badd is on next.' Then I walked off the stage.

"Didn't sing a word. But I didn't get booed either. Remember when you told me to 'control my mind' the first day you moved in with me, well, I'm telling you in business . . . 'control the situation.'"

"Yo, Jesse man, motherfucking JESSE! You see!!! That's what I'm talking about, motherfucker. That's what I'm talking about," SEAL says, as we get to the entrance of my office building.

1300

When we get up to my office, I ask SEAL if I can have some privacy for a moment. Usually he sits on the couch and watches me type emails during the day, but this afternoon I want to be alone. I want to just sit in my chair and think.

So, SEAL pulls up a chair and places it right in front of my office and closes the door. He sits in front of it like he is guarding the royal palace in London. If anyone has to ask me a question about Zico, well, they will have to get past SEAL first.

That fact that we took the morning off makes me feel like I'm on a week's vacation. I recline on my chair and start to think about all that has happened with SEAL. I'm reliving the past days in my mind when . . . zzzzzzzzzzzzzzzzzzz—I'm out. Like saliva-drooling-out-of-the-side-of-my-mouth asleep. Three hours later SEAL comes in and wakes me up.

"Let's get out of here," he says.

7:00 p.m.

As SEAL and I walk into my building's gym that evening, my twenty-four-year-old nephew, Yoni, is leaving. He uses the building gym often and I run into him like this from time to time. It's always nice to see him. Typically it's a slap of the hand, a hug, and a quick catch-up. "How's Lazer?" and "How's work?"

Yoni is in amazing shape. When he moved to New York from Florida eighteen months ago, he weighed 240 pounds. I don't know if it was the New York women or what, but something clicked in his brain and he decided to get in shape. He is now about 170 pounds and *ripped*. He has run several marathons and is a workout junkie.

"Come on, Yoni, join us," SEAL says. "We're doing push-ups."

"I wish. I already ran this morning and swam just now, but thanks."

SEAL whispers something in my nephew's ear. No idea what he says, but the expression on Yoni's face goes from happy-go-lucky to furrowed and pasty. Whatever SEAL said it manipulated my nephew. He decides to join us.

"This is what we're gonna do," SEAL says. "Twelve push-ups every forty-five seconds for twenty-two minutes, then fifteen pull-ups, two minutes rest. Then twenty push-ups, three pull-ups (five sets). Then a hundred flutter kicks."

"I should have left five minutes earlier," Yoni whispers.

After working out, we all grab a quick bite at the restaurant in our building. It's a bit fancy, but we grab a table in the back and order some light appetizers. The conversation is centered on Yoni and how far he has come with his training. It escalates.

SEAL somehow convinces Yoni that he should quit his "bullshit" job running social media for a big hotel chain and join the Navy. *And*...my cockamamie nephew has bought into it. It escalates even further. Now SEAL is convincing him he can pass the Navy SEAL training and become a SEAL. He is going over the requirements and the basic fit test. It escalates even further.

"Fuck this. Let's start this shit right now."

These two knuckleheads decide to head out for a run.

I go upstairs and about ninety minutes later SEAL returns to the apartment.

"Where's Yoni?"

"Not sure. He fell back about a hundred meters at mile four."

Ninety minutes later...

Yoni walks into the apartment. He looks like a pile of split fuck. He has vomit on his fleece and he is super pale. He looks dehydrated.

"I think I'm more of a social media guy," he says.

> **Workout totals: 364 push-ups, 30 pull-ups, 100 flutter kicks**

DAY 19

My Shoulders

You can always keep going.
—SEAL

New York City
28°
0700

We head out to the loop around Central Park. I really want to stay in bed and watch the beginning of the *Today* show with Sara, but I'm in a great rhythm with SEAL and don't want to let up. Plus, there is only about a week or so left of his time with me.

Today's goal sounds simple: 6.1 miles at a sub-eight-minute pace, with no mile over eight minutes.

Before I'm halfway through the run, though, my shoulders feel like I'm giving the rapper Fat Joe a piggyback ride. The pain is ridiculous. That's what thousands of push-ups in ten days will do. I literally (no BS) can't swing my arms as I run because my shoulders hurt so badly.

So I run the last three or so miles with my arms flailing. I look like the scarecrow in *The Wizard of Oz*. The slowest mile in the first five is 7:45. The last one is 8:08. SEAL looks at me like I left him on the battlefield.

Four hours later...

I have a meeting with the brass of a major hotel chain. I'm not really sure what the meeting is about, but my friend Kirk Posmantur set it up because he thought I could help the chain. Kirk owns a company called Axcess Luxury & Lifestyle, and he is the king of connecting dots. If Kirk says it's worth a meeting and exploring, then it's worth a meeting and exploring.

I ask SEAL to join.

There's no need to change, mostly because SEAL has nothing to change into. Rather, we throw on our ridiculous-looking weight vests (SEAL is again insisting on us wearing them) and we head to the meeting from the apartment. When we arrive, we are greeted by Kirk and four other guys in suits, and they look a lot smarter than me. I am definitely not prepared for the meeting. In fact, I'm a bit nervous.

"Nice vest," Kirk says.

"Oh, this old thing." I laugh. "I just threw it on."

They are so confused.

I immediately introduce SEAL and explain that he is living with me for a month and tailing my every move.

"Wait...like a Navy SEAL seal?" the Brooks Brother guy asks.

"What kind of training?" the Prada suit dude asks.

"Like lives in your house?" the sweater vest pipes in before I can answer any of the questions. All these guys want to do is talk about our workouts and why I hired SEAL. These guys are looking at me like I just invented the Internet. They're *blown away*. It's like when a stock on the New York Stock Exchange is halted and no business can be conducted. They're obsessed with our dynamic. They keep asking questions.

Two hours pass and it's a question-and-answer frenzy. At the end of the meeting they say to me "If you have any ideas for us, let us know, we want to do something with you."

It's like SEAL is a secret weapon. He's the best closer. I'm slowly realizing how appealing SEAL is to others. Men in suits are fascinated by a guy like SEAL. His work ethic. His workouts. His history. So...indirectly they are becoming more interested in me.

1900

Tonight is my company's holiday party. And of course SEAL is invited. I'm not sure if he wants to go, but he's coming. He deserves to be here; his mere presence practically signed Kevin Garnett for us. We all have a lot to celebrate. It's been a great year.

The party is a low-key dinner and all twelve employees attend. I'm worried a bit about how SEAL will interact in the social setting. I mean, there is a good chance he will sit there and not say a word. He can be like a sphinx. When he comes to work with me every day, he never talks to anyone. EVER. Never logs on to a computer. Never reads a paper. He just sits there until it's time to go. It's like having a piece of artwork in my office. I know he's trained to go off the grid, but it was wild. Not only to me but to everyone I work with. SEAL once told me that when he came back from a mission, when everyone would sit around and smoke and decompress, he would go running. After a twenty-four-hour mission, he would work out.

As it turns out, I don't have to worry about SEAL interacting with anyone tonight because he's on a food mission. I realize SEAL's eating habits are more complicated than I originally thought. For two weeks he hardly ate at all, except for his military-grade shakes. But at dinner this evening, he eats like a wood chipper. Steak, fish, fruits, vegetables, you name it—it goes down the hatch. Everything except dessert.

"Why would I want to waste the calories?" he says.

My employees seem a little looser than they usually are during the workday. Maybe it's the cocktails. They are all obsessed with SEAL. They ask him a million questions and get one-word answers back. They're intimidated and intrigued. It's like everyone wants to sit next to him, but nobody wants to sit next to him. Most of the people at the party have been following the blog. So they know what to ask but are afraid to ask it.

"Um, excuse me, do you mind telling me what you think has been the hardest workout so far?"

"I'm sorry to bother you, but can you explain what 1-18 is?"

"If you don't mind, would you tell me the Boston story?"

My employees are asking questions like we're in the conference room with a new potential client pitching us a product. It keeps going. And he keeps eating. When all is said and done, SEAL's food intake constitutes 75 percent of the dinner bill for the night.

Amazing.

On another note, we're serving sake at the party. I like sake.

I do a shot. Then another. And another. All the way to eight (well, maybe nine!).

It's on!

First drink(s) in eighteen days.

Best I've felt in eighteen days!

SEAL is totally cool with it. He is letting me do my thing and enjoying his hall pass as well.

The euphoria doesn't last.

When we get home, I definitely need to sleep. I was up at 6:00 a.m., worked out, had an eleven-hour workday followed by the party and all that alcohol. I'm toast. I can't wait to go to bed. My body and brain are both in agreement. The day should be over, but my gut tells me it isn't. It's sort of like when you're in third grade and look out at the one inch of snow that fell overnight. You *hope* school will be canceled, but you *know* better. So regardless of what my brain and body are rooting for, I make my way to my bedroom to get my shorts and sneakers.

SEAL smiles. "You know we gotta do it, right?"

"Yes."

I'm buzzed, and doing push-ups when you are buzzed is a whole different kind of thing. I actually think it may be easier at first. The first ones are funny. It's like you don't really know you're doing them, with the alcohol and the up-and-down push-up movement mixing to form a more intense buzz. But as you move on, that buzz turns to an I'm-fucked feeling.

I fight through the fucked feeling and we do ten push-ups on the minute for twenty minutes. That's another two hundred down. It's easy to write "two hundred" on paper, but it's another thing to do them. I have no idea how many push-ups the average forty-plus man can do, but I'm guessing around twenty at one shot. Doing two hundred is a *big* number. It is not easy.

I get into my bed and throw *SportsCenter* on. I'm fucked up.

> **Workout totals: 6 miles (sub-8-minute-mile pace) and 200 push-ups**

DAY 20

Start When the Second Hand Hits

If you're hungry, run faster. You'll be home quicker.
—SEAL

New York City
32°
0600

I get out of bed and head into the kitchen. It is pitch dark outside and cloudy. It looks brutally cold, but the thermometer says thirty-two degrees. I look out of my window onto Columbus Circle and there is nobody outside. It looks like an old barren movie set. SEAL is already in the kitchen sitting on a stool at our island. Just sitting.

"We are going to focus on the basics this morning. Push-ups and sit-ups. It all starts with the basics," SEAL says.

It's true.

My time with SEAL has convinced me the days of the

fancy gym memberships are numbered. Things like CrossFit and street workouts are going to prevail in the future. All you really need to do is get your push-up and sit-up routine consistent, and you can see amazing results.

I have another philosophy. You can be fit without being healthy, but you can't be healthy without being fit. Meaning…you can be in great shape on the outside, but if you don't eat great and don't take care of your insides, you aren't necessarily healthy. History shows us there were plenty of athletes who were in great shape but suddenly died of a heart attack. Balance is key.

I also believe being in really good shape takes a combination of many components. For starters, you have to be strong, but you also have to be explosive, flexible, capable of running stop-and-go sprints and running long distances. You need the full package.

So, back to basics.

I do ten push-ups followed by as many sit-ups as I can until the second hand on the clock hits 12 again. Then I start the push-ups and sit-ups again. We repeat that for thirty minutes nonstop. By the end of the workout, my core muscles, chest, and triceps are cooked. Plus my heart rate is up in the mid-150s.

The full package.

1300

My friend Bryan Fried comes over to hang out for a few hours. I've known Fried for a long time, and he is part of my

"Wonderful Wednesday" group, six friends who run together every Wednesday (hence the name). He is also a professional cyclist and in great shape. I think SEAL is in his room, but I told him I had a friend coming over, so I assume he'll come out to say hi.

"This beats your first apartment," Bryan says, getting comfortable on my couch.

"It does," I say. "But there was some charm to that place."

"When did you live there? Ninety-three?"

"Yeah."

It was on 60th between First and York. This was long before they renovated the 59th Street Bridge area. It was actually the mecca for transvestite prostitution. Every night coming home from the bars was an adventure. The first week living there I didn't even make eye contact. It only took a week or two for all of the prostitutes to know that Spit (my roommate) and I weren't looking for dates. Well, I should say we weren't looking for those kinds of dates. In no time we coexisted, but the crib wasn't exactly the Ritz-Carlton. We had to walk up 162 steps to get to our 150-square-foot apartment. The kitchen and bathroom were one room. There was no bedroom. I slept in a loft space with a six-foot ceiling. I couldn't sit up in bed and had to walk up these little steps to get to my mattress. I'd roll just to get into bed. And looking back, I had absolutely the best time living there. It was like sleeping on a ship. I paid $350 and Spit paid $417 a month. We lived there for two years.

My office then was the apartment living room.

I'd bought a television and it came in a huge cardboard

box. So I flipped the box upside down and that was my desk. It took up half the apartment. I'd write all of the phone numbers, dates, and appointments on the box. The only rule in the apartment was you couldn't drink on my desk. That box was my whole life. I had it forever. It was so organized. I knew where everyone's phone number was. I knew every appointment.

I loved living as a struggling artist; my mind-set was a creative eat what you kill. I was enjoying the fact that I was even in this position. I worked all day hitting the phone or studio if I had a job and then at night I was hitting the bars.

Just as Bryan and I are getting situated on the couch, laughing and talking, SEAL walks in the room to shake Bryan's hand. I think SEAL wants to show off his work on me to date as he says, "Let's knock out a quick five-minute round of push-ups."

Fried and I agree.

SEAL pulls out his watch and we begin. We do ten push-ups on the thirty-second dial. By the time we are three minutes into it, Fried is down to seven. I keep pace. Five minutes pass and we're done. I'm able to do them all. Fried is cooked. SEAL is proud of his student.

2100

SEAL pulls me off the couch where I am comfortably watching ESPN.

"Let's do a cooldown" are his exact words.

To SEAL, a cooldown is an eight-mile run. To me, a cooldown is the last thing I want to do. I put on all my shit and give Sara a kiss. Although we have been doing this for weeks, she can tell I'm tired and have already had multiple workouts today. She can tell I'm pissed. "Honey, this is really ridiculous. You're overdoing it."

We run through Central Park into Harlem up around 125th Street and start to head back.

There are three specific highlights from the run:

1. Three miles into the run I ask SEAL if he has $2 (the only words we have said to each other all run). He says, "For what?" I respond, "I haven't eaten all day. I need an energy bar or a banana." He says, "We have five miles left. If you are hungry, run faster. You'll be home quicker."

2. SEAL hears a dog nearby in the woods while we are running. I didn't hear a thing, but apparently SEAL has extrasensory hearing. SEAL says under his breath to himself and to the invisible dog, "Try me, mother-fucker. I mean it, try me." Let me be perfectly honest; he said it in a way where it sounded like he *wanted* the dog to attack him. The dog was smart; we never saw him.

3. There are millions of people in New York City. Literally millions. Yet tonight we only saw one other person running in all of Central Park. We're home at 10:25 p.m. At the doorstep to our building, SEAL says to me: "It's not what you do, it's when and how you do it. It's all about the conditions. Remember that."

Ten minutes later...

We have to hustle because we need to get to the airport and go down to Atlanta for a lightning-quick trip. Sara has a meeting in the morning and has asked us to keep her company. I want to stay in NYC and work, but SEAL reminds me, "You're not in control here, bro," and he's right. If my wife wants to roll to Atlanta...we roll to Atlanta. So we fly out at midnight. The plan is to go there and fly back in just twenty-four hours.

> **Workout totals: 8 miles, 400 push-ups, and 550 sit-ups**

White Van

I can sit still for hours. Waiting.
—SEAL

The next morning I see SEAL sitting absolutely still on the windowsill of our Atlanta house. The sun is still coming up. He's staring out at something. Maybe he's watching the sunrise, but I doubt it. He's dead silent. He doesn't even acknowledge me when I enter the kitchen. His eyes are locked onto the empty street outside. Staring…

I open the refrigerator and pour some juice into a glass. I intentionally make it noisy. No acknowledgment. Zero. He doesn't flinch. Staring…

"Everything cool?"

"Not really," SEAL says. Staring…

He pauses for a moment. He might see something.

"This shit is starting to get to me. Like it's makin' me uncomfortable. Real uncomfortable."

"What?"

"You tellin' me you haven't noticed?" SEAL asks. Still staring…

"No? What?"

"That white van?" he says.

I look outside. There's nothing. The street is empty, but it looks like it's going to be a nice day.

"Man, this van keeps driving by. It's like they are toying with me, bro. Like they're clowning me," SEAL says.

I look back out the kitchen window. I still don't see anything. "Where?"

"NO...NOT NOW. Usually around oh-two-hundred when I'm on lookout," he says.

"Lookout?"

"Yeah, lookout. Last time I was here at night I was sitting outside monitoring and the van creeped up. They were looking at the house. Fucking creepers."

SEAL continues to stare out the window. Not once does he look at me.

"I didn't get a read on the plate," he says. "But I'm onto them." SEAL ponders his thought. "By the way...you need to install an infrared camera at the west side of the driveway adjacent to the mailbox. IMMEDIATELY. It needs to be angled toward oncoming traffic. We can plant around it to make it blend with the bush. I got a guy that can install ASAP. That way we can't miss 'em. We've been breached, dude. Do not ignore this."

"Breached?"

"You've seen the van, right?"

"Actually, I haven't seen any cars in front of the house."

SEAL turns to me with a blank, cold, motionless face. He's pissed. *Really pissed.*

"It's a VAN, bro. It's not a car. It's a FUCKING VAN. The kind that looks like it's gonna do some shit it ain't supposed to be doing." SEAL stares back out the window again, at nothing. "Does the van think I'm some kinda fuckwad?"

I don't think I'm supposed to answer the question.

"I'm gonna camp out on this motherfucker," he says.

"Camp out?"

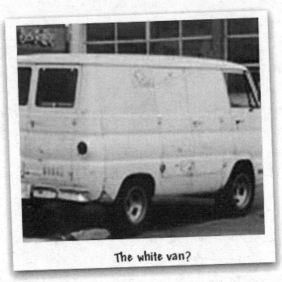

The white van?

"Fuck yeah! I'm gonna camp out and wait for his ass." SEAL pounds his fist against the wall.

"At night?"

"Not at night. EVERY NIGHT," he says. "I'll be out there on a lawn chair every night till that joker pulls up again. Then I'm gonna blast a high-beam light directly into his eyes and storm the vehicle. I'm gonna corner this fucker. I'm done playing defense."

SEAL pauses in thought, then says: "The thing is...he has no idea I'm even playing defense right now. He's probably thinking to himself, HO-HUM, the Itzlers are asleep. But NO HO-HUM. The Itzlers are NOT asleep. The goblins are awake in the Itzler house, bro." He cackles. "The goblins are WIDE AWAKE!"

And still staring...

DAY 21

One Rep at a Time

I don't like to talk to strangers. Actually,
I don't like to talk, period.
—SEAL

New York City
19°
0900

We're back in the city, and we head out to do a modified loop
in the park. SEAL tells me we are going to run ten miles
today in reverse order, meaning four miles this morning and
six miles at night. Usually we do a longer run in the morning
and a cooldown at night. Today we do the first four miles
at an eight-minute pace. Four-mile runs are becoming easy
breezy.

I've spent countless hours with SEAL running by now,
and we haven't spoken a word pounding the pavement for
days. Complete radio silence when we run. *Nothing ever
said*.

"Hey, SEAL, what do you think about when you run?"

"Finishing."

And he does. It's like he is able to block out all the clutter in his head and the world, for that matter, and just focus on the task at hand. Say what you want, but the dude has mastered the art of being present. There is something really cool about that.

As for me, I have a million things running through my brain…Sara, Lazer, work, meetings, Zico/Coke, training, the pipes freezing, blah blah blah. It's like there's a six-lane express highway running through my brain, and traffic is coming both ways. It's very hard for me to get my thoughts, worries, and ideas out my mind. It's a bit overwhelming and stressful.

However, with SEAL around, I am learning how to be more present. It's primarily because I have to. If I don't, there is no way I will be able to finish the tasks at hand. I just go one step at a time. One rep at a time. And when I'm done, I worry about the next step or rep. I'm finding that there's some crossover to my life as well. Now I finish the first thing on my list with 100 percent focus and then attack the next.

Thanks, SEAL.

2030

After a light meal of plain pasta with nothing on it, sliced carrots, cucumbers, and a glass of water, it's time for the second half of our reverse run. I would prefer to wait about an hour for my food to digest, but SEAL doesn't want to lose an hour of his life. So, we go.

As we ride the elevator down to the lobby of my building, I explain that I feel bloated. I like to run on an empty stomach and have a very hard time running with anything in me. That goes for races of any distance including marathons. Pre-marathons all I ever eat are bananas. So I ask SEAL how he approaches nutrition during his long races.

"I need calories when I'm running that long. I have trained myself to be able to eat while I'm running. I can take in six hundred to a thousand calories an hour, no problem. But it takes getting used to."

I hear the same thing from other ultra-marathon runners. They have become capable of eating large amounts of food during their races. Dean Karnazes, a legendary runner who put ultra-marathoning on the map, is famous for eating pizza during some of his longer runs. He actually orders and has the delivery guy meet him on the course so he can get the pizza and eat it during the race.

All that is good, but none of it is working for me as we start to run. I can feel the sustenance in my stomach bouncing. I'm belching every couple of strides. It's like the pasta, carrots, and cucumbers have set up a picket line in my belly and are protesting against one more step. We're not even at mile one yet and I feel heavy and sick. SEAL couldn't give three shits and keeps pace. In fact, I think he senses my discomfort and speeds the pace up a bit to make me feel even worse.

At around four miles I somehow figure out that if I breathe exclusively through my diaphragm, it feels a little better. I incorporate an unorthodox breathing style for the last two miles and make it home.

It takes about an hour for my stomach to settle down, but the run is in the books.

Another ten-mile day. Book it!

Workout totals: 10 miles @ 8-minute-mile pace

DAYS 22–23

Night Training

Be ready for anything at any time.
—SEAL

New York City to Connecticut
11° to 9°
1400

It's the Christmas holiday! New York City is lit up and beautiful. If you have never been to New York during this time, it really is special. The streets are quiet and all the stores are shut down as people prepare to spend the day with loved ones celebrating.

Our family, which now includes SEAL, decides to head back up to Connecticut. I love the holidays, especially with all the winter elements. There's something in the air that just makes me feel festive. Regardless of religion or beliefs, for the most part everyone is in the spirit of giving. Even SEAL.

SEAL and I head out for a quick six-mile run in the mountains. It is a maintenance run at an 8:30 clip. Meaning we are not getting better during this run, but we are not getting worse either. We are "maintaining our shit," he tells me. When we get back home, I shower up and change.

I meet Sara in the family room. As she and I exchange some Hannukah and Christmas gifts, SEAL comes into the room holding something in his hands. He's protecting it like a fullback would a football near the goal line.

"Your boy's got an inner toughness," SEAL says. "I wanted to capture that in a gift," and he hands a present to Lazer.

I'm wondering, Is it a toy truck? Blocks? Soccer ball? Nope. It's a miniature camouflage outfit, complete with hat. Real Army fatigues...a unique gift for a two-year-old!

Sara then gives SEAL a present from us. (She really wanted to.) And right after he opens it, she asks him to try it on. He politely declines. SEAL isn't big into receiving gifts. Most humans like gifts, SEAL looks at gifts like they are clutter. She asks again and he respectfully says, "Later." By the third time my wife is no longer asking, she's insisting. Even SEAL doesn't dare mess with her.

SEAL goes into the bedroom to change. But now he doesn't want to come out. But after a minute or two, he reluctantly appears.

Out walks SEAL in a very nice casual dress shirt. Your standard, light-blue button-down. It looks nice on him. But judging from SEAL's expression, you'd think he's wearing a straitjacket.

I hand Sara the gifts that I got her the other day at Barneys. She can tell by the size of the box that it's jewelry. She opens it up and puts the necklace around her neck.

"I love it, sweetie. But what I really love is that you went out of your way for me. Love you."

A for effort!

1900

It's frigid and snowy. The family is feeling good. We're all together. A typical late December in the Itzler household might be a fire in the fireplace, some blankets, and a movie once Lazer goes to bed. I'd usually vote for something with a little bit of edge to it, but Sara would lobby and win for a romantic comedy.

"It's bedtime," Sara says to Lazer.

He's on the floor playing with SEAL. They've got action heroes and Matchbox cars and are saving the world. Somehow SEAL has created a realistic village made up of blocks and tanks attacking from all directions. SEAL is barking orders like it's a real-life raid. He's taking it way too seriously, but Lazer is actually interested and looks like he's enjoying himself. Which alarms me.

0200

It's 2:00 a.m. and snowing like crazy. The door to my bedroom is locked and I'm sleeping when I hear what sounds like someone trying to pick the lock of my door. The door handle is making noises like it's being pulled and tugged from the other side of the door. Then the sound I hear is like when a dog is scratching to get into the room while the handle is being pulled and tugged some more.

I get out of my bed to check. I put my ear to the door to hear what's going on, but now I don't hear anything. Silence. So I bend down and get on all fours to look under the door crack to see if I see anything. Sure enough, I see SEAL's sneakers by the door. I stand up and pull open the door and SEAL is standing right there.

"It's time," he says.

SEAL tells me the plan is to run four miles every four hours for forty-eight hours!

Twelve runs of four miles each *every four hours*! He calls it the 4/4/48.

Are you kidding me?

Apparently, he's not. In fact, we're going to train for it by

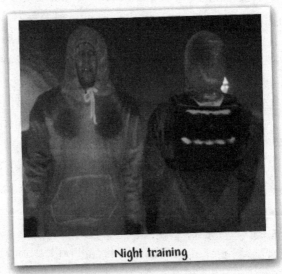

Night training

running 4.25 miles four times in twenty-four hours, or four runs every six hours.

I'm about to ask SEAL his logic behind this, but instead I just say, "Are you kidding me?"

0230

I open up my phone so I can get the light on it to shine and then I use it as a flashlight. I don't want to put the bedroom lights on because that might wake up Sara. She has been super cool about everything to date, but I'm not sure she would want me running in the snow at 2:00 a.m. in the mountains of Connecticut.

I go to my closet and quietly open up my drawers to get my gear. I feel like I'm sleepwalking, but I know that is wishful thinking. I layer up, tiptoe out of our bedroom, and head downstairs to the front door. SEAL is already outside.

I'm wearing a thermal, a hoodie, a hat, two pairs of gloves, and thermal pants. SEAL is in shorts, a hoodie, and gloves. It's freezing outside. Wet and freezing. We head out.

Every step feels like I'm about to fall off the earth. It's pitch black. I mean *pitch*. Five minutes into the run, SEAL turns to me and says, "Rough road ahead. Twenty meters."

Now, how could he possibly know that? I can't see one meter in front of me. In fact, I'm not sure I even know what a meter is. I mastered military time, but I'm not up on the metric system. Anyway, apparently, SEAL's eyesight isn't affected by darkness. It's like he has night vision without the night-vision goggles. He sees fine.

It's also bitter cold. My fingertips are completely numb. SEAL runs like he's in Anguilla, it's eighty degrees and sunny.

Meanwhile, the snow hits my frozen face like BB gun pellets. I'm squinting to see and closing my eyes for thirty seconds at a clip to keep the snow from pounding into my eyeballs. I'm no longer in the holiday spirit.

Soon we hit a patch of rough road. I say to myself, That must be how far twenty meters is. We move on.

We run 4.5 miles in exactly forty minutes. When we get home, we don't even turn the lights on. Our eyes are so adjusted to the dark that I can actually see fine in my pitch-dark house. Apparently SEAL's built in night-vision goggles have rubbed off on me.

I strip naked and put all of my clothing in the dryer. My skin has red blotches all over from the cold and I am freezing. I put on two sweatshirts and a ski hat and get into bed. Sara is sound asleep next to me.

Approximately four hours later...

My phone alarm goes off. I got about three hours of sleep. I get my clothes out of the dryer. If only they were still warm. SEAL is waiting at the front door. When we open the door, a bunch of snow falls into my foyer. It's twelve degrees outside.

We head out.

It's still as dark outside as when we got in from the last run, and it's still as cold and wet. It's like groundhog night. My muscles are super stiff from the cold (and the mileage), and my feet hurt when they hit the hard, snowy pavement. We do the same run as before in thirty-eight minutes. Brutal.

Four hours later...

19°

It's run number three in our twenty-four hours of runs every four hours. The hardest part so far has been the process of exerting myself, cooling down, and then having to start again. The restart is a bitch. SEAL throws me a bone and says if we do the loop in less than thirty-eight minutes, we don't have to run again in four hours. That's a bone I like!

Thus begins the great debate: Do we go out hard (the first mile is very tough with big elevation) or do we pace ourselves?

SEAL says, "Go hard."

"Let's go!" I say.

Out of a hundred runs on this mountain course, my fastest first mile *ever* is exactly 9:00. Trust me, this run is *hilly*. We do this one in 8:07! We are flying! I'm gasping for air. Literally. As we get to the top of the hill (1.1 miles) I feel like I'm cramping. I keep going and it gets worse. I can't run.

"Stop the clock for a second, something's off."

Groin pull?

It's so damn cold out I can't officially diagnose myself until we get home. We walk the one mile back. The sweat pours off of me. I guess SEAL was right, it's eighty and sunny, but with each step back, it feels like the temperature drops a degree. Then my body heat mixes with the cold and creates a thick, white vapor that rises from my skin. I'm a human chimney. After we get home and defrost, I confirm it. It is indeed my groin. I'm in abject pain. It's impossible to run.

"Push-ups instead," SEAL says.

We do ten sets of thirty (with a one-minute break in between). Drops of ice start to fall off my face as I go down and start the push-up routine.

"Is this the hardest forty-eight hours you've ever had?" SEAL asks.

"Physically, yeah," I say. "Then again, this is even harder than the Grant Hill shit."

"The basketball player?"

"Yeah," I say.

"You trained with him?"

"No."

"Then what the fuck are you talking about?"

One time Foot Locker hired me and my partner Kenny to do a national radio campaign. It was part of the work we were doing for our company Alphabet City. We were up against some other agencies, but we won the account because I promised them I could get Grant Hill to be in the commercial. Hill had been the NBA's Rookie of the Year and was a bona fide rising superstar. He was a big get. They wanted him and I promised we would get him.

"No problem," I said.

But, there was a problem—I didn't know Grant Hill.

After we signed Foot Locker to do the campaign, I learned Grant was making an appearance at a Foot Locker in Manhattan, so my plan was to approach him right at the event. All I needed to do was get Hill to say something like: "Hi, this is Grant Hill and I'm shopping at Foot Locker this holiday season," and then insert it into the radio spot. Then Foot Locker would give him a $500 gift certificate and I would be on my way.

Easy, right?

Except that I missed the event. I could go into a whole long explanation of what happened, but I'll save you the time. I just blew it. The next day the CEO of Foot Locker called me and asked if I got Grant Hill and I had to tell him no.

"You've got forty-eight hours," he said. "Or the deal's off."

I immediately got the NBA schedule and found out the Orlando Magic, Grant Hill's team, was playing the Hawks that night. I went straight to LaGuardia and headed for Atlanta. I got to the arena at 10:30 in the morning even though the game didn't tip-off until 7:30 at night. It was so early that I was able to walk right into the arena. Some marching band was rehearsing, and nobody questioned me because I was "with the band."

I knew that players typically showed up at 5:30 for a 7:30 game, so I had a lot of time to kill. I just walked around like I knew what I was doing. I just tried to look busy.

Though it seemed like forever, eventually some of the Orlando Magic began to show up. I stood at a payphone and pretended to make a call as I waited for Grant. And then I saw my mark. I walked right up to him as he came through the player entrance.

"Hey, Grant, it's Jesse from Foot Locker. I flew down and I'm here to get the audio clip I was supposed to get on Saturday," I said. "You ready now?"

"What audio clip?"

"Right. The audio clip from the Foot Locker event."

"Okay, let's talk about it after the game," he said, walking past me.

"No, no," I said. "I have to get it now and get back on the plane."

He kept walking into the locker room, so I leaned over and pulled his ear close to my mouth. "Grant, look into my eyes. I'm going to lose my job if I don't get this done. I can't go home without this. I flew down here on my own dime today to get this. I don't know what it is, but they need it. The CEO sent me."

Maybe he saw the genuine fear in my eyes or heard it in my plea. Whatever the case, he obliged.

"Okay," he said. "Follow me."

So I walked into the locker room with all of the players goofing off and starting to get ready for the game. I pull out my handheld recorder and hand him a script. BUT...it's too loud in the locker room, so I take him into the bathroom stall and close the door.

I hand Grant the script again and push record.

"Hey, this is Grant Hill, and this holiday season you can find me at Foot Locker. Foot Locker has got you covered."

Halfway through the third line he said, "Who are you again? And what is this being used for?"

"Grant, I've been on the phone with your agent all day. This is part of the Foot Locker package you did. They're running a holiday promotion." I was just throwing words at him. "It's the audio part." I was hoping he might pick up some buzzwords and think that I actually was supposed to be there.

"Okay, fine," he said, and he finished it and then I ran out.

As soon as I got out of the arena, I headed back to the airport and called Kenny from another payphone and played him the recording. The next day it was on national radio.

"That's some funny shit," Seal says without cracking a smile.

"Do you want to hear about the big red chicken now?"

"No."

3:00 p.m.

SEAL takes me down to the gym to do some push-ups. Our Connecticut house has a gym on the bottom floor. Adjacent to the gym is a steam room and a sauna. It's like a mini training facility, and I love hanging out down there.

I bought this house seven years ago and gutted the entire place right after the closing. At the time I was building Marquis Jet, and I wanted a place where I could entertain customers. One of the most important things I told the decorator was that I wanted a steam room that you never want to leave. Yeah, I picked out colors and approved floor plans, but I really only cared about the steam room. This gym and spa area are my personal retreat.

We do twenty sets of twenty push-ups with a one-minute break in between each set. Let me repeat...twenty sets of twenty push-ups!!! The first ten are actually fairly easy. But the second half starts to get the better of me. I push my way through it and get to the final set. I'm *jacked-up* sore.

"Finish up. GET THIS SHIT DONE, FUCKER."

I do. I have to hold a plank position in between reps for about twenty seconds on each of the last twenty push-ups, but I get it done.

That's seven hundred so far today including the three hundred we did earlier.

SEAL begs me to do three hundred more to get to a thousand push-ups. He begs me!

"I physically can't," I say.

And I mean it. I can't do one more push-up. I can't even hold a downward dog pose. I head upstairs with my arms dangling by my sides.

We call it a day and I relax on my couch. I grab the *Sports Business Journal* and get caught up on recent transactions. The few hours of downtime are like a vacation, and I'm feeling cozy.

Workout totals: 16.1 miles and 700 push-ups

DAY 24

Whiteout

The tougher the conditions, the more I like my odds.
—SEAL

Connecticut
5°
0600

We wake up to blizzard conditions. Sixteen inches of snow with 30-mph winds and –7 degrees with wind chill. Miraculously my groin feels better. Maybe it was just a cramp?

Repeatedly scrolling across the bottom of my television screen is an "EXTREME WEATHER WARNING." The local news in Connecticut is advising everyone to "STAY INSIDE UNLESS IT'S AN EMERGENCY."

"This is fucking perfect," SEAL says.

I guess he considers this an emergency.

He stares at the TV, bobbing his head like he's listening to Jay Z, only he's not wearing any headphones.

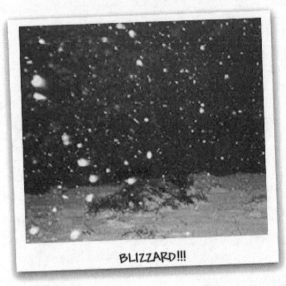

BLIZZARD!!!

Finally he says, "We gotta head out."

We run 3.5 miles in the mountains.

SEAL decides to wear the fifty-pound weight vest. He is *out of his mind*. I can't explain how hard this run is...in these conditions...with a fifty-pound weight vest on. When we get home, I think I'm frostbitten. My shirt is so cold and wet it hurts to take it off. In fact, my shirt is actually frozen. When I manage to get it off, it sits upright in my chair.

We do 144 push-ups, plus an extra ten for good measure.

2:00 p.m.

Sara goes outside to get the mail. The mailbox is at the end of our driveway, about fifty yards away once you walk out of the front door. The only obstacle or "threat" between our front door and getting our mail is the grass, which is covered by snow. The danger would be that someone slips on a patch of ice. What I mean is…getting the mail is not a high-wire act. It's not something on our radar as far as a thing to worry about.

Sara returns holding three envelopes and a fashion catalog. She begins to open the catalog.

SEAL is livid.

"Sara, you need to mix up your pattern."

"Pattern?"

"Yeah, your pattern. PATTERN. The time you get the mail. That's your pattern. It's the same every day. It's predictable."

"I get the mail after lunch," she says. "That's the most convenient time."

"Why after lunch?" SEAL asks baffled. "That seems common."

"Because that's when the mailman comes," she replies. "He delivers the mail after lunch."

"Exactly. You know that. And I know that. The mailman most definitely knows that. So I bet EVERYONE knows that. For sure your neighbors know that."

"But I'm just getting the mail…at my house…on our property," she says.

"Just do me a favor. Change up the pickup time. Go an hour or so later tomorrow. Break the pattern, Sara. Break the pattern."

2100

Sara and I have dinner before we put Lazer down for bed. Nothing fancy, just some veggie burgers and salad that we whipped up. Shortly after we get Lazer to sleep, we get into bed together to watch some TV. I'm fading into sleep land but can sense that Sara is still up and watching CNN.

At around 9:00 p.m. I feel Sara getting out of bed. She is doing it in a way not to wake me, but I'm slowly learning to be on alert. I'm awake.

"Where you going, sweetie?" I ask.

"I hear something in the basement. It sounds like our generator has kicked in."

"What are you talking about?"

Sara heads down before I can ask another question to check out the noise.

About eight minutes later Sara returns. She crawls back into bed and tells me, "No biggie." SEAL is on the stationary bike. He wants to "get some mileage in" and didn't want to "ride in the snow."

The next morning, we wake up at 7:00 a.m. and the generator sound is *still* making the same noise. This time I head downstairs. As I get closer I can hear the noise coming from the gym, and music is playing in the background. I open the door to the gym and a wave of hot air attacks me. It's like someone is holding a hair dryer on high and pointing it at my face. The room feels like a sauna and the windows are all fogged up. Straight ahead I see SEAL on the stationary bike with his shirt off and puddles of sweat on the floor. He doesn't look up. Clearly he knows I'm there, but he does *not* say a word. Not even a hello or good morning. He doesn't look happy—shocker, I know. He keeps riding.

He rode the entire night. Ten hours straight.

Workout totals: 3.5 miles and 154 push-ups

DAY 25

Get Your Balls Wet

Fear is one of the best motivators.
Anger is the other.
—SEAL

Connecticut
5°
0930

SEAL takes me on a five-mile run up Wanzer Hill. Wanzer Hill is the main road in my development, and it's so steep it's almost vertical. There should be double black diamonds on the street sign. Cars can't get up it in good weather. Other hills don't even want to be in the same neighborhood as Wanzer Hill, it's that intimidating. Plus, there's snow and black ice everywhere, making the run slower/harder/colder.

Didn't SEAL just ride a bike all night? WTF! He didn't stop.

When we get home after the run, I complain that the

tendon in my foot is killing me (recurring basketball injury) and my foot is swollen. Really swollen.

"I got a solution. Let's go into the lake and freeze your foot," SEAL says.

"Go into the lake? The lake's frozen."

"I'm not playing. Let's go," he says.

I know this is the dumbest idea ever, but there is something about it I like. I get excited. I've always wondered how cold the water under the top layer of ice in a frozen lake is. We run down the hill from my house to the lake in two feet of snow. I am in sneakers, socks, shorts, and a sweatshirt. It's about three hundred yards at a steady decline. I stumble twice and face-plant before I reach the bottom. SEAL descends flawlessly and effortlessly. When we arrive, he immediately takes off his shoes and finds a hole in the ice big enough to fit him.

And *jumps in*! The lake is frozen but not completely. Parts of the lake by the shore have thin patches of ice.

"Hold on to the floating ice," he says.

I swear this happened.

I crawl onto the frozen lake and inch my way toward the hole where SEAL jumped in.

"GET THE FUCK IN, MOTHERFUCKER. GET THE FUCK IN!"

He's lost his mind.

"NO. I can't. I'm sorry. I can't."

"Get the fuck in, motherfucker. Get the fuck in," he says again. His lips are blue. "You fucking pussy, Itzler, get the fuck in!"

I take off my shoes. I take off my socks. This is insane.

"Get in. Balls deep. GET IN, ITZLER."

I jump in up to my knees. It feels like someone is sawing off my legs. Or maybe it feels like I wish someone would saw off my legs.

"DEEPER," he yells. I inch my way deeper, up to my waist.

Then, all of a sudden, his expression changes. It's no longer taut with anger. Now it's furrowed and worried.

"We got five minutes till frostbite. GET OUT NOW!"

What?!

"Don't touch your skin to the ice as you get out, it'll stick," he yells.

"What?"

"Like that motherfucker in *Christmas Story*. Grab your sneakers and use them as gloves, climb out of the hole in the ice, and crawl across the ice with your BARE FEET sticking up," he yells.

It takes two minutes to get to land. My mind is counting down like MacGyver. We have about three minutes left until frostbite. We run up the hill toward my house, with shoes off, barefoot in the snow.

SEAL's yelling again, "WE HAVE TWO MINUTES... RUN."

Halfway up the hill, my body is fueled by fear. There isn't a coherent thought in my head other than to get up this hill. My toes are going to fall off. I can't feel one thing from my knees down. With each stride I take I feel like my legs could shatter like an antique teacup hitting the floor. This is bad.

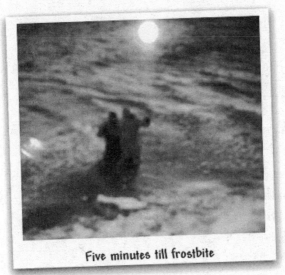

Five minutes till frostbite

Finally we reach the top. We go inside, peel off our wet clothing, dry off with towels and coats and anything we can grab.

Sara stands there, and I don't think I've ever seen her so angry. "That's the dumbest thing I've ever seen!" she yells.

"I'm sorry," I say.

"Sorry? You're a dad! Everyone knows not to go near ice on a *frozen lake.*"

She turns to SEAL. "And you!" she says to him. "You ought to be ashamed of yourself. Tell me what the medical benefit of jumping into a frozen lake is."

"There is none, Sara! This is what your husband SIGNED UP FOR!!! There's no benefit."

Fifteen minutes later...

SEAL comes and finds me and says, "We got to capitalize on this shit. We got to capitalize on this adrenaline."

What?

We do fifteen sets of fifteen push-ups on the minute (225 push-ups). The entire time I'm thinking to myself, Nobody would ever believe this. Nobody. But I'm so far into it I am now embracing the challenges. It's like I'm over the hump and I can't help but feel a little proud.

Twenty minutes later...

SEAL comes into my bedroom. I'm sitting with my feet elevated to ease my swollen ankle. "We only have four days left. We need to push our limits. Your work isn't done. You aren't ready to go back to the real world," SEAL says.

I pause and then realize...he's right. My life with SEAL isn't the real world. Then I think about him leaving. There's going to be a huge hole. These past twenty-five days have been unlike any other in my life. I didn't think this was possible, but I'm going to miss him. I'm going to miss the insanity. I'm going to miss the pain. I'm going to miss having him in charge.

"Let's make tacos tonight for dinner," I say.

"Tacos? Fuck the tacos," he says. "We're going to go into the steam room."

"The steam room?"

"Yeah, the fucking steam room. Setting that bitch at one hundred twenty-five degrees and we're in there for thirty minutes. No dumping water on our heads, no talking (obviously), and only twelve ounces of drinking water allowed in. I'm going to test your WILL."

SEAL sets the temp dial for 125 and we wait twenty minutes until it is properly heated. We strip to our undies and go in. To maximize the effect, SEAL tells me to sit on my hands and keep my arms locked straight. That will force our backs to be straight and our heads to be closer to the ceiling of the steam.

"Heat rises," he says.

NO KIDDING!

By keeping our heads up, we will get "maximum exposure," he repeats.

So, we go in.

Five minutes...okay.

Ten minutes...okay.

Twelve minutes...I drink all twelve ounces of water.

Fifteen minutes... okay.

Twenty minutes...Not so okay.

I hear a hissing sound.

It's hard for me to see with my eyeballs sweating.

I hope the hissing isn't coming out of me.

My heart rate is up and pounding. My skin looks like boiled chicken.

I'm overheating.

I'm nauseous.

SEAL sits in the opposite corner of the steam room, and I can barely make him out. I hear him whistling, and it is driving me mad. It sounds like a Beach Boys song. It can't be.

I'm hallucinating. *Only nine more minutes*, I tell myself. But it's not working. I try to think about baseball: Jeter's baseball average; Jason Kipnis's fielding percentage; Mariano Rivera's WHIP.

I'M LOSING MY MIND!

Now I know how a Hot Pocket feels inside a microwave.

One, two, three, four... I start counting to one hundred in my head. *Eleven, twelve, thirteen*...

I'm drifting into Faint City.

"I don't think I can do it," I say, finally breaking the twenty-one minutes of silence. "I'm sorry."

I don't wait for him to respond. I leap up and thrust open the door, almost breaking the glass.

SEAL follows me out, steam pouring into the room as the door stays open.

"Okay. Thirty-second rest and then back in."

I don't move. He looks closer.

"Whoa," he says, looking down at me crouched against the wall. "You don't look so good."

He looks blurry and his face is distorted like in a fun house mirror.

"Goarblogger rasootoootle," I respond.

"Man, we need to ABORT," he says.

Abort?

I sit in the chair outside my steam room for what feels like a day. Alone. SEAL does not come to check on me. My head is pounding. After thirty-five minutes, I finally begin to cool down. My heart rate is at 119. I'm sweating like I am in the desert in August. I down five Zicos, and it takes ninety minutes before I begin to feel remotely human.

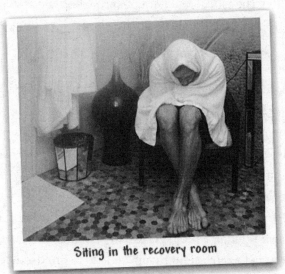

Sitting in the recovery room

Two hours later...

I have relocated to my bedroom and SEAL comes in. I'm under the covers watching CNN. He asks if I'm better.

"A little," I say.

"Good. Let's go."

Let's go?

"You don't even know what suffering is, motherfucker," he says with a look like he means it. He's right. I've lived a sheltered life.

He tells me to do a slow jog by myself outside "to loosen up my joints." (The ones that were fused together in the steam room or the ones that were frozen together in the lake?) He wants me to "understand myself better." He wants me to "feel the isolation." I'm not sure where he is going with this. In fact, I don't know what the hell he is talking about.

But I go outside.

Alone.

Before I leave, he hands me a flashlight because it is starting to get dark so early now. "Watch the black ice," he says.

"Thanks."

I do a 4.5-mile slow jog. When I come home, SEAL is waiting at the door. He is literally sitting outside by my front door in the snow eating a fucking apple.

"Nice work. You need that personal mind frame," he says. I still have no idea what he is talking about.

"Now get your strength up and do a hundred push-ups before you can come in the house. That's ten every thirty seconds. I'm not fucking around, man, this isn't sleep-away camp in upstate Fuckville."

Again, what?

But I get down and start to knock out the push-ups. SEAL disqualifies my first one.

"Start over. Your nose needs to touch the snow. We are past the make-believe shit."

2000

Fuck tacos is right. I heat up two veggie burgers. I'm obsessed with the MorningStar Grillers Prime and tonight I feel like I can eat the whole box. As soon as the microwave beeps indicating my meal is ready, in comes SEAL.

"You got a choice: Eat first and do 250 push-ups *or* eat after and choose to do what's behind curtain number two."

All of a sudden he is Bob Barker? I don't even ask a single question, I just say, "Give me door number two."

Well...*more push-ups*. We do twelve, then eight, then six, then four push-ups on the fifteen-second mark, followed by sit-ups, where we do as many as we can for sixty seconds. We rest one minute, then repeat for thirty minutes.

I'm a beaten man.

> **Workout totals: 9.5 miles, 775 push-ups, 125 sit-ups, 21-minute steam, frozen lake**

DAY 26

Primary Target

Know what's important to you and protect it
at all costs.
—SEAL

Connecticut
29°
0800

I'm fully recovered from the steam room incident. We're still
in Connecticut, and SEAL and I head out for the 4.5-mile
mountain loop near my house. I'm breathing just through my
nose. It feels like I'm flying. I check my time: 35:17. That's
three minutes faster than my previous personal best. Course
record for me! I'm feeling good.

We get home, shower, and meet in the den. I turn the
TV on.

Getting SEAL to watch television can be difficult. The
only thing I've seen him sit still for is sports. There are a few
college football bowl games on today so I'm hoping he won't

ask me to wear the fifty-pound weight vest in the second and fourth quarters. He seems fairly content on the couch. I wonder if he's thinking about leaving. The thought has been on my mind the last couple of days. At first, to be honest, I couldn't wait for the month to be over. But he's starting to grow on me. I appreciate his concern for my family's safety. It makes me wonder...

"Say, SEAL," I say. "What would you do if there was an intruder in the house?"

Slowly SEAL turns and looks at me. He holds me with an even, unemotional stare. Then he turns back to the TV without answering my question.

"No, really," I say. "What would you do?"

He shakes his head slowly.

"I think you know what I'd do," he says to the TV.

"Tell me."

"I would protect the primary."

"What's the primary?"

"That's the million-dollar question," he says. "What is your primary, Jesse? What would hurt you the most to lose? This big-screen TV? Those gold record awards you own? Jewelry? Cash? What do you hold most dear?"

"No," I say. "None of that."

"Well?" he asks.

"My wife and my son."

"Exactly, Jesse," he says. "They're your primary, and as long as I'm in this house they're my primary too. You asked me what I would do. I would protect my primary at any cost. And unfortunately for you, you're my third option."

At that moment I realize that despite all the time I have

spent with SEAL, he has always had an eye on Sara and Lazer. The plumber, the white van, the waiter…it's all been about protecting "us." Sure we have been training, but there is more to our relationship now. We have "primaries" to look after.

2100

I tell SEAL that I have to spend a few hours "closing the books" for the year, and I beg him not to interrupt me. He agrees.

"Go ahead and handle your shit, man."

I pull out all my notes and "to do" lists from this past year and take some personal inventory. I also make my annual donations and send out our holiday cards. It feels good to close out the year.

Once I come out from my office, he tells me, "We gotta get one in."

We go out for a five-mile run at top speed. I push, my body responds. Holy shit, I feel fit. Almost immortal. I feel up for anything! I think this is starting to pay off!

Workout totals: 9.5 miles

DAY 27

1,000 Push-ups

I don't celebrate victories but I learn from failures.
—SEAL

Connecticut
12°
0800

SEAL says "Today is goal day. Today all your hard work pays off. We are going to see if you can do one thousand push-ups."

I start the day off with ten quick sets of ten push-ups. We take a thirty-second rest in between sets. Feeling good. I rest.

Total: 100 push-ups

Two hours later...

First 1–18 push-ups and then one set of twenty-nine (8:58). Maybe I'm relying on muscle memory as I have done this already, but still feeling good. Rest again.

Total: 200 push-ups.

One hour later...

1–18 push-ups and then one set of twenty-nine (8:30). Now it's a struggle. I'm grinding these out. The last fifty I have to hold a plank position for a few seconds before I go down and up.

Total: 200 push-ups.

Three hours later...

1–18 push-ups and then one set of twenty-nine (8:30). Now I am getting into the REALLY HARD territory. I'm taking long breaks in between each push-up group. But, I'm doing it. My triceps are on FIRE.

Total: 200 push-ups.

1600

25, 25, 25, 25–1–18, 15, 14. These are BRUTAL. My arms are shaking like a leaf. My triceps feel like they have pins in them. It's a feeling I have never had before and I'm actually a bit concerned. SEAL tells me to "push through." My arms are trembling.

"Push through it," he yells.

I have to take a two-minute break before I complete the set of fifteen. Then I need a five-minute break before I can complete the last fourteen. But, once I'm close...there is no giving up!

Total: 300 push-ups.

In case you didn't count 'em, that's one thousand.

One thousand push-ups!

In one day. *Holy shit!* I take a seat on my couch by the steam room and smile. For the first time during this whole process, I'm truly proud of myself. Not because I did a thousand but because I stuck with the journey. I think back to the first day SEAL was here and the first set of push-ups we did. This proves to me that if you push the body, the body will respond.

1900

My body is inflated from all the push-ups. I feel like I'm wearing a wetsuit and someone has pumped air into it. I'm jacked up. But to SEAL, victories are short-lived. He tells me he never celebrates an accomplishment. Once his goal is done, it's time for his next goal. Our work is not done. It's time for our next goal.

SEAL and I head out for a 3.5-mile run.

When we get home, SEAL tells me to "get some shut-eye" and that "I earned it." I'm not sure, but I think that's a compliment. He is actually proud of me too. I go into my room and throw on ESPN to watch some Bowl highlights. SEAL heads to his room. He goes and continues to do twenty-five push-ups every ten minutes, 4:30 until midnight. He does twenty-five hundred for the day. *Superhuman.*

With fitness there's never a finish line. You can always do better. For me personally, I guess I probably have thirty or forty years left on earth. And how many of those am I going to be young enough and healthy enough to do things? I want to experience the best stuff I can. I've never jumped off a cliff—I should just jump off a cliff because I'm only here once. That's how I approach things now. That's how I feel about things. That's how I live my life.

A thousand push-ups is something I could never have imagined doing. It just shows that repetition and consistency equal results.

> **Workout totals: 3.5 miles and 1,000 push-ups!**

DAY 28

Up the Ante

If you don't challenge yourself, you don't know
yourself.
—SEAL

Connecticut
17°
0700

This morning we go for an 8.5-mile run up Leach Hollow
Road and back. Getting to Leach Hollow Road is not easy.
My friend Fish calls it "the Big Boy Run." It's a freak show.
Crazy hills, grueling course, and 8.5 miles is a good run
no matter how you slice it. I've run this course with many
friends, and only a select few have been able to complete it.

Anyway, I run it in 1:17:41 (an 8:57 average), with negative splits, which means clocking a better time the second
half of the run than the first. I'm two minutes faster on the
way back and I'm feeling psyched.

When we get home, the real fun begins.

"We have to up the ante," SEAL says.

"The lake?" I ask.

SEAL nods.

I begin to nod with him.

We stand there both understanding the mission and nodding together.

One little problem. This time there are no holes in the lake. It's frozen solid—six inches thick. There are even kids playing hockey on it.

"I have a plan," SEAL says.

"If you two knuckleheads even think about going through the ice again," Sara says, "don't bother coming back inside. It's frozen solid."

It's like my wife has a crystal ball or something. I didn't even see her standing there. She knows the nod. But I know Sara has a conference call later. So we wait.

When SEAL is sure my wife isn't watching, he sneaks down to the lake, grabs a boulder, and starts banging on the ice. And when I say boulder, I mean boulder, like from *The Flintstones*. This thing is huge, and SEAL has to bend down and lift with his legs and hold it with both hands before he can hoist it up. I look over at the kids skating and the game comes to an ice-spraying hockey stop. They are all watching SEAL.

SEAL pounds away: Boom-crackle crackle...Again... Boom-crackle crackle...Again...Boom-crackle crackle...

The hockey players head to solid ground.

The ice breaks. I think somewhere in SEAL's inner ear there's a tiny orchestra playing the theme song from *Rocky*. It's like he's at the top of the stairs of the Philadelphia

Museum of Art and he raises his arms in a victory pose. He gives a primal scream of "YESSSS!"

Socks off, shirt off…he's in!!!!

I start to hear the *Rocky* theme too.

I can do this…socks off, shirt off, I'm in!!!!

We repeat this twice and sprint up to my house to get warm.

I'm still freezing but feel: AMAZING!

Sara stands in the doorway. She glares at me but doesn't say a word. She gives the same stern look to SEAL. I feel like I'm seven. SEAL, who doesn't raise his eyes, looks like he's five.

My son is staring at my feet and looking puzzled. They have a reddish purple tint to them.

And SEAL…now he's on the TREADMILL!

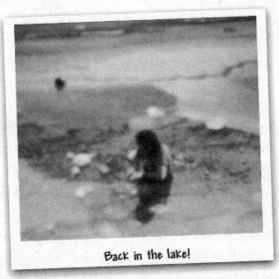

Back in the lake!

We're in the penalty box for about half the day. Sara wasn't really that mad, at least not at our houseguest. It's like she wanted to be mad, but she couldn't. Maybe it's because she knows all of this is coming to an end or perhaps she knows I'll probably never do this again. It's not safe.

5:00 p.m.... thirty minutes before dinner

We do ten push-ups on the thirty-second hand for ten sets (every five minutes).

That's a hundred total.

Then it's 1–10, 10–1, and three sets of thirty.

Another three hundred down!

8:00 p.m.

I'm in the bedroom with Sara, packing. We're going to Atlanta tomorrow but just staying overnight.

"What day is SEAL leaving again?" Sara asks.

"In two days," I say. "He'll come to Atlanta and then spend New Year's with us back here in Connecticut, but he's going home from there."

"I'm going to miss him," she says.

Sara had already told me that SEAL was the best houseguest we've ever had. She didn't have to tell him how to do anything or where anything was. He didn't need any instructions: He was spotless, thoughtful, and polite. But when SEAL really won her over is when Sara's grandmother, Nannie, stopped by one day in Atlanta. Nannie's right out of *The Andy Griffith Show*. SEAL was a total gentleman and did everything for her: carried her bags, made her breakfast, and walked with her on his arm. She adored him. When Nannie was around, I think she was SEAL's primary! Nannie kept referring to SEAL as "that nice young man." She would say, "Jesse, that nice young man...that friend of yours is just darling."

Sara seems to be very intently folding a blouse.

"I've been thinking," she says after a moment or two. "We should try and get SEAL to stay a bit longer."

As I'm looking at my wife packing it makes me realize what a difference a month can make. I know SEAL infinitely better than I did when he first showed up, but I still don't know him know him. But I think that's by design.

Sara snaps me back to present day with the toss of a diaper. I guess she knows something I don't. I catch the diaper and am about to make my way to Lazer when she looks at me.

"I've been giving it some thought. And I think I'd like to start a workout routine with SEAL too."

"Okay, sweetie. If that's what you really want, then ask him."

I'm acting cool, but I'm *psyched*!!!

"Just don't expect me to jump in the frozen lake," she says.

> **Workout totals: 8.5 miles, 300 push-ups, frozen lake**

DAY 29

Sloppy Seconds

I don't stop when I'm tired. I stop when I'm done.
—SEAL

Connecticut to Atlanta
36° to 88°
0900

We're leaving for a day trip to Atlanta this afternoon to do another check on the house, but first we head out on a 10.6-mile run in the rain and slush. It's warmed up a bit and the roads are sloppy.

"We gotta get one good one in before the flight," SEAL says.

The run is from my house to a diner on Route 22. I have no idea what the name of the diner is, but it is the *only* diner near us. I also know that when we drive up to the house from New York City, it's a marker for us. When we get to the diner, it's still a fifteen-minute drive. So the run is not going to be fun.

As predicted, it's lonely, miserable, hilly, and tough. I tell Sara we will be about an hour and a half and that we are running to the diner.

"You are going to run to the diner that we order takeout from? You *got to be kidding me.*"

"I kid you not," I reply.

"Can you pick me up some—" she says with a laugh.

SEAL must not have taken his patience pill when he took his handful of vitamins today because as soon as we start the run, he takes off. Every few straightaways he becomes visible for the first few miles, but then he completely disappears. He beats me there by eighteen minutes.

Time: 1:36:00.

Sara jumps in the car and picks us up at the diner ninety-five minutes after we leave the house.

Ninety minutes later...

It's noon. "We have to get to the airport in a few hours," I say to SEAL. "Sara will kill us if we are late."

Two minutes later he has me on the treadmill walking twenty minutes on a fifteen-degree incline at 3.6 pace.

"We'll get there," SEAL says.

Next it's three pull-ups every forty-five seconds for the next ten minutes.

"We gotta go."

"Relax."

We do ten push-ups on the thirty-second mark for another ten minutes.

Right before the last set SEAL says, "We clocked out. Let's go."

> **Workout totals: 10.6 miles, 20 minutes on treadmill on incline of 15, 100 push-ups, 30 pull-ups**

The Skinheads

I don't like assholes and I don't like bullies.
—SEAL

The weather in Atlanta is fantastic. The hot Georgia sun is pumping out punishing heat rays. I'm sitting alone at the pool in my backyard reading the paper when our cleaning lady approaches. She's flustered. Her English is good, but sometimes the words are hard for her to find.

"You come, Mr. Jesse," she says. "I concern. Two guys in front yard ask for owner. Something no right, Mr. Jesse."

So I throw on a shirt and go out front.

Sure enough, there are two guys, approximately twenty years old, in white T-shirts and jeans, and they're climbing over our small hedges and approaching the front door. Both are heavily tatted up. Both have shaved heads. Both reek of marijuana.

She's correct, "Something no right."

It's mostly a mix of doctors, lawyers, and young professionals who live in our Atlanta community. People go out for jogs in the neighborhood or ride expensive mountain bikes around the cul-de-sac. And everybody smiles.

From the street you can see our house quite clearly. Nothing spectacular. It has a well-groomed yard, better-than-average-size driveway, and a decent-size house. While we do have some surveillance cameras around the exterior, you'd have to look closely to notice them.

"Can I help you guys?" I say in my most laid-back voice.

"Sure can," says Skinhead Number One. "Can you tell me who the owner of this house is?"

"Well, what exactly do you guys need?"

"We just moved into the neighborhood, son," he says.

The guy calls me "son" and I'm at least twenty years older than him.

"We want to meet a thousand neighbors. Each and every one of 'em. If we do, we get points for college."

Number One smiles and shows me some bullshit pad on a clipboard.

"We already met Usher today. You know where Usher lives, dude? Well, we seen 'em."

I know Usher doesn't live anywhere near me. I really think these guys are casing out my house.

HOLY SHIT!

"Sorry, guys. I don't live here. I'm only a guest," I lie.

"Well then, can you get your daddy or the queen bee? We need to meet the actual owner," Number Two says.

He looks like a number two.

Did this guy really just tell me to get my daddy?

"You want me to get my dad?"

"Yeah! Or go get the queen bee." Number One laughs. "Just get someone in the house that lives here."

"No problem," I say. "Hang tight."

I walk into the kitchen. SEAL is making one of his military-grade shakes.

"We have a situation," I say, looking out through the window that faces the front lawn.

SEAL follows my stare. A smile spreads across his face

as he looks through the window. The skinheads start to leave as if they sense something isn't right. SEAL calmly finishes drinking his shake.

"Showtime," he says.

Twenty minutes later SEAL is back walking through the front door. He has his iPhone in his hand. He shows me a close-up photo of Number Two. His face is as red as his neck and his cheeks are puffed up like a blowfish. His eyes are stretched with fear.

"This him?" SEAL asks.

In the photo you can see SEAL's hand wrapped around the guy's neck. It reminds me of when Darth Vader picks the guy up by his neck in *Star Wars*.

"Yes! That's him."

SEAL puts the phone in his pocket and walks over to the sink. He takes the glass from which he was drinking the shake and washes it.

"Well?"

"I explained to them I was the homeowner and that I don't care for motherfuckers like them on my property and that if they ever came back, I would make sure they never walked again."

SEAL puts the glass back in the cupboard. "I really don't think they'll be back."

Resolutions

I don't want what you guys have.
—SEAL

It's the last day of the year. Most people make resolutions on New Year's Eve, and I finished mine on the plane back to Connecticut this a.m.

Sara and I are having a bunch of our friends up to the house for dinner. We'll go around the table and everybody will say their goals for the coming year before dessert. I pretty much have what I'm going to say in my head. It's more like bullet points in my head. I'm a big fan of winging it (obviously).

The whole "Wonderful Wednesday" clan is coming. A few years ago, we made it an annual thing that we would get together for New Year's up at the Connecticut house. Sara calls us the SuperFriends because we also like to run marathons and other races together. There's a lot of truth to the "super" part. I've met, worked, and hung around a lot of people over my years. But the friends I have now are friends for life. These are the guys and girls I want to be in a foxhole with.

The day and night goes like this: We all go for a nine-mile run up Wanzer Hill and then have dinner, wine, whatever, and everyone sleeps over.

During dinner the conversation shifts to the resolutions. I'm curious about what SEAL will say if he takes a turn. In fact, I think everybody here is wondering what SEAL will say, if anything. One friend wants to quit her job and start her own business. Another has decided he wants to move to California's Wine Country. When it's SEAL's turn the whole table quiets.

"I don't want the same shit you guys want. I'm not looking for anything else. I'm going to do the same shit I've been doing," he says, "only I'm going to do it better."

SEAL excuses himself and stands. He then goes downstairs to ride the stationary bike in the basement. When he returns later my friends start to ask him questions. They're drawn to him. A big circle has formed around SEAL in the living room. He is still sweating from the ride, but he has placed a towel on his lap to catch any dripping sweat that could potentially end up on our carpet. The alcohol has loosened everyone up a bit. He looks at us all. His armor has come down. It's as though he's sorry for coming on so strong at the dinner table.

"I just think you don't give your lives enough credit," he says softly.

DAY 30

Last Run

If you can see yourself doing something, you can do
it. If you can't see yourself doing something, usually
you can't achieve it.
—SEAL

New York City
40°
1230

It's after lunchtime and we just drove back to New York City.
SEAL gave me the morning off. I'm in the kitchen cleaning
up. Sara and SEAL are in the living room. Then I see my
wife in the doorway.

"How'd it go with asking SEAL to stay and train you?" I ask.

"He can only stay one more day," Sara says. "He's leaving
tomorrow."

My wife can be a very convincing woman. I'm surprised.

"Did he say why?"

"Business."

"Business?"

Sara shrugs.

"That's it?"

"That's it."

I'm both disappointed he's not staying and bursting with curiosity. I know better than to ask him though. Anyhow, I like the image I conjure of SEAL pulling off a midnight hostage rescue in Syria or something.

"Oh, he did say he'd come back to train me," Sara says.

"Really?"

"Yes, provided I do everything he says and *nothing* is off limits."

Just that moment, SEAL walks into the kitchen. He's wearing the biggest smile I've ever seen him wear.

"What's for dinner tonight?" Seal asks. "A big red chicken?" He cackles like it's the funniest thing anyone has ever said. We head out to Central Park for the 6.1-mile loop. It will be our last run.

My first run with SEAL in New York was thirty days ago. We ran the exact same loop. We did it in 56:04 (a 9:20-mile pace). After one month with SEAL training me, I'm running a 7:50 pace per mile.

As usual, we don't talk on the run, even though it was to be our last. There was no final test, no congratulatory conversation, nothing. Like two running partners who run every day. There wasn't anything unusual about the evening either. We had dinner together in the apartment. SEAL played with Lazer. Sara chatted with him. Although she tried not to show it, I could tell she was genuinely sad our time with SEAL was coming to a close. So was I.

Today's splits:

Mile 1: 8:02
Mile 2: 7:56
Mile 3: 7:26
Mile 4: 7:45
Mile 5: 7:43
Mile 6: 7:32
Total: 46:34 (average of 7:45)

Pre-SEAL I sometimes would be on the couch and not want to do whatever needed to be done and I'd be like "Fuck it," and blow it off. Procrastinate.

I don't think like that anymore. Just get off the couch and do it is what I remind myself. SEAL would never say, "Fuck it." He'd get off the couch and do it. Regardless of the time, the temperature, or how tired he was. I absorbed some of that just-get-it-done and there-are-no-excuses attitude. I'm grateful for that.

My perspective on time has changed too. I got so much more done when SEAL was here. I was much more efficient. Now if I have to drive a few hours in the car to get somewhere, I do not get frustrated. Rather, I think about how lucky I am to be sitting in a warm and comfortable environment. It's weird, maybe I became more present or maybe I'm more appreciative, but whatever it is, I view time differently. Maybe it is a newfound patience or maturity.

My will to not stop or quit has also changed...both in training and at work.

SEAL has an I-don't-give-a-shit attitude that really

makes him different. He's an African-American Navy SEAL, of which there aren't many, an African-American who competes in endurance sports that are dominated by Caucasians. He doesn't give a shit. SEAL does what SEAL wants to do. He doesn't live the way everyone tells him he's supposed to live. And he does it with purpose. I admire him for that. His normal has been abnormal. We have that in common.

The first day SEAL came to move in, he told me I needed to control my mind. I thought it was just a saying or a throwaway comment, but I think there might be more truth to it than I originally thought. Our minds sometimes tell us little lies about ourselves, and we believe them. We think we can't do this or that. It's not true.

I've never had a real résumé. I've always believed in a life résumé. I take a look at SEAL, who's writing in his logbook. He just wants to get better tomorrow. That's what I want now too.

Workout totals: 6 miles

DAY 31

A Sad Day

The only easy day was yesterday.
—SEAL

New York City
31°
0800

I wake up on my own at 8:00 a.m. and the house feels different; the energy has changed.

I go to SEAL's room, but there's no SEAL. He's gone. The room is spotless, and the bed is perfectly made with military corners. You could bounce a quarter off it. Everything is *exactly* the way it was before he arrived. It's like he was never even here. Eerie.

When I walk into the kitchen, I see a note.

It's from SEAL.

No big sendoff. No big good-bye. No big anything. Just three words:

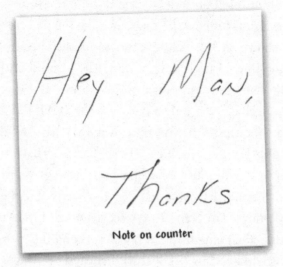

Note on counter

That's it. That's all he wrote. The guy woke me up at 5:00 a.m. for thirty days but didn't wake me up to say good-bye.

It starts to sink in that it's over. SEAL has returned to base.

Though SEAL left no trace in the bedroom, his finger-prints are all over the rest of the house. For example, every bedroom now has a fire extinguisher and a flashlight. Lazer, Sara, and I have full fire suits, in case we wake up one night and, God forbid, the place is an inferno. *And*, if the shit really hits the fan, behind our bar is an inflatable knapsack that turns into a life raft with oars and an attachable motor. It's there just in case some 9/11 shit happens. If anybody asks about it, I say what SEAL said to us: "It's our escape vehicle out of Manhattan, bitch." I also made a recent purchase at an outdoor furniture store in Atlanta, just in case I have to "camp out" on somebody.

SEAL also left an indelible mark on me. I've never been stronger, faster, or mentally tougher (take me to a frozen lake and I'll show you!). I can do a thousand push-ups in a day. I smoke the times I used to do around the Central Park Loop. I literally don't have an ounce of fat on me. But getting me in supreme shape was only a part of what SEAL did for me.

I have houses, a driver, fly privately. I have all of these things. SEAL has a military ID and cash. That's what he walks around with, just a backpack of belongings. He didn't want my life and I wanted his life. For starters, I'm going to simplify things. I'm going to try to get down to thirty items of clothing. I'm going through my closets and the extra shit in the garage and getting rid of stuff. I started deleting all of my emails, and it felt great. I started not answering people right away, and it felt fantastic.

SEAL clearly didn't want any part of our lives. I really admired how easy he lived his life. He didn't have to listen to others or have a team of people weigh in when making decisions. Part of that comes with the territory, and I get it. The simplicity that SEAL has is one of the most important things in life. He gets to do what he loves every day. He lives stress-free.

When SEAL broke both feet in the ultra-marathon with the twenty-thousand-foot climb, it wasn't the first time. He breaks his feet often when he runs grueling ultras. He has a hole in his aorta that surgeons can't seem to close. He's asthmatic.

And, he truly *hates to run*.

But he runs because he raises a lot of money for charity when he does to help the families of SEALs who died on the battlefield. One of the most emotional speeches I ever heard was Jimmy Valvano's at the ESPY Awards. Dying of cancer, with only months to live, he told the audience these important words. "Don't give up," he said. "Don't ever give up."

I hired SEAL because I wanted to get in the best shape of my life. I also hired him because I like the unexpected, and what better way to take a risk than having a Navy SEAL live with me for a month to train me? Finally, I hired him to get out of my routine, to shock the system, to mix things up so I could approach opportunities and challenges differently.

But I got much more than what I paid for.

"It's about protecting what you have," he said to me about being a SEAL. He might have been talking about defending democracy or freedom or saving us from terrorism. But I think he was talking about protecting something closer to home.

Now that SEAL is gone, I realize I don't need a lot of the crazy stuff in my life. These challenges I keep putting in front of myself to fulfill me. I'm not going to do any more of that. I'm staying put and focusing on the little things. I don't need manufactured adventures in my life to change me.

But maybe the most important thing I learned from SEAL was the level of appreciation he has for difficulty. The harder the training, the more courage it took to do and the more satisfaction was derived from it. SEAL taught me that you only get one shot at life and you should find out what's in your reserve tank. Coasting is for "pussies" as SEAL would say and it's when you dig deep that you feel the most alive. He lives his life that way. And some of that rubbed off on me.

EPILOGUE

A couple of months after SEAL moved out, Sara and I took a short vacation to the Bahamas. I invited SEAL to come down for a few days of R&R. It was going to be a quick trip, but I wanted to see if he was interested in joining us.

"Roger that," he said.

He brought *no luggage*, only his own bike and a stationary bike setup.

"I'm going to get a couple of hundred miles in," he said.

"On the island?"

"Nah, in my room."

We were there for three days, he put the PRIVACY sign on his doorknob, and he never left his room. The most beautiful setting in the world: girls, gambling, ocean the color of a Dodgers hat. He never went out. He just pushed his bed up against the wall so he could face the ocean and ride: Ocean Club, the Atlantis, twenty-seventh floor was SEAL's workout center. He said he was training for a bike ride across America.

One year later...

I'm in my office with Kish. The phone rings and she picks it up. She's smiling.

"It's for you," she says with her hand over the receiver.

"Who is it?" I whisper.

"SEAL," she whispers back.

"Hey, man. How are you?"

"Good," SEAL says.

"What's going on?"

"Just giving you a heads-up I'm in New York for some meetings today," he says.

"Cool," I say. "You wanna crash with us?"

"Nah, man, I don't want to impose on ya. Just wanted you to know I'm in town."

"Well, where are you going to stay?"

"I'm just going to sleep in Central Park," he says.

I look out the window of my office. It's snowing and my computer says fourteen degrees.

"Roger that," I say. "I'm thinking it's going to be seventy and sunny."

FIVE YEARS LATER

I think about what I need to be thinking about.
—SEAL

It's been five years since my SEAL experience. And a lot has changed since then—mostly the size of our family. Sara and I now have three more children and we're living in Atlanta full time. While my three new additions don't know SEAL (yet), Lazer still talks about him in the same light as a superhero. The other day our car wouldn't start, and Lazer, now six, came up with an instant solution:

"Dad, call SEAL! He can pick up the car with his bare hands and move it into the garage for us."

Roger that!

Sadly, SEAL didn't come flying down from the air to fix the car, AAA did. And in Lazer's eyes, that wasn't quite as cool. When SEAL left, it created a void in our family unit; for me especially. It was like I had a fitness hangover. I completely shut down. I didn't exercise for six weeks. As motivated as I was when he was there, it faded quickly when he left. It might be more appropriate to say it evaporated. It took months for me to get back on the program but after a while, a remarkable thing happened. I started to hear SEAL's voice in my ear. It was loud and clear like Obi-Wan Kenobi.

My Jedi Master was talking to me in my thoughts. I started consistently asking myself, "What Would SEAL Do?" or "#WWSD?" in each situation. I'd hear his voice on long runs ("Nah bro, you can't run without legs"), whispers in my office ("Burpee Test") and pretty much an echo all throughout the day ("Control your *mind*, Jesse"). I could picture his stone-faced expression in my thoughts. He saw me when I was sleeping; he knew when I was awake. He knew if I'd been bad or good so...you know how the rest of the song goes. It was some straight-up Santa Claus stalking.

Although he wasn't in my house, his presence was still there. And many of the life lessons SEAL taught me became part of my DNA. They were innate. I understood on a deeper level how SEAL trained my mind as much as my body. With his challenges of jumping in a frozen lake, the steam room episode, and all of the madness in between, what we were really doing was just exercising my most important muscle— my brain. Specifically, my mental toughness muscle. I learned that by constantly doing things that are hard and making myself uncomfortable, I improve my ability to handle obstacles. I get comfortable being uncomfortable—and that's real mental toughness.

The persistence and perseverance to achieve a long-term goal is a key driver to success. I've always had that blueprint, but SEAL helped me redefine success—Never Quit. And by constantly putting myself in situations that are challenging, I've created an environment in my head that makes me want to keep going even when things get ridiculously hard. In these situations, I have trained myself not to quit, but to attack. Thanks, SEAL.

One of the best things about having SEAL as your "Spirit Animal" is that you can take him everywhere you go, like the time he was in the Hudson River with me. It was a few years after he left. I was doing a thirty-mile, stand-up paddleboard race around Manhattan. The race started at Chelsea Piers, headed up past Columbia University, then crossed over to the East River before it ended down by Brooklyn. The currents were incredibly unpredictable and brutally challenging. The Hudson is a VERY difficult place to paddle. At times you could paddle as hard as humanly possible and not move ten yards. And then, when you stopped to rest, you'd get pushed forty feet in the opposite direction. It was both exhausting and demoralizing.

When I showed up at the race check-in, I knew I was in trouble. The competitors all looked like they were half Jeff Spicoli and half Thor. They acted as if paddleboarding was their full-time job. And...they'd been promoted every year! They had hydration systems attached to their deck pads. GUs and PowerBars were duct-taped to their boards and intricate navigation devices were installed on their aerodynamic stand-ups. Me? I had nothing except for the paddleboard I'd purchased online a week before the race. When I got to the starting area, I immediately noticed my board was way shorter than all the other boards, way heavier and *definitely* not aerodynamic. *Shit...* I should have brought my escape vehicle.

I wasn't sure if I'd get windburn or sunburn, because I was headed thirty miles directly into the wind. And it was hot—like 101 degrees hot. The currents were super strong and not in my favor. My board was built for a five-foot-ten male cruising around a recreational lake, or maybe a Budweiser commercial, but not for this type of distance and environment. I was fucked. I had to think. So, to make my board lighter, I decided to put all of my supplies (water, food, sunscreen, AND life jacket) on a canoe that my friends Mike and Rob Young rented. I'd be better off having them haul it than carrying it myself in a knapsack for ten hours.

"Just stay close to me," I told them. "You'll be my crew team."

As soon as the race started, one hundred paddlers took off and spread across the Hudson in a frenzy. About a hundred strokes into the rough water, I turned around and the Young brothers, my "crew" team, were nowhere to be seen. I looked...and looked...and looked...and they were NOWHERE. I finally spotted them back on shore. What were they doing? As it turned out, "the canoe wasn't suitable for the rough seas." Their words—not mine.

It was then that I realized I had to channel my inner SEAL. I had to gut out twenty miles alone on the Hudson with no water, food, or sunscreen. I created a SEAL mantra in my head...*Come on, motherfucker, come on*...I put it on loop.

And then there was a brief moment of shade at mile 20. I was under a bridge—I don't know, maybe it was the Throggs Neck. It sure looked as long as the Throggs Neck. As my board's tip entered into the sunlight again, I heard someone calling, "Itzler...Itzler!"

I looked up and there, way above me on the bridge, stood the Young Brothers.

"Dude, we got food for you," Young Brother Number One said.

He tossed a tuna sandwich and a bottle of ZICO in a plastic bag over the bridge. PLOP...I paddled over to and devoured the sandwich in three bites.

Come on, motherfucker, come on...

I don't know if I would have finished that race without my SEAL experience. He's gotten me through a lot. More challenging situations would continue to present themselves in my life—socially, at work, and personally. And each time I would think, "What would SEAL do?"

One day in 2012, I was putting some thoughts together to write a book. I wasn't sure what it was yet, so I started a folder. Over time, it got bigger and bigger. I had twenty or thirty different chapter ideas, but one kept calling to me. Every time I sat down to work I'd look at the SEAL chapter of my life. I'd relive those thirty-one days and beyond. Then it clicked. SEAL wasn't a chapter; SEAL was the book. I started to write. I used the blog that I started in 2010 to fact-check. Sara and I would compare notes at the breakfast table, laughing and reminiscing. I kept writing and, ironically, my workouts improved also.

And as I think about it, the book was a journey in itself. The reason I wrote it was because I wanted to share my experience with a wide audience in the hope that it'd bring some motivation (and humor)! I signed with an agent, Lisa Leshne; we crafted a proposal from my writing and shopped it for a book deal. Lisa brought me to Kate Hartson at Center Street, an imprint of Hachette Book Group, and the rest (as they say) is history. The process of writing the book was a new and exciting one for me, and I learned a ton along the way. But after the book was done, the cover was designed, and the marketing plan was in place, I realized I still hadn't shown it to SEAL. Whoops! So, I called my publisher and said we might have a slight delay. I needed to clear all of this with SEAL before we moved forward.

So, I texted SEAL...No response.

I emailed SEAL...No response.

I left voice mails...No response.

What the heck? Where the fuck was SEAL?

A few weeks later, my phone rang. It was him.

He gave me the feeling he was standing next to an angry hornet's nest and in a rush. So, of course, I jumped right into it.

"I wrote a book about our journey."

"What journey?"

"Our time together. When you lived with me."

"That wasn't a journey; I just lived with you."

I knew better than to debate. "I want your approval before I put it out."

"Put what out?"

"The book. The journey. Well, my journey."

Silence...

More silence...

"Man, well then just send me the fucking book."

My next stop was FedEx. As I popped the book in the envelope, I wondered what he'd think of it. Would he let me do it? How would I explain it to the publisher if he didn't sign off on it?

Weeks passed. Finally SEAL called.

"Hello."

His "hello" back could have scared an entire gang of Hells Angels. I almost pretended I was an answering machine so he could leave his message at the beep. I was afraid to speak.

"Um..."

"Yo, man, I read that shit. That BOOK."

"What'd you think?"

"Man, you made me sound dark. *Real* dark. You made me sound *angry*. Like an enraged angry. You made me sound like a fucking madman. Like someone who has thirty-nine marbles in his deck."

He paused for a bit and then said, "Man, you nailed it, motherfucker!"

SEAL: Revealed

In 2005, after being deployed to Iraq, SEAL was sent stateside for free-fall parachute training. During that time, he learned that a Chinook helicopter carrying several SEALs with whom he went through BUD/S training took on enemy fire in Kunar Province. Everyone on board was killed. These heroes were on their way to rescue four SEALs on a mission called "Operation Red Wings."

Soon after SEAL heard the news, he decided to raise money and consciousness for the families of the fallen soldiers. Rather than have a bake sale or host a golf outing, SEAL googled the ten most difficult athletic feats in the world. His plan was to compete in the world's toughest races for his cause. The organization SEAL chose to raise money for is the Special Operations Warrior Foundation, which gives college scholarships and grants to the children of fallen special operations soldiers.

SEAL's first race was the Badwater 135—the 135-mile race in Death Valley that I mentioned earlier in the book. When he called the race director to register, the race director insisted SEAL first run one hundred miles in twenty-four hours or less to qualify.

Four days later, SEAL was at the starting line of a twenty-four-hour race in San Diego. He had never run more than twenty miles in his life, but this was the only sanctioned race he could do in time to qualify for Badwater.

During the race, SEAL (who weighed over 250 pounds at the time) broke several metatarsals in both feet and suffered kidney failure due to his size and lack of nutrition. By mile 70, he was urinating blood and could barely walk. What did SEAL do? He got up off his chair and ran another thirty miles. He completed 101 miles in nineteen hours on his broken bones while experiencing kidney failure. He refused all medical attention after the race.

Three weeks later, with his feet not yet healed, he ran the Las Vegas Marathon in three hours and eight minutes, qualifying him for the Boston Marathon. Just weeks later, SEAL completed the HURT 100, one of the hardest hundred-mile trail races in the world. It was then that the Badwater race director granted him entry. Six months later, SEAL placed fifth in the toughest foot race in the world—Badwater 135 in Death Valley.

Four months after Badwater, SEAL completed the Ultraman World Championships in Hawaii. Whereas an IronMan is a 2.4-mile swim, 112-mile bike, and 26.2-mile run, the Ultraman is a 6.2-mile ocean swim, 261-mile bike ride, and a 52.4-mile run. WHAT? That is over a double IronMan! SEAL, who had not ridden a bike since childhood, flew to Hawaii for the race and rented a bike when he landed. Since the bike rental store on the island didn't offer a bike with clips for the clip-in bike shoes racers wear, SEAL rented a bike with cages for his shoes. He finished the race in second place.

Over the following years, SEAL competed in about fifty ultra-endurance races, and has had top five finishes in at least twenty of them. In 2007, he returned to Badwater and placed third. He started the IronMan in Kona by parachuting into the water. He's been on the covers of and profiled in *Runner's World* and *Outside Magazine*, the Navy has used him in recruiting commercials, and he made an appearance on NBC's *Today* where he tried to best the Guinness twenty-four-hour pull-up record of 4,021. He did 2,588 of them before tearing a muscle in his forearm. Four months later, in January 2013, SEAL set the Guinness World Record with 4,030 pull-ups completed in 17 hours. SEAL is widely considered to be "the toughest athlete on the planet."

His name is David Goggins.

Day	Miles Run	Push-Ups	Pull-Ups	Sit-Ups	Burpees	Jumping Jacks	Box Jumps	Flutter Kicks	Fireman Carries
1	6	0	100	0	0	0	0	0	0
2	12	0	0	0	0	0	0	0	0
Totals (Days 1 - 2)	18	0	100	0	0	0	0	0	0
3	14.3	0	0	0	0	0	0	0	0
Totals (Days 1 - 3)	32.3	0	100	0	0	0	0	0	0
4	6	100	36	0	0	0	50	0	0
Totals (Days 1 - 4)	38.3	100	136	0	0	0	50	0	0
5	0	150	0	0	0	0	0	0	0
Totals (Days 1 - 5)	38.3	250	136	0	0	0	50	0	0
6	12	300	0	0	100	0	0	0	0
Totals (Days 1 - 6)	50.3	550	136	0	100	0	50	0	0
7	17	275	0	0	0	0	0	0	0
Totals (Days 1 - 7)	67.3	825	136	0	100	0	50	0	0
8	6	0	0	0	0	0	0	0	0
Totals (Days 1 - 8)	73.3	825	136	0	100	0	50	0	0
9	6	0	10	100	0	0	0	0	0
Totals (Days 1 - 9)	79.3	825	146	100	100	0	50	0	0
10	2	171	30	0	0	0	0	0	0
Totals (Days 1 - 10)	81.3	996	176	100	100	0	50	0	0
11 - 12	8	484	0	132	0	0	0	0	0
Totals (Days 1 - 12)	89.3	1480	176	232	100	0	50	0	0
13	8	200	0	0	0	800	0	0	0
Totals (Days 1 - 13)	97.3	1680	176	232	100	800	50	0	0
14	6	0	0	0	100	0	0	0	14
Totals (Days 1 - 14)	103.3	1680	176	232	200	800	50	0	14
15	8	350	0	0	0	0	0	0	0
Totals (Days 1 - 15)	111.3	2030	176	232	200	800	50	0	14

(continued)

Day	Miles Run	Push-Ups	Pull-Ups	Sit-Ups	Burpees	Jumping Jacks	Box Jumps	Flutter Kicks	Fireman Carries
16	17	0	0	0	0	0	0	0	0
Totals (Days 1 - 16)	128.3	2030	176	232	200	800	50	0	14
17	3	465	0	50	0	0	0	50	0
Totals (Days 1 - 17)	131.3	2495	176	282	200	800	50	50	14
18	0	364	30	0	0	0	0	100	0
Totals (Days 1 - 18)	131.3	2859	206	282	200	800	50	150	14
19	6	200	0	0	0	0	0	0	0
Totals (Days 1 - 19)	137.3	3059	206	282	200	800	50	150	14
20	8	400	0	550	0	0	0	0	0
Totals (Days 1 - 20)	145.3	3459	206	832	200	800	50	150	14
21	10	0	0	0	0	0	0	0	0
Totals (Days 1 - 21)	155.3	3459	206	832	200	800	50	150	14
22 - 23	16.1	700	0	0	0	0	0	0	0
Totals (Days 1 - 23)	171.4	4159	206	832	200	800	50	150	14
24	3.5	154	0	0	0	0	0	0	0
Totals (Days 1 - 24)	174.9	4313	206	832	200	800	50	150	14
25	9.5	775	0	125	0	0	0	0	0
Totals (Days 1 - 25)	184.4	5088	206	957	200	800	50	150	14
26	9.5	0	0	0	0	0	0	0	0
Totals (Days 1 - 26)	193.9	5088	206	957	200	800	50	150	14
27	3.5	1000	0	0	0	0	0	0	0
Totals (Days 1 - 27)	197.4	6088	206	957	200	800	50	150	14
28	8.5	300	0	0	0	0	0	0	0
Totals (Days 1 - 28)	205.9	6388	206	957	200	800	50	150	14
29	10.6	100	30	0	0	0	0	0	0
Totals (Days 1 - 29)	216.5	6488	236	957	200	800	50	150	14
30	6	0	0	0	0	0	0	0	0
Totals (Days 1 - 30)	222.5	6488	236	957	200	800	50	150	14

Acknowledgments

I have always been a team sports guy. All great teams have outstanding teammates that are good at their positions. This book would not have been possible without the hard work of my core teammates: Jennifer Kish, my trusted right-hand woman who somehow manages to do the jobs of multiple people with grace and grit; Lisa Leshne, my tenacious literary agent who helped me shape the germ of an idea into a full-blown proposal and book deal and then promoted the hell out of it, and Turney Duff, my longtime friend and bestselling author who held my hand through the entire process. I'd also like to thank Rick Flynn, Marc Adelman, Adam Padilla, Bryan Black, Erica Jaffe, Marq Brown, Johnny "Photo," Joe Holder, Deana Levine, Stella Brown, Page Luther, and Chelsea Kardokus. I especially want to acknowledge the roles of my editor Kate Hartson, publisher Rolf Zettersten, Patsy Jones, Andrea Glickson, and the entire Center Street staff. Without them there is NO WAY this book would have come to fruition.

This book would obviously not have been possible without the support of my amazing wife, who let this outrageous stuff go on under her very own roof. Honey, I will NOT jump in a frozen lake again (fingers crossed).

Last, I wanted to thank SEAL for investing thirty-one days of his life to live with our family. The lessons I learned extend far beyond fitness. Thank you.

Great teammates believe in each other.

Roger that!

About the Author

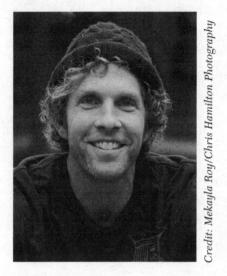

Credit: Mekayla Roy/Chris Hamilton Photography

JESSE ITZLER eats only fruit until noon, loves Run-D.M.C., and enjoys living life "out of the box." He cofounded Marquis Jet, the world's largest prepaid private jet card company, which he and his partner sold to Berkshire Hathaway/NetJets. Jesse then helped pioneer the coconut water craze with Zico coconut water, which was acquired by The Coca-Cola Company. He is a former rapper on MTV and he produced both the NBA's Emmy Award–winning "I Love This Game" music campaign and the popular New York Knicks anthem "Go NY Go." When he is not running ultra marathons or being a dad to his four kids, Jesse can be found at the NBA's

Atlanta Hawks games, where he is an owner of the team. He is married to Spanx founder Sara Blakely.

Find out more about Jesse Itzler:
Instagram: @the100mileman
Twitter: @the100mileman
www.the100mileman.com
The author is donating a portion of his proceeds to the Special Operations Warrior Foundation.

Stedman's

PLASTIC SURGERY/ ENT/DENTISTRY

WORDS

Stedman's

PLASTIC SURGERY/ ENT/DENTISTRY WORDS

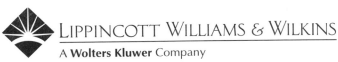

LIPPINCOTT WILLIAMS & WILKINS
A **Wolters Kluwer** Company
Philadelphia · Baltimore · New York · London
Buenos Aires · Hong Kong · Sydney · Tokyo

Series Editor: Maureen Barlow Pugh
Associate Managing Editor: Beverly J. Wolpert
Production Coordinator: Joan Scullin
Typesetter: Peirce Graphic Services, Inc.
Printer & Binder: Vicks Lithograph & Printing

Copyright © 1999 Lippincott Williams & Wilkins
351 West Camden Street
Baltimore, Maryland 21201–2436 USA

Printed in the United States of America

First Edition, 1993

Library of Congress Cataloging-in-Publication Data

Stedman's plastic surgery/ENT/dentistry words
     p.   cm. — (Stedman's word book series)
   Includes bibliographical references.
   ISBN 0-683-40460-1 (soft cover)
   1. Surgery, Plastic—Terminology. 2. Otolaryngology—Terminology.
3. Dentistry—Terminology.   I. Stedman, Thomas Lathrop, 1853–1938.
II. Series: Stedman's word books.
   [DNLM: 1. Surgery, Plastic terminology. 2. Otolaryngology terminology.
3. Dentistry terminology.   WO 15S8119-1999]
RD118.S745   1999
617.9'5'014—dc21
DNLM/DLC
for Library of Congress

                             98-33791
                                CIP
                             99-00
                    3 4 5 6 7 8 9 10

Contents

Acknowledgments

An important part of our editorial process is the involvement of medical transcriptionists—as advisors, reviewers and/or editors—and other members of the medical and scientific community.

We extend special thanks to Braden C. Stridde, MD, of Puget Sound Plastic Surgery, PS, in Federal Way, WA. A Diplomate of the the American Board of Plastic Surgery and the National Board of Medical Examiners, Dr. Stridde provided valuable assistance with the plastic surgery content of this book and its appendices.

Special thanks are also due Robert A. DeFilipps, Ph.D., of the Department of Botany at the Smithsonian Institution's National Museum of Natural History in Washington, DC. Dr. DeFilipps reviewed and verified the names of herbs in the appendix, enabling us to include the first authoritative listing of this kind in our reference series.

Immeasurable thanks to Ellen Atwood, who edited the new terms added to *Stedman's Plastic Surgery/ENT/Dentistry Words,* contributed much of the material for the appendices, and helped resolve many difficult content questions; to Anna Parr, CMT, who edited the manuscript at various stages; to Martha Richards, RRA, for reviewing and proofreading *Stedman's ENT Words* and *Stedman's Dentistry Words* (and for doing the necessary research involved with that large task); and to Helen Littrell, who also edited the manuscript and format.

Thanks to our *Stedman's Plastic Surgery/ENT/Dentistry Words* MT Editorial Advisory Board, including Alba DiGiovanni, CMT; Diana Rezac, CMT; Teresa Naleway; and Suzanne Taubert, CMT. These medical transcriptionists served as important contributors, editors, and advisors.

Other important contributors to this edition include Rose Berry; Jeanne Bock; Gail M. Hall; Alice Lazenby, CMT, ART, CVR; Pamela Maykulsky; Anna Sargent; Karen Thomas, CMT; Jenifer Walker; Tina Whitecotton; and Sandra Wideburg, CMT.

Barb Ferretti played an integral role in the process by reviewing the content files for format, updating the database, and providing a final quality check.

Acknowledgments

As with all our *Stedman's* word references, this resource incorporates the suggestions and expertise of our many contacts in the medical transcriptionist community. Thanks to all of our advisory board participants, reviewers, and editors; AAMT meeting attendees; and others who have written us with requests and comments—keep talking, and we'll keep listening.

Editor's Preface

Much is written and said about the explosion of technological and biochemical advances in medicine over the past decade, and rightly so. Miracles of lifelike restoration of appearance and function utilizing biomaterials that mimic or integrate with living tissues are becoming commonplace in plastic, reconstructive, ear, dental, and head and neck procedures and practices. Tissues destroyed or malformed through genetics, trauma, or infection can be made whole, functional, normal, and even attractive as never before. All of the major organs of sensation and communication, perception, and appearance involve the structures of the head and neck, and thus many of these new procedures are carried out by ENT, head, neck, dental, and plastic surgeons. Body parts are so frequently transposed, at times literally from one end to another, in reconstructive techniques that the burgeoning field of aesthetic, plastic, and reconstructive surgery demands intimate knowledge of all body systems and structures, not just those above the shoulders.

With novel procedures, reconstructive techniques, and anatomical substitutions, as well as changes in attitude and availability of cosmesis, even the very young and not-so-rich-and-famous are undergoing elective plastic or appearance-improving surgery and procedures. Formerly rare procedures have become commonplace, and all are accompanied by an ever-expanding vocabulary of medical terms. International connectivity via instant communication brings with it terminology based on languages other than standard Latin/Greek combinations and derivations. Creative advertising and naming conventions among suppliers of equipment and prostheses have resulted in a bewildering variety of spelling, capitalization, abbreviations, acronyms, and eponyms.

Physicians, dentists and other healthcare practitioners can elect to pursue a subspecialty as a means of containing the information explosion. As medical language specialists, however, medical transcriptionists are challenged continually to incorporate highly specialized words of anatomy, physiology, procedures, equipment, drugs, and materials relevant to disparate body systems. Beyond simple knowledge of these terms, we need to be able to apply them in relevant areas with the same kind of precision a microsurgeon applies to repair the most delicate of body tissues.

The sheer numbers of new words indicate that accessible, easily used, accurate, and reliable reference materials are more important than ever to ensure accurate medical reports and records. A reference book such as this one involves interaction and cooperation on many levels, and most important, input and participation by practicing medical transcriptionists. We hope that this effort has resulted in a reference book that is both informational and instructional, reflecting the needs of medical language specialists throughout the country and across many specialities in medicine.

Working on this project through the various phases and with the editors and staff at Lippincott Williams & Wilkins has certainly given me a new appreciation and understanding of the complexity, utility, and beauty of medical language.

Ellen Atwood

Publisher's Preface

Stedman's Plastic Surgery/ENT/Dentistry Words offers an authoritative assurance of quality and exactness to the wordsmiths of the healthcare professions—medical transcriptionists, medical editors and copy editors, health information management personnel, court reporters, and the many other users and producers of medical documentation.

For years we have received requests for a plastic surgery word book. Recently, we have also received requests for updates to *Stedman's ENT Words and Stedman's Dentistry Words*. As the requests continued, we realized that medical language professionals needed a comprehensive, current reference for plastic surgery, ENT, and dentistry terminology.

Users will find thousands of words encompassing congenital anomalies to esthetic surgery, appearance as well as function, instruments, anatomy, and biomaterials, in addition to the newest procedures and implants. This collection includes transplant terminology, along with autologous and other grafting materials. It also contains terminology related to reconstructive surgery and gender reassignment, as well as postsurgical reconstructive, postaccident, and posttrauma treatment. You will find sample reports for each specialty in the appendix; however, we included more for plastic surgery based on the recommendations of the editors, who felt that more were needed for this particular specialty, which presents medical transcriptionists with less common procedures not covered and/or not readily accessible in other sources.

This compilation in excess of 69,000 entries, fully cross-indexed for quick access, was built from a base vocabulary of more than 40,000 medical words, phrases, abbreviations and acronyms. The extensive A-Z list was developed from the database of *Stedman's Medical Dictionary* and supplemented by terminology found in current medical literature (please see list of References on page xvi).

We at Lippincott Williams & Wilkins strive to provide you with the most up-to-date and accurate word references available. Your use of this word book will prompt new editions, which we will publish as often as updates and revisions justify. We welcome your suggestions for improvements, changes, corrections, and additions — whatever will make this *Stedman's* product more useful to you. Please complete the postpaid card at the back of this book, and send your recommendations care of "Stedman's" at Lippincott Williams & Wilkins.

Explanatory Notes

Medical transcription is an art as well as a science. Both are needed to correctly interpret the dictation of a physician, whose language is a product of education, training, and experience. This variety in medical language means that there are several acceptable ways to express certain terms, including jargon. *Stedman's Plastic Surgery/ENT/Dentistry Words* provides variant spellings and phrasings for many terms. These elements, in addition to complete cross-indexing, make *Stedman's Plastic Surgery/ENT/Dentistry Words* a valuable resource for determining the validity of terms as they are encountered.

Alphabetical Organization

Alphabetization of main entries is letter by letter as spelled, ignoring punctuation, spaces, prefixed numbers, Greek letters, or other characters. For example:

acid-fast staining methods

acid formaldehyde hematin

α-acid glycoprotein

acid hematin

In subentry alphabetization, the abbreviated singular form or the spelled-out plural form of the noun main entry word is ignored.

Format and Style

All main entries are in **boldface** to expedite locating a sought-after term, to enhance distinction between main entries and subentries, and to relieve the textual density of the pages.

Irregular plurals and variant spellings are shown on the same line as the singular or preferred form of the word. For example:

scolex, pl. **scoleces**

curette, curet

Hyphenation

As a rule of style, multiple eponyms (e.g., Mears-Rubash approach) are hyphenated. Also, hyphens have been added between a manufacturer and one or more eponyms (e.g., Vital-Metzenbaum dissecting scissors). Please note that hyphenation is a question of style, not of accuracy, and thus is a matter of choice.

Possessives

Possessive forms have been dropped in this reference for the sake of consistency and conformance with the guidelines of the American Association for Medical Transcription (AAMT) and other groups. Please note, however, that retaining the possessive is a question of style, not of accuracy, and thus is a matter of choice. To form the possessive of a word, simply add the apostrophe or apostrophe "s" to the end of the word.

Cross-indexing

The word list is in an index-like main entry-subentry format that contains two combined alphabetical listings:

(1) A *noun* main entry-subentry organization, which is typical of the A-Z section of medical dictionaries like **Stedman's:**

access
   lexical a.
   translabial a.

lake
   lacrimal l.
   venous l.

(2) An *adjective* main entry-subentry organization, which lists words and phrases as you hear them. The main entries are the adjectives or modifiers in a multi-word term. The subentries are the nouns around which the terms are constructed and to which the adjectives or modifiers pertain:

bronchial
   b. adenocarcinoma
   b. adenoma
   b. respiration

coronal
   c. oblique projection
   c. plane
   c. projection

This format provides the user with more than one way to locate and identify a multi-word term. For example:

tissue
   connective t.

connective
   c. tissue

knife
 Cottle k.
 sickle k.

Cottle
 C. columella clamp
 C. knife

It also allows the user to see together all terms that contain a particular descriptor, as well as all types, kinds, or variations of a noun entity. For example:

tone
 complex t.
 t. deafness
 difference t.
 T. in Noise (TIN)

noise
 n. analyzer
 pink n.
 n. pollution
 Tone in N. (TIN)

tuning
 cochlear t.
 t. curve
 T. Fork Test

test
 T. of Adolescent Language
 articulation t.
 Tuning Fork T.

Wherever possible, abbreviations are separately defined and cross-referenced. For example:

CFM
 chemotactic factor for macrophage
chemotactic
 c. factor for macrophage (CFM)

macrophage
 chemotactic factor for m. (CFM)

References

In addition to the manufacturers' literature we gather at various medical meetings, scientific reports from hospitals, and the lists of our MT Editorial Advisory Board members (from their daily transcription work), we used the following sources for new words for *Stedman's Plastic Surgery/ ENT/Dentistry*:

Books

Agur AMR, Lee MJ. Grant's atlas of anatomy, 9th ed. Williams & Wilkins, 1991.

Dorland's illustrated medical dictionary, 28th ed. Philadelphia: WB Saunders Company, 1994.

Georgiade GS, Riefkohl R, Levin LS, editors. Plastic, maxillofacial and reconstructive surgery, 3rd ed. Baltimore: Williams & Wilkins, 1998.

Lance LL. Quick look drug book. Baltimore: Williams & Wilkins, 1998.

Nicolosi L, Harryman E, Kresheck J. Terminology of communication disorders, 4th ed. Baltimore: Williams & Wilkins, 1996.

Pyle V. Current medical terminology, 5th ed. Modesto: Health Professions Institute, 1994.

Sloane SB. The medical word book, 3rd ed. Philadelphia: WB Saunders Company, 1991.

Stedman's medical dictionary, 26th ed. Baltimore: Williams & Wilkins, 1995.

Zwemer TJ. Mosby's dental dictionary. St. Louis: Mosby, 1998.

Journals

Aesthetic Plastic Surgery. New York: Springer-Verlag, 1996.

American Journal of Speech-Language Pathology. Rockville, MD: American Speech-Language-Hearing Association, 1998.

Annals of Otology, Rhinology & Laryngology. St. Louis: Annals Publishing, 1995.

Annals of Plastic Surgery. Philadelphia: Lippincott-Raven, 1995–1996.

Archives of Otolaryngology—Head & Neck Surgery, 1996–1997.

Dental Surgery Products. Torrance, CA: Novicom, Inc., 1997–1998.

Dental Therapeutic Digest, 4th ed. Eastlake, OH: Odontos Publishing, Inc., 1997.

Hearing Instruments. Baltimore: Williams & Wilkins, 1995.

Implant Dentistry. Baltimore: Williams & Wilkins, 1995.

Journal of Endodontics. Baltimore: Williams & Wilkins, 1995–1997.

Journal of Oral and Maxillofacial Surgery. Philadelphia: WB Saunders, 1995–1998.

Journal of Oral Implantology. Alexandria, VA: International and American Associations for Dental Research, 1995.

Journal of the American Association for Medical Transcription. Modesto: American Association for Medical Transcription, 1995–1998.

MT Monthly. Gladstone, MO: Computer Systems Management, 1994–1998.

Otolaryngology-Head & Neck Surgery. St. Louis: Mosby, 1997–1998.

Perspectives on the Medical Transcription Profession. Modesto: Health Professions Institute, 1993–1998.

Plastic and Reconstructive Surgery. Baltimore: Williams & Wilkins, 1996–1998.

Plastic Surgery Products. Torrance, CA: Novicom, Inc., 1995–1998.

Stedman's WordWatcher. Baltimore: Williams & Wilkins, 1995–1997.

The Latest Word. Philadelphia: WB Saunders Company, 1994–1998.

A
> ampere
> apex
> apices
>> A and D ointment
>> A fiber
>> A point
>> A point chart

Å
> angstrom
> Ångström unit

AAC
> augmentative and alternative
> communication

AACI
> arachidonic acid cascade inhibitor

AB
> axiobuccal

ABA
> Apraxia Battery for Adults

abacterial

abatement

Abbe
>> A. flap
>> A. operation

Abbe-Estlander
>> A.-E. flap
>> A.-E. operation

Abbot paste

abbreviated rapid processing (ARP)

ABC
> aneurysmal bone cyst
> avidin-biotin-peroxidase complex
> axiobuccocervical

abdomen
>> globular a.
>> patulous a.
>> pendulous a.

abdominal
>> a. adipose tissue
>> a. apron
>> a. axial subcutaneous pedicle flap
>> a. binder
>> a. dermolipectomy
>> a. domain
>> a. flaccidity
>> a. pannus
>> a. sequela
>> a. wall insufficiency
>> a. washout
>> a. zipper

abdominal-diaphragmatic respiration

abdominoperineal resection

abdominoplasty
>> Callia a.

>> endoscopically assisted a.
>> French-line a.
>> Grazer a.
>> high-lateral-tension a.
>> male a.
>> Mladick a.
>> modified a.
>> muscle-access a.
>> partial subfascial a.
>> Pitanguy a.
>> a. procedure
>> Regnault a.

Abdopatch
>> A. Gel Z adhesive dressing
>> A. Gel Z self-adhesive scar
>> treatment

ABD pad

abduce

abducent
>> a. nerve

abduct

abduction
>> Gilbert stage shoulder a.

abductor
>> a. hallucis muscle
>> a. paralysis
>> a. pollicis longus muscle

Abelcet Injection

aberrant
>> a. breast tissue
>> a. cementosis
>> a. cementum
>> a. mongolian spot

ABG
> axiobuccogingival

ABI
> auditory brainstem implant

ability
>> central auditory a.'s
>> Flowers-Costello Test of Central
>> Auditory A.'s
>> Illinois Test of
>> Psycholinguistic A.'s (ITPA)
>> McCarthy Scales of Children's A.'s
>> Porch Index of
>> Communicative A.'s (PICA)
>> pretraining a.
>> a. test

ab initio

ABL
> axiobuccolingual

ABL520 blood gas measurement system

ablate

ablated skin

ablation
    procerus and corrugator a.
    tissue a.
    tumor a.
ablation-ligament (AL)
ablative procedure
ABLB
    alternate binaural loudness balance
ablution
abnormal
    a. airway resistance syndrome
    a. frenulum attachment
    ,a. frenum attachment
    a. occlusal relationship
    a. occlusal wear
    a. occlusion
    a. tooth mobility
abnormality
    clotting a.
    cutaneous vascular a.
    maxillofacial a.
    tympanomastoid a.
Abocath catheter
abocclusion
aboiement
aboral
abortus-equi
    Salmonella a.-e.
Aboulker stent
above-knee amputation (AKA)
ABR
    anterior band remover
    audiometric brainstem response
    auditory brainstem response
    ABR audiometry
abradant
abrade
abrasio dentium
abrasion
    acid a.
    betel nut a.
    bobby pin a.
    cervical a.
    corneal a.
    dentifrice a.
    denture a.
    gingival a.
    occupational a.
    a. resistance
    tobacco a.
    tooth a.
abrasive
    aluminum oxide a.
    diatomaceous silicon dioxide a.
    a. disk
    FF a.
    FFF a.
    flint a.
    garnet a.
    iron oxide a.
    a. point
    polishing a.
    quartz a.
    recrystallized kaolinite a.
    silicon carbide a.
    silicon dioxide a.
    sodium-potassium aluminum silicate a.
    a. strip
    zirconium silicate a.
abrasiveness
abrasor
abrupt topic shift
abscess
    acute apical a.
    acute periapical a.
    alveolar a.
    apical a.
    apical periodontal a.
    Bezold a.
    bicameral a.
    brain a.
    buccal space a.
    cerebellar a.
    chronic apical a.
    chronic periapical a.
    cold a.
    dental a.
    dental root a.
    dentoalveolar a.
    epidural a.
    extradural a.
    gingival a.
    inferior pole peritonsillar a.
    infraorbital space a.
    interradicular a.
    intramastoid a.
    laryngeal a.
    lateral a.
    lateral alveolar a.
    lateral periodontal a.
    lung a.
    masseter a.
    mastoid a.
    nasal septal a.
    nasopharyngeal a.
    orbital a.
    otic a.
    palatal a.
    parapharyngeal space a.
    parietal a.
    parotid gland a.
    periapical a.
    pericemental a.
    pericoronal a.
    periodontal a.

periodontal infrabony a.
periprosthetic breast a.
perisinus a.
peritonsillar a. (PTA)
phoenix a.
point of a.
prevertebral space a.
pterygomandibular space a.
pulp a.
pulpal a.
radicular a.
recrudescent a.
retrobulbar a.
retropharyngeal a.
root a.
stellate a.
subacute periapical a.
subdural a.
sublingual space a.
submandibular space a.
submasseteric space a.
submental space a.
subperiosteal a.
subperiosteal orbital a. (SPOA)
temporal fossa a.
temporal lobe a.
Tornwaldt a.
vestibular a.

absent
a. epiglottis
a. tooth

absolute
a. construction
a. pocket
a. quantity
a. threshold

absorbable
a. gelatin
a. gelatin sponge
a. suture

absorbefacient
absorbent
a. paper point
a. point

absorber
hyCURE hydrolyzed protein powder
and exudate a.

Absorbine
A. Antifungal
A. Antifungal Foot Powder
A. Jock Itch
A. Jr. Antifungal

Absorb-its material
absorption
a. lacuna
x-ray a.

abstraction
a. ladder

abulia
abuse
vocal a.

abusive vocal behavior
abutment
anatomically dimensioned
temporary a.
anterior a.
auxiliary a.
bombed a.
bridge a.
CeraOne a.
COC a.
Dalla Bona ball and socket a.
dovetail stress broken a.
a. groove
implant a.
a. implant substructure
intermediate a.
isolated a.
3i wide-diameter a.
low margin standard a.
multiple a.
multirooted a.
a. post
posterior bridge a.
primary a.
screw-type a.
secondary a.
Spectra-System a.
a. splint
splinted a.
subperiosteal implant a.
a. support
terminal a.
ThreadLoc non-cast-to a.
a. tooth
ZAAG a.

abutting consonant
AC
air conduction
alternating current
axiocervical

acacia
acalculia
Acanthamoeba

NOTES

acanthesthesia
acanthion
acantholysis
acanthomatous
    a. ameloblastoma
    a. pattern
acanthosis
acanthotic
acapnia
acarbia
Acarus
acatalasia, acatalasemia
acatamathesia
acataphasia
ACC
    adenoid cystic carcinoma
accelerated
    a. eruption
    a. speech
acceleration
    interverbal a.
    intraverbal a.
accelerator
    Becker a.
    A. II aspirator
    a. tip
accelerometer
accent
    foreign a.
acceptance
    a. approach
    Seal of A.
accepted
    A. Dental Therapeutics (ADT)
    a. dentifrice
access
    apical a.
    cavity a.
    a. cavity
    a. flap in osseous surgery
    a. form
    a. incision
    lexical a.
    a. opening
    palatal a.
    periapical a.
    a. preparation
    root canal a.
    translabial a.
Access-Blocker
accessibility
accessional teeth
accessory
    a. buccal cusp
    a. buccal root
    a. canal
    a. cusp
    a. feminizing operation

    a. mammary tissue
    a. maxillary ostium
    a. maxillary sinus ostium
    a. node
    a. ostium
    a. palatine canal
    a. root
    a. root canal
    a. salivary gland
    a. sinus
    a. tooth
ACCHN
    adenoid cystic carcinoma of head and
    neck
accident
    cerebrovascular a. (CVA)
    cochleovascular a.
accidental pulp exposure
accommodation
accordion graft
accretion
    a. line
ACCUJECT sterile disposable dental
  needle
Accu-line Products skin marker
Accu-Measure personal body fat tester
accuracy
    submillimetric a.
    timer a.
Accurate Surgical & Scientific
  Instruments (ASSI)
Accusat pulse oximeter
AccuSpan tissue expander
Accu-Spense cavity liner
Accutane
Accutorr bedside monitor
ACE
    Aerosol Cloud enhancer
    angiotensin-converting enzyme
    autologous-cultured epithelium
        ACE autografter bone filter
Ace
    A. Autografter
    A. bandage
    A. Bone Screw tack
    A. bone screw tacking kit
    A. wrap
acellular cementum
Ace/Normed osteodistractor
acentric
    a. glide
    a. occlusion
    a. relation
Acephen
Aceta
acetaminophen
    a., aspirin, and caffeine
    chlorpheniramine and a.

chlorpheniramine,
  phenylpropanolamine, and a.
a., chlorpheniramine, and
  pseudoephedrine
a. and codeine
a. and dextromethorphan
a., dextromethorphan, and
  pseudoephedrine
a. and diphenhydramine
hydrocodone and a.
hydrocodone bitartrate and a.
  10/325
a., isometheptene, and
  dichloralphenazone
oxycodone and a.
a. and phenyltoloxamine
phenyltoloxamine,
  phenylpropanolamine, and a.
propoxyphene and a.
a. and pseudoephedrine
Acetasol HC Otic
acetate
  cortisone a.
  Cortone A.
  cyproteron a.
  Hydrocortone A.
  m-cresyl a.
  medroxyprogesterone a.
  metacresyl a.
  paramethasone a.
acetazolamide
acetic
  a. acid
  a. acid, propylene glycol diacetate,
    and hydrocortisone
acetone
acetonide
  triamcinolone a.
acetylcholine
  a. receptor
acetylcholinesterase
acetylsalicylic acid (ASA)
acetylspiramycin
achalasia
achievable
  as low as reasonably a. (ALARA)
achievement
  a. age
  a. quotient (AQ)
Achillea millefolium
Achilles tendon
achlorhydric anemia

achondroplasia
Achromycin
  A. Ophthalmic
  A. Topical
acid
  a. abrasion
  acetic a.
  acetylsalicylic a. (ASA)
  alpha hydroxy a. (AHA)
  alphahydroxy a. (AHA)
  alpha-hydroxy a. (AHA)
  alphahydroxyl a. (AHA)
  aluminum acetate and acetic a.
  aminocaproic a.
  arachidonic a.
  ascorbic a.
  azelaic a.
  bicinchoninic a. (BCA)
  boric a.
  carbolic a.
  a. caustic
  cevitamic a.
  chondroitin sulfuric a.
  cis-retinoic a.
  citric a.
  5,8,11,14-eicosatetraynoic a. (ETYA)
  Epstein-Barr virus-encoded
    ribonucleic a. (EBER)
  a. etchant
  a. etch bonding technique
  a. etch cemented splint
  a. etching
  ethylenediaminetetraacetic a.
    (EDTA)
  folic a.
  gadolinium diethylamine triamine
    penta-acetic a. (Gd-DPTA)
  glacial phosphoric a.
  a. glutaraldehyde
  glycolic a.
  Gly Derm alphahydroxy a.
  Gly Derm glycolic a.
  hyaluronic a.
  hydrochloric a.
  hydrofluoric a.
  hydroperoxyeicosanoic a.
  hydroxyeicosanoic a.
  hydroxypropionic a.
  kojic a.
  lactic a.
  mefenamic a.
  a. mucopolysaccharide

NOTES

acid (continued)
- nalidixic a.
- nicotinic a.
- nordihydroguaiaretic a. (NDGA)
- orthophosphoric a.
- pantothenic a.
- phenolsulphonic a.
- a. phosphatase
- phosphoric a.
- podophyllin and salicylic a.
- polyacrylic a.
- polyglactic a.
- polyglycolic a. (PGA)
- polyhydroxy a. (PHA)
- polylactic a.
- poly-l-lactic a. (PLLA)
- pteroylglutamic a.
- retinoic a. (RA)
- ribonucleic a. (RNA)
- salicylic a.
- tannic a.
- tranexamic a.
- trichloroacetic a. (TCA)
- uric a.

acid-D-Phe-1
- indium 111-
- diethyltriaminepentaacetic a.-D.-P. (^{111}In-DTPA-D-Phe 1)

acid-etched restoration

acid-hematoxylin
- phosphotungstic a.-h. (PTAH)

acidogenic theory

acidophilic adenoma

acidophilus
- *Lactobacillus a.*

acidosis

acid-Schiff
- periodic a.-S. (PAS)
- a.-S. staining

acidulated
- a. fluoride
- a. phosphate fluoride
- a. phosphate-fluoride gel

acinar
- a. cell
- a. lumen

Acinetobacter

acini (pl. of acinus)

acinic
- a. cell carcinoma
- a. cell tumor

acinous cell carcinoma

acinus, pl. acini
- serous a.

Ackerman
- A. bar
- A. bar joint

Ackerman-Proffitt
- A.-P. classification
- A.-P. classification of malocclusion
- A.-P. orthogonal analysis acoustic coupler

Acland clamp

aclarubicin

ACLC
- Assessment of Children's Language Comprehension

Aclovate Topical

aclusion

Acme articulator

ACMI light source connector

acnes
- *Propionibacterium a.*

"A" company appliance

acor
- apex cornea

ACORDE bur

acorn
- a. carver

Acorn II nebulizer

acouesthesia

acoupedic method

acoupedics

acoustic
- a. agnosia
- a. analysis
- a. aphasia
- a. contralateral reflex
- a. energy
- a. feedback
- a. gain
- a. gain control
- a. immittance measurement
- a. impedance
- a. impedance probe
- a. impedance test
- a. ipsilateral reflex
- a. macula
- a. meatus
- a. method
- a. nerve
- a. neurilemoma
- a. neurinoma
- a. neuroma (AN)
- a. notch
- a. phonetics
- a. pressure
- a. reference level
- a. reflex amplitude
- a. reflex decay
- a. reflex latency
- a. reflex pattern
- a. reflex threshold
- a. rhinometry (AR)
- a. schwannoma

a. spectrum
a. stapedial reflex
a. stria
a. tolerance
a. trauma deafness
a. tumor
acoustica
hyperesthesia a.
acoustically
a. modified speech
a. specified neutral reference
acoustical streaming
acoustic-amnestic aphasia
acousticofacial
a. nerve
a. nerve bundle
acousticopalpebral reflex
acoustics
ACPS
acrocephalopolysyndactyly
acquired
a. aphasia
a. centric
a. centric relation
a. cholesteatoma
a. cuticle
a. defect
a. eccentric jaw relation
a. eccentric relation
a. enamel cuticle
a. immunodeficiency syndrome (AIDS)
a. immunoglobulin A deficiency
a. myotonia
a. nasopharyngeal stenosis
a. pellicle
acral lentiginous melanoma
acrivastine
a. and pseudoephedrine
acroangiodermatitis
acrocephalia
acrocephalopolysyndactyly (ACPS, ACS)
acrocephalosyndactylia,
  acrocephalosyndactyly (ACS)
acrocephaly
acrochordon
acrodont
acrodynia
acrokeratosis paraneoplastica
acrolect
acromegalic face
acromegaly

acronym
acrosclerosis
acrospiroma
eccrine a.
across-speech task
Acrotorque hand engine
acrylic
a. bite wafer
a. block
a. color correction kit
a. denture
a. ear splint
fast-setting a.
a. interocclusal splint
a. jig
a. monomer
a. overlap
a. overlay
a. overlay splint
a. paint
a. plastic
a. polymer
a. resin
a. resin base
a. resin bite-guard splint
a. resin and copper band appliance
a. resin dental cement
a. resin denture
a. resin tooth
a. resin tray
self-curing pink a.
Soft Denture Reline a.
a. veneer crown
a. veneer facing
ACS
acrocephalopolysyndactyly
acrocephalosyndactylia
act
biological a.
sensorimotor a.
speech a.
Actagen
A.-C
A. Syrup
A. Tablet
ACTH
adrenocorticotropic hormone
Acthar
Actiderm
Actifed
A. Allergy Tablet (Day)
A. Allergy Tablet (Night)

NOTES

actin
Actinex Topical
actinic
 a. cheilitis
 a. damage
 a. keratosis
Actinobacillus actinomycetemcomitans
Actinomyces
 A. bovis
 A. israelii
 A. naeslundii
 A. viscosus
actinomycetemcomitans
 Actinobacillus a.
actinomycin
actinomycosis
 cervicofacial a.
actinophytosis
 staphylococcal a.
action
 bacteriolytic a.
 centripetal a.
 a. current
 a. potential
 rasping a.
action-locative
action-object
Actisite periodontal fiber tetracycline
Activair battery
activate
activated
 a. dermis
 a. resin
activation
 a. moment
activator
 Andresen a.
 Andresen-Häupl a.
 a. appliance
 bow a.
 functional a.
 a. headgear appliance
 Klammt a.
 a. modification
 Nuva-Lite ultraviolet a.
 Schwarz a.
 a. therapy
active
 a. appliance therapy
 a. bilingualism
 a. caries
 a. eruption
 a. filter
 a. immunity
 a. range of motion (AROM)
 a. reciprocation
 a. voice

activity
 a. of daily living (ADL)
 enzyme a.
Actron
ACU-dyne
acuity
 auditory a.
 olfactory a.
 a. test
 visual a.
Acular Ophthalmic
acuminatum
 condyloma a.
acupuncture
acusis
Acuspot
 710 A.
 Sharplan Laser 710 A.
ACUSTAR I neurosurgical localization system
acusticus
 porus a.
acute
 a. apical abscess
 a. diffuse external otitis
 a. disseminated histiocytosis X
 a. follicular adenoiditis
 a. frontal sinusitis
 a. herpetic gingivostomatitis
 a. hordeolum
 a. infectious arthritides
 a. infectious gingivostomatitis
 a. inflammation
 a. laryngitis
 a. localized external otitis
 a. maxillary sinusitis
 a. necrotizing gingivitis
 a. necrotizing ulcerative gingivitis (ANUG)
 a. otitis media (AOM)
 a. periapical abscess
 a. periodontitis
 a. phoneme
 a. primary keratotic gingivostomatitis (APKG)
 a. pulpalgia
 a. pulpitis
 a. radiation syndrome
 a. respiratory disease
 a. rhinitis
 a. streptococcal stomatitis
 a. submandibular sialadenitis
 a. suppurative parotitis
 a. supraglottic laryngitis
 a. tubular necrosis
 a. ulcerating gingivitis
 a. ulceromembranous gingivitis

Acutrim
A. 16 Hours
A. II, Maximum Strength
A. Late Day
Acutronic AMS 1000 automatic jet ventilator
acyclovir
AD
Alzheimer disease
anterior displacement
auris dexter
axiodistal
adamantina
membrana a.
prismata a.
substantia a.
adamantine
a. layer
a. membrane
a. prism
a. substance
adamantinoblastoma
adamantinocarcinoma
adamantinoma
Adamount pocket mounts
Adams
A. ball
A. clasp
A. saw
Adam's apple
adaptation
auditory a.
a. effect
epithelial a.
marginal a.
masticatory a.
a. test
vestibular a.
adapter, adaptor
a. band
band a.
Luer-Lok a.
power a.
Adaptic
A. gauze
adaptive
a. behavior
a. immunity
A. Speech Alignment (ASA)
a. temporomandibular joint remodeling
adaptor (*var. of* adapter)

ADC
axiodistocervical
ADCC
antibody-dependent cellular cytotoxicity
ADD
angled delivery device
attention deficit disorder
ADD side-directed probe
Addison disease
addisonian crisis
additional canal
addition type
adduct
adduction
adductor
a. longus muscle
a. magnus muscle
a. paralysis
a. spasmodic dysphonia
adenitis
tuberculous a.
adenoadipose flap
adenoameloblastoma
adenocarcinoma
bronchial a.
gastrointestinal a.
mucinous cell a.
papillary a.
pleomorphic a.
polymorphous low-grade a. (PLGA)
prostatic a.
adenoid
a. cystic carcinoma (ACC)
a. cystic carcinoma of head and neck (ACCHN)
a. cystic tumor
a. facies
lateral trim of the a.
a. squamous carcinoma
adenoidal pad
adenoidal-pharyngeal-conjunctival (A-P-C)
adenoidectomy
lateral a.
power-assisted a.
tonsillectomy and a. (T&A)
adenoiditis
acute follicular a.
follicular a.
hyperplastic a.
hypertrophic a.
recurrent bacterial a.

NOTES

adenolymphoma
adenolymphomatosum
adenoma
 acidophilic a.
 apocrine a.
 basal cell a.
 basaloid monomorphic a. (BMA)
 bronchial a.
 canalicular a.
 carcinoma ex pleomorphic a.
 duodenal a.
 ectopic a.
 malignant pleomorphic a.
 monomorphic a.
 oncocytoma a.
 oxyphilic a.
 parathyroid a.
 parotid-derived pleomorphic a.
 pituitary a.
 pleomorphic a.
 recurrent pleomorphic a. (RPA)
 sebaceous a.
 a. sebaceum
 thyroid a.
 tracheal a.
adenomastectomy
adenomatoid
 a. ameloblastoma
 a. odontogenic tumor (AOT)
adenomatous
 a. goiter
 a. hyperplasia
 a. polyp
adenopapillary carcinoma
adenosine
 cyclic a. 3′,5′-monophosphate
 (cAMP)
 a. triphosphatase
 a. triphosphate (ATP)
adenotonsillar
 a. hemorrhage
adenotonsillectomy
 same-day a.
adenovirus
 a. virus
adequate crown
Aderer
 A. "C" bridge
 A. No. 3 Bridge gold
 A. No. 20 clasp
ADG
 axiodistogingival
ADHD
 attention deficit hyperactivity disorder
Ad-hear cerumen guard
adherence
 immune a.

adherens
 macula a.
 zonula a.
adherent
 a. cementicle
 a. denticle
adhering junction
adhesion
 a. bridge
 fibrous a.
 sublabial a.
adhesive
 Benefit denture a.
 biologic fibrogen a.
 a. bonding
 Cel Touch a.
 a. cement
 dental a.
 denture a.
 Durafill a.
 Enamelite 500 a.
 Endur a.
 a. foil
 Fotofil a.
 Mammopatch gel self a.
 microfilled a.
 no-mix a.
 a. otitis
 a. otitis media
 residual a.
 resin a.
 a. resin-bonded bridge
 a. resin bonded cast restoration
 Secure-on-Touch a.
 silicone a.
 a. system
 Tisseel biologic fibrogen a.
 visual light-polymerized a.
 a. wax
ADI
 axiodistoincisal
adiadochokinesis
adipectomy
adipo aspirate
adipocyte
adipodermal graft
adipofascial
 a. axial pattern cross-finger flap
 a. flap
 a. sural flap procedure
 a. turnover flap
adipose
 a. tissue
adiposus
 panniculus a.
adjacent
 a. odontoblasts
 a. root

adjunctive
adjustable
    a. anterior guide
    a. articulator
    a. axis face-bow
    a. external suture
    a. occlusal pivot
    a. orthodontic band
    a. saline breast implant
    a. screw
adjusted occlusion
adjustment
    incisal guide a.
    occlusal a.
    a. occlusion
    postretention a.
adjuvant chemotherapy
ADL
    activity of daily living
ad libitum
Adlone Injection
admaxillary
administration
    buccal a.
    Food and Drug A. (FDA)
    Occupational Safety and Health A.
      (OSHA)
admixture
adnexa
    ocular a.
    tooth a.
adnexal skin tumor
ADNR
    anterior displacement no reduction
ADO
    axiodisto-occlusal
ADOD
    arthrodentosteodysplasia
adolescent
    Fullerton Language Test for A.'s
    A. Language Screening Test
    a. voice
Adolph Gasser camera system
adoral
Adprin-B
    Extra Strength A.-B.
Adrenalin
adrenalin
adrenal insufficiency
α-adrenergic
    α-a. receptor

β-adrenergic
    β-a. receptor
adrenocorticotropic hormone (ACTH)
Adriamycin
    A. PFS
    A. RDF
Adson
    A. forceps
    A. suction
Adson-Brown forceps
Adsorbocarpine Ophthalmic
Adsorbotear Ophthalmic Solution
adsorption
ADT
    Accepted Dental Therapeutics
adult
    a. acquired micrognathia
    Apraxia Battery for A.'s (ABA)
    a. Chiari malformation
    a. rhinosinusitis
    Slosson Intelligence Test for
      Children and A.'s
AdultPatch
    Trans-Ver-Sal A.
adult-type well-differentiated liposarcoma
adumbration
advance
    a. cochlear echo technique
Advanced beta 200 otoscope
advancement
    a. flap
    galea-frontalis a.
    a. genioplasty
    hyoid a.
    lip border a.
    mandibular a.
    mandibular osteotomy-
      genioglossus a.
    maxillofacial skeletal a.
    transcranial monobloc frontofacial a.
    volar flap a.
    V-Y a.
    V-Y lip roll mucosal a.
adventitia
    tunica a.
adventitious
    a. deafness
    a. dentin
Advil
    A. Cold & Sinus Caplets
ADWR
    anterior displacement with reduction

NOTES

Aeby muscle
AED
    aerodynamic equivalent diameter
AERA
    average evoked response audiometry
aeration
Aeroaid
aerobe
aerobic
    a. bacteria
AeroBid
    A.-M Oral Aerosol Inhaler
    A. Oral Aerosol Inhaler
aerodigestive
    a. tract
    a. tumor
Aerodine
aerodontalgia
    primary a.
    secondary a.
aerodontia
aerodontics
aerodynamic
    a. analysis
    a. equivalent diameter (AED)
aerodynamics
aerophagia
Aeroseb-Dex
aerosialophagy
aerosinusitis
aerosol
    bacterial a.
    A. Cloud enhancer (ACE)
    dental a.
    Fluro-Ethyl A.
    Nasalide Nasal A.
aerosolization
AeroSonic personal ultrasonic nebulizer
aerotitis media
aerotolerant anaerobe
aeruginosa
    Pseudomonas a.
Aesculus hippocastanum
aesthesioneuroblastoma
aesthetic (*var. of* esthetic)
Aesthetica C topical vitamin C skin
    care product
aesthetics (*var. of* esthetics)
AE surgical contra-angle 20:1 press-
    button chuck
AF
    apical foramen
        Diprolene AF
        SSD AF
AFDC
    Aid to Families with Dependent Children
affected dentin
affective function

afferent
    a. feedback
    a. lymphatic
    a. motor aphasia
    a. nerve
    a. neuron
afferent-efferent pathway
affix
afflux
affricate
affrication
affricative
AFH
    angiomatoid fibrous histiocytoma
    anterior facial height
afibrillar cementum
Afrin
    A. Children's Nose Drops
    A. Sinus
    A. Tablet
AFS
    allergic fungal sinusitis
Aftate
    A. for Athlete's Foot
    A. for Jock Itch
aftercondensation
after-glide
afterperception
after root amputation restoration
aftersensation
aftersound, after-sound
aftertaste, after-taste
afunctional
    a. occlusion
    a. ulatrophy
AG
    axiogingival
agalactiae
    Streptococcus a.
agar
    a. hydrocolloid
    a. hydrocolloid conditioner
    a. hydrocolloid impression material
    a. impression
    a. impression material
agar-alginate
    a.-a. impression
    a.-a. impression material
agate burnisher
age
    achievement a.
    basal a.
    chronological a. (CA)
    developmental a.
    educational a. (EA)
    mental a. (MA)
aged
    a. tooth

Agee
>A. carpal tunnel release
>A. device
>A. sign

agenesis
>corpus callosum a.
>penile a.
>tracheal a.
>vaginal a.

agenitive

agent
>alkylating a.
>All-Bond 2 dentin bonding a.
>anesthetic a.
>anti-inflammatory a.
>antineoplastic a.
>antipseudomonal a.
>bleaching a.
>bonding a.
>cavity lining a.
>chelating a.
>chemotactic a.
>chemotherapeutic a.
>disclosing a.
>enamel-bonding a.
>endogenous algogenic a.
>ganglionic blocking a.
>Gluma dentin bonding a.
>hydrolytic a.
>hypotensive a.
>immunosuppressive a.
>infectious a.
>Karisma carbamide peroxide bleaching a.
>keratolytic a.
>lipotropic a.
>luting a.
>myoneural blocking a.
>Nite White carbamide peroxide bleaching a.
>Opalescence carbamide peroxide bleaching a.
>oxidizing agent polishing a.
>paralytic a.
>ProBond dentin bonding a.
>Proxigel carbamide peroxide bleaching a.
>sclerosing a.
>silane coupling a.
>vasoconstrictive a.
>vasodilating a.
>wetting a.

agent-action

agent-object

ageusia, ageustia

Agfa
>A. Dentus M2 comfort intraoral radiograph film
>A. Dentus RP 6 blue-sensitive extraoral radiograph film
>A. Dentus ST8 G green-sensitive extraoral radiograph film

agger
>a. nasi
>a. nasi cell

agglutinate
>vasoactive a.

agglutination
>latex a.

aggregate
>mineral trioxide a. (MTA)

aggressive lesion

aging
>a. pulp
>vector of a.

agitolalia

agitophasia

aglossia

aglossia-adactylia syndrome

aglutition

agminated blue nevus

agnathia

agnosia
>acoustic a.
>auditory a.
>auditory verbal a.
>finger a.
>tactile a.
>visual a.
>visual-verbal a.

agomphious

agomphosis, agomphiasis

agonist

agrammatica

agrammatism

agrammatologia

agranular reticulum

agranulocytic ulceration

agranulocytopenia

agranulocytosis

agraphia
>pure a.

Agropyron repens

NOTES

AHA
  alpha-hydroxy acid
  alphahydroxy acid
  alpha hydroxy acid
  alphahydroxyl acid
Ahern knot
AHH
  arylhydrocarbon hydroxylase
AHI
  apnea-hypopnea index
AHO
  Albright hereditary osteodystrophy
AH-26 silver-free sealer
A-hydroCort
AI
  axioincisal
Aiache technique
Aicardi syndrome
aid
      air-conduction hearing a.
      Argosy Cameo CIC hearing a.
      binaural hearing a.
      body hearing a.
      bone-anchored hearing a. (BAHA)
      bone conduction hearing a.
        (BCHA)
      canal hearing a.
      Canal-Mate hearing a.
      CIC hearing a.
      completely-in-the-canal hearing a.
      compression hearing a.
      digital hearing a.
      hearing a.
      interoral speech a.
      in-the-ear hearing a.
      ITE hearing a.
      linear hearing a.
      Maico Gamma hearing a.
      monaural hearing a.
      pseudobinaural hearing a.
      Servox electronic speech a.
      Servox Inton speech a.
      SolarEar hearing a.
      Tactaid hearing a.
      Trilogy I hearing a.
      Tru-Canal hearing a.
      Ultra Voice speech a.
      Unitron Esteem CIC hearing a.
      vibrotactile hearing a.
      Y-cord hearing a.
aided augmentative communication
Aid to Families with Dependent
  Children (AFDC)
AIDS
  acquired immunodeficiency syndrome
    AIDS dementia complex
AIDS-related
      A.-r. complex (ARC)

      A.-r. cryptococcal meningitis
      A.-r. virus (ARV)
AIM 7 thermocouple input module
Ainsworth punch
air
      a. cell
      complemental a.
      a. conduction (AC)
      a. embolism
      a. embolus
      a. firing
      a. flow
      high-efficiency particulate a.
        (HEPA)
      a. injection
      ionized a.
      a. pollutant
      a. pollution
      a. PTA
      reserve a.
      residual a.
      a. space
      supplemental a.
      a. syringe
      a. threshold
      tidal a.
      a. wastage
air-bearing turbine handpiece
air-blade sound
air-bone gap
airbrasive technique
air-conduction
      a.-c. hearing aid
      a.-c. receiver
Airdent
Aire-Cuf tracheostomy tube
airflow
      a. bisymmetry
      a. management
air-iodinated contrast
AirLITE support pad
airstream
      nasal a.
air/water syringe tubing
airway
      Combitube a.
      laryngeal mask a. (LMA)
      a. management
      nasal a.
      a. obstruction
      upper a.
AK
      AK-Chlor Ophthalmic
      AK-Cide Ophthalmic
      AK-Dex Ophthalmic
      AK-Dilate Ophthalmic Solution
      AK-Homatropine Ophthalmic
      AK-Nefrin Ophthalmic Solution

AK-Neo-Dex Ophthalmic
AK-Pentolate
AK-Poly-Bac Ophthalmic
AK-Pred Ophthalmic
AK-Spore H.C. Ophthalmic
Ointment
AK-Spore H.C. Ophthalmic
Suspension
AK-Spore H.C. Otic
AK-Spore Ophthalmic Solution
AK-Sulf Ophthalmic
AK-Taine
AK-Tracin Ophthalmic
AK-Trol

AKA
above-knee amputation
Akarpine Ophthalmic
AKBeta
Akne-Mycin Topical
AKPro Ophthalmic
Akros mattress
AKTob Ophthalmic
Akwa Tears Solution
AL
ablation-ligament
axiolingual
AL reconstruction
ALA, Ala
axiolabial
ala, pl. alae
Burkitt lymphoma of nasal a.
nasal a.
a. nasi
thyroid a.
ala-facial groove
ALAG, ALaG
axiolabiogingival
ALAL, ALaL
axiolabiolingual
alalia
alalic
alar
a. area
a. base
a. base reduction
a. batten graft
a. cartilage
a. crease
a. dome and cartilage
a. facial groove
a. fascia
a. flutter

a. muscle
a. reconstruction
a. rim
a. rim collapse
a. rim excision
a. suspension stitch
a. wedge excision
ALARA
as low as reasonably achievable
ALARA principle
alar-columella relation
alar-facial junction
alaryngeal
a. communication
a. speech
a. voice
A-Lastic thread
alba
linea a.
lingua a.
lingua villosa a.
materia a.
pachymucosa a.
terra a.
Albacer
Albalon-A Ophthalmic
Albalon Liquifilm Ophthalmic
albendazole
Albers-Schönberg disease
albicans
Candida a.
Albrecht syndrome
Albright
disseminated form A. syndrome
A. hereditary osteodystrophy (AHO)
A. syndrome
albuginea
tunica a.
albumin
a. test
albus
Staphylococcus a.
ALC
axiolinguocervical
Alcaine
alcalescens
Veillonella a.
Alcian
A. blue
A. blue stain
Alcide
alclometasone

NOTES

alcohol
    ethyl a.
    isopropyl a.
    a. sniff test (AST)
Alconefrin Nasal Solution
ALD
    Appraisal of Language Disturbance
    assistive listening device
alder
    red a.
aldolase
aldosterone
alendronate
Alert Label
Aleve
Alexander
    A. attachment
    A. deafness
alexandrite laser
alexia
    auditory a.
    pure a.
    visual a.
ALEXlazr
    Candela A.
    A. laser
Alezzandrini syndrome
alfalfa
Alfenta Injection
alfentanil
ALG
    axiolinguogingival
alganesthesia
algesia
algesimetry
alginate
    calcium a.
    Coe a.
    hard set a.
    a. hydrocolloid
    Hydro-Jel a.
    a. impression
    a. impression material
    sodium a.
Algipore Picasso visual transmission system
Algo-1, -2 automated auditory brainstem response device
algogenesis
algogenic
    a. pain fiber
Algo-2 hearing screening device
algorithm
    bone a.
aliesterase
alignment, alinement
    Adaptive Speech A. (ASA)
    arch a.

    beam a.
    a. curve
    tooth a.
aliquot
alkali caustic
alkaline
    a. hypochlorite
    a. perborate
    a. peroxide
    a. phosphatase
    a. phosphatase test
alkaloids
    chlorpheniramine, phenylephrine, phenylpropanolamine, and belladonna a.
    opium a.
Alka-Seltzer
    A.-S. Plus Cold Liqui-Gels Capsules
    A.-S. Plus Flu & Body Aches Non-Drowsy Liqui-Gels
alkylating agent
All Access laser system
Alladin InfantFlow nasal continuous positive air pressure
allantoin
    a. vaginal cream
All-Bond 2 dentin bonding agent
Alldress multilayered wound dressing
Allegra
Allen
    A. root pliers
    A. test
    A. traction system
Aller-Chlor
Allercon Tablet
Allerest
    A. Eye Drops
    A. 12 Hour Capsule
    A. 12 Hour Nasal Solution
    A. Maximum Strength
    A. No Drowsiness
Allerfrin
    A. Syrup
    A. Tablet
    A. w/Codeine
Allergan Ear Drops
allergen
allergic
    a. coryza
    a. fungal sinusitis (AFS)
    a. gingivitis
    a. gingivostomatitis
    a. mucin
    a. reaction
    a. rhinitis
    a. salute
    a. sialadenitis

allergy
AllerMax Oral
Allerphed Syrup
AllHear cochlear implant
alligator forceps
Allis
    A. clamp
    A. hemostat
    A. tissue forceps
Allison forceps
alliteration
Allium
    A. cepa
    A. sativum
allochiria
AlloDerm
    A. acellular dermal graft
    A. cellular dermal graft
    A. preserved human dermis
alloderm
allogenic, allogeneic
    a. bone
    a. bone crib
    a. crib
    a. graft
    a. keratinocyte graft
allogenically vascularized prefabricated
  flap
allograft
    decalcified freeze-dried bone a.
     (DFDBA)
    demineralized freeze-dried bone a.
     (DFDBA)
    Proplast a.
    Silastic a.
    a. wound covering
alloimplant
allolalia
allomorph
allophasis
allophone
alloplast
alloplastic
    a. AMA
    a. augmentation
    a. chin augmentation
    a. crib
    a. graft
    a. graft material
    a. implant
    a. plate
    a. prosthesis

    a. reconstruction
    a. transplant
alloplasty
all-or-none phenomenon
allotransplantation
allotriodontia
alloy
    6AI/4V ELI a. implant material
    amalgam a.
    a. backing
    base metal a.
    base metal crown and bridge a.
    Bridge III-C dental casting gold a.
    Bridge Partial IV-D dental casting
     gold a.
    Caulk Micro II a.
    Caulk Optaloy II a.
    Caulk spherical a.
    ceramic a.
    ceramo-metal a.
    chromium base casting a.
    chromium-cobalt a.
    chromium-cobalt-molybdenum a.
    chromium-cobalt-nickel base a.
    chromium-iron a.
    cobalt base a.
    cobalt-chromium a.
    cobalt-chromium-molybdenum a.
    comminuted a.
    Crown Hylastic gold wire a.
    cut amalgam a.
    dental amalgam a.
    dental casting gold a.
    dental gold a.
    Dentillium CB a.
    dispersed phase a.
    dispersion a.
    dispersion phase a.
    dispersion system a.
    Dispos-A-Cap amalgam a.
    Electraloy a.
    eutectic a.
    Forticast a.
    Gemini a.
    gold a.
    gold-based a.
    gold-copper a.
    gold-palladium a.
    high-copper a.
    high-gold a.
    high-noble a.
    high-palladium a.

NOTES

alloy *(continued)*
    Jelenko Durocast gold a.
    Jelenko Modulay gold a.
    Jel-Span a.
    Knapp gold a.
    Linc a.
    Line a.
    low-copper a.
    low-fusing a.
    Maxigold a.
    Midas a.
    Midigold a.
    Minigold a.
    Ney gold color elastic gold
      wire a.
    Ney-Oro elastic No. 4 gold
      wire a.
    Ney-Oro gold a.
    nickel a.
    nickel-chromium a.
    nickel titanium a.
    Noble gold a.
    nonprecious a.
    Nürnberg gold a.
    Optaloy amalgam a.
    Optaloy II copper a.
    palladium-copper a.
    palladium-silver a.
    Par-Cast gold a.
    porcelain-fused-to-gold a.
    powdered gold-calcium a.
    preamalgamated a.
    a. restoration
    Royal a.
    Shofu spherical a.
    silver a.
    silver-copper a.
    silver-tin a.
    Speyer dental casting gold a.
    spherical amalgam a.
    Sterngold dental casting gold a.
    Sterngold Supercast dental casting
      gold a.
    Suteraloy a.
    Sybraloy high-copper a.
    Ticonium 44, 50, 100 a.
    Ticonium dental casting gold a.
    Tytin high-copper a.
    Velvalloy amalgam a.
    Vitallium a.
    white gold a.
    Wilkinson dental casting gold a.
    Williams gold wire a.
    Wironium casting a.
    Wiron S crown and bridge a.
    X-12 a.
    zinc-free a.

alloy-forming metal
alloy-mercury ratio
All-Pro automatic film developer
Allskin marker
allusion
almond
ALO
    axiolinguo-occlusal
Al_2O_3
    aluminum oxide
aloe
    Cortaid with a
    Dermtex HC with a
alogia
Alomide Ophthalmic
alopecia
    a. areata
    traumatic a.
Alor 5/500
Alpha
    A. fiberoptic pocket otoscope
alpha
    a. fibers
    a. hydroxy acid (AHA)
    a. rhythm
    a. wave
alphabet
    initial teaching a.
    International Phonetic A. (IPA)
    International Standard Manual A.
    manual a.
    phonetic a.
Alphagan
alpha-hydroxy acid (AHA)
alphahydroxy acid (AHA)
alphahydroxyl acid (AHA)
AlphaNine SD
Alphatrex
Alport syndrome
ALPS
    Aphasia Language Performance Scale
AL-R
ALS
    amyotrophic lateral sclerosis
Alström syndrome
Alta
    A. femoral bolt
    A. femoral plate
    A. intramedullary rod
alteration
    bone a.
    periapical tissues a.
    periodontium a.
altered passive eruption
Alternaria
    A. antigen
    A. *tenuis*

alternate
    a. binaural loudness balance (ABLB)
    a. binaural loudness balance test
    a. forms reliability coefficient
    a. monaural loudness balance (AMLB)
    a. motion rate (AMR)
alternating
    a. current (AC)
    a. pulse
alternative
    a. communication
    a. communication device
Althaea officinalis
altitude chamber
Alton Deal pressure infusor
alumina
alumina-reinforced porcelain crown
aluminoceramic crown
aluminous porcelain
aluminum
    a. acetate and acetic acid
    a. chloride hexahydrate
    a. crown
    a. filter
    a. foil
    a. oxide (Al_2O_3)
    a. oxide abrasive
    a. oxide disk
    a. phosphate
Alupent
Aluwax
alveoalgia, alveolalgia
alveodental suppuration
alveoform
    A. binder
    a. biograft
Alveograf binder
alveolabial sulcus
alveolalgia (*var. of* alveoalgia)
alveolar
    a. abscess
    a. angle
    a. arch
    a. arch derangement
    a. area
    a. artery
    a. assimilation
    a. atrophy
    a. body
    a. bone

a. bone defect
a. bone density
a. bone graft
a. bone radiography
a. border
a. border of mandible
a. border of maxilla
a. canal
a. carcinoma
a. cavity
a. cleft
a. cleft graft
a. consonant
a. crest
a. crest fiber
a. dehiscence
a. fiber
a. fistula
a. foramina
a. gingiva
a. grafting
a. height
a. hemorrhage
a. hyperventilation
a. hypoventilation
a. index
a. limbus of mandible
a. limbus of maxilla
a. margin
a. margin of mandible
a. mucosa
a. nerve
a. osteitis
a. periosteum
a. plate fenestration
a. point
a. point-basion line
a. point meatus plane
a. point-nasal point line
a. point-nasion line
a. process
a. process crater
a. process fracture
a. process of mandible
a. process of maxilla
a. profile angle
a. ridge
a. ridge augmentation
a. ridge mucosa
a. septum
a. sinus
a. socket

NOTES

alveolar *(continued)*
a. socket wall fracture
a. soft part sarcoma (ASPS)
a. support
a. supporting bone
a. surface
a. surface of mandible
a. surface of maxilla
alveolaris
arcus a.
processus a.
alveolate
alveolectomy
partial a.
alveoli (*gen. and pl. of* alveolus)
alveolingual
a. groove
a. sulcus
alveolitis
a. sicca dolorosa
alveolobasilar line
alveoloclasia
alveolocondylar
alveolocondylean
alveolodental
a. ligament
a. membrane
a. osteoperiostitis
a. periostitis
a. protrusion
a. retrusion
alveologingival
a. fiber
alveololabial
alveololabialis
alveololingual
alveolomerotomy
alveolonasal
a. line
alveolopalatal
alveoloplasty
interradicular a.
intraseptal a.
alveoloschisis
alveolotomy
alveolus, gen. and pl. alveoli
buccal a.
canine a.
cleft a.
dental a.
alveoli dentales
a. dentalis
distobuccal a.
first premolar a.
lingual a.
mandibular a.
maxillary a.
maxillary first molar a.

mesiobuccal a.
mucous a.
salivary gland a.
second premolar a.
septum alveoli
serous a.
supramentale mandibular a.
tapetum alveoli
alveolysis
alveoplasty
Alvogyl surgical dressing
ALZET continuous infusion osmotic pump
Alzheimer disease (AD)
AM
amplitude modulation
axiomesial
AMA
augmentation of the mandibular angle
alloplastic AMA
Amalcap-plus
amalgam
a. alloy
a. burnisher
a. carrier
a. carver
Caulk Optaloy a.
Class I a.
a. condensation
a. condenser
copper a.
a. core
cut a. alloy
dental a.
a. die
Dispersalloy a.
gold a.
Kerr Spher-A-Caps a.
Kerr Spheraloy a.
marginal integrity of a.
a. matrix
a. mixer
Mowrey 695 a.
occlusal a.
a. pigmentation
pin a.
pinned a.
pin-retained a.
pin-supported a.
a. plugger
a. restoration
retrograde a.
scrap a.
silver a.
spherical a.
a. squeeze cloth
a. strip
a. tattoo

Toraloy dental a.
Tytin high copper a.
amalgamate
amalgamation
amalgamator
Crown a.
mechanical a.
Amalgambond
amaranth
green a.
amaurosis
consecutive a.
a. corticalis
a. fugax
Ambenyl Cough Syrup
ambidextrous
ambient noise
ambiguity
inferential a.
lexical a.
linguistic a.
ambiguous
a. word
ambiguus
nucleus a.
ambilaterality
Ambi Skin Tone
ambisyllabic
ambivalence
ambiversion
AMC
arthrogryposis multiplex congenita
axiomesiocervical
amcinonide
Amcort
AMD
axiomesiodistal
amebic infection
Ameflow device
ameloblast
Tomes process of a.
ameloblastic
a. adenomatoid tumor
a. carcinoma
a. fibrodentinoma
a. fibroma
a. fibro-odontoma
a. fibrosarcoma
a. layer
a. odontoma
a. sarcoma

ameloblastoma
acanthomatous a.
adenomatoid a.
desmoplastic a.
intraosseous a.
luminal a.
mural a.
peripheral a.
pigmented a.
unicystic a.
amelocyte
amelodental junction
amelodentinal
a. junction
amelogenesis
a. imperfecta
amelogenic
amelogenin
amelo-onychohypohidrotic syndrome
Amen Oral
amentia
Americaine
A. otic
A. Otic ear drops
American
A. Board of Medical Specialties
A. cockroach
A. Dental Association Uniform Code on Dental Procedures and Nomenclature
A. elm
A. ginseng
A. Gold "B" bridge
A. Gold "C" partial extra hard
A. Gold "M-H" inlay
A. Gold "M" inlay
A. Gold "T" bridge
A. Gold "T" bridge hard
A. Indian Sign Language (AMERIND)
A. leishmaniasis
A. Medical Source laparoscopic equipment
A. Sign Language (Ameslan, ASL)
A. Society for Testing and Materials
A. style forceps
AMERIND
American Indian Sign Language
Ameslan
American Sign Language
Ames plastic porcelain

NOTES

A-methaPred Injection
AMG
  axiomesiogingival
Amgenal Cough Syrup
AMI
  axiomesioincisal
Amicar
Amici disk
amikacin
Amikin Injection
amimia
amine
    quaternary a.
amine-accelerated sealant
aminocaproic acid
aminoglycoside
Amino-Opti-E
aminopeptidase
aminopterin
Ami-Tex LA
amitriptyline
AMLB
  alternate monaural loudness balance
amlexanox
ammonia
  a. inhalant
ammonium
  a. chloride
  hydrocodone, phenylephrine,
    pyrilamine, phenindamine,
    chlorpheniramine, and a.
  a. phosphate
Ammons Full Range Picture
  Vocabulary Test
amnesia
  localized a.
  posttraumatic a. (PTA)
  retroactive a.
amnesic, amnestic
  a. aphasia
amnion
  a. graft
  human a.
amniotic
  a. band disruption sequence
  a. band syndrome
AMO
  axiomesio-occlusal
amodiaquine
Amoeba
  A. buccalis
  A. coli
  A. dentalis
amorphous calcification
amoxicillin
  a. and clavulanate potassium
Amoxil

amperage
ampere (A)
amphicrine carcinoma
amphoric voice sound
Amphotec
amphotericin
  a. B
  a. B colloidal dispersion
  a. b lipid complex
  a. B topical
ampicillin
  a. sodium
  a. and sulbactam
amplification
  compression a.
amplifier
amplify
amplitude
  acoustic reflex a.
  a. distortion
  a. domain
  effective a.
  maximum a.
  a. modulation (AM)
  prephonatory a.
  a. shimmer
  zero a.
ampudontology
ampulla
  membranaceous a.
  osseous a.
ampullaris
  crista a.
ampullary
  a. crest
  a. nerve
ampullofugal stimulation
ampullopetal direction
amputated tooth
amputation
  above-knee a. (AKA)
  avulsion a.
  below-knee a.
  Chopart a.
  degloved a.
  labiomaxilloseptocolumellar a.
  labiomental a.
  labiopalatal a.
  modified Chopart a.
  a. neuroma
  nipple-areolar a.
  pulp a.
  root a.
AMR
  alternate motion rate
amusia
amylacea
  corpora a.

amylase
α-a. ptyalin
amyloid
a. macroglossia
a. tongue
amyloidosis
amyotonia
amyotrophic lateral sclerosis (ALS)
AN
acoustic neuroma
ANA
antinuclear antibody
anachoresis
anachoretic pulpitis
Anacin
anaclasis
anacusis, anacousis, anakusis
anaerobe
aerotolerant a.
anaerobic
a. bacteria
a. culture
a. streptococcus
anaerobius
Peptostreptococcus a.
anákhré
anakusis (*var. of* anacusis)
analgesia
local a.
analgesic
analog
long-acting somatostatin a.
stomatostatin a.
testosterone a.
analogon
resin a.
analogy
anal verge
analysis, pl. **analyses**
acoustic a.
aerodynamic a.
anteroposterior a.
arch perimeter a.
arch width a.
auditory a.
automatic voice a.
bite a.
Bolton a.
cephalometric a.
Cohen a.
counterpart a.
densitometric a.

distinctive feature a.
Downs a.
Downs cephalometric a.
energy dispersed x-ray a. (EDXA)
euclidean distance matrix a.
(EDMA)
facial a.
Fourier a.
grammatical a.
immunoradiometric a. (IRMA)
Jarabak a.
kinesiographic a.
kinesthetic a.
kinetic a.
Mantel-Haenszel a.
mixed dentition a.
morphometric a.
morphometric video a.
nasofacial a.
natural process a.
occlusal a.
occlusal cephalometric a.
occlusion a.
orthogonal a.
perceptual a.
phonemic a.
phonetic a.
phonological a.
phonological process a.
proportional facial a.
segmental a.
sound a.
spectrophotometric a.
substitution a.
suprasegmental a.
task a.
tooth size a.
total space a.
traditional a.
Tweed method of dentofacial a.
a. of variance (ANOVA)
vector a.
Vocal Profiles A. (VPA)
analytic
a. method
Analytic Technology pulp tester
analyzer
noise a.
octave band a.
analyzing rod
Anamine Syrup
anamnesis

NOTES

anamnestic response
anaphoric pronoun
anaphylactic
> a. hypersensitivity
> a. shock

anaphylactoid
> a. reaction

anaphylatoxin
anaphylaxis
> eosinophil chemotactic factor of a. (ECF-A)
> slow-reacting substance of a. (SRS-A)

anaplastic
> a. carcinoma

anaplasty
Anaplex Liquid
Anaprox
anarthria
Anaspaz
anastomosed graft
anastomosis, pl. anastomoses
> arteriovenous a. (AVA)
> cricotracheal a.
> dog ear of a.
> end-to-end a. (EEA)
> end-to-end microvascular a.
> end-to-end venous a.
> end-to-side a.
> end-to-side venous a.
> Galen a.
> glossolaryngeal a.
> Hyrtl a.
> lymphaticovenous a.
> microvascular a.
> nerve a.
> Roux-en-Y a.
> small-vessel a.
> suspension a.
> venous-to-venous a. (VVA)

anatomic
> a. crown
> a. form
> a. impression
> a. occlusion
> a. repair
> a. ridge
> a. root
> a. snuff box
> a. teeth

anatomical
> a. crown
> a. dead space
> a. Tobin malar prosthetic implant

anatomically dimensioned temporary abutment

anatomy
> dental a.
> gingival a.

Anatuss
> A. DM

Anbesol
> Maximum Strength A.
> A. Maximum Strength

Ancef
anchor
> a. band
> endosteal implant a.
> implant a.
> Kurer a.
> Mitek a.
> Mitek GII suture a.
> Mitek Mini GII a.
> a. molar
> Radix a.
> a. splint
> a. suture
> a. tooth
> a. washer
> ZAAG implant a.
> Zest A. Advanced Generation (ZAAG)
> Zest implant a.

anchorage
> Baker a.
> a. bend
> cervical a.
> a. control
> cranial a.
> dynamic a.
> extramaxillary a.
> extraoral a.
> a. force
> intermaxillary a.
> intramaxillary a.
> intraoral a.
> major a.
> maxillomandibular a.
> minimal a.
> multiple a.
> occipital a.
> precision a.
> reciprocal a.
> reinforced a.
> a. resistance
> a. saver
> simple a.
> a. space-to-save chart
> stationary a.

anchoring fibril
ancient schwannoma
Ancobon
anconeus muscle
Ancorvis hinge

Andemann syndrome
Anderson-Hynes pyeloplasty
Andresen
    A. activator
    A. monobloc appliance
    A. removable orthodontic appliance
Andresen-Häupl activator
Andrews
    A. bar
    A. bridge
    A. six keys to normal occlusion
    A. spinal surgery table
Andrews-type nonorthodontic normal
  crown angulation
Androcur
androgen insensitivity syndrome
androsterone sulfate
Andy Gump deformity
anechoic
    a. chamber
anemia
    achlorhydric a.
    aplastic a.
    Cooley a.
    pernicious a.
anemometer
    warm-wire a.
anesthesia
    Bier block a.
    block a.
    a. cartridge
    cocaine a.
    conscious a.
    dental a.
    dilute local a.
    Diprivan a.
    general a.
    Hunstad system for tumescent a.
    infiltrative local a.
    intracavitary a.
    intraligamentary a.
    intrapulpal a.
    jet insufflation a.
    laryngeal a.
    ligamental a.
    local a.
    local infiltrative a. (LIA)
    methohexital a.
    periodontal a.
    periodontal ligament a.
    pressure a.
    propofol a.

    regional a.
    selective a.
    topical a.
    tumescent a.
anesthesiologist
anesthetic
    a. agent
    eutectic mixture of local a.'s
      (EMLA)
    Fluoro-Ethyl topical a.
    Frigiderm topical a.
    local a.
    low-flow a.
    a. needle
    Orajel Brace-Aid Oral A.
    Silverstein tetracaine base
      powder a.
aneurysm
    aortic a.
    basilar artery a.
    carotid a.
    false a.
    posterior fossa artery a.
    tuberculous a.
aneurysmal
    a. benign fibrous histiocytoma
    a. bone cyst (ABC)
    a. fibrous histiocytoma
aneurysmectomy
Anexate
Anexsia
Angelica sinensis
angina
    a. diphtheritica
    Ludwig a.
    necrotic a.
    a. pectoris
    Plaut a.
    pseudomembranous a.
    a. scarlatinosa
    Vincent a.
anginosus
    Streptococcus a.
angioblast
angiofibroma
    juvenile a.
    juvenile nasopharyngeal a.
    nasopharyngeal a.
angiofollicular lymph node hyperplasia
angiogenesis
    HBO-induced a.
    hyperbaric oxygen-induced a.

NOTES

angiogenic factor
angiography
    magnetic resonance a. (MRA)
    spiral computed tomography a.
angiokeratoma
angioleiomyoma
    laryngeal a.
angiolipoma
    subcutaneous a.
angioma
    cherry a.
angiomatoid
    a. fibrous histiocytoma (AFH)
    a. myosarcoma
angiomatous
    a. lymphoid hamartoma
    a. neoplastic tissue
angioneurotic edema
angiopathy
    giant cell hyaline a.
angioplasty
angiosarcoma
angiosomal flap
angiosome
angiospasm
    labyrinthine a.
angiotensin-converting enzyme (ACE)
angle
    alveolar a.
    alveolar profile a.
    augmentation of the mandibular a.
      (AMA)
    auriculocephalic a.
    auriculomastoid a.
    axial line a.
    A. band
    basal mandibular a.
    A. basic E arch appliance
    Bennett a.
    a. bisection technique
    buccal a.
    bucco-occlusal a.
    bucco-occlusal line a.
    cavity a.
    cavity line a.
    cavosurface a.
    cerebellopontine a. (CPA)
    cerebropalatine a.
    cervicomental a.
    A. classification of malocclusion
    conchal-mastoid a.
    cosine a.
    cricothyroid a.
    cusp a.
    distal a.
    distobuccal line a.
    distobucco-occlusal point a.
    distoclusal point a.

distolabial line a.
distolabioincisal point a.
distolingual line a.
distolinguoincisal point a.
distolinguo-occlusal point a.
facial a.
facial plane a.
a. former
Frankfort mandibular a. (FMA)
Frankfort mandibular incisor a.
  (FMIA)
Frankfort mandibular plane a.
gonial a.
incisal a.
incisal guidance a.
incisal mandibular plane a. (IMPA)
intergonial a.
interincisal a.
labial a.
labioincisal line a.
lateral incisal guide a.
line a.
lingual a.
linguoincisal line a.
linguo-occlusal line a.
mandibular a.
mandibular plane a.
maxillary a.
mesial a.
mesiobuccal line a.
mesiobucco-occlusal point a.
mesiolabial line a.
mesiolabioincisal point a.
mesiolingual line a.
mesiolinguoincisal point a.
mesiolinguo-occlusal point line a.
mesio-occlusal line a.
nasofrontal a.
nasolabial a.
occlusal plane a.
occlusal rest a.
piriform a.
point a.
prophy a.'s
prophylactic a.'s
protrusive incisal guide a.
Ranke a.
rest a.
sella-nasion-subspinale a. (SN_A, S-N-A, SNA)
sella-nasion-supramentale a. (SN_B, S-N-B, SNB)
sinodural a.
A. splint
tooth a.
Trautmann a.
visor a.

W & H Endodontic Contra A.
Z a.

angled
a. cannula
a. delivery device (ADD)
a. elevator
a. scissors
a. telescope

angstrom (Å)
Ångström unit (Å)
angular
a. artery
a. cheilitis
a. elevator
a. facial vein
a. gyrus
a. incision
a. nasal artery
a. position of the ramus
a. vestibular nucleus

angularis
dens a.

angulate
angulated
ASSI breast dissector a.
a. buccal tube
a. cell

angulation
Andrews-type nonorthodontic normal
  crown a.
bracket a.
bracket slot a.
built-in a.
horizontal a.
lower incisor a.
upper incisor a.
vertical a.

anhydrase
carbonic a.

anhydride
methacryloxyethyl trimellitic a.
  (META)

animal graft
animate
animation
facial a.

anise
anisocoria
anisognathous
ankle strategy

ankyloglossia
a. superior
a. superior syndrome

ankylosed tooth
ankylosing spondylitis
ankylosis
bony a.
cricoarytenoid a.
dental a.
fibro-osseous a.
fibrous a.
glossopalatine a.
juxta-articular a.
temporomandibular joint a.
TMJ a.
a. of tooth
zygomatic-coronoid a.

anneal
annealing
a. furnace
a. lamp
a. tray

annotation
annual bluegrass
annulare
granuloma a.

annular ligament
annulus
bony a.
tympanic a.
a. tympanicus

anode
anodontia
partial a.

anodontism
Anodynos-DHC
anomalous
a. tongue position

anomaly, pl. anomalies
cleft a.
craniofacial a.
dental a.
dentofacial a.
dysgnathic a.
eugnathic a.
fourth branchial a.
gestant a.
hemifacial microsomia a.
kleeblattschädel a.
laryngeal a.
maxillofacial a.
oral a.

NOTES

anomaly *(continued)*
> pragmatic a.
> temporal bone a.
> third branchial a.

anomia

anomic
> a. aphasia

anoplasty

anosmia

anosmic

anosognosia

anotia

ANOVA
> analysis of variance
> ANOVA method

anoxia
> cerebral a.
> pulpal a.

ANS
> anterior nasal spine

ansa, pl. **ansae**
> a. galeni
> a. hypoglossi
> a. hypoglossus muscle

Ansaid
> A. Oral

anserinus
> pes a.

Anspach 65K instrument system

ant
> black a.
> fire a.
> red a.

Antaeos C file

antagonist
> narcotic a.

antagonistic muscle

Antazoline-V Ophthalmic

antecedent
> a. event

antecubital fossa

antegonial
> a. notch
> a. notching

antegrade
> a. approach
> a. blood flow
> a. island flap

anterior
> a. abutment
> a. active mask rhinomanometry
> a. arch length
> a. arch width
> a. axillary line
> a. band
> a. band remover (ABR)
> a. chamber hyphema
> a. clinoid process

a. commissure
a. component
a. component of force
a. condylar vein
a. cranial fossa
a. craniectomy
a. cricoid split
a. crossbite
a. determinants of cusp occlusion
a. diastema
a. displacement (AD)
a. displacement no reduction (ADNR)
a. displacement with reduction (ADWR)
a. divergence
a. ethmoid
a. ethmoidal air cell
a. ethmoidal artery
a. ethmoidal foramen
a. ethmoidal nerve
a. ethmoidal ostium
a. ethmoidectomy
a. facial height (AFH)
a. facial vein
a. flared tooth
a. force
a. fracture
a. guide
a. hairline incision
a. helical rim free flap
a. inferior cerebellar artery
a. mallear fold
a. mallear ligament
a. mandibular posturing
a. mandibulectomy
a. middle meatus
a. naris
a. nasal spine (ANS)
a. nasal valve
a. occlusion
a. palatal bar
a. palatal major connector
a. palatine groove
a. palatine suture
a. partial laryngectomy
a. pillar tumor
a. port scalp excision
a. rectus capitis
a. retraction archwire
rhinitis sicca a.
a. rhinoscopy
a. scaler
a. scoring technique
a. septum
serratus a. (SA)
a. skull base
a. subperiosteal implant

a. superficialis muscle
a. superior iliac spine (ASIS)
a. surface
a. surface of maxilla
a. surface of premolar and molar teeth
a. suspension of hyoid bone
a. suspensory ligament
a. teeth
a. tympanic artery
a. vertical canal
a. view
anterior-posterior
a.-p. discrepancy
a.-p. otoplasty
anteroclusion
anterolateral
a. thigh flap
anteroposterior
a. analysis
a. correction
a. dysplasia
a. facial dysplasia
anterosuperior quadrant
anteversion
anthelix (*var. of* antihelix)
Anthony quadrisected minigraft dilator
anthrax
anthrolith
anthropological linguistics
anthropometer
anthropometric measurement
anthropometry
antiandrogen treatment
antibacterial
a. mouthwash
a. protein
Antibenzil
AntibiOtic
A. Otic
antibiotic
corticosteroid a.
endovenous a.
intraluminal a.
intravenous a.
nonpenicillin a.
oral a.
a. prophylaxis
a. tongue
antibody
antiductal a.
antinuclear a. (ANA)

anti-Ro a.
collagen a.
herpes simplex virus a.
monoclonal a.
radiolabeled a.
salivary gland a.
smooth muscle a.
thyroglobulin a.
antibody-dependent cellular cytotoxicity (ADCC)
anticariogenic
anticarious
anticholinergic
anticholinesterase
anticipatory
a. behavior
a. coarticulation
a. emotion
a. reaction
a. and struggle behavior theories
anticoagulant
anticonvulsive drug
anticurvature filing
anticus
isthmus tympani a.
antidepressant
antiductal antibody
anti-expectancy
antifungal
Absorbine A.
Absorbine Jr. A.
Breezee Mist A.
antigen
Alternaria a.
Bermuda grass a.
carcinoembryonic a.
cat epithelium a.
Cladosporium herbarium a.
common ragweed a.
Dermatophagoides farinae a.
dog epithelium a.
elm tree a.
English plantain a.
epithelial membrane a. (EMA)
fungal a.
grasses a.
Helminthosporium halodes a.
hepatitis B core a. (HBcAg)
hepatitis B e a. (HBeAg)
hepatitis B surface a. (HBsAg)
house dust mite a.
human lymphocyte a.'s (HLA)

NOTES

antigen *(continued)*
 June grass a.
 mountain cedar a.
 oak a.
 pecan tree a.
 perennial a.
 proliferating cell nuclear a.
  (PCNA)
 a. receptor
 Ro intracellular a.
 seasonal a.
 short ragweed a.
 super a.
 timothy grass a.
 tumor-specific a.
 Ulex europaeus a.
 white oak a.
antigenic
antigenicity
antigen-presenting cell (APC)
antihelical fold
antihelix, anthelix
 superior crus of a.
antihemorrhagic stent
Antihist-1
antihistamine
Antihist-D
antihormonal therapy
anti-inflammatory agent
anti-inflammatory-antibiotic combination
Antilirium
antimesenteric
antimetabolite
antimicrobial
 a. barrier
antimitotic
anti-Monson curve
antineoplastic agent
antinuclear antibody (ANA)
antiodontalgic
antioxidant eye treatment
antipseudomonal agent
antipyrine and benzocaine
antirejection drug therapy
antiresonance
antiretroviral therapy
anti-Ro antibody
antisepsis
antiseptic
antiserum
 trivalent botulinum a.
antisialagogue
antisialic
antitetanus booster
antitragohelicina
 fissura a.
antitragus
antitrismus

antituberculous drug
Antivert
antiviral
 a. prophylactic
Antoni
 A. A, B areas
 A. A, B tissue
 A. classification of schwannoma
  morphology
antral
 a. carcinoma
 a. cell
 a. irrigation
 a. lavage
 a. mucosal cyst
 a. mycosis
 a. polyp
 a. sarcoma
antrectomy
Antrizine
antrobuccal
antrochoanal polyp
antrodynia
antrolith
antroscope
antroscopy
antrostomy
 Caldwell-Luc maxillary a.
 inferior meatal a.
 intraoral a.
 middle meatal a.
 nasal a.
antrotomy
antrum
 bipartite a.
 Highmore a.
 mastoid a.
 maxillary a.
 a. punch forceps
ANUG
 acute necrotizing ulcerative gingivitis
anus
 imperforate a.
anvil
Anxanil
anxiety
AO
 axio-occlusal
 AO mandibular system
 AO reconstruction plate
 AO rigid fixation
AO/ASIF titanium craniofacial system
AOM
 acute otitis media
aorta
aortic
 a. aneurysm
 a. body

aortobiprofunda femoral bypass
aortoenteric fistula formation
aortofemoral
    a. bypass graft
    a. bypass grafting
AOT
    adenomatoid odontogenic tumor
AO-Titanium microplate
AP
    axiopulpal
Apacet
apathy
apatite crystal
A-P-C
    adenoidal-pharyngeal-conjunctival
APC
    antigen-presenting cell
Apdyne phenol applicator kit
aperiodic
    a. fibril
    a. wave
aperiodicity
Apert
    A. disease
    A. syndrome
aperta
    pulpitis a.
    rhinolalia a.
apertognathia
    compound a.
    infantile a.
    simple a.
apertognathism
aperture
    eye a.
    pyriform a.
apex, gen. apicis, pl. apices (A)
    a. blunderbuss
    closed a.
    a. cornea (acor)
    a. cuspidis
    flaring a.
    a. locator
    a. nasi
    open a.
    orbital a.
    a. pin
    a. radicis dentis
    radiographic a.
    retropapillary a.
    root a.
apexification

apexigraph
Apexit
    A. calcium hydroxide root canal
    sealer
apexogenesis
APF gel
Apgar score
aphagia
aphallia
aphasia
    acoustic a.
    acoustic-amnestic a.
    acquired a.
    afferent motor a.
    amnesic a.
    anomic a.
    associative a.
    auditory a.
    Bedside Evaluation and Screening
    Test of A.
    Broca a.
    central a.
    childhood a.
    A. Clinical Battery I
    conduction a.
    developmental a.
    dynamic a.
    efferent motor a.
    executive a.
    expressive a.
    expressive-receptive a.
    fluent a.
    global a.
    infantile a.
    International Test for A.
    isolation a.
    jargon a.
    kinesthetic motor a.
    kinetic motor a.
    Language Modalities Test for A.
    A. Language Performance Scale
    (ALPS)
    Minnesota Test for Differential
    Diagnosis of A.
    motor a.
    nominal a.
    nonfluent a.
    pragmatic a.
    pure a.
    receptive a.
    semantic a.
    sensory a.

NOTES

aphasia *(continued)*
 simple a.
 speech reading a.
 subcortical motor a.
 syntactic a.
 Token Test for Receptive Disturbances in A.
 transcortical sensory a.
 verbal a.
 Wernicke a.
aphasic
 a. phonological impairment
aphasiologist
aphasiology
aphemia
 pure a.
aphonia
 conversion a.
 functional a.
 hysterical a.
 intermittent a.
 a. paralytica
 psychogenic a.
 syllabic a.
aphonic
 a. episode
aphonous
aphrasia
 pure a.
aphtha, pl. aphthae
 Bednar aphthae
 herpetiform aphthae
 aphthae major
 Mikulicz aphthae
 aphthae minor
 periadenitis a.
 recurrent a.
 recurrent scarring a.
Aphthasol
aphthoid
aphthosis
aphthous
 a. stomatitis
 a. ulcer
 a. ulitis
aphysiologic
 a. sway
apical
 a. abscess
 a. access
 a. area
 a. base
 a. cell
 a. cementum
 a. cochlea
 a. curettage
 a. curve
 a. cyst

 a. delta
 a. dental ligament
 a. dentin
 a. elevator
 a. fenestration
 a. fiber
 a. foramen (AF)
 a. fragment ejector
 a. fragment forceps
 a. granuloma
 a. infection
 a. pathosis
 a. pericementitis
 a. periodontal abscess
 a. periodontal cyst
 a. periodontitis
 a. pick
 a. puncture
 a. radicular cyst
 a. radiolucency
 a. ramification
 a. root perforation
 a. root resorption
 a. seal
 a. space
 a. transportation
 a. width
 a. zip
 a. zone
apicalization
apically repositioned flap in mucogingival surgery
apicectomy
 petrous a.
apiceotomy *(var. of* apicotomy*)*
apices *(pl. of* apex*)* **(A)**
apicis *(gen. of* apex*)*
apicitis
 petrous a.
apicoectomy
apicolocator
apicostome
apicostomy
apicotomy, apiceotomy
apicurettage
Apit electronic apex locator
Apium graveolens
API universal foam chin strap
APKG
 acute primary keratotic gingivostomatitis
aplasia
 cochlear a.
 condylar a.
 a. of dentition
 enamel a.
 enamel and dental a.
 labyrinthine a.

müllerian duct a.
salivary gland a.
aplastic anemia
Aplicap
Espe Ketac-Bond A.
Espe Photac-Bond A.
apnea
central a.
deglutition a.
obstructive a.
obstructive sleep a. (OSA)
peripheral a.
polysomnography-proven obstructive
sleep a. (PSG-proven OSA)
sleep a.
apnea-hypopnea index (AHI)
apneic method
apocrine
a. adenoma
a. gland
a. hidrocystoma
aponeurectomy
aponeurosis, pl. aponeuroses
Denonvilliers a.
external oblique a.
fibrovascular a.
internal oblique a.
musculotendinous a.
palatal a.
rhomboid a.
transversus abdominis a.
aponeurotica
galea a.
lateral galea a.
aponeurotic galea
apoplexy
apoptosis
apoptotic pathway
apoxemena
apoxesis
subgingival a.
apparatus, pl. apparatus
attachment a.
branchial a.
dental a.
Golgi a.
masticating a.
masticatory a.
silverplating a.
vestibular a.
appearance
bizarre giant-cell a.

blown-out a.
chamois yellow a.
cotton-wool a.
cyst-like a.
eggshell a.
esthetic a.
glued-on ear a.
gray a.
hair-on-end a.
honeycomb a.
lamina dura-like a.
micrognathic a.
onion-peel a.
Paget disease-like mosaic a.
pigtail a.
punched-out a.
soap-bubble a.
sunken-eye a.
sunray a.
worm-eaten a.
appendage
auricular a.
appendiciforme
radiculum a.
appendix of laryngeal ventricle
apperception
applanation tonometry
apple
Adam's a.
appliance
"A" company a.
acrylic resin and copper band a.
activator a.
activator headgear a.
Andresen monobloc a.
Andresen removable orthodontic a.
Angle basic E arch a.
Begg fixed orthodontic a.
Begg light wire a.
Bimler removable orthodontic a.
biphasic pin a.
Bowles multiphase a.
Case a.
chin cup extraoral orthodontic a.
craniofacial a.
Crozat removable orthodontic a.
Denholz a.
differential force a.
edgewise fixed orthodontic a.
expansion plate a.
extraoral a.
extraoral fracture a.

NOTES

appliance (*continued*)
    extraoral orthodontic a.
    finger-sucking re-education a.
    finishing a.
    fixed orthodontic a.
    flange guide a.
    flexible finishing a.
    four-stage light wire a.
    Fränkel removable orthodontic a.
    functional a.
    Griffin a.
    habit-breaking a.
    Hawley retaining orthodontic a.
    hay rake fixed orthodontic a.
    Herbst a.
    holding a.
    Hyrax a.
    intraoral fracture a.
    intraoral orthodontic a.
    jacket a.
    jackscrew a.
    Jackson a.
    Johnson twin wire a.
    jumping-the-bite a.
    Kesling a.
    Kingsley a.
    Kloehn cervical extraoral
      orthodontic a.
    labiolingual fixed orthodontic a.
    Latham-Georgiade pin-retained
      presurgical orthopaedic a.
    Level Anchorage a.
    light round wire a.
    light wire a.
    lip habit a.
    mandibular advancement a. (MAA)
    Mayne muscle control a.
    a. modification
    monobloc a.
    mouthstick a.
    Muhlmann a.
    multibanded a.
    multiphase a.
    Nord a.
    obturator a.
    Ormco a.
    orthodontic a.
    palatal expansion a.
    palate-splitting a.
    pin and tube fixed orthodontic a.
    prefinishing a.
    prosthetic a.
    Proxi-Floss cleaning a.
    regulating a.
    removable orthodontic a.
    retaining orthodontic a.
    ribbon arch a.
    Roger-Anderson pin fixation a.
    sagittal a.
    Schwarz a.
    space retaining a.
    split plate a.
    Stage I a.
    straight wire fixed orthodontic a.
    surgical a.
    therapeutic a.
    thumb-sucking a.
    tongue-thrust a.
    tooth movement a.
    twin-wire fixed orthodontic a.
    Unitek a.
    universal fixed orthodontic a.
    vinyl palatal a.
    visceral deglutition a.
    visceral swallowing a.
    Walker a.

application
    arch bar a.
    topical a.

applicator
    root canal a.

applied
    a. linguistics
    a. phonetics

apposition
    compensatory periosteal bone a.
    soft-tissue a.

appraisal
    A. of Language Disturbance (ALD)
    Wits a.

approach
    acceptance a.
    antegrade a.
    axillary subpectoral a.
    bicoronal a.
    bicoronal subperiosteal a.
    buttonhole a.
    cochleovestibular a.
    conjunctival a.
    embryological a.
    endonasal a.
    errant a.
    extended frontal a.
    external pharyngotomy a.
    extralaryngeal a.
    extraoral a.
    infralabyrinthine a.
    infratemporal fossa a.
    intraoral a.
    Kaye minimal-incision anterior a.
    lingual a.
    mandibular swing a.
    middle fossa a.
    nonexcisional anterior a.
    otomicrosurgical transtemporal a.
    retrograde a.

A

retrolabyrinthine a.
retroseptal transconjunctival a.
retrosigmoid a.
Risdon a.
subciliary a.
sublabial a.
sublabial transsphenoidal a.
suboccipital a.
supratentorial a.
transantral a.
transblepharoplasty a.
transcanine a.
transcervical a.
transcochlear a.
transconjunctival a.
translabyrinthine a.
transmandibular a.
transmastoid a.
transmaxillary a.
transmeatal a.
transpalatal a.
transpalpebral a.
transseptal a.
transsphenoidal a.
vertical midline a.
Walsh-Ogura transantral a.
yawn-sigh a.
approach-avoidance
a.-a. theory
appropriate reduction
approximate
approximation
successive a.
a. suture
vocal fold a.
word a.
wound a.
approximator
a. clamp
nerve a.
Neuromeet soft tissue a.
APQ
average perturbation quotient
APR
auropalpebral reflex
apraclonidine
apratropium bromide
apraxia
A. Battery for Adults (ABA)
constructional a.
developmental articulatory a.
ideational a.

ideomotor a.
oral a.
speech a.
verbal a.
apraxic
a. impairment
apricot
aprismatic enamel
Aprodine
A. Syrup
A. Tablet
A. w/C
apron
abdominal a.
a. band
a. flap
a. flap procedure
lead a.
leaded protective a.
lingual a.
redundant abdominal a.
rubber dam a.
aprosody
aprotinin
apsithyria
aptitude
Hiskey-Nebraska Test of
Learning A.
a. test
AQ
achievement quotient
Nasacort AQ
Vancenase AQ
Aqua
A. Brites ear plug
A. Glycolic cream
A. Glycolic skin care product
Aquacare Topical
AquaMEPHYTON Injection
AquaNot swim mold
Aquaplast
A. alloplastic material
A. dressing
A. nasal splint
A. rapid setting splint material
AquaSens
AquaSite Ophthalmic Solution
Aquasol E
aqueduct
cerebral a.
cochlear a.

NOTES

aqueduct *(continued)*
    hypodevelopment of vestibular a.
    vestibular a.
aqueous
    a. humor
    a. methyl cellulose
    penicillin G, parenteral, a.
    a. synthetic dual phenolic
      disinfectant
AR
    acoustic rhinometry
arabinosyl
    cytosine a.
arachidic bronchitis
arachidonic
    a. acid
    a. acid cascade inhibitor (AACI)
arachnoid
    a. cyst
    a. space
    a. trabeculation
    a. villi
arbitrary block-out
arborescens
    lipoma a.
arborize
arbor vitae
ARC
    AIDS-related complex
arc
    reflex a.
    sensorimotor a.
    a. welding
arcade
    capillary a.
    mesenteric a.
arcading effect
arch
    a. alignment
    alveolar a.
    a. bar
    a. bar application
    a. bar cutter
    basal a.
    blue Elgiloy upper utility a.
    branchial a.
    collapse of dental a.
    continuous a.
    continuous ribbon a.
    A. of Cupid
    deep plantar a.
    dental a.
    dentulous dental a.
    digitopalmar a.
    a. discrepancy
    edentulous dental a.
    expansion a.
    expansion of the a.

filtral a.
Force 9 a.
a. form
glossopalatine a.
Gothic a.
high labial a.
horseshoe-shaped a.
hyoid branchial a.
inferior dental a.
labial a.
labial and lingual a.'s
a. length
a. length deficiency
lingual a.
lower a.
malar a.
mandibular a.
mandibular visceral a.
maxillary a.
Mershon a.
Nitinol a.
oral a.
oval a.
ovoid a.
palatal a.
palatine a.
palatoglossal a.
palatomaxillary a.
partially edentulous dental a.
passive lingual a.
a. perimeter
a. perimeter analysis
pharyngeal a.
pharyngopalatine a.
premandibular a.'s
prescription a.
removable lingual a.
residual dental a.
ribbon a.
rounded square a.
square a.
stacked a.
staggered a.
stationary lingual a.
steel anchorage a.
superficial palmar a.
superior dental a.
tapering a.
torque a.
trapezoidal a.
upper a.
U-shaped a.
utility a.
visceral a.
V-shaped a.
W a.
a. width
a. width analysis

Wilson bimetric a.
a. wire
wire a.
zygomatic a.
arch form
Roth a. f.
architectural disturbance
architecture
gingival a.
neural a.
tissue a.
archwire
anterior retraction a.
continuous a.
double keyhole loop a.
Elgiloy a.
finishing a.
helical loop a.
Jarabak-type a.
leveling a.
multiple loop a.
reverse a.
Siamese twin a.
spiral a.
Stage I, II, III, IV a.
straight a.
tie-back loop a.
T loop a.
twisted a.
Arcon semiadjustable articulator
Arctium lappa
Arctostaphylos uva-ursi
arcuata
eminentia a.
zona a.
arcuate
a. eminence
a. fasciculus
a. line
arcus, pl. arcus
a. alveolaris
a. alveolaris mandibulae
a. alveolaris maxillae
a. dentalis
a. dentalis inferior
a. dentalis superior
a. glossopalatinus
a. marginalis
a. senilis
a. zygomaticus
area, pl. areae
alar a.

alveolar a.
Antoni A, B areas
apical a.
articulation a.
auditory a.
auriculomastoid a.
basal seat a.
bilabial a.
Broca a.
Brodmann areas
Brodmann a. 41
Brodmann a. 44
contact a.
denture-bearing a.
denture foundation a.
denture-supporting a.
glottal a.
hinge a.
impression a.
interplacodal a.
intertriginous a.
Kiesselbach a.
labiodental a.
linguoalveolar a.
linguodental a.
Little a.
lowlight a.
mesial contact a. (MCA)
motor a.
nasal cross-sectional a.
palatal a.
parasymphysis a.
parotid-masseteric a.
pear-shaped a.
petroclival a.
postauricular a.
post dam a.
posterior palatal seal a.
postpalatal seal a.
prelacrimal a.
pressure a.
proximal subcontact a. (PSCA)
relief a.
rest a.
rest seat a.
retention a.
root-end surface a.
somesthetic a.
stress-bearing a.
stress-supporting a.
subglottic a.
supporting a.

NOTES

area *(continued)*
    surgically denervated a.
    thalamocortical a.
    tissue-bearing a.
    total body surface a. (TBSA)
    velar a.
    visual a.
    Warthin a.
    Wernicke a.
areata
    alopecia a.
Aredia
areflexia
    caloric a.
areola
    coning of a.
areolar
    a. demarcation
    a. gingiva
    a. grafting
    a. reconstruction
    a. tissue
areolomammary complex
argentaffin
    a. cell
    a. stain
argentum, pl. **argenti**
Argesic-SA
argon
    a. gas
    a. green laser
    a. tuneable dye laser
Argosy Cameo CIC hearing aid
Argyle
    A. anti-reflux valve
    A. silicone Salem sump
argyria
    local a.
argyrophilic
    a. collagen fiber
    a. fibril
argyrosis
arhinia malformation
Arie-Pitanguy
    A.-P. mammaplasty
    A.-P. operation
Aristocort
    A. A
    A. Forte
Arizona
    A. Articulation Proficiency Scale
    A. ash
    A. cypress
    A./Fremont cottonwood
Arkansas stone
arm
    bar clasp a.
    circumferential clasp a.
    a. clasp
    clasp a.
    dynein a.
    endosteal implant a.
    engine a.
    A. & Hammer Dental Care
    reciprocal a.
    retentive a., retention a.
    retentive circumferential clasp a.
    stabilizing a.
    stabilizing circumferential clasp a.
    T clasp a.
    Y clasp a.
armamentarium
    endodontic a.
    occlusal adjustment a.
    periodontal a.
    preprosthetic reconstructive a.
Armand Frappier strain
A.R.M. Caplet
Armitage-Cochran test
Armstrong prosthesis
Army-Navy retractor
Arnica montana
Arnold-Bruening syringe
Arnold-Chiari malformation
Arnold nerve
AROM
    active range of motion
AROSupercut scissors
ARP
    abbreviated rapid processing
arrangement
    tooth a.
array
    electrode a.
arrested dental caries
arresting consonant
arrhizus
    Rhizopus a.
arrow
    a. blade
    a. clasp
ARROWgard central venous catheter
arrowhead clasp
arrow-point
    a.-p. tracer
    a.-p. tracing
arrowroot
arsenic
Artecoll
arterial
    a. flap
    a. hemorrhage
    a. loop
    a. plexus
arterialized flap
arteriography

arteriole
>2° feeding a.
>main a. (MA)
>terminal a. (TA)

arterioplasty
arteriorrhaphy
arteriosclerosis
arteriovenous (AV)
>a. anastomosis (AVA)
>a. fistula (AVF)
>a. hemangioma
>a. malformation (AVM)
>a. shunt
>a. shunting

arteritis
>cranial a.
>giant cell a.
>temporal a.

artery
>alveolar a.
>angular a.
>angular nasal a.
>anterior ethmoidal a.
>anterior inferior cerebellar a.
>anterior tympanic a.
>ascending palatine a.
>ascending pharyngeal a.
>auditory a.
>auricular a.
>auriculotemporal a.
>axillary a.
>basilar a.
>buccal a.
>buccinator a.
>caroticotympanic a.
>carotid a.
>circumflex iliac a.
>circumflex scapular a.
>closed disruption of digital a.
>cochlear a.
>common carotid a.
>cricothyroid a.
>cubital a.
>deep inferior epigastric a.
>dental a.
>descending palatine a. (DPA)
>dorsalis pedis a.
>dorsal lingual a.
>a. of Drummond
>ectatic vertebral a.
>epigastric a.
>ethmoidal a.

external carotid a. (ECA)
facial a.
first dorsal metatarsal a. (FDMA)
frontal a.
gastroepiploic a.
greater palatine a.
inferior laryngeal a.
inferior thyroid a.
inferior tympanic a.
infrahyoid a.
infraorbital a.
innominate a.
intercostal a.
interdental a.
internal auditory a.
internal carotid a. (ICA)
internal maxillary a.
interradicular a.
labial a.
labyrinthine a.
laryngeal a.
lateral tarsal a.
lesser palatine a.
lingual a.
mammary a.
mandibular a.
masseteric a.
maxillary a.
medullary a.
meningeal a.
mental a.
middle meningeal a.
nasal a.
nasal accessory a.
occipital a.
ophthalmic a.
palatine a.
palpebral a.
perforating alveolar a.
petrosal a.
pharyngeal a.
postauricular a.
posterior auricular a.
posterior ethmoidal a.
posterior inferior cerebellar a.
>(PICA)
posterior palatine a.
posterior septal a.
posterior superior alveolar a.
posterior tympanic a.
posterolateral nasal a.
profunda femoris a. (PFA)

NOTES

artery *(continued)*
 radial a.
 ranine a.
 retroauricular a.
 septal a.
 sphenopalatine a.
 spiral a.
 stapedial a.
 stylomandibular a.
 stylomastoid a.
 sublingual a.
 submental a.
 subscapular a.
 superficial petrosal a.
 superficial temporal a.
 superior alveolar a.
 superior auricular a.
 superior laryngeal a.
 superior pharyngeal a.
 superior thyroid a.
 superior tympanic a.
 supratrochlear a.
 temporal a.
 thoracoacromial a.
 thoracodorsal a.
 thyroid a.
 thyroid ima a.
 tonsillar a.
 transnasal ligation of internal
  maxillary a.
 transverse cervical a.
 transverse facial a.
 trigeminal a.
 tympanic a.
 vertebral a.
 vestibulocochlear a.
 vidian a.
artery-nerve conflict
Artha-G
arthralgia
 temporomandibular a.
arthritis, pl. arthritides
 acute infectious arthritides
 A. Foundation Pain Reliever
 A. Foundation Pain Reliever,
  Aspirin Free
 rheumatic a.
 rheumatoid a.
arthrocentesis
arthrodentosteodysplasia (ADOD)
arthrodesis
 cricoarytenoid a.
 joint a.
 Sauve Kapandji a.
arthrogram
arthrography
arthrogryposis
 a. multiplex congenita (AMC)

Arthropan
arthropathy
 Charcot a.
arthroplastic implant
arthroplasty
 interpositional gap a.
 intracapsular temporomandibular
  joint a.
arthroscopic lysis and lavage
arthroscopy
 dual-port a.
 temporomandibular a.
arthrosis, pl. arthroses
 septic arthroses
 temporomandibular a.
arthrotomographic image
Arthur Adaptation of the Leiter
 International Performance Scale
artichoke
articular
 a. disk
 a. eminence
 a. eminence of temporal bone
 a. fossa of mandible
 a. surface of mandibular fossa
 a. tubercle
 a. tubercle of temporal bone
articulare
articulate
articulated
 a. chin prosthesis
 a. partial denture
articulating paper
articulation
 a. area
 articulator a.
 Assessment Link Between
  Phonology and A.
 balanced a.
 Bryngelson-Glaspey Test of A.
 compensatory a.
 confluent a.
 cranial coronal ring a.
 a. curve
 Deep Test of A.
 dental a.
 deviant a.
 a. disorder
 a. error
 external ligament of mandibular a.
 external ligament of
  temporomandibular a.
 Goldman-Fristoe Test of A.
 a. index
 lateral ligament of
  temporomandibular a.
 mandibular a.
 place of a.

point of a.
Predictive Screening Test of A.
a. programming
scapholunate a.
Screening Deep Test of A.
secondary a.
Templin-Darley Tests of A.
temporomandibular joint a.
a. test
vomerosphenoidal a.
articulation-gain function
articulation-resonance
articulator
Acme a.
adjustable a.
Arcon semiadjustable a.
a. articulation
Balkwell a.
Bergström a.
Bonwill a.
Christensen a.
complex a.
Denar a.
dental a.
Dentatus a.
Evans a.
Gariot a.
Granger a.
Gysi a.
Hanau 130-21 a.
hinge a.
Ney a.
non-arcon a.
plain-line a.
semi-adjustable a.
Stuart a.
Walker a.
Whip-Mix a.
articulatory
a. basis
a. phonetics
a. specified neutral reference
Articulose-50 Injection
articulostat
artifact
background a.
trigeminal nerve a.
artificial
a. classification cavity
a. crown
a. dentition
a. ear

a. fistulation
a. larynx
a. mastoid
a. method
a. root
a. saliva
a. sound generator
a. sphincter
a. tears
a. tooth
a. vagina
a. velum
artifistulation
Artista II Tempera paint
artistic biases
ARV
AIDS-related virus
aryepiglottic
a. fascia
a. fold
a. muscle
arylhydrocarbon hydroxylase (AHH)
arylsulfatase
arytenoid
a. cartilage
a. muscle
a. perichondritis
arytenoidectomy
arytenoiditis
arytenoidopexy
AS
auris sinister
A.S.
Crysticillin A.S.
ASA
acetylsalicylic acid
Adaptive Speech Alignment
Lortab ASA
A.S.A.
asapholalia
asbestos
a. liner
ascending
a. palatine artery
a. pharyngeal artery
a. pitch break
a. process
a. ramus
a. ramus of the mandible
a. technique
a. technique audiometry
Ascher syndrome

NOTES

Asclepias tuberosa
ascorbate
    sodium a.
ascorbic acid
Ascorbicap
Ascriptin
asemasia, asemia
asepsis
aseptic
    a. necrosis
    a. technique
ash
    Arizona a.
    A. forceps
    green a.
    Oregon a.
    white a.
Asher high-pull face-bow
Asian ginseng
ASIS
    anterior superior iliac spine
ASL
    American Sign Language
as low as reasonably achievable (ALARA)
Asnis 2 guided screw
ASP
    automatic signal processing
asparagus
A-Spas S/L
aspect
    buccal a.
    inferomedial a.
    linguistic a.
    speech a.
aspen
aspera
    linea a.
aspergillosis
Aspergillus
    A. *flavus*
    A. *fumigatus*
    A. *niger*
    A. otomastoiditis
asphyxia
aspirate
    adipo a.
aspiration
    a. biopsy cytology
    a. cannula
    fine-needle a. (FNA)
    foreign body a.
    lipoma a.
    needle a.
    permucosal needle a.
    suction a.
    a. tube

aspirator
    Accelerator II a.
    Cavitron ultrasonic surgical a.
    dental a.
    Frazier a.
    Frazier suction tip a.
    General A. Q
    Hu-Friedy suction tip a.
    A. II+
    A. III
    LySonix 250 a.
    suction a.
    surgical a.
    ultrasonic surgical a.
    ULTRA ultrasonic a.
aspirin
    Bayer Buffered A.
    carisoprodol and a.
    a. and codeine
    Extra Strength Bayer Enteric 500 A.
    hydrocodone and a.
    methocarbamol and a.
    oxycodone and a.
    propoxyphene and a.
    Regular Strength Bayer Enteric 500 A.
    St Joseph Adult Chewable A.
Aspirin Free Anacin Maximum Strength
Aspirin-Free Bayer Select Allergy Sinus Caplets
asplenia
A-splint
Asprimox
ASPS
    alveolar soft part sarcoma
assay
    enzyme-linked immunosorbent a. (ELISA)
    Maximal Static Response A. (MSRA)
assembly
    malleostapedial a.
    malleus-footplate a.
    malleus-stapes a.
assessment
    A. of Children's Language Comprehension (ACLC)
    Compton-Hutton Phonological A.
    developmental a.
    A. of Intelligibility of Dysarthric Speech
    Interpersonal Language Skills and A. (ILSA)
    A. Link Between Phonology and Articulation
    metalinguistic a.

Performance A. of Syntax Elicited and Spontaneous (PASES)
A. of Phonological Processes
System of Multicultural A. (SOMA)
System of Multicultural Pluralistic A. (SOMPA)
Assess peak flowmeter
Assézat triangle
ASSI
Accurate Surgical & Scientific Instruments
ASSI breast dissector angulated
ASSI breast dissector spatulated
ASSI forceps
ASSI nasal and sinus instruments
ASSI Polar-Mate bipolar coagulator
ASSI Super-Cut scissors
assimilated nasality
assimilation
alveolar a.
double a.
labial a.
nasal a.
a. phonological process
progressive vowel a.
reciprocal a.
regressive a.
velar a.
assistant
extended function dental a. (EFDA)
Registered Dental A. (RDA)
assistive
a. listening device (ALD)
a. technology device
association
auditory-vocal a.
CHARGE a.
sound-symbol a.
associative aphasia
assonance
AST
alcohol sniff test
Astelin
A. nasal spray
astemizole
astereognosis
asteroid body
asteroides
Nocardia a.
asthenopia

asthma
bronchial a.
Millar a.
asthmatoid wheeze
astomia
Aston
A. cartilage reduction system
A. nasal retractor
A. submental retractor
Astra
A. dental cartridge
A. Tech dental implant
Astramorph PF Injection
astringent
a. mouthwash
asymmetric maxillomandibular growth
asymmetry
facial a.
forehead a.
gingival a.
olfaction and sensory a.
tumofactive a.
asynergic
asynergy, asynergia
Atarax
ataxia
Friedreich a.
ataxic
a. dysarthria
a. and spastic dysarthria
ataxiophemia
atelectasis
atelectatic otitis
Atgam
athetosis
athetotic
athymic
atlantoaxial
a. instability
a. subluxation
ATL-HDL color flow Doppler scanner
Atolone
atomic absorption spectrophotometry
atonia
atopic
a. dermatitis
a. rhinitis
ATP
adenosine triphosphate
atraumatic
a. bowel clamp
a. needle

NOTES

atresia
    aural a.
    bony a.
    choanal a.
    esophageal a.
    laryngeal a.
    meatal a.
    oral a.
    a. plate
    tracheal a.
    vaginal a.
atretic outflow tract
Atrisorb bioabsorbable barrier
Atrohist Plus
Atropa belladonna
Atropair
atrophic
    a. facial acne scar
    a. glossitis
    a. lichen planus
    a. pharyngitis
    a. pulp
    a. pulposus
    a. rhinitis
    a. scar
    a. senile gingivitis
    a. ulatrophy
atrophied
    a. papilla
atrophy
    alveolar a.
    dermal a.
    diffuse alveolar a.
    gingival a.
    glandular a.
    hemifacial a.
    horizontal a.
    myofiber a.
    periodontal a.
    precocious advanced alveolar a.
    presenile a.
    pressure a.
    progressive hemifacial a.
    pulp a.
    reticular pulp a.
    Romberg hemifacial a.
    senile a.
    spinal muscular a. (SMA)
atropine
    A.-Care
    Isopto A.
    a. sulfate
atropinoid
Atropisol
Atrovent
A/T/S Topical
attached
    a. cementicle

    a. cranial section
    a. craniotomy
    a. denticle
    a. gingiva
    a. gingiva extension
    a. gingival cuff
    a. island
attaching material implant
superstructure
attachment
    abnormal frenulum a.
    abnormal frenum a.
    Alexander a.
    a. apparatus
    ball-and-socket a.
    Ballard stress equalizer a.
    bar a.
    bar clip a.
    bar-sleeve a.
    Bowles multiphase a.
    Ceka a.
    Chayes a.
    C & L a.
    Clark a.
    Closed Chain Exercise A.
    C & M 637 a.
    Conex a.
    Crismani a.
    CSP a.
    Cu-Sil a.
    a. cuticle
    Dalbo extracoronal a.
    Dalbo stud a.
    Dalla Bona a.
    Dolder bar joint a.
    dowel rest a.
    edgewise a.
    epithelial a.
    a. epithelium
    extracoronal a.
    friction a.
    Gerber a.
    gingival a.
    Gottlieb epithelial a.
    Hade-ring a.
    Hart-Dunn a.
    high frenum a.
    Hruska a.
    a. implant superstructure
    implant superstructure a.
    internal a.
    intracoronal a.
    Ipsoclip a.
    key a.
    key-and-keyway a.
    keyway a.
    lingual a.
    McCollum a.

A

multiphase a.
Neurohr spring-lock a.
O-ring a.'s
orthodontic a.
parallel a.
pericemental a.
Pin-Dalbo a.
pinledge a.
a. plaque
precision a.
Pressomatic a.
projection a.
ribbon arch a.
Roach a.
Roach ball precision a.
Rothermann a.
Schatzmann a.
Schubiger a.
Scott a.
semiprecision a.
Sherer a.
slotted a.
Stabilex a.
Steiger a.
Steiger-Boitel a.
Stern a.
Stern G/A a.
Stern gingival latch a.
Stern G/L a.
Stern stress-breaker a.
stress-breaker a.
stud a.
superstructure a.
Tach-E-Z a.
Tasserit shoulder a.
twin-wire a.
universal orthodontic a.
Zest anchor system a.
attack
glottal a.
hard glottal a.
transient ischemic a. (TIA)
vocal a.
attention
auditory a.
a. deficit disorder (ADD)
a. deficit hyperactivity disorder (ADHD)
Flowers Test of Auditory Selective A.
a. span
attenuated media raphe

attenuation
interaural a.
attenuator
attenutation number
attical cholesteatoma
atticotomy
attribute-entity
attrition
attritional occlusion
A-type reamer
atypia
cytologic a.
epithelial a.
melanocytic a.
atypical
a. articulatory contact
a. carcinoid tumor
a. cleft
a. facial neuralgia
a. gingivitis
a. gingivostomatitis
a. mycobacterium
AU
auris uterque
Auclair operation
AuD
doctorate of audiology
audibility threshold
audible
a. range
audile
auding
audioanalgesia
audiogenic
audiogram
a. configuration
pure tone a.
speech a.
audiologic
a. habilitation
audiological evaluation
audiologist
audiology
clinical a.
diagnostic a.
doctorate of a. (AuD)
educational a.
experimental a.
geriatric a.
pediatric a.
rehabilitative a.

NOTES

audiometer
> automatic a.
> Békésy a.
> Crib-O-Gram a.
> group a.
> GSI 16 a.
> limited range a.
> Madsen OB822 clinical a.
> narrow range a.
> pure-tone a.
> Rudmose a.
> speech a.
> wide range a.

audiometric
> a. brainstem response (ABR)
> a. test
> a. zero

audiometrist

audiometry
> ABR a.
> ascending technique a.
> auditory brainstem response a.
> automatic a.
> average evoked response a. (AERA)
> BAER a.
> behavioral observation a. (BOA)
> Békésy a.
> brainstem auditory evoked response a.
> brainstem evoked response a.
> brief tone a. (BTA)
> BSER a.
> CAER a.
> cardiac evoked response a. (CERA)
> conditioned orientation reflex a.
> COR a.
> cortical auditory evoked response a.
> delayed feedback a. (DFA)
> descending technique a.
> diagnostic a.
> Doppler a.
> electric response a. (ERA)
> electrodermal a. (EDA)
> electrodermal response test a. (EDRA)
> electroencephalic a. (EEA)
> electroencephalic response a. (ERA)
> electrophysiologic a.
> evoked response a. (ERA)
> galvanic skin response a. (GSRA)
> group a.
> high-frequency a.
> identification a.
> impedance a.
> industrial a.
> LAER a.

> late auditory evoked response a.
> live voice a.
> monitored live voice a.
> monitoring a.
> play a.
> psychogalvanic skin response a. (PGSRA)
> pure-tone a.
> reduced screening a.
> screening a.
> speech a.
> tangible reinforcement of operant conditioned a. (TROCA)
> threshold a.
> Visual Reinforcement A.
> Weber a.

audiovisual

audition
> chromatic a.

audito-oculogyric reflex

auditory
> a. acuity
> a. adaptation
> a. agnosia
> a. alexia
> a. analysis
> A. Analysis Test
> a. aphasia
> a. area
> a. artery
> a. attention
> a. blending
> a. brain mapping
> a. brainstem implant (ABI)
> a. brainstem response (ABR)
> a. brainstem response audiometry
> a. brainstem response test
> a. canal
> a. closure
> a. comprehension
> a. comprehension impairment
> a. cortex
> a. cue
> a. differentiation
> a. discrimination
> a. discrimination test
> a. disorder
> a. evoked potential
> a. evoked response
> a. fatigue
> a. feedback
> a. field
> a. figure-ground
> a. figure-ground discrimination
> a. flutter
> a. flutter fusion
> a. function
> a. imperception

a. localization
a. memory
a. memory span
a. method
a. middle latency response
a. modality
a. nerve
a. oculogyric reflex
a. oculogyric response
a. ossicle
a. pathway
a. pattern
a. perception
a. phonetics
A. Pointing Test
a. process
a. processing disorder
a. selective listening
a. sequencing
a. skill
a. synthesis
a. teeth
a. threshold
a. training
a. training units
a. tube
a. vein
a. verbal agnosia
a. vertigo
auditory-vocal
a.-v. association
a.-v. automaticity
Aufrecht
A. point
A. sign
augmentation
alloplastic a.
alloplastic chin a.
alveolar ridge a.
autologous a.
breast a.
calf a.
camouflage a.
cheek a.
chin a.
connective tissue a.
Farrior graft a.
Fomon graft a.
a. genioplasty
gingival a.
Gore-Tex lip a.
a. graft

Hogan and Converse graft a.
hydroxyapatite ridge a.
lip a.
Longacre graft a.
malar alloplastic a.
malar facial a.
malar shell a.
a. mammaplasty
a. of the mandibular angle (AMA)
mastopexy-breast a.
midface alloplastic a.
Millard graft a.
Musgrave and Dupertuis graft a.
permanent lip a.
PermaRidge alveolar ridge a.
pharyngeal wall a.
premandible alloplastic a.
premandibular a.
preprosthetic a.
ridge a.
silicone lip a.
subantral a.
subglandular a.
submandibular a.
subpectoral a.
temporary lip a.
transaxillary breast a.
vocal fold a.
augmentation/mastopexy
augmentative
a. and alternative communication (AAC)
a. communication
a. communication device
a. communication system
augmented feedback
Augmentin
augnathus
aura
Aurafil resin
aural
a. atresia
a. fullness
a. myiasis
a. pressure
a. rehabilitation
a. vertigo
Auralgan
aural-oral technique
Aureobasidium
Aureomycin
A. ointment

NOTES

aures (*pl. of* auris)
aureus
    methicillin-resistant
      Staphylococcus a. (MRSA)
    Staphylococcus a.
auricle
    supernumerary a.
auricula, gen. and pl. **auriculae**
    concha auriculae
auricular
    a. appendage
    a. artery
    a. cartilage
    a. cartilage graft
    a. composite graft
    a. muscle
    a. nerve
    a. point
    a. prosthesis
    a. reflex
    a. repositioning
    a. trauma
    a. tubercule
auriculare, pl. **auricularia**
auriculocephalic angle
auriculoinfraorbital plane
auriculomastoid
    a. angle
    a. area
auriculopalpebral reflex
auriculotemporal
    a. artery
    a. nerve
    a. neuralgia
    a. syndrome
auris, pl. **aures**
    a. dexter (AD)
    incisura terminalis a.
    a. sinister (AS)
    a. uterque (AU)
aurium
    susurrus a.
    tinnitus a.
Auro Ear Drops
Aurolate
auropalpebral
    a. reflex (APR)
Auroto
auscultation
Austin
    A. knife
    A. retractor
    A. Spanish Articulation Test
Australian
    A. pine
    A. Special Plus wire
autism
    infantile a.

    primary a.
    secondary a.
autistic
autoallergic disease
autocastration
autoclave
    a. sterilization
autoclaving
autoclitic operant
auto-cured resin
autocystoplasty
autodermic
    a. graft
autogeneic graft
autogenetic, autogenic
autogenous
    a. bone graft
    a. cartilage graft
    a. composite tissue
    a. corneal protector
    a. corticocancellous graft
    a. fascia lata sling procedure
    a. fat graft
    a. grafting
    a. nerve graft
    a. tooth transplantation
    a. union
autograft
    bone a.
    cultured a.
Autografter
    Ace A.
autografting
autoimmune
    a. disease
    a. hearing loss
    a. inner ear disease
    a. response
    a. sialadenitis
    a. sialopathy
autoimmunity
autoinflate
autoinflation
Autologen
autologous
    a. augmentation
    a. blood
    a. bone
    a. donor
    a. fat
    a. fat graft
    a. fat injection
    a. iliac crest bone graft
    a. implant
    a. rib
    a. rib bone graft
autologous-cultured epithelium (ACE)
autolysis

automallet
automatic
    a. audiometer
    a. audiometry
    a. condenser
    a. gain control
    a. language
    a. plugger
    a. processing
    a. signal processing (ASP)
    a. speech
    a. vibrator
    a. voice analysis
    a. volume control (AVC)
automaticity
    auditory-vocal a.
automatism
automaton
automobile
    a. airbag impulse noise
    a. exhaust
autonomic
    a. control
    a. nervous system
autophagocytosed cellular material
autophony
autoplast
autoplastic
    a. graft
    a. suture
autoplasty
autoplugger
autopolymer
    a. resin
autopolymerizing
    a. acrylic resin
autoradiographic film
autoradiography
autosomal
autosome
autotransplant
autotransplantation
Autovac autotransfusion system
auxiliary
    a. abutment
    a. canal
    a. cone
    dental a.
    expanded duty dental a. (EDDA)
    a. implant rest
    modal a.
    a. occlusal rest

    a. rest implant substructure
    a. spring
    torquing a.
    a. verb
    a. wire
AV
    arteriovenous
    AV fistula
AVA
    arteriovenous anastomosis
available arch length
avascular
    a. necrosis (AVN)
    a. scaphoid necrosis
AVC
    automatic volume control
    AVC Cream
    AVC Suppository
Avellis syndrome
average
    a. evoked response audiometry
    (AERA)
    a. perturbation quotient (APQ)
    preoperative pure tone a.
    pure-tone a. (PTA)
averaging
    signal a.
AVF
    arteriovenous fistula
    transcatheter embolization of AVF
aviation otitis
aviator's ear
avidin-biotin-peroxidase complex (ABC)
avidum
    Propionibacterium a.
Avitene
avium
    Mycobacterium a.
avium-intracellulare **complex**
    Mycobacterium a.-i.
Avlosulfon
AVM
    arteriovenous malformation
    transcatheter embolization of AVM
AVN
    avascular necrosis
avoidance
avoiding zip
avulsed tooth
avulsion
    a. amputation
    a. injury

NOTES

avulsion *(continued)*
    mechanical a.
    a. of portion of finger
    ring a.
    tooth a.
awareness
    speech a.
axes *(pl. of* axis)
axetil
    cefuroxime a.
axial
    a. anchor screw
    a. flap
    a. inclination
    a. line angle
    a. loading
    a. pattern vascularized skin flap
    a. plane
    a. projection
    a. rotation joint
    a. spillway
    a. stress
    a. surface
    a. surface cavity
    a. temporoparietal fascial flap
    a. wall
    a. wall of the pulp chambers
    a. walls of the pulp chamber
axial-based flap
axilla, pl. axillae
    pterygium axillae
axillary
    a. artery
    a. breast tissue
    a. catheter
    a. hidradenitis
    a. hidradenitis suppurativa
    a. node dissection
    a. prolongation
    a. subpectoral approach
    a. tail of Spence
    a. vein
axiobuccal (AB)
axiobuccocervical (ABC)
axiobuccogingival (ABG)
axiobuccolingual (ABL)
    a. plane
axiocervical (AC)
axiodistal (AD)
axiodistocervical (ADC)
axiodistogingival (ADG)
axiodistoincisal (ADI)

axiodisto-occlusal (ADO)
axiogingival (AG)
axioincisal (AI)
axiolabial (ALA, Ala)
axiolabiogingival (ALAG, ALaG)
axiolabiolingual (ALAL, ALaL)
    a. plane
axiolingual (AL)
axiolinguocervical (ALC)
axiolinguogingival (ALG)
axiolinguo-occlusal (ALO)
Axiom
    A. drain
axiomesial (AM)
axiomesiocervical (AMC)
axiomesiodistal (AMD)
    a. plane
axiomesiogingival (AMG)
axiomesioincisal (AMI)
axiomesio-occlusal (AMO)
axio-occlusal (AO)
axiopulpal (AP)
axioversion
axis, pl. axes
    beam rotation a.
    central neuronal a.
    condylar a.
    hinge a.
    long a.
    mandibular a.
    neutral a. of straight beam
    opening a.
    orthogonal a.
    ring finger a.
    rotational a.
    sagittal a.
    subscapular a.
    Tessier cleft a.
    tooth of a.
    transverse horizontal a.
    vertical a.
    Y a.
axolemma
axon
    a. crossover
    myelinated a.
    nonmyelinated a.
    a. regeneration
    a. terminal
axonal sprouting
axoneme
axonotmesis
axonotmetic injury
axon-to-axon contact
axoplasmic prolapse
Axostim
Aygestin
Ayurveda philosophy

Ayurvedic total wellness
azatadine
    a. and pseudoephedrine
azathioprine
Azdone
azelaic
    a. acid
    a. acid cream
azelastine HCl

Azelex
    A. cream
azidothymidine (AZT)
azithromycin
AZT
    azidothymidine
Aztec ear
Azzolini technique

NOTES

β (*var. of* beta)
B
    bone
        B cell
        B fiber
        B lymphocyte
        B point
B1
    bifurcation of root
B-1, B-2 reamer
BA
    buccoaxial
Babbitt metal
babble
    vowel-to-consonant b.
babbled speech
babbling
    canonical b.
    nonreduplicated b.
    reduplicated b.
    social b.
Babcock
    Endo-grasper by B.
    B. Endo-grasper
Babee Teething
Babinski reflex
baby
    b. bottle syndrome
    b. bottle tooth decay
    b. talk
    b. tooth
BAC
    buccoaxiocervical
bacampicillin
Bachelor
    B. of Dental Science (BDSc)
    B. of Dental Surgery (BDS)
Baciguent Topical
bacille
    B. bilié de Calmette-Guérin (BCG)
    B. Calmette-Guérin vaccine
Bacillus
    B. fusiformis
    B. stearothermophilus spore
    B. subtilis spore
bacillus, pl. bacilli
    b. Calmette-Guérin (BCG)
    tubercle b.
    von Frisch b.
bacitracin
    b. irrigation
    b., neomycin, and polymyxin B
    b., neomycin, polymyxin B, and hydrocortisone
    b., neomycin, polymyxin B, and lidocaine

    b. ointment
    b. and polymyxin B
bacitracin,
back
    b. consonant
    b. cut incision
    b. phoneme
    b. table
    b. teeth
    b. vowel
back-action
    b.-a. clasp
    b.-a. condenser
    b.-a. plugger
back-and-forth septoplasty
backbiting
    b. bone punch
    b. forceps
back-filing
background
    b. artifact
    b. noise
    b. radiation
Backhaus towel clip
backing
    alloy b.
    b. to velar
backplug
backward
    b. caries
    b. coarticulation
    b. masking
    b. position
backward-biting ostrum punch
BacStop checkvalve
bacteremia
    transient b.
bacteria
    aerobic b.
    anaerobic b.
    black-pigmented b. (BPB)
    coccoid b.
    gram-positive b.
    vegetative b.
bacterial
    b. aerosol
    b. culture
    b. endocarditis
    b. filter
    b. flora
    b. infection
    b. keratoconjunctivitis
    b. meningitis
    b. plaque

B

bacterial *(continued)*
    b. pseudomycosis
    b. sialadenitis
bactericidal
bacteriolytic action
bacteriosis
    granular b.
bacteriostatic
Bacteroides
    B. endodontalis
    B. forsythus
    B. fucci
    B. gingivalis
    B. intermedius
    B. melaninogenicus
    B. oralis
Bactocill
BactoShield Topical
Bactrim
    B. DS
Bactroban
BADGE
    Békésy Ascending-Descending Gap
    Evaluation
badge
    film b.
    radiation film b.
**Baek musculocutaneous pedicle
technique**
BAEP
    brainstem auditory evoked potential
BAER
    brainstem auditory evoked response
    BAER audiometry
BAG
    buccoaxiogingival
bag
    B. Balm
    cheek b.
    malar b.
    Politzer b.
    trauma induced saddle b.
bag-gel implant
BAHA
    bone-anchored hearing aid
Bahia grass
Baillarger syndrome
Bailyn classification
**Baird Electric System 5000 Power Plus
electrosurgical unit**
Bair Hugger patient warming blanket
Bakamjian flap
baked porcelain
Baker
    B. anchorage
    B. capsular contracture
    B. class IV contracture
    B. composite graft

    B. grade
    B. inlay
    B. P&S Topical
    B. self-sumping tube
    B. velum
balance
    alternate binaural loudness b.
    (ABLB)
    alternate monaural loudness b.
    (AMLB)
    binaural alternate loudness b.
    (BALB)
    Clinical Test for Sensory
    Interaction of B.
    b. mechanism
    occlusal b.
    occlusion b.
    spacial b.
    spatial b.
balanced
    b. articulation
    b. bite
    b. force technique
    b. occlusion
    phonetically b. (PB)
    b. salt solution (BSS)
balanced-force instrumentation technique
balancing
    b. contact
    b. occlusal surface
    b. side
    b. side condyle
balanic hypospadias
balanoplasty
BALB
    binaural alternate loudness balance
    BALB test
bald
    b. cypress
    b. tongue
Baldex
baldness
    Juri II, III degree of male
    pattern b.
    male-pattern b.
Balkwell articulator
ball
    Adams b.
    b. burnisher
    fatty b. of Bichat
    b. forceps
    b. and socket joint
ball-and-socket attachment
Ballard stress equalizer attachment
ballistic
    b. energy generator
    b. movement

B

balloon
  Brandt cytology b.
  b. dissection
  endovascular b.
  b. expansion
  nasomaxillary b.
  b. occlusion
  Origin PDB 1000 b.
  b. tamponade
balm
  Bag B.
  lemon b.
  Post Laser B.
balsam
  Canada b.
  b. of Peru
Balshi packer
banana
  b. roll
Bancap HC
band
  b. adapter
  adapter b.
  adjustable orthodontic b.
  anchor b.
  Angle b.
  anterior b.
  apron b.
  b. and bar space maintainer
  Bünger b.
  calciotraumatic b. (CTB)
  copper b.
  b. and crib space maintainer
  critical b.
  fibrous b.
  b. frequency
  Hunter-Schreger b.'s
  iliotibial b.
  incisal b.
  lip furrow b.
  matrix b.
  mentalis b.
  molar b.
  orthodontic b.
  palatoglossal b.
  platysmal b.
  b. pliers
  posterior b.
  preformed b.
  premolar b.
  b. pusher
  b. remover

  sagittal b.
  Schreger b.
  seamless b.
  b. seater
  Simonart b.
  b. spectrum
  b. and spur retainer
  stainless steel b.
  synechial b.
  tourniquet b.
  vocal b.
bandage
  Ace b.
  Barton b.
  Coban b.
  Esmarch b.
  four-tailed b.
  Gibson b.
  Tubi-Grip circumferential elastic b.
bandelette plate
banding
  tooth b.
Band-Lok orthodontic band cement
band-pass filter
band-removing pliers
band-soldering pliers
bandwidth
Banicide
Bank
  The Pacific Coast Tissue B.
banked freeze-dried bone
banking the fork
Bankson Language Screening Test
Banner flap
Banophen
  B. Decongestant Capsule
  B. Oral
Banthine
bar
  Ackerman b.
  Andrews b.
  anterior palatal b.
  arch b.
  b. attachment
  Bill b.
  Brookdale b.
  buccal b.
  b. clasp
  clasp b.
  b. clasp arm
  b. clip attachment
  connector b.

NOTES

bar *(continued)*
>distal terminal b.
>Dolder b.
>double lingual b.
>Dynamic Mesh craniomaxillofacial pre-angled connecting b.
>Erich dental arch b.
>fixable-removable cross arch b.
>Gaerny b.
>Gilson fixable-removable b.
>Goshgarian transpalatal b.
>Hader implant b.
>horseshoe b.
>hyoid b.
>I b.
>Jelenko arch b.
>b. joint
>b. joint denture
>Kazanjian T b.
>Kennedy b.
>labial b.
>lingual b.
>mesostructure b.
>mesostructure conjunction b.
>occlusal rest b.
>palatal b.
>Passavant b.
>retention b.
>RP-I b.
>silver b.
>Steiger-Boitel b.
>terminal b.
>T b. of Kazanjian
>transpalatal b. (TPB)
>Winter arch b.

Bárány
>B. caloric test
>B. chair
>B. sign

barbaralalia
barbed broach
barberry
Barbita
barbiturate
barbula hirci
Barclay-Baron disease
Bardach cleft rhinoplasty
Bard-Parker
>B.-P. blade
>B.-P. handle

barium
>b. sulfate

Barkann technique
Barker-Gordon phenol
barley
Barlow disease
barn dust
barnsdahl wax

baroreceptor
baroreflex dysfunction (BRD)
barosinusitis
barotitis media
barotrauma
>otic b.
>sinus b.

barred tooth
barrel bur
Barrett ulcer
barrier
>antimicrobial b.
>Atrisorb bioabsorbable b.
>histoincompatibility b.
>b. membrane
>b. protection
>space-maintaining b.
>b. technique

Barry Five Slate System
Barsky alar cartilage relocation
bar-sleeve attachment
Bartholin
>B. cyst
>B. duct

Barton bandage
basal
>b. age
>b. arch
>b. bone
>b. bunching suture
>b. cell
>b. cell adenoma
>b. cell carcinoma (BCC)
>b. cell nevus syndrome
>b. fluency
>b. ganglion
>b. infolding
>b. lamella
>b. lamina
>b. layer
>b. mandibular angle
>b. pitch
>b. ridge
>b. seat
>b. seat area
>b. seat outline
>b. surface
>b. surface of denture
>b. turn cochlea

basale
>stratum b.

basaloid
>b. monomorphic adenoma (BMA)
>b. tumor

base
>acrylic resin b.
>alar b.
>anterior skull b.

apical b.
cavity preparation b.
cement b.
cheoplastic b.
b. component
denture b.
extension b.
b. of flap
b. former
free-end b.
high-strength b.
intermediary b.
low-strength b.
mandibular b.
b. material
metal b.
b. metal alloy
b. metal crown and bridge alloy
occult malformation of the skull b.
osteomyelitis of the skull b.
b. paste
b. plane
plastic b.
b. plate
Plexiglas b.
polyether rubber b.
polysulfide rubber b.
processed denture b.
record b.
b. rule
saddle connector b.
saddle denture b.
shellac b.
silicone rubber b.
skull b.
sprue b.
stabilized b.
b. structure
temporary b.
tinted denture b.
tissue-supported b.
tissue-tissue-supported b.
b. of tongue (BOT)
tooth-borne b.
trial b.
b. word
Basedow disease
baseline
basement
    b. membrane
    b. membrane zone
    b. membrane zone injury

baseplate
    gutta-percha b.
    b. material
    permanent b.
    stabilized b.
    b. wax
basialveolar length
basic
    B. Concept Inventory
    b. fibroblastic growth factor (bFGF)
    B. Language Concepts Test
    b. plate
    b. skill
basicranial sagittal growth
basilar
    b. artery
    b. artery aneurysm
    b. artery migraine
    b. impression
    b. index
    b. kyphosis
    b. membrane
    b. pit
    b. prognathism
basilect
basin
    catch b.
basion
basis
    articulatory b.
basket crown
basophilic concretion
basosquamous carcinoma (BSC)
Bass
    B. brush
    B. method
    B. method of toothbrushing
    B. technique
    B. toothbrush
Bassen-Kornzweig syndrome
basting suture
BAT
    bilateral advancement transposition
    BAT procedure
bat
    b. ear correction
Bates decision
batten
    lateral b.
battered buttock syndrome

B

NOTES

battery
>Activair b.
>Children's Language B.
>Duracell Activair hearing aid b.
>Environmental Pre-language B.
>Goldman-Fristoe-Woodcock Auditory Skills B.
>Panasonic hearing aid b.
>Renata b.
>Right Hemisphere Language B. (RHLB)
>test b.
>vocal capability b.
>Western Aphasia B. (WAB)
>Woodcock Language Proficiency B., English Form

batting
>Dacron b.

Battle sign
Batt tip
Baudens wiring
Bauer retractor
Bauhin gland
Baume classification
Baumgartner needle holder
Bauschinger effect
Baxter
>B. method of burn treatment
>B. V. Mueller laparoscopic instrumentation

bayberry
Bayer
>B. Buffered Aspirin
>B. Low Adult Strength
>B. Select Chest Cold Caplets
>B. Select Head Cold Caplets
>B. Select Pain Relief Formula

Bayley Scales of Infant Development
bayonet
>b. canal
>b. condenser
>b. curve
>b. root tip forceps

bayonet-curved canal
Bazex syndrome
BC
>Bilhaut-Cloquet
>bone conduction
>buccal cusp
>buccocervical
>>BC procedure

BCA
>bicinchoninic acid

BCC
>basal cell carcinoma

BCG
>Bacille bilié de Calmette-Guérin
>bacillus Calmette-Guérin

BCG-itis
BCHA
>bone conduction hearing aid

BCI
>blunt carotid injury

BCL
>Békésy comfortable loudness

BCR
>buccal cervical ridge

BD
>behavior disorder
>brain dysfunction
>buccodistal

B-D
>B.-D. gun
>B.-D. Luer syringe

BDG
>buccal developmental groove

BDS
>Bachelor of Dental Surgery

BDSc
>Bachelor of Dental Science

bead
>hydropolymer b.'s
>hydroxyapatite b.
>b. sterilizer
>b. technique filling

beading
beak
>cutaneous polly b.
>fibrous polly b.
>polly b.

beam
>b. aligning holder
>b. alignment
>cantilever b.
>CO_2 b.
>continuous b.
>electron b.
>helium neon b.
>HeNe b.
>neutral axis of straight b.
>restrained b.
>b. rotation axis
>simple b.
>b. size
>b. splitter
>x-ray b.

bean
>castor b.
>green b.
>green coffee b.
>kidney b.
>lima b.

navy b.
string b.

BEAR
brainstem evoked auditory response
bearberry
bearing
central b.
Beaver miniblade
beaver-tail
b.-t. burnisher
b.-t. retractor
becaplermin
Bechterew nucleus
Becker
B. accelerator
B. dissector cannula
B. flat dissector tip
B. Greater Grater dissecting cannula
B. implant
B. nevus
B. round dissector tip
B. scissors
B. tip
B. twist dissector tip
B. vibrating cannula system
Becker-Parkin pliers
Beckwith-Wiedemann syndrome
beclomethasone
b. dipropionate
b. dipropionate, monohydrate
Beconase AQ Nasal Inhaler
bed
Fluid-Air Plus b.
granular b.
Kinn-Air b.
nail b.
pigmented lesion of nail b.
thyroid b.
Bednar aphthae
Bedside Evaluation and Screening Test of Aphasia
bee
sweat b.
b. venom
beech
Beechwood pellet
beef
beefy tongue
Beepen-VK
Beer law
beeswax

beet
sugar b.
b. tongue
Begg
B. fixed orthodontic appliance
B. light wire appliance
B. light wire differential force technique
B. paralleling
B. slots
B. straight-wire combination bracket
B. theory
B. torquing
behavior
abusive vocal b.
adaptive b.
anticipatory b.
b. disorder (BD)
incompatible b.
b. modification
operant b.
phonological b.
social b.
terminal b.
behavioral
b. criterion
b. objective
b. observation audiometry (BOA)
b. semantics
behaviorism
Behçet
B. disease
B. syndrome
behind-the-ear (BTE)
b.-t.-e. listening device
Békésy
B. Ascending-Descending Gap Evaluation (BADGE)
B. audiometer
B. audiometry
B. comfortable loudness (BCL)
B. Forward-Reverse Tracing
B. tracing type
bel
belch
Belgium ultrasound (B.U.S.)
Belix Oral
BELL
Benelli-Eng-Little
BELL flap
Bell
B. palsy

B

NOTES

Bell *(continued)*
    B. phenomenon
    B. reflex
    B. Visible Speech
bell
    b. crown
    b. flap
    b. flap nipple reconstruction
    b. stage
belladonna
    b. and opium
    b., phenobarbital, and ergotamine
    tartrate
    phenobarbital with b.
bell-crowned
Bellergal
    B.-S
bellows
    chest b.
bell-shaped
    b.-s. crown
    b.-s. curve
Bellugi-Klima Language Comprehension
    Test
belly
    muscle b.
    posterior b.
below-knee amputation
Bel-Phen-Ergot S
belt
    compression b.
Bemis suction canister
Benadryl
    B. Decongestant Allergy Tablet
    B. Injection
    B. Oral
Ben-Allergin-50 Injection
bend
    anchorage b.
    first order b.
    second order b.
    third order b.
    V b.
Bendick polish
bending
Benefit denture adhesive
Benelli-Eng-Little (BELL)
Benelli technique
benign
    b. cellular blue nevus
    b. cementoblastoma
    b. chondroma
    b. cystic teratoma
    b. epidermal pigmented lesion
    b. epithelial neoplasm
    b. epithelial odontogenic tumor
    b. fibroosseous process
    b. fibrous histiocytoma

    b. intracranial hypertension
    b. intraepithelial dyskeratosis
    b. lipoblastoma
    b. lipoblastomatosis
    b. lymphoepithelial lesion (BLL)
    b. mesenchymal neoplasm
    b. mesenchymal tumor
    b. migratory glossitis
    b. mixed tumor
    b. mucous membrane pemphigoid
    (BMMP)
    b. necrotizing otitis externa
    (BNOE)
    b. nevus
    b. paroxysmal positional vertigo
    (BPPV)
    b. paroxysmal postural vertigo
    b. pemphigus
    b. periapical fibroma
    b. positional vertigo (BPV)
    b. triton tumor
Benjamin
    B. binocular slimline laryngoscope
    B. pediatric operating laryngoscope
    B. tube
Benjamin-Havas fiberoptic light clip
Benjamin-Lindholm microsuspension
    laryngoscope
Ben-Jet tube
Bennett
    B. angle
    B. movement
bent film
Benza
benzalkonium chloride
Benzaquen-Chajchir extraction/reinjection
    system
benzathine
    penicillin G b.
Benzedrex
benzocaine
    antipyrine and b.
    cetylpyridinium and b.
    b., gelatin, pectin, and sodium
    carboxymethylcellulose
    Orabase With B.
Benzocol
Benzodent
Benzoin
benzol-arginine naphthylamide
benzoyl
    b. peroxide
Berberis vulgaris
Bergström articulator
beriberi
Berko Test
Berlin tulip flap

Bermuda
- B. grass
- B. grass antigen
- B. smut

Bernard-Burow technique
Bernoulli
- B. effect
- B. law
- B. principle

Bernstein test
berry
- chaste tree b.
- hawthorn b.
- juniper b.'s
- B. ligament
- B. syndrome

Berry-Talbott Language Test
beryllium
Besnier-Boeck-Schaumann disease
beta, β
- b. fibril
- B. Glucan skin care system
- b. rhythm
- transforming growth factor b. (TGF-β)
- b. wave

Betachron E-R Capsule
betacism
Betadine
- B. First Aid Antibiotics + Moisturizer
- B. 5% Sterile Ophthalmic Prep Solution

Betagan Liquifilm
Betagen
beta-glucuronidase (BG)
betamethasone
Betapen-VK
Betasept
Betatrex
Beta-Val
betaxolol
betel nut abrasion
bethanechol
- b. chloride

Betimol Ophthalmic
Betoptic
- B. S Ophthalmic

Better Hearing Institute
Beuren syndrome
bevel
- cavosurface b.

- chamfer b.
- facial b.
- marginal b.
- reverse b.
- standing b.

beveled septal cartilage
beveling
- b. root

Bexophene
Bezold
- B. abscess
- B. mastoiditis
- B. perforation
- B. sign
- B. symptom
- B. triad

bFGF
- basic fibroblastic growth factor

BG
- beta-glucuronidase
- buccal groove
- buccogingival

BGCF
- buccal groove of central fossa

BHI
BHN
- Brinell hardness number

bias, pl. **biases**
- artistic biases
- cultural biases

Biaxin
bibeveled
- b. cutting instrument
- b. drill

bibliotherapy
bicameral abscess
bicanaled
- b. root

bicanalicular silicone tubes
bicanine
- b. breadth
- b. width

Bichat
- B. fat pad
- fatty ball of B.
- B. fossa
- B. protuberance
- B. tunic

Bicillin
- B. C-R 900/300 Injection
- B. L-A

bicinchoninic acid (BCA)

NOTES

biconcave
  b. washer
Bicon dental implant
biconvex
bicoronal
  b. approach
  b. incision
  b. ridge
  b. scalp flap
  b. subperiosteal approach
bicortical
  b. iliac bone block
  b. superior border screw
BICROS
  bilateral contralateral routing of offside signals
bicuspid
  mandibular b.
  maxillary b.
  b. tooth
bicuspidal
bicuspidate
bicuspidization
bicuspidus
  dens b.
bicuspoid
bicycle ergometer
bidental
bidentate
BIEF
  bilateral inferior epigastric artery flap
Bier block anesthesia
Biermer sign
bifid
  b. epiglottis
  b. nose
  b. tongue
  b. uvula
bifidity
Bifidobacterium bifidum
bifrontal craniotomy
bifurcate
bifurcated canal
bifurcation
  b. involvement
  b. of root (B1)
bigonial
  b. breadth
bijaw
  b. osteotomy
  b. segmental dentoalveolar setback osteotomy
bikini
  disposable b.
  b. incision
bilabial
  b. area
  b. consonant

bilaminar zone
bilateral
  b. abductor paralysis
  b. acoustic neurofibromatosis
  b. adductor paralysis
  b. advancement transposition (BAT)
  b. asymmetric turbinate volume reduction
  b. balanced occlusion
  b. canthopexy
  b. cleft-lip-associated nose
  b. cleft lip and palate
  b. cleft palate
  b. contralateral routing of offside signals (BICROS)
  b. coronal synostosis reoperation
  b. coronoidectomies
  b. distoclusion
  b. fronto-orbital modeling
  b. gluteus maximus transposition
  b. hypesthesia
  b. inferior epigastric artery flap (BIEF)
  b. laryngeal paralysis
  b. malposition
  b. mandibular sagittal split osteotomy
  b. masseteric hypertrophy
  b. McKissock reduction mammaplasty
  b. mesioclusion
  b. neck dissection
  b. partial denture
  b. sagittal split advancement osteotomy (BSSO)
  b. sagittal split osteotomy (BSSO)
  b. temporal neurotomy
  b. vestibular deafferentation
bilberry
bi-leaflet
bi-level chisel
Bilhaut-Cloquet (BC)
BiliBlanket phototherapy system
bilingual
  B. Syntax Measure (BSM)
bilingualism
  active b.
  passive b.
biliptysis
Bill bar
Billeau wax curette
billet
bilobed
  b. transposition flap
bilophodont
Bilson fixable-removable cross arch bar splint
bilumen implant

bimaxillary
- b. dentoalveolar protrusion
- b. prognathism
- b. protrusion
- b. protrusive occlusion
- b. trusion

bimeter gnathodynamometer

Bimler
- B. elastic plate
- B. removable orthodontic appliance
- B. stimulator

bimodal method

bimolar
- b. breadth
- b. width

binangle
- b. chisel

binary
- b. principle

binaural
- b. alternate loudness balance (BALB)
- b. alternate loudness balance test
- b. CROS
- b. fusion
- b. hearing aid
- b. integration
- b. resynthesis
- b. separation
- b. summation

binauralis
- diplacusis b.

binder
- abdominal b.
- Alveoform b.
- Alveograf b.
- compression b.
- Dale abdominal b.
- B. implant
- Orthomatrix b.
- Osteograf b.
- B. syndrome
- Velcro b.

Bing
- B. bridge
- B. Test

Bing-Siebenmann malformation

binocular
- b. loupe
- b. microscopy

bioacoustics

bioactive glass

biobarrier
- b. membrane

BioBarrier membrane guided tissue regeneration system

Biobrane
- B. dressing
- B. sheet
- B. wound covering

bioburden
- denatured b.

Biocef

Biocell
- B. anatomical reconstructive mammary implant
- B. textured silicone
- B. texture implant

biocidal

Biocide

biocompatibility

biocompatible
- b. spacing material

biodegradable polymer scaffold

BioDIMENSIONAL
- B. saline-filled implant
- B. system

Biodine

bioelectric

bioengineering

Bio-Esthetic abutment system

bioexcretable gel

biofeedback
- electromyographic relaxation b.
- laryngeal image b.
- palatographic visual b.
- visual b.

bioflavonoid

bioform porcelain shade

Biogel
- B. Sensor surgical glove
- B. surgeons' gloves

Bio-Gide resorbable barrier membrane

Bioglass
- B. bone substitute material
- B. synthetic bone
- B. synthetic bone graft particulate

biograft
- alveoform b.

BioGran
- B. resorbable synthetic bone graft
- B. synthetic graft

biohazard label

Biohist-LA

NOTES

bioimplant
>DynaGraft b.

biolinguistic theory

biologic
>b. creep of skin
>b. fibrogen adhesive
>b. response modifier
>b. width

biological act

biology
>oral b.

Biolux 521

biomaterial
>polymeric b.

biomechanical
>b. cleansing

biomechanics
>dental b.

BioMedic
>B. MicroEncapsulated retinol cream

BioMend
>B. membrane
>B. periodontal material

biomodulation

Bio-Modulator

Biomox

Bionater

BIONIQ skin care product

Bionix disposable nasal speculum

Bion Tears Solution

BIO-OSS
>B.-O. freeze-dried demineralized bone
>B.-O. maxillofacial bone filler

biophysics
>dental b.

Bioplant
>B. hard tissue replacement synthetic bone
>B. HTR synthetic bone
>B. HTR-24 synthetic bone replacement

Bioplastique
>B. augmentation material
>B. polymer

Bioplate
>B. screw fixation system

bioprogressive technique

biopsy
>core needle b.
>diagnostic excisional b.
>directed fine-needle aspiration b.
>excisional b.
>fine-needle b.
>fine-needle aspiration b. (FNAB)
>FNA b.
>b. forceps
>incisional b.

>needle localization breast b.
>punch b.
>b. punch
>second-look b.
>shave b.
>small incisional b.
>total b.
>transoral open b.
>ultrasound-guided b.
>vertical lip b.
>wide resection b.

Bioquant histomorphometry system

bioresorbability

bioresorbable
>b. guided tissue membrane

bioresorption

Bioseal

Biospan anatomical tissue expander

biosynthetic wound covering

Bio-Tab Oral

biotechnologic method

Bio-Vent implant

Biovert
>B. ceramic implant
>B. implant material

Biozyme-C

B.I.P.
>Breast Implant Protector

bipartite antrum

bipartition
>transcranial facial b.

bipedicled
>b. delay flap
>b. TRAM flap

bipedicle flap

bipennate muscle

bipenniform morphological pattern

biphalangeal thumb

biphase
>external pin fixation, b.
>Hall-Morris b.
>b. pin fixation

biphasic
>b. pin
>b. pin appliance
>b. stridor

Bi-Phasic exfoliator

biplanar forehead lift

bipolar
>b. cautery
>b. cautery dissection tonsillectomy
>b. electrosurgical unit
>b. forceps
>b. neuron

Bipolaris

bipupital plane

Birbeck granule

birch
    red b.
    river b.
bird-beak jaw
bird face
bird-face retrognathism
bird's-eye view
birth
    b. cry
    b. defect
birthmark
    port wine stain b.
    vascular b.
Birt-Hogg-Dube syndrome
biscuit
    b. bite
    hard b.
    high b.
    low b.
    medium b.
    soft b.
biscuit-bake
biscuit-firing
biscuiting
biscuspidized tooth
bisected
    b. angle radiograph
    b. minigraft dilator
bisecting
    b. angle cone position
    b. angle technique
bisecting-the-angle technique
bisensory method
Bisfil M, P
bis-GMA
    bisphenol A-glycidyl methacrylate
    phosponated bis-GMA
    bis-GMA resin
Bishop
    B. collar deformity
    B. retractor
bismuth
    b. gingivitis
    b. gingivostomatitis
    b. ingestion
    b. line
    b. pigmentation
    b. subgallate
bisphenol
    b. A glycidyl dimethacrylate
    b. A-glycidyl methacrylate (bis-GMA)

bisque
    hard b.
    soft b.
bisque-baked prosthesis
bistoury
bisyllable
bisymmetry
    airflow b.
bite
    b. analysis
    balanced b.
    biscuit b.
    b. block
    close b.
    closed b.
    compound open b.
    cross b.
    deep b.
    dual b.
    edge-to-edge b.
    end-to-end b.
    b. force
    b. force measurement
    b. force transducer
    b. fork
    b. gauge
    b. guard
    jumping the b.
    locked b.
    mature b.
    mush b.
    normal b.
    open b.
    phasic b.
    pitviper b.
    b. plane
    b. plane therapy
    b. plate
    posterior open b.
    raising b.
    b. registration wax
    rest b.
    b. rim
    scissors b.
    skeletal deep b.
    skeletal open b.
    b. stick
    Sunday b.
    tonic b.
    underhung b.
    unsustained b.
    wax b.

B

NOTES

bite *(continued)*
    working b.
    X-b.
biteblock, bite-block
bitegauge
bitelock
bitemporal
    b. bossing
    b. width
biteplate, bite plate
bite-rim
bitewing, bite-wing
    b. film
    b. intraoral radiography
    b. loop
    b. radiograph
    b. technique
bithermal-caloric test
biting
    cheek b.
    b. force
    lip b.
    b. pressure
    b. strength
    tongue b.
bitter dock
bivalve nasal splint implant
Bivona-Colorado voice prosthesis
bizarre
    b. giant-cell appearance
Bjork
    B. flap tracheostomy
    B. polygon
Björnstad syndrome
BL
    buccolingual
black
    b. ant
    B. classification
    b. cohosh
    b. copper cement
    b. dentin
    B. English
    b. eschar
    b. fly
    B. formula
    b. hairy tongue
    b. hatchet
    b. locust
    b. mulberry
    b. pepper
    B. retractor
    b. stain
    b. stone
    b. tongue
    b. walnut
    B. wiring

blackberry
black-pigmented bacteria (BPB)
bladder
    gel-filled b.
    b. mucosa
bladderwrack
blade
    arrow b.
    Bard-Parker b.
    carving b.
    EDGE coated b.
    endosteal implant b.
    b. endosteal implant
    jigsaw b.
    lancet b.
    Lite b.
    Otocap myringotomy b.
    Personna prep b.'s
    ramus b.
    Rubin b.
    scalpel b.
    scapular b.
    Sharpoint b.
    Sharptome crescent b.
    sickle b.
    Supercut b.
    b. of tongue
    tongue b.
    Typhoon cutter b.
    X-Acto b.
blade-form
    b.-f. device
    b.-f. implant
blade-type holder
Blade-Vent implant system
Blainville ears
Blair-Brown graft
Blair knife
Blake
    B. drain
    B. silicone drain
Blakesley
    B. forceps
    B. grasper
Blakesley-Weil upturned ethmoid forceps
Blakesley-Wilde forceps
blanche
blanching
    gingival b.
Blandin
    B. ganglion
    B. gland
    B. and Nuhn glands
Blandin-Nuhn cyst
blanket
    Bair Hugger patient warming b.
    mucous b.

Blaskovics
> B. eyelid shortening technique
> B. operation

blast
> b. energy induced trauma
> stoma b.

blaster
> shell b.

blastomycosis
> laryngeal b.
> South American b.

Blauth type II hypoplastic thumb
bleach
> walking b.

bleaching
> b. agent
> coronal b.
> mouthguard b.
> night guard vital b. (NGVB)
> nonvital b.
> thermo-photocatalytic b.

bleb
bleed
> silicone b.
> silicone gel b.

bleeder disease
bleeding
> gastrointestinal b.
> gingival b.
> b. index
> oral b.
> b. pocket
> b. tendency

blend
> consonant b.

blending
> auditory b.
> sound b.

blennorrhea
> Stoerk b.

Blenoxane
bleomycin (BLM)
Bleph-10 Ophthalmic
blephamide
Blephamide Ophthalmic
blepharochalasis
> b. syndrome

blepharoperiorbitoplasty
blepharophimosis syndrome
blepharoplasty
> CO$_2$ laser b.
> combined upper b.

> laser incisional b.
> laser lower lid transconjunctival b.
> long-skin flap b.
> b., modified Loeb and de la Plaza technique
> b. procedure
> skin/muscle flap b.
> transconjunctival b. (TCB)
> transconjunctival lower lid b.

blepharoptosis
blepharospasm
> essential b.

blind
> b. alley phenomenon
> b. nasotracheal intubation
> b. osteotomy

blindness
> cerebral b.
> odor b.
> transient b.
> word b.

Blissymbolics
Blis-To-Sol
BLL
> benign lymphoepithelial lesion

BLM
> bleomycin

bloc
> en b.

Blocadren Oral
Bloch-Sulzberger syndrome
block
> acrylic b.
> b. anesthesia
> bicortical iliac bone b.
> bite b.
> clonic b.
> Dembone demineralized cortical dental b.
> disposable styrofoam b.
> G$_1$ b.
> Greco cutting b.
> inferior alveolar nerve b.
> infraorbital b.
> b. injection
> Lell bite b.
> local nerve b.
> mandibular b.
> metal and rubber b.
> nerve b.
> b. osteotomy
> peridural b.

NOTES

block *(continued)*
    plastic b.
    Plexiglas tissue equivalency b.
    rubber b.
    silicone b.
    stellate ganglion b.
    tonic b.
    wood b.
blocker
    calcium channel b. (CCB)
    ganglionic b.
block-out, blockout
    arbitrary b.-o.
    b.-o. material
    parallel b.-o.
    shaped b.-o.
    b.-o. wax
Blom-Singer
    B.-S. tracheoesophageal prosthesis
    B.-S. valve
    B.-S. voice prosthesis
blood
    autologous b.
    b. product
    b. vessel
    b. worm
blood-borne
    b.-b. macrophage
    b.-b. pathogen
blood-free cylinder
bloodroot
blood-stained pattern
bloodstream
bloomer
    late b.
blossom
    orange b.
blow-in fracture
blowing
    maximum duration of sustained b.
blown-out appearance
blow-out fracture
blowpipe
blowtorch
    gas-air b.
blue
    Alcian b.
    b. cohosh
    b. Elgiloy upper utility arch
    b. flag iris
    b. line
    b. mantle
    methylene b.
    b. nevus
    B. Peel chemical method
    B. Peel chemical peel
    b. rubber bleb nevus
    b. sclera

    b. stone
    Swiss b.
    toluidine b.
    b. tooth
bluegrass
    annual b.
    Canada b.
    Kentucky b.
blue-lining
bluish hue
blunderbuss
    apex b.
    b. apical canal
blunt
    b. bullet-tip cannula
    b. carotid injury (BCI)
    b. dissection
    b. lacrimal probe
    b. suction-assisted lipoplasty
    b. suction lipectomy
BM
    buccomesial
BMA
    basaloid monomorphic adenoma
BMMP
    benign mucous membrane pemphigoid
BMP
    bone morphogenetic protein
    bone morphogenic protein
BMP-2
    bone morphogenic protein-2
    BMP-2 protein
BMT
    bone marrow transplant
BNOE
    benign necrotizing otitis externa
BO
    bucco-occlusal
BOA
    behavioral observation audiometry
board
    communication b.
    conversation b.
    direct selection communication b.
    encoding communication b.
    scanning communication b.
    Targa+ image capture b.
    Workers' Compensation B. (WCB)
Bobath method
bobby pin abrasion
Bödecker index
bodily
    b. movement
    b. movement of tooth
    b. trusion
body
    alveolar b.
    aortic b.

asteroid b.
b. baffle effect
carotid b.
crystalloid b.
b. dysmorphic disorder
B. Dysmorphic Disorder
  Examination
B. Dysmorphic Disorder
  Modification of Yale-Brown
  Obsessive-Compulsive Scale,
  McLean version
foreign b.
b. hearing aid
hypoplastic mandibular b.
b. image
b. image disorder
b. image dissatisfaction
b. image disturbance
b. language
multivesicular b.
nasal swell b.
phagocytized dense b.'s
pharmacoradiologic disimpaction of
  esophageal foreign b.'s
rice b.'s
Rushton b.'s
b. sculpting
sense of foreign b.
swell b.
b. of tongue
tracheobronchial foreign b.
trapezoid b.
Verocay b.'s
body-contour surgery
Boehm
  B. Test of Basic Concepts-
    Preschool
  B. Test of Basic Concepts-R
Boehringer Autovac autotransfusion
  system
Boerhaave syndrome
Boettcher tonsil scissors
bogginess
boggy
Bohn nodules
boil
boilermaker's deafness
Boley gauge
Bolk paramolar root
Bollinger granule
bolster
  muscular b.

b. suture
tie-over b.
bolt
Alta femoral b.
denture b.
Pullen-Warner b.
Bolton
  B. analysis
  B. point
  B. triangle
bolus
standardized constant b.
bombarding
bombed abutment
bombesin
bonded
  b. cast restoration
  b. pontic
  b. retainer
  b. space maintainer
Bondek
  B. absorbable suture
Bondeze resin
bonding
  adhesive b.
  b. agent
  bracket b.
  chemical b.
  dentin b.
  direct b.
  enamel b.
  enamel-dentin b.
  indirect b.
  Panavia b.
  porcelain-metal b.
  tooth b.
bond strength
bone (B)
  b. algorithm
  allogenic b.
  b. alteration
  alveolar b.
  alveolar supporting b.
  anterior suspension of hyoid b.
  articular eminence of temporal b.
  articular tubercle of temporal b.
  b. autograft
  autologous b.
  banked freeze-dried b.
  basal b.
  Bioglass synthetic b.

NOTES

bone *(continued)*
    BIO-OSS freeze-dried
      demineralized b.
    Bioplant hard tissue replacement
      synthetic b.
    Bioplant HTR synthetic b.
    bundle b.
    b. bur
    calvarial b.
    cancellous b.
    cancellous cellular b. (CCB)
    b. carpentry
    cheek b.
    b. chisel
    chondroid b.
    b. collector
    compact b.
    b. conduction (BC)
    b. conduction hearing aid (BCHA)
    b. conduction level
    b. conduction threshold
    cortical b.
    corticocancellous b.
    b. crater
    crestal b.
    b. cutter
    b. cyst
    decalcified freeze-dried cortical b.
      (DFDCB)
    b. defect
    Dembone demineralized human b.
    Dembone freeze dried b.
    demineralized b. (DMB)
    demineralized freeze-dried b.
      (DFDB)
    b. deposition
    embryonic b.
    endochondral b.
    ethmoid b.
    facial b.
    b. file
    b. flap
    b. forceps
    freeze-dried demineralized b.
      (FDDB)
    frontal b.
    b. graft
    b. grafting
    haversian b.
    hemiseptum of interalveolar b.
    horizontal plate of palatine b.
    hyoid b.
    immature b.
    inferior maxillary b.
    inferior turbinated b.
    interproximal b.
    intrajugular process of temporal b.

    invasive fungal infection of
      temporal b.
    jaw b.
    jugal b.
    lacrimal b.
    Lambone demineralized laminar b.
    Lambone freeze dried b.
    lamellar b.
    lamellated b.
    laminar b.
    lateral mastoid b.
    lateral surface of zygomatic b.
    lingual b.
    b. liquefaction
    lunate b.
    malar b.
    malar surface of zygomatic b.
    b. margin
    marginal process of malar b.
    marginal tubercle of zygomatic b.
    b. marrow
    b. marrow exposure guideline
    b. marrow transplant (BMT)
    b. marrow transplantation
    masticatory b.
    b. matrix
    maxillary b.
    maxillary process of zygomatic b.
    maxillary surface of perpendicular
      plate of palatine b.
    medial turbinated b.
    meiopragic b.
    metatarsal b.
    monocortical b.
    b. morphogenetic protein (BMP)
    b. morphogenic protein (BMP)
    b. morphogenic protein-2 (BMP-2)
    nasal b.
    b. nipper
    occipital b.
    Osteomin freeze dried b.
    Paget disease of b.
    palate b.
    palatine b.
    palatomaxillary groove of
      palatine b.
    parietal b.
    petrous b.
    b. plate
    Pneumocystis carinii in temporal b.
    prefrontal b.
    pyramidal tuberosity of palatine b.
    b. rasp
    b. recession
    b. remodeling
    b. resection
    b. resorption
    b. sequestrum

B

sphenoid b.
sphenoidal turbinated b.'s
b. spicule
spine of sphenoid b.
spongy b.
squama of temporal b.
superior maxillary b.
superior surface of horizontal plate
  of palatine b.
superior turbinated b.
supporting b.
supraorbital rim of frontal b.
supreme turbinated b.
synthetic b.
b. tack system
temporal b.
temporal process of zygomatic b.
temporal surface of frontal b.
temporal surface of zygomatic b.
thickened b.
b. threshold
b. trabecula
trabecular b.
turbinated b.'s
vaginal process of the sphenoid b.
vascular bundle implantation
  into b.
b. wax
b. window
woven b.
xenogeneic b.
zygomatic b.
zygomatic process of frontal b.
zygomatic process of temporal b.
bone-anchored hearing aid (BAHA)
bone-conduction
　　b.-c. oscillator
　　b.-c. receiver
　　b.-c. vibrator
bonelet
BoneSource hydroxyapatite cement
Bonfil primer
Bonine
Bonwill
　　B. articulator
　　B. crown
　　B. triangle
Bonwill-Hawley chart
bony
　　b. ankylosis
　　b. annulus
　　b. atresia

b. atretic plate
b. caval opening
b. chin button
b. crater
b. destruction
b. impaction
b. kyphos
b. labyrinth
b. mobilization
b. palate
b. pogonion
b. protuberance
b. rasping
b. reconstruction
b. regeneration
b. septation
b. septum
b. vault collapse
Böök syndrome
boomerang rectus abdominis
　　musculocutaneous free flap
boomerang-shaped skin paddle
booster
　　antitetanus b.
booth
　　double-walled audiometric test b.
borate
　　epinephryl b.
border
　　alveolar b.
　　alveolar b. of mandible
　　alveolar b. of maxilla
　　b. cell
　　denture b.
　　lateral upper lip vermilion b.
　　mandibular b.
　　b. molding
　　pulp b.
　　ruffled b.
　　b. seal
　　striated b.
　　b. structure
　　b. tissue
　　b. tissue movement
　　tragal b.
　　vermilion b.
Bordetella pertussis
bore
Borg
　　B. dizziness index
　　B. scale
boric acid

NOTES

Borrelia vincentii
borrowing
Bosker
> B. TMI Reconstruction system
> B. TMI surgery
> B. transmandibular reconstructive surgical system

bossing
> bitemporal b.
> frontal b.
> tip b.

Boston
> B. Diagnostic Aphasia Examination
> B. University Speech Sound Discrimination Test

B&O Supprettes
BOT
> base of tongue

Botox
botryoid odontogenic cyst
Botryomyces
botryomycoma
botryomycosis
bottom pocket
bottom-shaped nose
botulinum
> *Clostridium b.*
> b. toxin
> b. toxin type A

botulism
> wound b.

bouche de tapir
Bouchut tube
bougie
> Hurst b.
> Jackson steel-stem woven filiform b.
> Maloney b.
> Plummer b.
> Tucker b.

bougienage
bounce
bound
> b. morpheme
> upper b.

boundary
> language b.

boutonniere
> b. deformity

bovine
> b. cartilage
> b. collagen

bovine-derived bone filler
bovis
> *Actinomyces b.*
> *Mycobacterium b.*

bow
> b. activator

Cupid's b.
Logan b.
b. spring

bowed vocal fold
Bowen
> B. cavity primer
> B. disease
> B. resin

Bowen-Chalfant Receptive Language Inventory
bowenoid papulosis
bowing
> vocal cord b.

bowl
> conchal b.
> ear b.
> b. of ear
> mastoid b.

Bowles
> B. bracket
> B. multiphase appliance
> B. multiphase attachment
> B. technique

Bowman
> B. glands

box
> anatomic snuff b.
> b. elder maple

boxer's ear
boxing
> b. of nipple
> b. strip
> b. wax

Box technique
Boyce position
boydii
> *Pseudallescheria b.*

Boyer cyst
Bozzolo sign
BP
> buccopulpal
> BP Cuff pressure infuser

BPB
> black-pigmented bacteria

BPM
> breaths per minute

BPPV
> benign paroxysmal positional vertigo

BPV
> benign positional vertigo

BR
> buccal root

brace
> invisible b.
> jaw b.

braces

B

brachial
    b. dermolipectomy
    b. fascia
    b. plexitis
    b. plexus
brachialis muscle
brachioradialis muscle
brachycephalic
brachycephalofrontonasal dysplasia
brachycephaly
brachycheilia
brachydactyly
    Haws type b.
    b. type C
brachyesophagus
brachyfacial
brachyglossal
brachygnathia
brachygnathous
brachymetacarpia, brachymetacarpalia
    cryptodontic b.
brachyodont
brachyprosopic
brachyrhinia
brachyrhynchus
brachystaphyline
brachysyndactyly
brachytelephalangia
brachytherapy
brachyuranic
bracing
bracket
    b. angulation
    Begg straight-wire combination b.
    b. bonding
    Bowles b.
    Broussard b.
    ceramic b.
    curved base Lewis b.
    curved base twin b.
    Cusp-Lok b.
    edgewise b.
    Hanson speed b.
    Lewis b.
    ligatureless b.
    metal b.
    metal frame reinforced plastic b.
    b. modification
    molar b.
    multiphase b.
    orthodontic b.
    plastic b.

    ribbon arch b.
    Siamese twin b.
    single width b.
    b. slot
    b. slot angulation
    square b.
    steel-slotted plastic b.
    Steiner b.
    torqued slot b.
    twin edgewise b.
    universal b.
    vertical slot Lewis b.
Brackett probe
Brackman
    B. grade
bradyarthria
bradycardia
bradyglossia
bradykinesia
bradykinesthetic
bradykinin
bradylalia
bradylogia
bradyphagia
bradyphasia
bradyphemia
braided wire
brain
    b. abscess
    b. dysfunction (BD)
    b. mapping
    b. tumor
brainstem
    b. auditory evoked potential (BAEP)
    b. auditory evoked response (BAER)
    b. auditory evoked response audiometry
    b. evoked auditory response (BEAR)
    b. evoked response (BSER)
    b. evoked response audiometry
    b. stroke
Bramante technique
branch
    buccal b.
    cervical b.
    cochlear b.
    facial nerve b.'s
    frontal b.
    genital b.

NOTES

73

branch *(continued)*
  marginal mandibular b.
  nerve b.
  zygomatic b.
branchial
  b. apparatus
  b. arch
  b. arch syndrome
  b. cleft cyst
  b. cleft sinus
  b. cyst
  b. fistula
  b. nerve
  b. pouch cyst
branching
  b. canal
  b. steps
  b. tree diagram
branchiogenic
  b. carcinoma
  b. cyst
Brandt cytology balloon
Brand tendon repair
brandy
  b. nose
  B. scalp stretcher II, front closure
  B. scalp stretcher I, rear closure
Brånemark
  B. implant
  B. implant system
  B. restorative protocol
Branhamella catarrhalis
Brännström hydrodynamics theory
brasiliensis
  Nocardia b.
brassiere
  skin b.
brass wire
brassy cough
brawny
  b. edema
  b. induration
Brazil
  B. nut
  B. wax
braziliana
  bubas b.
Brazilian rubber
brazing
BRD
  baroreflex dysfunction
breadth
  bicanine b.
  bigonial b.
  bimolar b.
  b. of mandible
  b. of mandibular ramus
  maxilloalveolar b.

  midfacial b.
  b. of palate
  zygomatic b.
break
  ascending pitch b.
  descending pitch b.
  phonation b.
  pitch b.
breakdown theory
breaker
  hinge stress b.
  stress b.
breast
  b. augmentation
  b. cancer
  b. contour
  b. hypertrophy
  hypoplastic tuberous b.
  b. implant
  B. Implant Protector (B.I.P.)
  b. lift
  b. ptosis
  b. reconstruction
  b. reduction
  shaping of the b.
  b. strap
breath
  b. chewing
  b. stream
  b. support
breathiness
breathing
  b. disorder
  donkey b.
  glossopharyngeal b.
  b. method
  mouth b.
  opposition b.
breaths per minute (BPM)
breathy voice
Breda disease
Bredall amalgam plugger
bredouillement
Breezee Mist Antifungal
bregma
bregma-menton
  b.-m. extraoral radiography
  b.-m. projection
  b.-m. radiograph
brephoplastic graft
Breschet canal
Breslow thickness
brevis
  extensor digitorum b. (EDB)
bridge
  b. abutment
  Aderer "C" b.
  adhesion b.

B

adhesive resin-bonded b.
American Gold "B" b.
American Gold "T" b.
Andrews b.
Bing b.
cantilever b.
cast metal b.
cast perforated b.
ceramo-metal implant b.
complex b.
compound b.
Conquest crown and b.
cross b.
dental b.
dentin b.
etched cast resin bonded b.
extension b.
fixed b.
fixed-fixed b.
fixed-movable b.
Hollywood b.
B. III-C dental casting gold alloy
impedance b.
b. impression
intercellular b.
Lang b.
Maryland b.
palmar skin b.
b. partial IV-D
B. Partial IV-D dental casting gold
  alloy
porcelain finished b.
removable b.
resin-bonded b.
Rochette b.
simplex b.
b. splint
spring b.
stationary b.
three-unit b.
Ticonium 44, 50, 100 nickel-
  chromium base metal crown
  and b.
bridgework
fixed b.
removable b.
brief tone audiometry (BTA)
Brigham 1x2 teeth forceps
brightener
C-Brite nonchemical skin b.
Brilliant Lux
Brill-Symmers disease

brimonidine
Brinell
B. hardness
B. hardness indenter point
B. hardness number (BHN)
B. hardness test
B. scale
Brinker tissue retractor
Brink PeriPyriform implant
Briquet syndrome
Brissaud-Marie syndrome
bristle
b. brush
hard b.
natural b.
nylon b.
soft b.
b. wheel
Brite
Ultra B.
brittle
b. bone disease
b. material
broach
barbed b.
endodontic b.
b. holder
pathfinder b.
root canal b.
smooth b.
broad
b. centric
b. forehead
b. transcription
Broadbent-Bolton transparency
Broadbent registration point
Broca
B. aphasia
B. area
B. plane
broccoli
Broders classification
Brodmann
B. area 41
B. area 44
B. areas
Brofed Elixir
broken-down tooth
broken-stress
b.-s. partial denture
b.-s. space maintainer
Bromaline Elixir

NOTES

Bromanate
    B. DC
    B. Elixir
Bromanyl Cough Syrup
Bromarest
Bromatapp
Brombay
bromegrass
Bromfed
    B. Syrup
    B. Tablet
bromfenac
    b. sodium
Bromfenex
bromide
    apratropium b.
    methantheline b.
    potassium b.
bromidrosis, bromhidrosis
bromodiphenhydramine and codeine
bromopnea
Bromotuss w/Codeine Cough Syrup
Bromphen
    B. DC w/Codeine
    B. Tablet
brompheniramine
    b. and phenylephrine
    b. and phenylpropanolamine
    b., phenylpropanolamine, and
      codeine
    b. and pseudoephedrine
bronchi (pl. of bronchus)
bronchial
    b. adenocarcinoma
    b. adenoma
    b. asthma
    b. respiration
bronchiectasis
bronchiolar carcinoma
bronchiolitis
bronchitis
    arachidic b.
bronchoesophagology
bronchoesophagoscopy
bronchogenic
    b. carcinoma
    b. cyst
bronchography
bronchopharyngoesophagoscopy
bronchoplasty
bronchopneumonia
bronchoprovocation
bronchoscope
    Dumon-Harrell b.
    Holinger b.
bronchoscopic
    b. sponge
    b. sponge carrier
    b. telescope

bronchoscopy
    flexible fiberoptic b.
bronchostomy
bronchus, pl. bronchi
Brookdale bar
Brooke tumor
broom
    butcher's b.
Brophy operation
Brotane
Broussard bracket
brow
    b. lift
    b. ptosis
brow-forehead lift
browlift, brow-lift
    open coronal b.
brown
    b. adipose tissue
    B. and Brenn stain
    B. electric dermatome
    B. and McDowell alar cartilage
      relocation
    b. pellicle
    B. sign
    b. stain
    b. striae
    B. test
Brown-Adson side-grasping forceps
Brown-Brenn staining method
Brown-Gruss provocation
brownian
    b. motion
    b. movement
browpexy
brow-upper lid complex
Broyle ligament
brucellosis
Brudzinski sign
Bruhn method
bruising
bruit
brush
    Bass b.
    bristle b.
    denture b.
    interproximal b.
    Oral-B soft foam interdental b.
    Plak-Vac oral suction b.
    polishing b.
    sable b.
    b. technique filling
    tooth b.
Brushfield spot
brushing
    paint b.
brushite

Brussel sprouts
bruxing
bruxism
bruxomania
Bryngelson-Glaspey Test of Articulation
BSC
    basosquamous carcinoma
BSER
    brainstem evoked response
        BSER audiometry
BSM
    Bilingual Syntax Measure
BSS
    balanced salt solution
BSSO
    bilateral sagittal split advancement
      osteotomy
    bilateral sagittal split osteotomy
BTA
    brief tone audiometry
BTE
    behind-the-ear
        BTE listening device
BTR
    buccal triangular ridge
bubas
    b. braziliana
bucca
    b. cavioris
    b. cavum oris
buccae
    Prevotella b.
buccal
    b. administration
    b. alveolar plate
    b. alveolus
    b. angle
    b. artery
    b. aspect
    b. bar
    b. branch
    b. caries
    b. cavity
    b. cervical ridge (BCR)
    b. commissure
    b. contour
    b. cortex
    b. cortical plate
    b. crossbite
    b. curve
    b. cusp (BC)
    b. cyst

b. defect
b. developmental groove (BDG)
b. embrasure
b. envelope flap
b. epithelium
b. fat
b. fat extractor
b. fat extractor tip
b. fat pad
b. flange
b. frenum
b. gingiva
b. gland
b. groove (BG)
b. groove of central fossa (BGCF)
b. interdigitation
b. lamina
b. lymph node
b. mucosa
b. mucosa graft
b. mucosal flap
b. mucous gland
b. muscle
b. musculomucosal flap
b. nerve
b. neuralgia
b. notch
b. object rule
b. occlusion
b. ostectomy
b. peak
b. pit
b. region
b. restoration
b. ridge
b. root (BR)
b. shelf
b. space
b. space abscess
b. speech
b. splint
b. sulcus
b. surface
b. teeth
b. tooth tip
b. triangular ridge (BTR)
b. tube
b. vestibule
b. view
b. whisper
buccale
    Treponema b.

B

NOTES

buccalis
    Amoeba b.
    Leptotrichia b.
    linea alba b.
buccal-lingual alveolar diameter
buccal or upper lingual of lower
  (BULL)
buccinator
    b. artery
    b. crest
    b. muscle
    b. myomucosal flap
    b. nerve
    b. plication
    b. space
buccoangular
buccoaxial (BA)
buccoaxiocervical (BAC)
buccoaxiogingival (BAG)
buccocervical (BC)
    b. ridge
buccoclination
buccodistal (BD)
buccogingival (BG)
    b. lamina
    b. ridge
buccoglossopharyngitis
buccolabial
buccolingual (BL)
    b. curvature
    b. diameter
    b. dimension
    b. plane
    b. relation
    b. relationship
    b. stress
buccolingually
buccomaxillary
buccomesial (BM)
bucco-occlusal (BO)
    b.-o. angle
    b.-o. line angle
buccopalatal
    b. height
    b. width
buccopharyngeal
    b. space
buccoplacement
buccopulpal (BP)
buccoversion
Buck
    B. deep penile fascia
    B. fascia
    B. knife
    B. wax curette
buck
    b. tooth
Buckley formocresol

buckling
buckthorn
buckwheat
Bucladin-S Softab
buclizine
bud
    B. bur
    gustatory b.
    limb b.
    b. stage
    taste b.
    tooth b.
budesonide
    b. nasal inhaler
    b. powder
Buerger disease
buffered mouthwash
Bufferin
Buffex
buff-puff
building
    b. solder
    voice b.
build-up
    composite b.-u.
    core b.-u.
built-in angulation
bulb
    hair b.
    hollow b.
    jugular b.
    olfactory b.
    saphenous b.
    speech b.
bulbar
    b. paralysis
bulbi
    proptosis b.
bulbosa
    myringitis b.
bulbous
    b. internal auditory canal
    b. nasal tip
bulge
    periocular b.
bulk pack technique
BULL
    buccal or upper lingual of lower
bulla, pl. **bullae**
    ethmoidal b.
    b. ethmoidalis
    frontal b.
    intrabasilar b.
    sub-basilar b.
    suprabasilar b.
bulldog
    vascular b.
bullet-shaped cannula

bullosa
    concha b.
    epidermolysis b.
bullous
    b. lichen planus
    b. myringitis
    b. pemphigoid
bullous/erosive disease
bumblebee
bumper
    lip b.
bundle
    acousticofacial nerve b.
    b. bone
    extravelar muscle b.
    b. fiber
    fiber b.
    inferior alveolar neurovascular b.
    nerve b.
    nerve fiber b.
    neurovascular b.
    olivocochlear b.
    orbital neurovascular b.
    principal fiber b.
    sensory nerve fiber b.
    vascular b.
Bünger band
Bunnell suture
bunodont
bunolophodont
bunoselenodont
Bunsen burner
buphthalmia, buphthalmos
bupivacaine
Buprenex
buprenorphine
bur, burr
    ACORDE b.
    barrel b.
    bone b.
    Bud b.
    carbide b.
    carbide finishing b.
    cone b.
    countersink b.
    cross-cut straight fissure b.
    cross-cut tapered fissure b.
    cutting b.
    cylinder b.
    dentate straight fissure b.
    dentate tapered fissure b.
    denture vulcanite b.

    diamond b.
    diamond finishing b.
    b. drill
    end-cutting b.
    end-cutting fissure b.
    endodontic b.
    excavating b.
    Feldman b.
    finishing b.
    fissure b.
    flame b.
    fluted finishing b.
    Gates-Glidden b.
    GPX b.
    handpiece round b.
    high-speed diamond three-tiered
      depth cutting b.
    high-speed diamond wheel b.
    high-speed tungsten carbide b.
    high-speed two-grit b.
    b. hole
    intramucosal insert base-
      preparing b.
    inverted cone b.
    Lindeman b.
    low-speed Christmas tree
      diamond b.
    low-speed tapered carbide b.
    Masseran trepan b.
    narrow fissure b.
    b. neck
    oval b.
    Parapost b.
    pear b.
    plug-finishing b.
    pointed cone b.
    pure end-cutting b.
    round b.
    rounded b.
    safe-tipped b.
    b. shank
    Shannon b.
    spiral fluted tungsten carbide b.
    S.S. White J-Notch surgical
      handpiece b.
    S.S. White 100 K surgical
      handpiece b.
    Starlite Omni-AT b.
    straight fissure b.
    Supercut diamond b.
    surgical b.
    tapered fissure b.

NOTES

B

bur *(continued)*
    tungsten carbide b.
    wheel b.
burden
    tumor b.
burdock
buried
    b. de-epithelialized local flap
    b. free forearm flap transfer
    b. penis
Burkitt
    B. lymphoma
    B. lymphoma of nasal ala
Burlew
    B. disk
    B. wheel
burn
    chemical b.
    laryngeal b.
    slag b.
    thermal b.
burner
    Bunsen b.
burning tongue
burnisher
    agate b.
    amalgam b.
    ball b.
    beaver-tail b.
    fishtail b.
    fissure b.
    flat b.
    gold b.
    straight b.
burnishing
burnout, burn-out
    inlay b.
    b. procedure
    b. wax
    wax b.
Burns Uni-File
Burow
    B. operation
    B. procedure
    B. solution
    B. triangle
    B. triangle deformity
burr *(var. of* bur)
burrobrush
    white b.

bursa
    nasopharyngeal b.
    pharyngeal b.
    Tornwaldt b.
burst
    staccato b.
Burton
    B. line
    B. sign
    B. vitalometer
burweed
B.U.S.
    Belgium ultrasound
    B.U.S. Endotron-Lipectron ultrasonic
      scalpel
bush
    iodine b.
    rabbit b.
butadiene-styrene rubber
butalbital compound and codeine
butcher's broom
Butler stimulator
butoconazole
butorphanol
butt
    b. joint
button
    bony chin b.
    Groningen b.
    implant b.
    lingual b.
    stoma b.
    b. suture
buttonhole approach
buttonholing
    b. of skin
buttress
    maxillary b.
    nasomaxillary b.
    pterygomaxillary b.
    b. reconstruction
    zygomatic b.
    zygomaticomaxillary b.
buttressing
butyl methacrylate
bypass
    aortobiprofunda femoral b.
    b. conduit
Byzantine arch palate

C
cathode
celsius
centigrade
C fiber
C & L attachment
C & L retainer
C & M 637 attachment
C sliding osteotomy

CA
cervicoaxial
chronological age

Ca
cathode

cabbage

cable
ESI Lite-Pipe fiberoptic c.
c. graft
c. tie

CaCO₃
calcium carbonate

cacodontia

cacogeusia

cacosmia

cactus

cadaverine

CAD/CAM
computer assisted design/computer assisted manufacture

CADL
Communicative Abilities in Daily Living

caecoidosis

CAER
cortical auditory evoked response
CAER audiometry

Cafatine

café
c. au lait
c. au lait macule
c. au lait spot
c. coronary

Cafergot

CAFET
computer-aided fluency establishment trainer

Cafet
C. for Kids software
C. system

Cafetrate

caffeine
acetaminophen, aspirin, and c.
orphenadrine, aspirin and c.

Caffey-Silverman disease

Cagot ear

Cairns maneuver

Calasept
C. medicament delivery system
C. sealer
C. sterile calcium hydroxide paste

calcic ulatrophy

calcifediol

calcific
c. degeneration
c. hematoma
c. metamorphosis
c. pulposis
c. regression of pulp

calcificate

calcification
amorphous c.
c. of breast implant
capsular c.
diffuse c.
diffuse pulp c.
dystrophic c.
intratubular c.
c. line
c. lines of Retzius
pulp c.
c. of pulp chamber
root canal c.
soft-tissue c.
c. zone

calcified
c. canal
c. cementum
c. cephalhematoma
c. dentin
c. lymph node
c. nodule
c. oil cyst

calciform papillae

calcifying
c. cyst
c. epithelial odontogenic tumor
c. epithelioma of Malherbe
c. and keratinizing odontogenic cyst
c. odontogenic cyst

Calcimar Injection

Calciobiotic root canal sealer

calciotraumatic
c. band (CTB)
c. line

calcite

Calcitek
C. drill
C. implant system
C. Integral ThreadLoc implant
C. retaining screw

Calcitite hydroxyapatite coating
calcitonin
calcium
    c. alginate
    c. alginate gel
    c. carbonate ($CaCO_3$)
    c. channel blocker (CCB)
    c. deposit
    c. hydroxide (CH)
    c. hydroxide cement light-cured
    c. hydroxide cement self-cured
    c. hydroxide paste
    c. hydroxide root canal sealer
      (CRCS)
    c. oxalate crystal
    c. phosphate ceramic implant
    c. pyrophosphate dihydrate
    c. pyrophosphate dihydrate deposit
      (CPDD)
    c. salt
    c. sulfate
    c. tungstate crystal
calcium-binding protein
α-calcium sulfate hemihydrate
β-calcium sulfate hemihydrate
calcospherite mineralization
calculation
calculi (*gen. and pl.* of calculus)
calculous disease
Calculus
calculus, gen. and pl. calculi
    dental c.
    hard c.
    hematogenetic c.
    C. Index, Simplified (CI-S)
    c. inhibitor
    invisible c.
    nasal c.
    pharyngeal c.
    c. pocket
    pulp c.
    radiopaque c.
    salivary c.
    serumal c.
    subgingival c.
    supragingival c.
    C. Surface Index (CSI)
    tonsillar c.
    visible c.
Caldecort
    C. Anti-Itch Spray
Calderol
Caldwell-Luc
    C.-L. incision
    C.-L. maxillary antrostomy
    C.-L. operation
    C.-L. window procedure
Caldwell view

calendula
Calendula officinalis
calf augmentation
calibrate
calibrated
    c. electrical stimulation
    c. probe
calibration overshoot
calibrator
California
    C. Consonant Test
    C. hatchet
    C. peppertree
caliper
    Castroviejo c.
    digital c.
    Mitutoyo Digimatic c.
    Vernier c.
Callahan
    C. method
    C. root canal filling method
Callia abdominoplasty
calling
    word c.
callosal disconnection syndrome
callosum
    corpus c.
Calmette-Guérin
    Bacille bilié de C.-G. (BCG)
    bacillus C.-G. (BCG)
Calm-X Oral
calor
caloric
    c. areflexia
    c. irrigation
    c. nystagmus
    c. test
calvarectomy
calvarial
    c. bone
    c. bone graft
    c. defect
    c. repair
calvarium
Calxyl calcium hydroxide paste
CAM
    cell adhesion molecule
Cama Arthritis Pain Reliever
Cameco syringe pistol
camera
    charge-coupled device video c.
    Dental Pro II c.
    Dine Digital Macro c.
    gamma c.
    immersible video c.
    c. lucida
    5 lux color video c.
    MLR+ c.

OralVision intraoral c.
Reveal MLR+ c.
Reveal single lens reflex c.
Yashica Dental Eye II c.
Cameron elevator
CAML
  Coarticulation Assessment in Meaningful
  Language
camouflage
  c. augmentation
  c. cosmetic
  c. make-up
  orthodontic c.
cAMP
  cyclic adenosine 3′,5′-monophosphate
Camper
  C. line
  C. plane
Campho-Phenique
camphorated
  c. mono-parachlorophenol (CMCP)
  c. phenol
camphor, menthol, and phenol
camptodactyly
Campylobacter rectus
Canada
  C. balsam
  C. bluegrass
canal
  accessory c.
  accessory palatine c.
  accessory root c.
  additional c.
  alveolar c.
  anterior vertical c.
  auditory c.
  auxiliary c.'s
  bayonet c.
  bayonet-curved c.
  bifurcated c.
  blunderbuss apical c.
  branching c.
  Breschet c.
  bulbous internal auditory c.
  calcified c.
  c. cap
  carotid c.
  carpal c.
  collateral pulp c.
  common c.
  completely-in-the-c. (CIC)
  c. configuration

c. crack
C-shaped c.
c. curvature
curved c.
c. debridement
c. debris
defalcated root c.
dehiscent mandibular c.
dental c.
dentinal c.
dilacerated c.
Dorello c.
ear c.
external auditory c. (EAC)
facial c.
fallopian c.
filling c.
C. Finder system
furcation c.
greater palatine c.
gubernacular c.
Guyon c.
haversian c.
c. hearing aid
Hirschfeld c.'s
horizontal c.
Huguier c.
Hunter c.
hypoglossal c.
identifying c.
incisal c.
incisive c.
inoperable c.
interdental c.'s
internal auditory c. (IAC)
c. irrigation
large c.
lateral c.
locating c.
mandibular c.
mandibular neurovascular c.
C. Master drills
C. Master instrumentation technique
C. Master rotary instrument
maxillary c.
mesiobuccal c.
nutrient c.
c. obturation
optic c.
overfilled c.
palatine c.
palatomaxillary c.

C

NOTES

canal *(continued)*
    palatovaginal c.
    perforating c. of Zuckerkandl
    posterior semicircular c. (PSC)
    posterior vertical c.
    pulp c. (PC)
    radicular c.
    c. resonance response (CRR)
    retrosigmoid/internal auditory c. (RSG/IAC)
    ribbon-shaped c.
    Rivinus c.'s
    root c.
    c.'s of Scarpa
    semicircular c.
    sickle-shaped c.
    sphenopalatine c.
    straight c.
    Sucquet-Hoyer glomus c.
    supplementary c. (SC)
    supraorbital c.
    Tourtual c.
    Type I, II, III, IV c.
    vestibular c.
    vidian c.
    c. wall-down mastoidectomy
    c. wall-down tympanoplasty
    c. wall-up mastoidectomy
    zipped c.
    Zuckerkandl perforating c.
    zygomaticofacial c.
    zygomaticotemporal c.
canal-down procedure
canalicular
    c. adenoma
    c. system
canaliculi of cementocyte
canaliculus
    c. of chorda tympani
    cochlear c.
    intercellular c.
canalithiasis
canalith repositioning procedure
Canal-Mate hearing aid
canaloplasty
Canals-N root canal filling material
Canals root canal filling material
canal-wall-down
    c.-w.-d. cavity
    c.-w.-d. procedure
canal-wall-up technique
canary grass
cancellation
cancellous
    c. bone
    c. cellular bone (CCB)
    c. cellular bone graft
    c. cellular marrow

cancer
    breast c.
    claypipe c.
    differentiated thyroid c.
    glottic c.
    head and neck c.
    laryngeal c.
    oral c.
    oral cavity c. (OCC)
    smoker's c.
cancerization
    field c.
cancrum
    c. nasi
    c. oris
    c. oris (noma) noma trismus
Candela
    C. ALEXlazr
    C. laser
    C. ScleroLaser
candelilla
    c. wax
Candida
    C. albicans
candidiasis
    esophageal c.
    isolated laryngeal c.
    oral c.
candy
    c. cane cannula
    c. cane cannula style I
    c. cane cannula style II
Canfield facial plastics garment
canine
    c. alveolus
    c. crowding
    c. eminence
    c. fossa
    maxillary c.
    c. muscle
    c. prominence
    c. smile
    c. tooth
canine-to-canine
    c.-t.-c. bonded retainer
    c.-t.-c. lingual splint
caniniform
caninus, pl. canini
    dens c.
    dentes canini
canister
    Bemis suction c.
    Lipovacutainer c.
    reusable Sorensen 2000 cc c.
    Sep-T-Vac suction c.
canker
    c. sore

Cannon
white sponge lesion of C.
cannula
angled c.
aspiration c.
Becker dissector c.
Becker Greater Grater dissecting c.
blunt bullet-tip c.
bullet-shaped c.
candy cane c.
candy cane c. style I
candy cane c. style II
cobra c.
Coleman aspiration c.
Coleman infiltration c.
Concorde c.
curved c.
four-pronged liposuction c.
Goddio disposable c.
golf tee hollow titanium c.
Gonzalez specialized dissecting c.
Illouz c.
infusion/infiltration c.
Karman c.
Klein c.
Leon cobra c.
liposuction c.
Mercedes c.
Pinto superficial dissection c.
pyramid c.
Rabinov c.
Robles cutting point c.
Rosenberg dissecting c.
shark-mouth c.
single-lumen c.
small-bore c.
suction c.
c. tip
Toledo V-dissector c.
Toomey angled c.
Toomey G-bevel c.
Toomey standard c.
TriEye c.
Unitech Toomey c.
Unitri c.
cannulation
duct c.
canonical babbling
CANS
central auditory nervous system

CANS
computer assisted neurosurgical
navigational system
cant
occlusal c.
c. of occlusal plane of mandible
cantaloupe
cantholysis
inferior c.
superior c.
canthopexy
bilateral c.
lateral c.
canthoplasty
inferior retinacular lateral c.
lateral c.
medial c.
c. procedure
canthotomy
lateral c.
canthus
lateral c.
medial c.
Cantil
cantilever
c. beam
c. bridge
c. fixed partial denture
c. graft
c. partial denture
c. space maintainer
cantilevered bone graft
cantilevering
canting
occlusal c.
canyon ragweed
cap
canal c.
chin c.
enamel c.
germinal c.
c. splint
c. stage
c. technique
capacitance
capacitor
capacity
functional residual c. (FRC)
inspiratory c. (IC)
lung c.
respiratory c.

C

NOTES

capacity *(continued)*
  total lung c. (TLC)
  vital c. (VC)
Capdepont-Hodge syndrome
Capdepont syndrome
capelike distribution
capillary
  c. arcade
  c. bed shunt
  c. hemangioma
  c. hyperemia
  lymph c.
  c. lymphangioma
  lymphatic c.
  c. plexus
  c. vascular malformation
Capital and Codeine
capitate papillae
capitis
  anterior rectus c.
  lateral rectus c.
capitium
capitonnage
capitulum mandibulae
Caplet
  Advil Cold & Sinus C.'s
  A.R.M. C.
  Aspirin-Free Bayer Select Allergy
    Sinus C.'s
  Bayer Select Chest Cold C.'s
  Bayer Select Head Cold C.'s
  Dimacol C.'s
  Dimetapp Sinus C.'s
  Dristan Cold C.'s
  Dristan Sinus C.'s
  TripTone C.'s
  Tylenol Extended Release C.'s
capnography
capping
  direct pulp c.
  indirect pulp c.
  pulp c.
  c. technique
capriloquism
caproate
  hydroxyprogesterone c.
caprylate
  penicillin, bacitracin,
    streptomycin, c. (PBSC)
  sodium c.
Caps
  Drixoral Cough & Congestion
    Liquid C.
  Drixoral Cough & Sore Throat
    Liquid C.
  Feverall Sprinkle C.
  Sudafed Cold & Cough Liquid C.
Capsella bursa-pastoris

capsicum
Capsicum frutescens
capsular
  c. calcification
  c. contracture
  c. flap pyeloplasty
  c. mineralization
capsulatum
  Histoplasma c.
capsule
  Alka-Seltzer Plus Cold Liqui-
    Gels C.'s
  Allerest 12 Hour C.
  Banophen Decongestant C.
  Betachron E-R C.
  Dapacin Cold C.
  Dimetapp 4-Hour Liqui-Gel C.
  Duadacin C.
  fibrous c.
  Glisson c.
  Intal Inhalation C.
  Kadian C.
  lateral c.
  nasal c.
  Ordrine AT Extended Release C.
  otic c.
  parotid c.
  periprosthetic fibrous c.
  Poly-Histine-D C.
  Rescaps-D S.R. C.
  salivary gland c.
  c. of temporomandibular joint
  temporomandibular joint c.
  tumor c.
  Tuss-Allergine Modified T.D. C.
  Tussogest Extended Release C.
capsulectomy
capsulitis
capsulopalpebral fascia
capsuloplasty
capsulotomy
  closed c.
  open c.
captopril
caput
  c. angulare quadratus labii
    superioris
  c. malleus
Carabelli
  cusp of C.
  C. tubercle
caramiphen and phenylpropanolamine
carat, karat
  24 c. gold
carbachol
carbamazepine
carbamide peroxide (CP)
Carbastat Ophthalmic

carbenicillin
carbide
    c. bur
    c. finishing bur
    multifluted c.
    power cut/tungsten c. (PC/TC)
    silicon c. (SiC)
    tungsten c. (TC)
carbinoxamine
    c. and pseudoephedrine
    c., pseudoephedrine, and
      dextromethorphan
Carbiset
    C. Tablet
    C.-TR Tablet
Carbocaine
Carbodec
    C. DM
    C. Syrup
    C. TR Tablet
carbogen
carbohydrate moiety
carbolic acid
carbon
    c. dioxide (CO_2)
    c. dioxide laser
    c. dioxide snow
    c. dioxide snow method
    c. dioxide snow test
carbonate
    calcium c. ($CaCO_3$)
    sodium c.
    zinc c.
carbonic anhydrase
carbonization
carboplatin
Carboptic Ophthalmic
carborundum
    c. disk
    c. wheel
carboxymethylcellulose
    benzocaine, gelatin, pectin, and
      sodium c.
carcinoembryonic antigen
carcinogenesis
carcinogenic
carcinogenicity
carcinoid
    laryngeal c.
    oncocytoid c.
    c. tumor

carcinoma
    acinic cell c.
    acinous cell c.
    adenoid cystic c. (ACC)
    adenoid squamous c.
    adenopapillary c.
    alveolar c.
    ameloblastic c.
    amphicrine c.
    anaplastic c.
    antral c.
    basal cell c. (BCC)
    basosquamous c. (BSC)
    branchiogenic c.
    bronchiolar c.
    bronchogenic c.
    central mucoepidermoid c. (CMEC)
    clear cell c.
    cribriform salivary c. of the
      excretory duct (CSCED)
    c. cuniculatum
    cystogenic c.
    ductal c.
    EME c.
    epidermoid c.
    epithelial-myoepithelial c.
    c. ex pleomorphic adenoma
    follicular c.
    follicular thyroid c.
    gastrointestinal c.
    glottic c.
    glottic squamous cell c.
    glottic-subglottic squamous cell c.
    head and neck squamous cell c.
      (HNSCC)
    Hürthle cell c.
    hypopharyngeal squamous cell c.
    infiltrating c.
    infraglottic squamous cell c.
    intraepithelial c.
    intraosseous c.
    invasive lobular c.
    keratinizing squamous cell c.
    laryngeal c.
    laryngeal neuroendocrine c.
    lingual thyroid c.
    lobular c.
    maxillary sinus c.
    Merkel cell c.
    metastatic c.
    metastatic basal cell c.
    microcystic adnexal c.

C

NOTES

carcinoma *(continued)*
    moderately differentiated neuroendocrine c.
    morpheaform basal cell c.
    mucoepidermoid c. (MEC)
    mucus-producing adenopapillary c. (MPAPC)
    nasopharyngeal c. (NPC)
    c. of nasopharynx
    c. of nasopharynx type a, b, c
    neuroendocrine c.
    nonkeratinizing c.
    oat cell c.
    oral squamous c.
    oral squamous cell c. (oral SCC)
    pancreatic c.
    papillary thyroid c.
    parotid c.
    postcricoid c.
    postcricoid squamous cell c.
    primary intraosseous c.
    pseudosarcomatous c.
    recurrent squamous cell c.
    renal cell c.
    salivary duct c. (SDC)
    salivary gland c. (SGC)
    Schmincke-Regaud lymphoepithelial c.
    sebaceous c.
    c. in situ
    small cell c.
    small cell neuroendocrine c.
    spindle cell c.
    squamous cell c. (SCC)
    subglottic squamous cell c.
    subungual squamous cell c.
    supraglottic c.
    supraglottic squamous cell c.
    terminal duct c.
    thyroid c.
    tonsillar c.
    transglottic squamous cell c.
    transitional cell c.
    undifferentiated c.
    unresectable squamous cell c.
    verrucous c.
    well-differentiated c.
card
    Speech Improvement C.'s
Cardec DM
Cardec-S Syrup
Carden bronchoscopy tube
cardiac
    c. evoked response audiometry (CERA)
    c. gland
Cardiff electrode

cardinal
    c. tongue
    c. vowel
carding
    c. wax
cardiopulmonary
    c. resuscitation (CPR)
cardiovascular disease
carditis
care
    Arm & Hammer Dental C.
    GraftCyte system for wound c.
    Hymed therapeutic skin c.
    palliative c.
    prosthodontic c.
    wound c.
careless weed
Carhart notch
caries
    active c.
    arrested dental c.
    backward c.
    buccal c.
    cemental c.
    cementum c.
    central c.
    cervical c.
    c. classification
    compound c.
    contact c.
    dental c.
    dentinal c.
    distal c.
    enamel c.
    fissure c.
    furcation c.
    healed dental c.
    incipient dental c.
    interdental c.
    internal c.
    interproximal c.
    lateral c.
    mesial c.
    necrotic c.
    nursing bottle c.
    occlusal c.
    pit c.
    pit and fissure c.
    postirradiation dental c.
    primary c.
    proximal dental c.
    c. pulpitis
    radiation c.
    rampant dental c.
    recurrent dental c.
    residual dental c.
    root c.
    secondary c.

senile dental c.
sicca c.
smooth surface c.

carina

carinii

    Pneumocystis c.

cariogenesis
cariogenic
cariogenicity
cariology
cariosity
cariostatic
carious

c. dentin
c. dentin softener
c. pulp exposure
c. restoration margin
c. tooth

carisoprodol

c. and aspirin
c., aspirin, and codeine

Carlens mediastinoscope
C-arm

Siremobil C.-a. unit

Carmault hemostat
Carmichael crown
Carmody-Batson operation
Carmol

C.-HC Topical
C. Topical

carmustine
carnassial

c. tooth

carnauba

c. wax

Carnoy mixture
Carol Gerard screw
caroticotympanic artery
carotid

c. air cell
c. aneurysm
c. artery
c. body
c. body tumor
c. canal
c. genu
c. isolation
c. sheath
c. sheath type parapharyngeal
    schwannoma
c. space

carotid-cavernous sinus fistula (CCSF)

carotodynia, carotidynia
carpal

c. canal
c. tunnel decompression
c. tunnel release (CTR)
c. tunnel release system (CTRS)
c. tunnel release system device
c. tunnel syndrome (CTS)

Carpenter syndrome
carpentry

bone c.

carp mouth
carpometacarpal (CMC)
carposcope
Carpue method
Carpule
Carrell Discrimination Test
carrier

amalgam c.
bronchoscopic sponge c.
foil c.
lentula c.
lentula paste c.
lentula spiral c.
miniature c.
paste c.
c. phrase
Thermafil plastic c.
vascular c.

carrot
Carrow

C. Auditory-Visual Abilities Test
C. Elicited Language Inventory
    (CELI)

carryover

c. coarticulation

carteolol
cartilage

alar c.
alar dome and c.
arytenoid c.
auricular c.
beveled septal c.
bovine c.
conchal c.
condylar c.
corniculate c.
costal c.
cricoid c.
cuneiform c.
dentinal c.
c. edge

C

NOTES

cartilage *(continued)*
 gingival c.
 c. graft
 hyaline c.
 hyoid c.
 irradiated homologous costal c.
 c. island
 laryngeal c.
 lateral c.
 lower lateral c.
 mandibular c.
 Meckel c.
 morselized c.
 quadrangular c.
 septal c.
 c. spike
 splayed alar c.
 thyroid c.
 tragal c.
 upper lateral nasal c.
 vomeronasal c.
 Wrisberg c.
cartilaginous
 c. autologous thin septal (CATS)
 c. autologous thin septal graft
 c. graft
cartilago triticea
cartridge
 anesthesia c.
 Astra dental c.
Cartrol Oral
cartwheel motion
caruncle
 Stensen duct c.
 submaxillary c.
caruncula sublingualis
carver
 acorn c.
 amalgam c.
 cleoid c.
 discoid c.
 Gritman No. 6. c.
 Hollenback c.
 LeCron c.
 porcelain c.
 Roach c.
 Shooshan A c.
 Vehe c.
 wax c.
carving
 c. blade
cascade
 clotting c.
 complement c.
cascading effect
cascara sagrada
case
 C. appliance

C. enamel cleaver
 c. grammar
 c. relation
 weeping c.
caseation
casei
 Lactobacillus c.
caseosa
 coryza c.
 ozena c.
 rhinitis c.
caseous
 c. necrosis
 c. purulent rhinorrhea
cashew
cassette
 Kodak X-Omatic C-1 c.
Cassia senna
cast
 c. bar splint
 c. buccal tube
 c. clasp
 c. core
 c. core and crown
 dental c.
 diagnostic c.
 diagnostic implant c.
 c. glass ceramic
 c. glass ceramic crown
 gnathostatic c.
 c. gold inlay
 c. gold onlay
 implant c.
 investment c.
 c. investment
 master c.
 c. material
 c. metal bridge
 modified c.
 c. perforated bridge
 preextraction c.
 preoperative c.
 refractory c.
 silverplated c.
 c. support
 working c.
Castanares face lift scissors
casting
 centrifugal c.
 ceramo-metal c.
 dental c.
 direct c.
 c. flask
 gold c.
 c. investment
 c. machine
 c. model
 c. mold

porous c.
c. ring
c. sprue
superstructure c.
vacuum c.
c. wax
Castleman lymphoma
Castone
castor bean
Castorway
castration
Castroviejo
    C. caliper
    C. forceps
CAT
  computed axial tomography
  computerized axial tomography
    CAT scan
cat
    c. cry syndrome
    c. dander
    c. epithelium antigen
    c. scratch disease
    c. sneer exercise
catabolic
    c. steroid
Cataflam Oral
catalase
catalogia
Catamaran swim plug
cataphasia
catarrh
    nasal c.
    tubal c.
catarrhal
    c. deafness
    c. disease
    c. gingivitis
    c. otitis media
    c. stomatitis
catarrhalis
    Branhamella c.
    Moraxella c.
    Neisseria c.
catastrophic response
catch
    c. basin
    glottal c.
catecholamine
category
    grammatical c.
    lexical c.

catenary curve
catenate
catenative
caterpillar flap
catgut suture
catheter
    Abocath c.
    ARROWgard central venous c.
    axillary c.
    eustachian c.
    fine-bore c.
    Fogarty c.
    Fogarty adherent clot c.
    Foley c.
    Hickman c.
    nasotracheal c.
    pectoral c.
    sialographic c.
    silicone epistaxis c.
    transoral c.
catheterization
cathode (C, Ca)
Catrix
    C. cream
    C. lip saver
    C. 10 ointment
CATS
  cartilaginous autologous thin septal
    CATS graft
cat's paw retractor
Cattel Scale
cattle dander
cauda
    c. equina
    c. helicis
caudad
caudal
    c. platyrrhinia
    c. rotation
caudalis
    subnucleus c.
caudolateral
Caulfield retriever
cauliflower
    c. ear
Caulk
    C. impression paste
    C. Micro II alloy
    C. Optaloy amalgam
    C. Optaloy II alloy
    C. spherical alloy

C

NOTES

Caulk (*continued*)
    C. Syntrex F cement
    C. varnish
Caulophyllum thalictroides
causalgia
    facial c.
    genitofemoral c.
    c. neuralgia
causality
caustic
    acid c.
    alkali c.
    c. ingestion
    c. substance
cauterization
    phenol c.
cautery
    bipolar c.
    Colorado tip c.
    c. knife
cava (*pl. of* cavum)
cave
    Meckel c.
cavernosa
    corpora c.
cavernosum
    corpus c.
cavernous
    c. hemangioma
    c. lymphangiohemangioma
    c. lymphangioma
    c. sinus
    c. sinus thrombosis
    c. tissue
    c. voice sound
CAVHD
    continuous arteriovenous hemodialysis
caviar lesion
Cavidentin sealer
Cavidry base liner
Cavi-Endo
    C.-E. ultrasonic system
Cavilax
Cavi-Line cavity varnish
cavitas, pl. **cavitates**
    c. dentis
cavitation
Cavitec cement
Cavit G
**Cavi-Trol acidulated phosphate fluoride
topical gel**
Cavitron
    C. ultrasonic surgical aspirator
    C. ultrasonic system
cavit temporary
cavity
    access c.
    c. access

alveolar c.
c. angle
artificial classification c.
axial surface c.
buccal c.
canal-wall-down c.
c. classification
c. cleaner
complex c.
compound c.
crippling of oral c.
c. debridement
dental c.
distal c.
DO c.
endodontic c.
eosinophilic ulcer of oral c.
fissure c.
gingival c.
heterotrophic gastrointestinal mucosa
    of oral c.
idiopathic bone c.
incisal c.
labial c.
c. line angle
c. liner
lingual c.
c. lining
c. lining agent
c. margin
mastoid c.
MO c.
MOD c.
nasal c.
neovaginal c.
nonseptate c.
occlusal c.
open c.
oral c.
pit and fissure c.
c. preparation
c. preparation base
c. preparation form
prepared c.
c. primer
progressive bone c.
proximal c.
pulp c.
c. seal
smooth surface c.
Stafne idiopathic bone c.
c. test
toilet of c.
c. toilet
c. of tooth
tympanic c.
c. varnish

vitreous c.
c. wall
cavosurface
c. angle
c. bevel
c. margin
cavum, pl. **cava**
c. conchae
c. conchal cartilage graft
c. dentis
c. tympani
Cawthorne-Day procedure
cayenne
c. pepper
CB
Dentillium CB
CB Erbium/2.94 laser
CBA No. 9080 cement
C-Brite nonchemical skin brightener
CCB
calcium channel blocker
cancellous cellular bone
CCB graft
CCD
charge-coupled device
CCG
costochondral graft
CCL cell
CCMS
cerebrocostomandibular syndrome
CCNU
cyclohexylchloroethylnitrosurea
CCOT
clear cell odontogenic tumor
C-Cream
pHaze 16 C.-C.
CCRN
congenital cartilaginous rest of the neck
C-Crystals
CCSF
carotid-cavernous sinus fistula
CD
Ceclor CD
CDDP
cis diaminedichloroplatinum diamine
cisplatin
CDF
color flow Doppler
CDG
central developmental groove
CDI
communicative development inventory

cDNA probe
CDP
computerized dynamic posturography
CDPP
computerized dynamic platform
posturography
CDT
Certified Dental Technician
CDTADA
CE-3000 video technology
Cebid Timecelles
Ceclor
C. CD
Cecon
cecum
foramen c.
vestibular c.
cedar
Japanese c.
mountain c.
red c.
salt c.
Cedax
CeeNU
Ceepryn
cefaclor
cefadroxil
Cefadyl
cefamandole
cefazolin
cefepime
cefixime
Cefizox
cefmetazole
Cefobid
cefonicid
cefoperazone
Cefotan
cefotaxime
cefotetan
cefoxitin
cefpodoxime
c. proxetil
cefprozil
ceftazidime
ceftibuten
Ceftin
C. Oral
C. tablet
ceftizoxime
ceftriaxone

NOTES

C

cefuroxime
>   c. axetil
>   c. sodium

Cefzil

ceiling

CEJ
>   cemento-enamel junction

Ceka attachment

Cel
>   C. Touch adhesive
>   C. Touch white indicator powder

Celay
>   C. InCeram crown
>   C. milling unit
>   C. system
>   C. Tech light curing resin

celery

Celestin tube

Celestone

CELF
>   Clinical Evaluation of Language
>   Functions

CELI
>   Carrow Elicited Language Inventory

celiac syndrome

celiotomy
>   staged c.

cell
>   acinar c.
>   c. adhesion molecule (CAM)
>   agger nasi c.
>   air c.
>   angulated c.
>   anterior ethmoidal air c.
>   antigen-presenting c. (APC)
>   antral c.
>   apical c.
>   argentaffin c.
>   B c.
>   basal c.
>   border c.
>   carotid air c.
>   CCL c.
>   centrocyte-like c.
>   chief c.
>   chondroblastic c.
>   chondroid c.
>   chondroprogenitor c.
>   ciliated c.
>   c.'s of Claudius
>   cochlear hair c.
>   connective tissue c.
>   cover c.
>   cuboidal c.
>   cultured periosteal c.
>   c. cycle
>   defense c.
>   dendritic c.

dentin c.
dentinoblastic c.
dentin-producing c.
desquamated epithelial c.
differentiated c.
duboid c.
end c.
endothelial c.
epithelial c.
epithelioid c.
epitympanic air c.
ethmoid air c.'s
ethmoidal c.'s
ethmoidal labyrinth c.
fibroblastic c.
fibrous histiocytic c.
follicular dendritic c. (FDC)
frontoethmoidal c.
ganglionic nerve c.
giant c.
goblet c.
granular c.
hair c.
Haller c.
c.'s of Hansen
Hürthle c.
hyaline c.
immunocompetent c.
inflammatory c.
infralabyrinthine air c.
infundibular c.
interdigitating dendritic c. (IDC)
K c.
killer c.
Langerhans c.'s
Langhans c.'s
Langhans-type giant c.'s
leprae c.
lymphoid wandering c.
lymphokine-activated killer c.
   (LAK)
macular hair c.
malpighian c.
mast c.
mastoid tip c.
medial wall of agger nasi c.
memory c.
meningothelial c.
Merkel c.
mesenchymal c.
microvillar c.
Mikulicz c.'s
monocytoid c.
mucous c.
mucus-secreting c.
multinucleated dentinoblastic c.
multinucleated giant c.
myoepithelial c.

natural killer c. (NK)
nerve c.
c. nest
Neumann c.
neural crest c.
odontoprogenitor c.
olfactory c.
oncocytic epithelial c.
Onodi c.
osteoclastic c.
osteoclast-like giant c.
osteocompetent c.
osteoprogenitor c.
Paneth c.
paraganglion c.
parenchymal c.
periaqueductal air c.
peripheral blood mononuclear c. (PBMC)
phagocytic c.
physaliphorous c.
plasma c.
pluripotential c.
pluripotential primordial germ c.
polygonal c.
polygonal fat c.
postcarotid air c.
posterior ethmoidal c.
posterior wall of agger nasi c.
postmitotic c.
precarotid air c.
precochlear c.
prickle c.
progenitor c.
red blood c. (RBC)
Reed-Sternberg c.
reserve c.
resorption c.
resorptive c.
restructured c.
retrofacial c.
retrofacial air c.
Schwann c.
secretory c.
serous c.
serous demilune c.
SG c.
sinus group of air c.
smooth muscle c.
special c.
spindle c.
spinous c.

substantia gelatinosa c.
subtubal air c.
supporting c.
supracarotid air c.
supracochlear air c.
supraorbital air c.
sustentacular c.
synthetic c.
T c.
taste c.
Tc c.
TDTH c.
telangiectatic c.
T-helper c.
thyroid C c.
transmission c.
tympanic c.
Tzanck c.
undifferentiated c.
undifferentiated mesenchymal c.
vacuolated Hurler c.
zygomal c.

CellCept
Cellex-C
cell-free zone
cell-mediated
 c.-m. immune response
 c.-m. immunity
cell-poor zone
cell-rich zone
cellular
 c. cementum
 c. and complex-mediated immune response
 c. pleomorphism
cellulite
 Chesterfield sofa c.
 c. phenomenon
cellulitis
 facial and cervical c.
 orbital c.
 periorbital c.
 peritonsillar c.
 preseptal c.
 submaxillary c.
 synergistic necrotizing c.
cellulocutaneous flap
celluloid
 c. matrix
 c. strip
 c. strip crown

NOTES

C

95

cellulose
    aqueous methyl c.
    hydroxyethyl c.
    hydroxypropyl c.
    nitrated c.
    oxidized c.
celsius (C)
cement
    acrylic resin dental c.
    adhesive c.
    Band-Lok orthodontic band c.
    c. base
    black copper c.
    BoneSource hydroxyapatite c.
    calcium hydroxide c. light-cured
    calcium hydroxide c. self-cured
    Caulk Syntrex F c.
    Cavitec c.
    CBA No. 9080 c.
    composite dental c.
    composite resin luting c.
    copper c.
    copper dental c.
    copper phosphate c.
    c. corpuscle
    CR inlay c.
    cyanoacrylate c.
    dental c.
    dental base c.
    Dentemp ZOE temporary c.
    dimethacrylate c.
    Durelon c.
    Dycal c.
    EBA c.
    Elite c.
    endodontic c.
    Fleck c.
    Fluoro-Thin c.
    glass ionomer c.
    glass ionomer c. light-cured
    glass ionomer c. self-cured
    Grip c.
    Harvard-C.
    hydrophosphate c.
    inorganic dental c.
    Justi resin c.
    Kent zinc c.
    Ketac Fil c.
    Ketac Silver c.
    Ketac-Silver glass-ionomer c.
    Kirkland c.
    Kryptex dental c.
    c. line
    luting c.
    modified zinc oxide-eugenol c.
    MQ c.
    My-Bond Carbo c.

    Mynol c.
    organic dental c.
    oxyphosphate c.
    periodontal c.
    polycarboxylate c.
    polymer-reinforced zinc oxide-eugenol c.
    polymethyl methacrylate c.
    porcelain c.
    pseudocopper c.
    red copper c.
    resin c.
    root canal c.
    sealer c.
    silicate c.
    silicate zinc c.
    siliceous dental c.
    silicophosphate c.
    Smith resin c.
    Smith zinc c.
    c. spatula
    Sultan C. UP
    SuperEBA c.
    Surgical Simplex P bone c.
    temporary c.
    Temrex zinc oxide-eugenol c.
    Tenacin zinc phosphate c.
    tooth c.
    unmodified zinc oxide-eugenol c.
    Vitrebond c.
    Zapit c.
    zinc oxide c.
    zinc oxide-eugenol c.
    zinc oxide-eugenol dental c.
    zinc oxide-eugenol c. Type IV
    zinc oxyphosphate c.
    zinc phosphate c.
    zinc polyacrylate c.
    zinc polycarboxylate c.
    zinc silicophosphate c.
cemental
    c. caries
    c. crack
    c. cuticle
    c. dysplasia
    c. fiber
    c. fracture
    c. gingiva
    c. lamella
    c. lesion
    c. ligament
    c. line
    c. repair
    c. resorption
    c. spicule
    c. spike
    c. tear

cementation
    final c.
    trial c.
cemented
    c. gingiva
    c. pin
cementicle
    adherent c.
    attached c.
    embedded c.
    free c.
    interstitial c.
cementification
cementifying fibroma
cementing
    c. line
    c. substance
cementitis
cementoblast
cementoblastoma
    benign c.
cementoclasia
cementoclast
cementocyte
    canaliculi of c.
    lacuna of c.
cementodentinal
    c. junction
cemento-enamel junction (CEJ)
cementogenesis
cementogenic
    c. layer
    c. theory
cementoid
    c. tissue
cementoma
    first-state c.
    gigantiform c.
    gigantiform monstrous c.
    true c.
cement-on-crown (COC)
cementopathia
cementoperiostitis
cementoproximal
cementosis
    aberrant c.
cement-retained prosthesis
cementum
    aberrant c.
    acellular c.
    afibrillar c.
    apical c.

    calcified c.
    c. caries
    cellular c.
    coronal c.
    c. crystal
    decalcified c.
    c. fracture
    c. hyperplasia
    hyperplastic c.
    hypertrophic c.
    c. hypertrophy
    incremental lines of c.
    intermediate c.
    lamellar c.
    necrotic c.
    periapical c.
    primary c.
    c. resorption
    root c.
    secondary c.
    c. tear
    uncalcified c.
Cenafed
    C. Plus Tablet
Cencit
    C. facial scanner
    C. imaging system
Cenolate
center
    dentary c.
    germinal c.
    c. of gravity (COG)
    gustatory c.
    Instrument Recirculation C. (IRC)
    language c.
    c. of ridge
    swallowing c.
    taste c.
center-action forceps
centering
    c. drill
    c. genioplasty
centigrade (C)
Centra 28
central
    c. aphasia
    c. apnea
    c. auditory abilities
    c. auditory disorder
    c. auditory function
    c. auditory nervous system (CANS)
    c. auditory perception

C

NOTES

central *(continued)*
  c. auditory process
  c. bearing
  c. caries
  c. cementifying fibroma
  c. cementifying/ossifying fibroma
  c. cusp
  c. deafness
  c. developmental groove (CDG)
  c. facial paralysis
  c. fibroma
  c. fibromatosis
  c. fossa (CF)
  c. giant cell granuloma
  c. giant cell reparative granuloma
  c. giant cell tumor
  c. granular cell odontogenic tumor
    (CGCOT)
  c. groove of central fossa (CGCF)
  c. hearing
  c. hearing loss
  c. hemangioma
  c. incisor
  c. incisor tooth
  c. language disorder (CLD)
  c. language imbalance
  c. masking
  c. mucoepidermoid carcinoma
    (CMEC)
  c. nervous system (CNS)
  c. neurogenic neoplasm
  c. neuronal axis
  c. occlusion
  c. odontogenic fibroma
  c. ossifying fibroma
  c. pit (CP)
  c. ray
  c. resorption
  c. speech range
  c. sulcus
  c. tendency
  c. trunk
  c. vermilion
  c. vertigo
  c. vowel
  c. zone
  c. zone inflammation
central-bearing
  c.-b. point
  c.-b. tracing device
centration
Centrax bipolar system
centric
  acquired c.
  broad c.
  c. checkbite
  c. contact
  habitual c.

  c. interocclusal record
  c. jaw relation
  long c.
  c. maxillomandibular record
  c. mounting
  Myo-Monitor c.
  c. occluding relation
  c. occluding relation record
  c. occlusion
  point c.
  c. position
  power c.
  c. relation-centric occlusion
    (CR/CO)
  c. relation occlusion
  retruded c.
  slide in c.
centrically balanced occlusion
centrifugal
  c. casting
centrifugation
centrifuge
  c. test
centriole
centripetal action
Centrix-type syringe
centrocyte-like cell
centrofacial
Cēpacol Anesthetic Troche
Cēpastat
cephalad
cephalexin
cephalgia
  histamine c.
  Horton histamine c.
cephalhematoma
  calcified c.
cephalic
  c. index
cephalicus
  herpes zoster c.
cephalogram
  digitized lateral c.
  submental vertex c.
cephalography
cephalometer
  radiographic c.
cephalometric
  c. analysis
  c. correction
  c. laminagraphy
  c. landmark
  c. protractor
  c. radiograph
  c. radiography
  c. roentgenogram
  c. tracing
cephalometrics

cephalometry
cephalophore
cephalopolysyndactyly syndrome
cephalosporin
Cephalosporium
cephalostat
cephalothin
cephaloxerogram
cephapirin
Ceptaz
CERA
    cardiac evoked response audiometry
Ceramco porcelain
CeraMed
    C. bone grafting material
ceramic
    c. alloy
    c. bracket
    cast glass c.
    chairside economical restorations of
      esthetic c.'s (CEREC)
    dental c.'s
    c. dentistry
    c. enamel
    c. endosseous implant
    c. endosteal implant
    glass c.
    c. inlay
    machineable apatite-free glass c.
    c. onlay
    c. orthoclase
    c. restoration
    c. veneer
ceramic-metal crown
ceramodontics
ceramo-metal, ceramometal
    c.-m. alloy
    c.-m. casting
    c.-m. implant bridge
    c.-m. margin
    c.-m. restoration
CeraOne
    C. abutment
    C. abutment implant
    C. implant system
cerclage wire technique
cerebellar
    c. abscess
    c. speech
    c. vein
cerebellopontine (CP)
    c. angle (CPA)

c. angle collision tumor
c. angle syndrome
cerebellum
    flocculus of c.
cerebral
    c. anoxia
    c. aqueduct
    c. blindness
    c. cortex
    c. dominance
    c. dominance and handedness
      theory
    c. edema
    c. localization
    c. palsy
    c. palsy symptomatology
    c. reference line
    c. thumb
cerebri
    falx c.
    pseudotumor c.
    tinnitus c.
cerebriform tongue
cerebrocostomandibular syndrome
    (CCMS)
cerebropalatine angle
cerebrospinal
    c. fluid (CSF)
    c. fluid leak
    c. fluid otorrhea
    c. fluid rhinorrhea
cerebrovascular accident (CVA)
cerebrum
CEREC
    chairside economical restorations of
      esthetic ceramics
      CEREC system
ceresin
cerin
Cerose-DM
cerosin
Certified Dental Technician (CDT)
cerumen
    impacted c.
    c. inspissatum
Cerumenex Otic
ceruminal
ceruminolytic
ceruminoma
ceruminosis
ceruminous

NOTES

C

cervical
- c. abrasion
- c. anchorage
- c. branch
- c. caries
- c. clamp
- c. convergence
- c. cyst
- c. diverticulum
- c. enamel
- c. esophagostomy
- c. esophagus
- c. fascia
- c. flap
- c. ganglion
- c. hydrocele
- c. hygroma
- c. hyperesthesia
- c. line (CL)
- c. loop
- c. margin
- c. metastasis
- c. midline pterygium
- c. muscle contraction
- c. plexus
- c. skin replacement
- c. soft tissue
- c. sympathectomy
- c. sympathetic nerve
- c. sympathetic schwannoma
- c. thymus
- c. vertebra
- c. vertigo
- c. vessel
- c. zone
- c. zone of tooth

cervical-occipital roll
cervices (pl. of cervix)
cervicis (gen. of cervix)
cervicoaxial (CA)
cervicobregmatic diameter
cervicobuccal
cervicodynia
cervicofacial
- c. actinomycosis
- c. rhytidectomy procedure
- c. sling
- c. trunk

cervicofacioplasty
cervicolabial
cervicolingual
cervicolinguoaxial
cervicomastoid region
cervicomental angle
cervico-occipital
cervico-oculo-acoustic syndrome
cervicopectoral flap

cervicoplasty
cervix, gen. cervicis, pl. cervices
- c. dentis
- implant c.

Cesead
C-Esta
Cetamide Ophthalmic
Cetapred Ophthalmic
Cetavlon
- ethylenediaminetetraacetic acid C. (EDTAC)

cetirizine
- c. HCl

cetylpyridinium
- c. and benzocaine

Cevalin
Cevi-Bid
Ce-Vi-Sol
cevitamic acid
CF
- central fossa
  - Guiatuss CF
  - Robafen CF

CFFR
- crevicular fluid flow rate

CFM
- chemotactic factor for macrophage

C-form osteotomy
CGCF
- central groove of central fossa

CGCOT
- central granular cell odontogenic tumor

CH
- calcium hydroxide

Chaetomium
Chagas-Cruz disease
Chagas disease
chain
- glycosaminoglycan c.
- ossicle c.
- ossicular c.
- polypeptide c.
- polysaccharide molecular c.

chaining
chair
- Bárány c.
- computerized rotary c.
- rotational c.
- video fluoroscopic imaging c.

chairside
- c. economical restorations of esthetic ceramics (CEREC)
- c. economical restorations of esthetic ceramics system

Chajchir dissector
chalazion
- c. forceps

chalinoplasty

chalk
chamber
    altitude c.
    anechoic c.
    axial walls of the pulp c.
    calcification of pulp c.
    echo c.
    ion-collecting c.
    ionization c.
    no-echo c.
    packing c.
    pulp c. (PCH)
    relief c.
chamfer
    c. bevel
    c. preparation
chamois
    c. yellow appearance
chamomile
Champy
    C. miniplate
    C. miniplate, rigid fixation system
change
    cushingoid c.
    dimensional c.
    oncocytoid c.
    phylogenetic c.
    thermal dimensional c.
    volumetric dimensional c.
changer
channels
    ectatic capillary c.
channel shoulder pin technique
chaparral
character
characteristic
    sexual c.'s
characterization
    denture c.
Charcot
    C. arthropathy
    C. vertigo
Charcot-Marie-Tooth disorder
chard
    Swiss c.
char-free carbon dioxide laser
CHARGE
    coloboma of iris, heart deformities,
    choanal atresia, retarded growth, genital
    and ear deformities
        CHARGE association

charge-coupled
    c.-c. device (CCD)
    c.-c. device video camera
Charisma resin
charley horse
Charlie-M syndrome
Charlin syndrome
chart
    anchorage space-to-save c.
    A point c.
    Bonwill-Hawley c.
    dental c.
    Hawley c.
    Northampton c.'s
    periodontal c.
    Snellen Eye C.
    Troyer Patient Education Series c.
Charters
    C. method
    C. method of toothbrushing
    C. technique
chaste tree berry
Chausse
    C. III projection
    third projection of C.
Chayes
    C. attachment
    C. method
checkbite, check-bite
    centric c.
    eccentric c.
    lateral c.
    protrusive c.
checkpoint
    G_1 c.
check-rein effect
checkvalve
    BacStop c.
cheek
    c. advancement flap
    c. augmentation
    c. bag
    c. biting
    c. bone
    cleft c.
    collapsed c.
    c. implant
    c. mucous-muscle flap
    c. muscle
    c. pad
    postmaxillectomy collapsed c.
    c. pouch

C

NOTES

cheek *(continued)*
    c. retractor
    c. rotation flap
    c. tone
    c. and tongue retractor
    c. tooth
    vestibule of c.
cheek-lip flap
cheese
    Swiss c.
cheilalgia
cheilectomy
cheilectropion
cheilion
cheilitis
    actinic c.
    angular c.
    commissural c.
    c. glandularis
    c. granulomatosa
    granulomatous c.
cheilitis-glossitis-gingivitis syndrome
cheiloalveoloschisis
cheiloangioscopy
cheilocarcinoma
cheilognathoglossoschisis
cheilognathopalatoschisis
cheilognathoprosoposchisis
cheilognathoschisis
cheilognathouranoschisis
cheilophagia
cheiloplasty
cheilorrhaphy
cheiloschisis
cheilosis
cheilostomatoplasty
cheilotomy
cheirology
cheiroplasty
chelate
chelating agent
chelation
chelonei
    Mycobacterium c.
chemical
    c. bonding
    c. burn
    c. denervation
    c. face peeling
    c. labyrinthectomy
    c. peel
    c. shift
    c. substance
    c. vapor sterilization
chemically
    c. activated system
    c. cured composite resin
chemicoparasitic theory

chemoactivation
chemodectoma
chemoexfoliation
chemokine
chemoreceptor
chemosis
chemosurgery
    Mohs c.
chemosurgical
    c. gingivectomy
    c. superficial dermatologic peel
chemotactic
    c. agent
    c. factor
    c. factor for macrophage (CFM)
chemotaction
chemotaxis
chemotherapeutic agent
chemotherapy
    adjuvant c.
    combination c.
    intra-arterial c.
    neoadjuvant c.
Chenopodium
cheoplastic
    c. base
    c. tooth
cheoplasty
cherry
    c. angioma
    c. hemangioma
    wild c.
cherubism
chessboard graft
chest
    c. bellows
    c. flap
    c. pulse
    c. voice
    c. wall
Chesterfield sofa cellulite
chestnut
    horse c.
chevron
    c. incision
    c. marking technique
chew-in
    c.-i. record
    c.-i. technique
chewing
    breath c.
    c. cycle
    c. force
    c. method
CHI
    closed head injury
Chiaie tooth

Chiari
> C. type I, II, III, IV malformation
> C. type I malformation with
>   syringomyelia

chiasm
> optic c.

chicken
> c. feather dander
> c. feathers

chickenpox
Chick patient transfer device
chief cell
childhood
> c. aphasia
> progressive spinal muscular atrophy
>   of c.
> c. psychosis
> c. schizophrenia

children
> Aid to Families with
>   Dependent C. (AFDC)
> Halenol C.'s
> Kaufman Assessment Battery
>   for C.
> Porch Index of Communicative
>   Abilities in C. (PICAC)
> Short Test for Use with Cerebral
>   Palsy C.
> Test of Language Competence
>   for C. (TLC-C)
> Token Test for C.
> Women, Infants, and C. (WIC)

Children's
> C. Advil Oral Suspension
> C. Dynafed Jr
> C. Hospital Medical Center
>   sarcoma chemotherapy protocol
> C. Language Battery
> C. Language Processes
> C. Motrin
> C. Motrin Oral Suspension
> C. Silapap
> C. Silfedrine

chilitis
chiloplasty
chilopodiasis
chilorrhaphy
chiloschisis
chilosis
chilostomatoplasty
chilotomy

chin
> c. augmentation
> c. cap
> c. cup extraoral orthodontic
>   appliance
> extended anatomical c.
> galoche c.
> c. muscle
> c. point
> c. rest
> c. spasm
> c. support
> c. tuck
> witch's c.

chincap
Chinese
> C. elm
> C. flap

chink
> glottal c.
> glottic c.

chin-nose view
chip
> Dembone demineralized
>   cancellous c.'s
> Dembone demineralized cortical c.'s
> Dembone demineralized
>   corticocancellous c.'s
> c. graft
> c. syringe

chip-blower
chipped tooth
chirology
chiroplasty
chisel
> bi-level c.
> binangle c.
> bone c.
> contra-angle c.
> curved c.
> enamel c.
> monoangle c.
> periodontal c.
> posterior c.
> c. scaler
> Sorensen c.
> straight c.
> c. tip
> unibevel c.
> Wedelstaedt c.

chi-square test
chive

NOTES

Chlamydia trachomatis
Chlo-Amine
chloasma
Chlorafed Liquid
chloral hydrate
chlorambucil
chloramphenicol
    c., polymyxin B, and hydrocortisone
    c. and prednisolone
Chloraseptic
    C. Oral
    Vicks Children's C.
Chlorate
chlordiazepoxide
chlorhexidine
    c. digluconate
    c. gluconate (CHX)
chloride
    ammonium c.
    benzalkonium c.
    bethanechol c.
    edrophonium c.
    ethyl c.
    polyvinyl c. (PVC)
    sodium c.
    strontium c.
chlorin
    m-tetra(hydroxyphenol) c. (*m*-THPC)
chlorine
    c. dioxide
    c. dioxide disinfectant
chloroform
Chloromycetin
chloropercha
    c. method
    c. sealer
chloroprocaine
Chloroptic-P Ophthalmic
Chloro-Thymonol root canal dressing
Chlorphed
Chlorphed-LA Nasal Solution
chlorpheniramine
    c. and acetaminophen
    c., phenindamine, and phenylpropanolamine
    c. and phenylephrine
    c., phenylephrine, and codeine
    c., phenylephrine, and dextromethorphan
    c., phenylephrine, and methscopolamine
    c., phenylephrine, and phenylpropanolamine
    c., phenylephrine, phenylpropanolamine, and belladonna alkaloids
    c., phenylephrine, and phenyltoloxamine
    c. and phenylpropanolamine
    c., phenylpropanolamine, and acetaminophen
    c., phenylpropanolamine, and dextromethorphan
    c. phenyltoloxamine, phenylpropanolamine, and phenylephrine
    c. and pseudoephedrine
    c. pseudoephedrine, and codeine
    c. pyrilamine, and phenylephrine
    c. pyrilamine, phenylephrine, and phenylpropanolamine
chlorpheniramine,
Chlor-Pro
chlorpromazine
Chlor-Rest Tablet
chlortetracycline
    c. ointment
Chlor-Trimeton
    C.-T. 4 Hour Relief Tablet
chlorzoxazone
choana, pl. choanae
choanal
    c. atresia
    c. opening
    c. polyp
    c. stenosis
chocolate
choke
    c. vessel
cholangiography
cholangiopancreatography
    endoscopic c.
choledochoplasty
cholelithiasis
    occult c.
cholesteatoma
    acquired c.
    attical c.
    congenital c.
    iatrogenic c.
    c. pearl
    rhinitis c.
cholesterol
    c. cleft
    c. crystal
    c. granuloma
    c. granuloma cyst
    c. slits
choline
    c. magnesium trisalicylate
    c. salicylate
cholinergic
chondrectomy
chondritis

chondroblast
chondroblastic
  c. cell
  c. osteosarcoma
chondroblastoma
chondrocranium
chondrocutaneous flap for ear
  reconstruction
chondrocyte
  c. proliferation
chondroectodermal dysplasia
chondroethmoidal junction
chondrogenesis
chondrogenic sarcoma
chondroglossus muscle
chondroid
  c. bone
  c. cell
chondroitin
  c.-4 sulfate
  c.-6 sulfate
  c. sulfate
  c. sulfuric acid
chondroma
  benign c.
  condylar c.
  juxtacortical c.
  laryngeal c.
  malignant c.
  nasal c.
  periosteal c.
  tracheal c.
  true c.
chondromalacia
  generalized c.
  c. of larynx
  systemic c.
chondromatosis
  synovial c. (SCM)
chondromatous growth
chondromucosal graft
chondromyxoidfibroma
chondronectin
chondro-osteoplastica
  tracheopathia c.-o.
chondroplasty
chondroprogenitor cell
chondroradionecrosis
  laryngeal c.
chondrosarcoma
  extraosseous c.
  extraskeletal c.

  mesenchymal c. (MC)
  synovial c. (SCS)
chondrosternoplasty
chondrosulfatase
chondrotomy
Chopart
  C. amputation
  C. level
choral
  c. reading
  c. speaking
chorda
  c. tympani
  c. tympani nerve
chordee
  correction of c.
  c. release
  residual c.
chorditis
  c. nodosa
  c. tuberosa
  c. vocalis inferior
chordoid
chordoma
  craniocervical c.
  dedifferentiated c.
  sacrococcygeal c.
  skull base c.
  vertebral c.
chorea
  laryngeal c.
choreoathetosis
choriomeningitis
  lymphocytic c.
chorioretinitis
  cytomegalovirus c.
choristoma
  neuromuscular c.
choristomatic cyst
Christensen articulator
chroma
chromatic audition
chromation
  nuclear c.
chromatography
  high-performance liquid c. (HPLC)
chrome
chrome-cobalt alloy pin
chrome-cobalt-molybdenum material
Chromel-Alumel thermocouple
chromic suture
chromium base casting alloy

C

NOTES

chromium-cobalt alloy
chromium-cobalt-molybdenum alloy
chromium-cobalt-nickel base alloy
chromium-iron alloy
chromogranin
Chromolaena odorata
chromophore
    cutaneous c.
chromosome 21-trisomy syndrome
chronaxie, chronaxy
chronic
    c. active hepatitis
    c. apical abscess
    c. atrophic polychondritis
    c. atrophic senile gingivitis
    c. cholesteatomatous otitis media
    c. cicatricial laryngeal stenosis
    c. desquamative gingivitis
    c. diffuse external otitis
    c. diffuse sclerosing osteomyelitis
    c. endemic dental fluorosis
    c. endemic fluorosis
    c. ethmoiditis
    c. fatigue syndrome
    c. fibrotic tonsillitis
    c. focal sclerosing osteomyelitis
    c. frontal sinusitis
    c. granulation otitis media
    c. hyperplastic laryngitis
    c. hyperplastic pulpitis
    c. hypertrophic rhinosinusitis
    c. inflammation
    c. interstitial salpingitis
    c. laryngitis
    c. lingual papillitis
    c. maxillary sinusitis
    c. mononucleosis syndrome
    c. otitis media (COM)
    c. otitis media with effusion
    (COME)
    c. perforating pulp hyperplasia
    c. periapical abscess
    c. periapical periodontitis
    c. pulpalgia
    c. pulpitis
    c. recurrent multifocal osteomyelitis
    (CRMO)
    c. recurrent parotitis
    c. rhinitis
    c. sialadenitis
    c. stenosing external otitis
    c. subglottic laryngitis
    c. suppurative otitis media (CSOM)
    c. suppurative pericementitis
    c. ulcerative pulpitis
chronological age (CA)
Chronotabs
    Disophrol C.

Chrysanthemum parthenium
Chrysosporium
chuck
    AE surgical contra-angle 20:1
      press-button c.
    EA surgical contra-angle 10:1
      press-button c.
    E/200 contra-angle 1:5 press-
      button c.
    E/KM surgical contra-angle 40:1
      press-button c.
    press-button c.
chunking
Churg-Strauss vasculitis
CHX
    chlorhexidine gluconate
chyle
    c. fistula
    c. leak
chylomicron
Ciaglia percutaneous tracheostomy
  introducer set
Cibacalcin Injection
CIC
    circulating immune complex
    completely-in-the-canal
    CIC hearing aid
    CIC listening device
    Little Secret CIC
Cica-Care silicone gel sheeting
cicatricial
    c. ridge
    c. stenosis
cicatrix
cicatrization
    epithelial c.
ciclopirox
Cidex
    C. 7
    C. liquid chemical sterilization
cidofovir
cigarette smoke
cilastatin
    imipenem and c.
cilia (*pl. of* cilium)
ciliary
    c. ganglion
    c. highway
    c. immobility
    c. motion
    c. pathway
ciliastatic
ciliated cell
ciliotoxicity
cilium, pl. cilia
    olfactory c.
    respiratory c.
    rudimentary c.

Ciloxan Ophthalmic
cimetidine
Cimicifuga racemosa
cinch suture
cine-esophagogram
cinefluorography
cinefluoroscopy
cinematography
cineradiography
cineroentgenography
cingula (*pl. of* cingulum)
cingulate
cingule
cingulum, gen. cinguli, pl. cingula
    c. dentis
    c. modification
    c. rest
    c. of tooth
cinnamon
Cipro
    C. HC otic
    C. HC Otic suspension
    C. Injection
    C. Oral
ciprofloxacin
    c. HCl/hydrocortisone
circle of Willis
CircOlectric bed frame
Circon/ACMI endoscope
circuit
    convergence c.
    divergence c.
    feedback reduction c. (FRC)
    neuronal c.
    nociceptive c.
    telephone booster c.
circular
    c. dental ligament
    c. fiber
    c. subcutaneous island flap
    c. trepanation
    c. with Passavant ridge pattern of closure
circulating immune complex (CIC)
circulation
    cutaneous c.
    pulpal c.
circulator
circumalveolar fixation
circumaural
    c. hearing protection device
circumaxillary

circumdentinal wire
circumferential
    c. clasp
    c. clasp arm
    c. esophageal reconstruction
    c. filing
    c. lamella
    c. retention
    c. stroke
    c. suture tie
    c. tearing of skin
    c. wiring
circumflex
    c. iliac artery
    c. scapular artery
    c. scapular flap
    c. scapular pedicle
    c. scapular vessel
circumlocution
circummandibular
    c. fixation
    c. wiring
circumoral
circumpulpal dentin
circumscribed labyrinthitis
circumscriptum
    lymphangioma c.
circumvallate papillae
circumzygomatic
    c. fixation
    c. wiring
cirrhosis
    Laënnec c.
CI-S
    Calculus Index, Simplified
CIS-2 system
cis diaminedichloroplatinum diamine (CDDP)
cisplatin (CDDP)
cis-retinoic acid
cistern
cisternal portion
cisternography
Citanest
citrate
    dibasic sodium c.
    sodium c.
citric
    c. acid
    c. acid cycle
    c. acid-ferric chloride/4 META

NOTES

CL
cervical line
Cladosporium
    C. herbarium antigen
Claforan
Clagett procedure
clam
clamp
    Acland c.
    Allis c.
    approximator c.
    atraumatic bowel c.
    cervical c.
    Cottle columella c.
    D'Assumpcão c.
    David-Baker c.
    David-Baker lip c.
    Ferrier 212 gingival c.
    c. forceps
    gingival c.
    Gomco c.
    Hatch c.
    Hatch gingival c.
    c. holder
    ivory c.
    ivory rubber dam c.
    Joseph c.
    Khan-Jaeger c.
    Lahey c.
    Millard c.
    nerve-approximating c. (NAC)
    pedicle c.
    plate-holding c.
    root rubber dam c.
    rubber dam c.
    rubber dam retainer c.
    shape memory c.
    S.S. White c.
Clapton line
Clarion cochlear implant
clarithromycin
Claritin
    C.-D
    C.-D 24-Hour
Clark
    C. attachment
    C. level
    C. Picture Phonetic Inventory
    C. polarographic oxygen electrode
    C. rule
Clarke-Fournier glossitis
Clark-Madison Test of Oral Language
clasp
    Adams c.
    Aderer No. 20 c.
    arm c.
    c. arm
    arrow c.

    arrowhead c.
    back-action c.
    c. bar
    bar c.
    cast c.
    circumferential c.
    combination c.
    continuous lingual c.
    Crozat c.
    c. denture
    embrasure c.
    extended c.
    flexibility c.
    flexure c.
    formed c.
    c. guideline
    hairpin c.
    half-and-half c.
    infrabulge c.
    lingual c.
    mesiodistal c.
    movable-arm c.
    multiple c.
    reciprocal arm c.
    retentive c.
    retentive circumferential arm c.
    reverse-action c.
    ring c.
    Roach c.
    stabilizing circumferential arm c.
    stress-breaking c.
    c. torsion
    wrought c.
clasp-adjusting pliers
clasp-bending pliers
class
    closed c.
    C. I amalgam
    C. V cervical matrix
    c. II distoclusion
    c. I, II, III malocclusion
    c. III mesioclusion
    c. I molar and canine occlusion
    C. V Multiple Step Build-up
      technique
    c. I, II, III occlusion
    open c.
    c. III ring avulsion injury pattern
    C. I, II stone
    word c.
    c. word
classical conditioning
classification
    Ackerman-Proffitt c.
    Angle c. of malocclusion
    Bailyn c.
    Baume c.
    Black c.

Broders c.
caries c.
cavity c.
cleft palate c.
c. of cleft palate
Coombs c.
Cummer c.
denture c.
Gell c.
Gustilo soft tissue c.
House c.
House-Brackman c.
Kazangia and Converse facial
  fracture c.
Kazangia and Converse mandibular
  fracture c.
Kennedy c.
Pell and Gregory c.
Regnault c.
Sassouni c.
Schuknecht c.
Schwarz c.
Seddon c.
sentence c.
Skinner c.
Spaulding c.
Stark c.
Sunderland c.
Tessier c.
tongue thrust c.
tympanogram c. Feldman model
tympanogram c. Jerger model
Veau c.
Winter c.

Claudius
cells of C.

clausa
pulpitis c.
rhinolalia c.

clause terminal

clavicular
c. respiration

claw
devil's c.

Clayette

claypipe cancer

CLD
central language disorder

cleaner
cavity c.
dentin c.
denture c.

enamel c.
Everbest Prosonic c.
Proxi-Floss interproximal c.

cleaning
ultrasonic c.

cleanser
denture c.
Kleenite denture c.
Prevacare no-rinse personal c.
Shick Sonic-Action denture c.
Shick Ultrasonic denture c.
SilqueClenz skin c.
StainAway Plus denture c.
Whirl-a-Dent denture c.

cleansing
biomechanical c.
interdental c.

Clean-Wheel disposable neurological pinwheel

clear
C. Away Disc
c. cell carcinoma
c. cell hidradenoma
c. cell odontogenic tumor (CCOT)
C. Eyes
c. sterile MB premium
c. sterile premium tubing
c. sterile tubing
c. zone

clearance
interocclusal c.
occlusal c.

Clearcut II with smoke eater tube

Clearfill
C. CR inlay
Photo C.

ClearSite wound dressing

cleat

cleavage
enamel c.
c. plane

cleaver
Case enamel c.
enamel c.
Orton enamel c.

CLEF-P
Clinical Evaluation of Language
Function-Preschool

cleft
alveolar c.
c. alveolus
c. anomaly

C

NOTES

cleft *(continued)*
atypical c.
c. cheek
cholesterol c.
congenital earlobe c.
c. crista galli
c. earlobe
facial c.
Facial Impairment Scales for c.'s
gingival c.
gluteal c.
incomplete c.
interdental c.
intergluteal c.
isolated naso-ocular c.
c. jaw
labial c.
laryngeal c.
laryngotracheoesophageal c.
c. lip
c. lip deformity
c. lip nose
c. lip and palate (CLP)
c. lip/palate syndrome
c. margin flap
median facial c.
median maxillary anterior
  alveolar c.
mesenchymal c.
middle ear c.
c. muscle of Veau
naso-ocular c.
natal c.
non-Hodgkin lymphoma of middle
  ear c.
nose c.
oblique facial c.
olfactory c.
operated c.
c. palate
c. palate classification
c. palate impression
c. palate and lateral synechia
  syndrome (CPLS)
c. palate prosthesis
c. palate repair
palatomaxillary c.
pharyngeal c.
postalveolar c.
postoperated c.
prealveolar c.
rare c.
soft palate c.
stenotic c.
Stillman c.
submucous c.
Tessier c.
c. tongue

tracheoesophageal c.
type II earlobe c.
unoperated c.
c. uvula
clefting
facial c.
midline cranio-orbital c.
cleidocranial
c. dysostosis
c. dysplasia
Cleland ligament
clemastine
c. and phenylpropanolamine
clenching
Cleocin
C. HCl
C. Pediatric
C. Phosphate
cleoid
c. carver
Clerf-Arrowsmith safety pin closer
click
glottal c.
temporomandibular joint c.
clicker
click-evoked otoacoustic emission
clicking
c. tinnitus
climate
occlusal c.
clindamycin
clinica
corona c.
radix c.
clinical
c. audiology
c. crown
c. crown ratio
c. eruption
C. Evaluation of Language
  Function-Preschool (CLEF-P)
C. Evaluation of Language
  Functions (CELF)
C. Probes of Articulation
  Consistency (CPAC)
c. root
c. root ratio
C. Test for Sensory Interaction of
  Balance
clinician
language c.
speech and language c.
voice c.
clinodactyly
clinoid process
Clinoril
clip
Backhaus towel c.

Benjamin-Havas fiberoptic light c.
Hader bar c.
microvascular c.
Raney c.
Zimmer c.

Cliplamp
Mini C.
Clip-Lite clip-on headlight
clipped
c. speech
c. word
clipping
peak c.
clitoris
clitoromegaly
clitoroplasty
clivus
C. L. Jackson
C. L. J. head-holding forceps
C. L. J. head-holding forceps
C. L. J. pin-bending costophrenic forceps
C. L. J. pin-bending costophrenic forceps
cloacal membrane
clobetasol
c. propionate
Clocort Maximum Strength
clocortolone
Cloderm Topical
clofazimine
Clomycin
clonal proliferation
clonic
c. block
clonus
Clorox
Clorpactin WCS-90
closable
close
c. bite
c. transcription
c. vowel
closed
c. apex
c. bite
c. capsulotomy
C. Chain Exercise Attachment
c. class
c. degloving injury
c. disruption of digital artery
c. head injury (CHI)

c. juncture
c. median diastema
c. mouth impression
c. osteotomy
c. pulpitis
c. reduction
c. spring
c. syllable
c. tympanoplasty
closed-bite malocclusion
closed-coil nickel titanium spring
closer
Clerf-Arrowsmith safety pin c.
closing stroke
clostridia
c. gangrene
clostridial syndrome
Clostridium
C. botulinum
C. perfringens
C. subterminali
C. tetani
closure
auditory c.
circular with Passavant ridge pattern of c.
compression skull cap c.
cyma (ogee) c.
Dorrance c.
early hard palate c.
facial compression finger c.
facial compression skull cap c.
flask c.
floor-of-mouth c.
Furlow c.
glottic c.
Gore-Tex c.
grammatic c.
inconsistent velopharyngeal c.
Marlex mesh c.
maxillary antrum c.
palatopharyngeal c.
Prolene mesh c.
sinus c.
supraglottic c.
SutureStrip Plus wound c.
twisting c.
velopharyngeal c.
visual c.
von Langenbeck palatal c.
V-Y c.
V to Y fashion c.

NOTES

closure *(continued)*
    watertight c.
    watertight skin c.
clot
cloth
    amalgam squeeze c.
clothesline injury
clotrimazole
clotting
    c. abnormality
    c. cascade
    c. system
cloud-like shadow
clove oil
clover
    red c.
cloverleaf skull
cloves
    oil of c.
cloxacillin
Cloxapen
CLP
    cleft lip and palate
CLR 2940 erbium laser
club
    Lost Cord C.
    Nu Voice C.
clubfoot
clubhand
cluster
    consonant c.
    c. headache
    c. reduction
cluttering
clysis
CMC
    carpometacarpal
    CMC joint
CMCP
    camphorated mono-parachlorophenol
CMD
    craniomandibular dysfunction
CMEC
    central mucoepidermoid carcinoma
CMP
    cross-modal priming
CMS AccuProbe 450 system
CMV
    cytomegalovirus
CNAP
    cochlear nerve action potential
CNS
    central nervous system
CNT
    could not test
CO_2
    carbon dioxide
    CO_2 beam

CO_2 laser
CO_2 laser blepharoplasty
Coach incentive spirometer
coagulase-negative staphylococcus
coagulate
coagulation
    cutaneous protein c.
    cutaneous proteinaceous c.
    laser c.
    c. necrosis
    c. test
coagulator
    ASSI Polar-Mate bipolar c.
coagulopathy
    diffuse intravascular c.
Coakley tenaculum
coalescence
coalescent mastoiditis
coaptation
coarse
    c. disk
    c. facial feature
coarticulation
    anticipatory c.
    backward c.
    carryover c.
    forward c.
Coarticulation Assessment in Meaningful Language (CAML)
coast sage
coat
    fuzzy c.
    mucosal c.
coated
    c. tongue
    c. Vicryl Rapide suture
coater
    Hummer V Sputter c.
coating
    Calcitite hydroxyapatite c.
    c. material
    Polyglyd suture c.
cobalt 60
cobalt base alloy
cobalt-chromium alloy
cobalt-chromium-molybdenum alloy
Coban
    C. bandage
    C. wrap
cobblestone tongue
cobblestoning
Cobra
    C. K+ tip
    C. K tip
    C. + tip
cobra
    c. cannula
cobra-head drill

COC
cement-on-crown
COC abutment
cocaine
c. anesthesia
coccidioidomycosis
c. tenosynovitis
coccoid bacteria
cochlea
apical c.
basal turn c.
fenestra c.
cochlear
c. aplasia
c. aqueduct
c. artery
c. branch
c. canaliculus
c. duct
c. echo
c. hair cell
c. hearing loss
c. hydrops
c. implant
c. microphonic
c. nerve
c. nerve action potential (CNAP)
c. nerve stretching
c. nucleus
c. outer hair cell function
c. partition
c. prosthesis
c. reflex
c. reserve
c. stereocilia
c. tuning
c. vein
c. window
cochleariformis
processus c.
cochleariform process
cochleo-orbicular
c.-o. reflex
cochleopalpebral
c. reflex (CPR)
cochleosacculotomy
cochleostapedial reflex
cochleostomy
cochleovascular accident
cochleovestibular
c. approach
c. nerve

c. neurectomy (CVN)
c. system
cockatiel feather dander
cocked hat procedure
cocklebur
cockleshell ear
cockroach
American c.
German c.
cocoa
cocontraction
coconut
Codafed Expectorant
Codamine
C. Pediatric
code
language c.
multipeak cochlear stimulation c.
Codehist DH
codeine
acetaminophen and c.
aspirin and c.
bromodiphenhydramine and c.
brompheniramine,
  phenylpropanolamine, and c.
butalbital compound and c.
Capital and C.
carisoprodol, aspirin, and c.
chlorpheniramine, phenylephrine,
  and c.
chlorpheniramine, pseudoephedrine,
  and c.
Deproist Expectorant with C.
Empirin With C.
Fiorinal With C.
guaifenesin, pseudoephedrine, and c.
Phenaphen With C.
Phenergan VC With C.
Pherazine VC w/ C.
promethazine, phenylephrine, and c.
Promethist with C.
Prometh VC with C.
triprolidine, pseudoephedrine, and c.
Tylenol With C.
Codesco topical fluoride phosphate
  anticaries gel
codfish
Codoxy
Coe
C. alginate
C.-Cide
C.-Comfort

C

NOTES

Coe *(continued)*
>C.-Cure
>C.-Flex
>C.-Flo
>C.-Pack
>C.-Pak paste
>C.-Soft

Coecal

coefficient
>alternate forms reliability c.
>comparable forms reliability c.
>c. of correlation
>linear thermal expansion c.
>penetration c.
>reliability c.
>split half reliability c.
>test-retest reliability c.

coffee

Coffin
>C. split plate
>C. spring

Coffin-type transpalatal wire

COG
>center of gravity

Cogan syndrome

Cogent Micro Illumination technology

Co-Gesic

cognate
>c. confusion

cognition

cognitive
>c. development
>c. development stage
>c. dissonance
>c. distancing
>c. evoked potentials to speech and tonal stimulus
>c. impairment
>c. mapping
>c. style

Cohen
>C. analysis
>C. syndrome

Coherent
>C. UltraPulse laser

cohesion
>lexical c.

cohesive
>c. device
>c. failure
>c. gold
>c. gold foil
>c. site density

Co-Hist

cohosh
>black c.
>blue c.

coil
>embolization c.
>helical c.
>induction c.
>platinum embolization c.
>c. spring
>c. spring space regainer
>steel embolization c.

coiled tubing

co-infection

coin test

col

cold
>c. abscess
>C. & Allergy Elixir
>c. beam laser
>c. bend test
>common c.
>c. cure resin
>c. dissection
>c. gutta-percha
>c. in the head
>c. intolerance
>c. ischemic time
>c. light
>rose c.
>c. sterilization
>Sudafed Severe C.
>c. test
>c. therapy
>c. welding

cold-curing
>c.-c. plastic
>c.-c. resin

cold-knife dissection

Coldlac-LA

Coldloc

Coldrine

cold-running
>c.-r. speech

Cold-Running Speech Test

Coleman
>C. aspiration cannula
>C. infiltration cannula
>C. microinfiltration system

Cole uncuffed endotracheal tube

Colgate PerioGard oral rinse

coli
>*Amoeba c.*
>*Escherichia c.*

colic
>salivary c.

Colin STBP-780 stress test blood pressure monitor

colistimethate sodium

colistin
>c., neomycin, and hydrocortisone

colla (*pl. of* collum)

CollaCote
    C. bovine collagen
    C. wound dressing
collagen
    c. antibody
    bovine c.
    CollaCote bovine c.
    dentin c.
    c. deposition
    c. disease
    c. fiber
    Fibrel c.
    c. fibril
    c. implant
    c. injection
    microfibrillar c.
    c. molecule
    pulp c.
    pulpal c.
    purified bovine c.
    purified fibrillar c. (PFC)
    c. septum
    c. synthesis
    c. type IV
    Zyderm I, II injectable c.
    Zyplast injectable c.
collagenase
    interstitial c.
    C. Santyl
collagenous
    c. fiber
    c. tissue
collagen-vascular disease
CollaPlug wound dressing
collapse
    alar rim c.
    bony vault c.
    c. of dental arch
    inspiratory laryngeal c.
    nasal valve c.
collapsed cheek
collar
    c. crown
    gingival c.
    c. incision
    mucosal c.
    shower c.
    thyroid c.
Collastat OBP microfibrillar collagen hemostat material
CollaTape wound dressing

collateral
    c. ligament
    c. pulp canal
collecting
    c. vein (CV)
    c. venule
collection
    globular c.
    saccular c.
    c. trap
collective monologue
collector
    bone c.
    parotid c.
Colles
    C. fascia
    C. fracture
Collet-Sicard syndrome
colli
    fibromatosis c.
    hydrocele c.
    pterygium c.
colliculus
    inferior c.
collimation
    rectangular c.
collimator
    cylinder c.
    lead c.
collinear
colliquative necrosis
collision tumor
collograft
colloid
    c. impression material
    c. infusion
colloidal
colloquial
colloquialism
collum, pl. colla
    c. dentis
    c. mandibulae
collutory
    Miller c.
Collyrium Fresh Ophthalmic
coloboma, pl. colobomata
    c. of iris, heart deformities, choanal atresia, retarded growth, genital and ear deformities (CHARGE)
    c. lobuli
colo-cecum

C

NOTES

colocolpopoiesis
colonic interposition
colon interposition vaginoplasty
colony-stimulating factor (CSF)
color
 C. Bar Schirmer strip
 extrinsic c.
 c. flow Doppler (CDF)
 gingival c.
 c. hearing
 intrinsic c.
 c. modifier
 tone c.
 c. toner
 c. wheel
Colorado
 C. electrocautery tip
 C. MicroDissection needle
 C. MicroNeedle needle electrode
 C. tip cautery
coloration
colored indicator spray
colorimetric caries susceptibility test
coloring
 extrinsic c.
 intrinsic c.
Coloured Progressive Matrices
colovaginoplasty
colpocystoplasty
colpoperineoplasty
colpoplasty
colpopoiesis
Coltene
 C. inlay/onlay
 C. inlay system
 C. oven
Coltoflax polysiloxane impression
coltsfoot
Columbia
 C. curette
 C. Mental Maturity Scale
 C. retractor
 C. scaler
columella, pl. columellae
 hanging c.
columellar
 c. deformity
 c. flap
 c. jut of nose
 c. reconstruction
 c. repair
 c. strut
 c. subluxation stabilization
columnar
 c. dentinoblast
Coly-Mycin S Otic Drops
COM
 chronic otitis media

coma
 diabetic c.
Combi-40 cochlear implant
combination
 anti-inflammatory-antibiotic c.
 c. chemotherapy
 c. clasp
 corticosteroid-antibiotic c.
 multiword c.
 c. restoration
 c. surgery
 TCB/TCA c.
 transconjunctival
  blepharoplasty/trichloroacetic
  acid c. (TCB/TCA)
combinatorial/thematic play
combined
 c. gingivitis
 c. method
 c. operation
 c. palsy
 penicillin G benzathine and
  procaine c.
 c. upper blepharoplasty
combined-flow lesion
Combison 530 3D sonographer
Combitube airway
COME
 chronic otitis media with effusion
comedocarcinoma
comedone
Comfort
 C. Ophthalmic
 C. Tears Solution
comfrey
Comhist
 C. LA
comitans, pl. comitantes
 vena c.
Command
 C. Ultrafine
 C. Ultrafine resin
COM/MAND mandibular fixation
 system
commando
 c. operation
 c. procedure
commercially
 c. pure (CP)
 c. pure titanium
comminuted alloy
comminution
 c. of alveolar socket
 mandibular symphysis c.
commissural
 c. cheilitis
 c. inhibition
 c. pit

commissure
anterior c.
buccal c.
labial c.
lateral oral c.
oral c.
posterior c.
c. repair
commissuroplasty
oral c.
common
c. blue nevus
c. canal
c. carotid artery
c. cold
c. facial vein
c. ragweed antigen
c. reed
commotio retinae
commune
crus c.
communicating junction
communication
C. Abilities Diagnostic Test and Screen
aided augmentative c.
alaryngeal c.
alternative c.
augmentative c.
augmentative and alternative c. (AAC)
c. board
c. disorder
Evaluating Acquired Skills in C. (EASIC)
facilitated c.
c. failure theory
nonoral c.
nonvocal c.
oral c.
oroantral c.
oronasal c.
c. science
C. Screen
total c.
unaided augmentative c.
communicative
C. Abilities in Daily Living (CADL)
c. competence
c. development inventory (CDI)
c. disorder

c. gesture
c. intent
c. interaction
c. technique
communicologist
communicology
community
c. dentistry
dialect speech c.
speech c.
compact
c. bone
c. phoneme
compactability
compacted gutta-percha
compaction
direct filling gold c.
gold foil c.
compactor
McSpadden c.
Micro-Flow c. (MFC)
comparability
comparable forms reliability coefficient
comparative
c. linguistics
c. research
compartment
c. syndrome
visceral c.
Compat enteral feeding pump
compatibility
pulpal c.
Compazine
compensated edentia
compensating curve
compensation
c. technique
worker's c.
compensational frontal plagiocephaly
compensatory
c. articulation
c. bone resorption
c. movement
c. periosteal bone apposition
c. wear
competence
communicative c.
Evaluating Communicative C.
Fisher-Logemann Test of Articulation C.
linguistic c.
Test of Language C. (TLC)

NOTES

competence *(continued)*
    Tests of Minimal Articulation C.
    velopharyngeal c. (VPC)
competency
    lip c.
    velopharyngeal c.
competing
    c. messages
    c. messages integration
complement
    c. cascade
    objective c.
    c. system
complemental air
complementary
    c. distribution
    c. gesture
    c. hue
complete
    c. bilateral deformity
    c. cleft lip
    c. cleft palate
    c. crown
    c. cutaneous syndactyly of all four limbs
    c. denture
    c. denture impression
    c. denture prosthesis
    c. denture prosthetics
    c. facial rejuvenation
    c. prosthodontics
    c. pulpectomy
    c. pulpotomy
    c. recruitment
    c. stress-breaker
    c. subject
    c. subperiosteal implant
    c. syndactyly
    c. veneer crown
complete-arch blade endosteal implant
completely-in-the-canal (CIC)
    c.-i.-c. hearing aid
    c.-i.-c. listening device
Completing Sentence Test (CST)
completion thyroidectomy
complex
    AIDS dementia c.
    AIDS-related c. (ARC)
    amphotericin b lipid c.
    areolomammary c.
    c. articulator
    avidin-biotin-peroxidase c. (ABC)
    c. bridge
    brow-upper lid c.
    c. cavity
    circulating immune c. (CIC)
    craniofacial c.
    DAE c.

    dentofacial c.
    Diluent C. V
    disseminated *Mycobacterium avium* c. (DMAC)
    c. filling
    forehead-brow c.
    Golgi c.
    hyperkeratosis c.
    immune c.
    junctional c.
    lemon bioflavonoid c.
    levator c.
    major histocompatibility c. (MHC)
    malar ligament c.
    maxillozygomatic c.
    modified junctional c.
    Mycobacterium avium c. (MAC)
    Mycobacterium avium-intracellulare c. (MAC)
    nipple-areola c. (NAC)
    c. noise
    nuclear c.
    c. odontoma
    olivary c.
    ostiomeatal c.
    periodontitis c.
    c. phenol
    c. pocket
    c. polysyndactyly
    post-cervix-crown c.
    c. predentinal nerve fiber
    pulpodentinal c.
    Robin c.
    c. sentence
    sicca c.
    sling ring c.
    c. SMAS
    C. Speech Sound Discrimination Test
    c. superficial musculoaponeurotic system rhytidectomy
    superior olivary c.
    c. syllabic
    c. of symptoms
    c. tone
    triangular fibrocartilage c. (TFCC)
    trigeminal nuclear c.
    c. wave
    c. word
    zygomatic malar c. (ZMC)
    zygomatic maxillary c. (ZMC)
    zygomaticomaxillary c. (ZMC)
compliance
complication
    implant related c.'s (IRC)
    neurotologic c.
component
    anterior c.

anterior c. of force
base c.
c. of force
grammatical c.
linguistic c.
c. of mastication
morphophonemic c.
c. of occlusion
secretory c.
composite
    c. bilateral infrastructure
      maxillectomy
    c. build-up
    c. chondrocutaneous flap
    c. core
    c. dental cement
    dentin-bonded resin c.
    c. filling
    fine particle c.
    FluoroCore resin c.
    hybrid based c.
    c. impression
    c. inlay
    c. inlay antral and nasal bone
      graft
    c. mandibular reconstruction
    c. material
    microfilled c.
    ML-c.
    c. odontoma
    c. onlay
    c. osteomyocutaneous preformed
      flap
    c. plastic
    c. radiograph
    c. resection
    c. resin
    c. resin color modifier
    c. resin color opaquer
    c. resin finishing disk
    c. resin luting cement
    c. resin restoration
    Retroplast resin c.
    c. rhytidectomy
    visible light-polymerizing c.
composition
    lexical c.
    modeling c.
compound
    c. apertognathia
    c. bridge
    c. caries

c. cavity
c. composite odontoma
c. cone
c. consonant
Darvon c. 65
dental c.
dihydrocodeine c.
c. filling
c. flap
c. fracture
c. heater
c. heater tray
impression c.
Microfil silicone-rubber injection c.
modeling c.
c. nevus
N-nitroso c.
nominal c.
c. odontoma
c. open bite
pentazocine c.
platinum-iron c.
c. pocket
Prema enamel microabrasion c.
c. restoration
c. sentence
Soma C.
Talwin C.
tray c.
C. W
c. word
compound-complex sentence
comprehension
    Assessment of Children's
      Language C. (ACLC)
    auditory c.
    c. span
comprehension-production gap
compressed speech
compressibility
compressible
compression
    c. amplification
    c. belt
    c. binder
    c. bone conduction
    esophageal c.
    c. garment
    c. girdle
    c. hearing aid
    c. molding
    nerve c.

C

NOTES

compression *(continued)*
  neurovascular cross c. (NVCC)
  c. plate
  c. plating
  c. skull cap closure
  c. splint
  c. switch
  tissue c.
  tracheal c.
  variable release c.
  c. vest-male
  wide dynamic range c. (WDRC)
compressive
  c. force
  c. plastic splint
  c. strength
  c. stress
Compton-Hutton Phonological Assessment
Compton Speech and Language Screening Evaluation
compulsion
computed
  c. axial tomography (CAT)
  c. tomography (CT)
computer
  c. assisted design/computer assisted machining
  c. assisted design/computer assisted manufacture (CAD/CAM)
  c. assisted neurosurgical navigational system (CANS)
  c. imaging
  c. language
computer-aided fluency establishment trainer (CAFET)
computerized
  c. axial tomography (CAT)
  c. dynamic platform posturography (CDPP)
  c. dynamic posturography (CDP)
  c. morphometric system
  c. pattern generator (CPG)
  c. rotary chair
  c. speech lab (CSL)
Comspan
Comtrex Maximum Strength Non-Drowsy
concatenation
concavity
  macroscopic c.
concentrated
  c. force
  c. mouthwash
concept
  Boehm Test of Basic C.'s-Preschool
  Boehm Test of Basic C.'s-R

critical band c.
C. CTS Relief Kit for carpal tunnel release
disease c.
Kronfeld mountain pass c.
object c.
self-role c.
symptom c.
conceptual disorder
conceptualization
concha, pl. conchae
  c. auriculae
  c. bullosa
  cavum conchae
  cymba conchae
  inferior c.
  inferior nasal c.
  medial nasal c.
  middle nasal c.
  nasal c.
  sphenoidal nasal conchae
  superior nasal c.
  supreme nasal c.
conchal
  c. bowl
  c. cartilage
  c. cartilage graft
  c. contraction
  c. crest of maxilla
  c. mucosa
  c. pocket
  c. retrodisplacement
  c. show
  c. surgery
conchal-mastoid angle
Concise resin
concomitant
  c. injection
  c. turbinectomy
Concorde cannula
concrement
concrescence
concrete operations period
concretion
  basophilic c.
concretism
concurrent validity
concussion
condensation
  amalgam c.
  filling material c.
  gold foil c.
  heavy c.
  lateral c.
  porcelain c.
  pressure c.
  resin c.
  spatulation c.

c. type
vibration c.
warm c.
whipping c.

condense

condensed gutta-percha

condenser
amalgam c.
automatic c.
back-action c.
bayonet c.
electromallet c.
foil c.
foot c.
gold c.
hand c.
Hollenback c.
long-handled foil c.
McShirley electromallet c.
mechanical c.
parallelogram c.
pneumatic c.
c. point
point c.
reverse c.
root canal filling c.
round c.
stepping c.

condensing
c. force
c. osteitis

condition
focal spot c.

conditioned
c. disintegration theory
c. orientation reflex (COR)
c. orientation reflex audiometry
c. reinforcer
c. response
c. stimulus

conditioner
agar hydrocolloid c.
Nuva-System tooth c.
tissue c.
tooth c.

conditioning
classical c.
counter c.
c. denture
instrumental c.
operant c.
pavlovian c.

phonological c.
prepeel c.
respondent c.
tangible reinforcement of operant c.

conductance

conduction
air c. (AC)
c. aphasia
bone c. (BC)
compression bone c.
distortional bone c.
inertial bone c.
osteotympanic bone c.
sensory acuity level bone c.
c. velocity

conductive
c. deafness
c. hearing loss

conductivity
thermal c.

conduit
bypass c.
polyglycolic acid c.

condylar
c. aplasia
c. axis
c. cartilage
c. chondroma
c. deformation
c. dysplasia
c. emissary vein
c. guidance
c. guidance inclination
c. guide
c. guide inclination
c. hinge position
c. hyperplasia
c. hypoplasia
c. lag screw plate
c. neck
c. neck retractor
c. process fracture
c. process fracture axial anchor
  screw fixation
c. span
c. translation

condyle
balancing side c.
c. cord
c. head
lateral c.
c. of mandible

C

NOTES

condyle *(continued)*
    mandibular c.
    native c.
    neck of c.
    occipital c.
    orbiting c.
    c. path
    protrusive c.
    c. rod
    rotating c.
    working side c.
condylectomy
condylion
condylodiskal
condyloid process
condyloma acuminatum
condyloplasty
condylotomy
cone
    auxiliary c.
    c. bur
    compound c.
    cutting c.
    c. cutting radiography
    gutta-percha c.
    intraoral c.
    lead-lined c.
    c. of light
    long c.
    master c.
    open-end c.
    Politzer luminous c.
    silver c.
-cone
cone-cutting
coned heparin tip
cone-socket instrument
Conex
    C. attachment
conference
configuration
    audiogram c.
    canal c.
    morning glory c.
    word c.
confirmation
    intraoperative spatial c.
conflict
    artery-nerve c.
    vessel-nerve c.
confluent articulation
confocal microscope
conformer
confused language
confusion
    cognate c.
congenita
    arthrogryposis multiplex c. (AMC)

    cutis aplasia c.
    dyskeratosis c.
    fistula auris c.
    fistula colli c.
    pachyonychia c.
congenital
    c. alveolar synechia syndrome
    c. cartilaginous rest of the neck (CCRN)
    c. cholesteatoma
    c. deafness
    c. defect
    c. discoloration
    c. dysosmia
    c. earlobe cleft
    c. ectodermic dysplasia syndrome
    c. epulis of newborn
    c. facial diplegia
    c. luetic labyrinthitis
    c. malformation
    c. myotonia
    c. nevus
    c. oral teratoma
    c. polycystic disease
    c. pseudoarthrosis
    c. stridor
    c. subglottic hemangioma
    c. syphilis
    c. torticollis
    c. tympanic plate dehiscence
Congess
    C. Jr
    C. Sr
Congestac
Congestant D
congestion
    nasal c.
    nasal mucosal c.
    Vicks 44D Cough & Head C.
conical
    c. flap
    c. tooth
-conid
conidiobolae
    entomophthoramycosis c.
coning of areola
coniotomy
conjoined twins
conjoiner
conjoint extensor digitorum brevis muscle and dorsalis pedis osteocutaneous island flap
conjunction
conjunctival approach
conjunctivodacryocystorhinostomy
    c. procedure
conjunctivomullerectomy
conjunctivoplasty

conjunctivorhinostomy
Conley incision
connate tooth
Connaught strain
connected speech
connection
    internal hex-thread c.
    vestibulocerebellar c.
connective
    c. tissue
    c. tissue augmentation
    c. tissue cell
    c. tissue graft
    c. tissue neoplasm
connector
    ACMI light source c.
    anterior palatal major c.
    c. bar
    cross arch bar splint c.
    c. implant superstructure
    implant superstructure c.
    Karl Storz light source c.
    lingual bar major c.
    linguoplate major c.
    Machida light source c.
    major c.
    minor c.
    nonrigid c.
    Olympus light source c.
    palatal c.
    Pentax light source c.
    posterior palatal major c.
    rigid c.
    saddle c.
    secondary lingual bar major c.
    Steiger c.
    subocclusal c.
    superstructure c.
    Y-port c.
connotation
    lexical c.
Conquest crown and bridge
conscious anesthesia
consecutive amaurosis
consensual reflex
consent
    informed c.
consequence
conservation
    hearing c.
    speech c.
    c. surgery

conservative subtraction-addition
    rhinoplasty (CSAR)
consistency
    Clinical Probes of Articulation C.
    (CPAC)
    doughy c.
    c. effect
    gingival c.
    object c.
    perceptual c.
consonance
consonant
    abutting c.
    alveolar c.
    arresting c.
    back c.
    bilabial c.
    c. blend
    c. cluster
    compound c.
    deletion of final c.
    deletion of initial c.
    devoicing of final c.
    double c.
    flap c.
    fortis c.
    front c.
    glottal c.
    c. inventory
    lax c.
    lenis c.
    nasal c.
    c. position
    prevocalic voicing of c.
    releasing c.
    syllabic c.
    velar c.
    velarized c.
    vibrant c.
    voiced c.
    voiceless c.
    c. voicing
    c.-vowel (CV)
    c.-vowel-consonant (CVC)
    weakness of pressure c.
consonantal
consonant-injection method
consonant-vowel preference
constancy
constant force
constellatus
    Streptococcus c.

C

NOTES

constituent
  immediate sentence c.
  sentence c.
  c. sentence
constraint
  fetal head c.
  semantic c.
constricted
  c. ear
  c. vocal production
constriction
  nares c.
  vocal c.
constrictor
  inferior pharyngeal c.
  middle pharyngeal c.
  c. pharyngeal muscle
  superior pharyngeal c.
construct
  reconstructive cell/polymer c.
  tissue-engineered c.
  c. validity
construction
  absolute c.
  costochondral graft mandibular
    ramus c.
  endocentric c.
  exocentric c.
  single denture c.
  wireloop/Gelfoam c.
constructional apraxia
contact
  c. allergic stomatitis
  c. area
  c. area point
  c. area zone
  atypical articulatory c.
  axon-to-axon c.
  balancing c.
  c. caries
  centric c.
  deflective occlusal c.
  c. dermatitis
  faulty c.
  faulty interproximal c.
  c. granuloma
  c. hypersensitivity
  indirect c.
  initial c.
  initial occlusive c.
  interceptive occlusal c.
  c. lens
  light c.
  linguapalatal c.
  c. point
  point of proximal c.
  premature c.
  proximal c., proximate c.

  retruded c. (RC)
  c. surface of tooth
  c. ulcer
  weak c.
  working c.
contagiosum
  molluscum c.
containment
  c. equipment
contaminant
contaminated
  c. laundry
  c. needlestick
  c. sharps
  c. waste
contamination
content
  language c.
  c. validity
  c. word
contentive word
context
  phonetic c.
  plausible c.
context-specific nasal emission
contiguity disorder
contiguous
contingency management
contingent
continuant
continuity of speech
continuous
  c. arch
  c. archwire
  c. arteriovenous hemodialysis
    (CAVHD)
  c. bar retainer
  c. beam
  c. clasp splint
  c. clip forceps
  c. eruption
  c. gum denture
  c. gum technique
  c. lingual clasp
  c. loop wire
  c. loop wiring
  c. positive airway pressure (CPAP)
  c. reinforcement schedule
  c. ribbon arch
  c. running suture
  c. sling suture
  c. wave laser
contour
  breast c.
  buccal c.
  c. defect
  c. deformity
  equal loudness c.

flange c.
gingival c.
gingival denture c.
gum c.
height of c.
intonation c.
c. line
c. lines of Owen
mandibular c.
C. Profile Natural saline breast
  implant
proximal c.
c. restoration
restoration c.
terminal c.
tooth c.
contourer
prosthesis c.
contouring
facial c.
implant c.
occlusal c.
c. pliers
contra-angle
c.-a. chisel
c.-a. handpiece
c.-a. head
c.-a. portepolisher
contra-aperture
contrabevel
contraction
cervical muscle c.
conchal c.
ECM c.
extracellular matrix c.
false muscle c.
c. gap
muscle c.
stapes tendon c.
wound matrix c.
contracture
Baker capsular c.
Baker class IV c.
capsular c.
fibrous capsular c.
flexion c.
joint c.
scar c.
soft tissue c.
spastic c.
spherical c.
Volkmann ischemic c.

contraindication
contralateral
c. face
c. frontalis injection
c. musculature
c. routing of offside signals
  (CROS)
contrast
air-iodinated c.
long-scale c.
maximal c.
minimal c.
c. radiograph
short-scale c.
c. study
contrastive
c. distribution
c. linguistics
control
acoustic gain c.
anchorage c.
automatic gain c.
automatic volume c. (AVC)
autonomic c.
disordered speech motor c.
gain c.
c. group
humoral c.
Hunstad Handle flow c.
locoregional c.
manual volume c.
musculoaponeurotic c.
plaque c.
c. problem
rate c.
resonant peak c.
tone c.
volume c.
controlled water added technique
contrusion
contusion
Contuss
C. XT
conus elasticus
convenience
c. form
c. jaw relation
c. occlusion
c. point
conventional
c. method
c. SMAS face-lift

NOTES

C

convergence
> cervical c.
> c. circuit
> c. theory

convergent

conversation
> c. board
> spontaneous c.

conversational postulates

Converse
> C. flap
> C. retractor
> scalping flap of C.
> C. scissors
> C. technique

conversion
> c. aphonia
> c. deafness
> c. hysteria
> c. reaction
> sex c.
> c. trismus

convex
> c. forehead

convolute

convolution

convulsion

cooing

coolant
> tooth c.

Cool Comfort cold pack

Cooley anemia

Coombs classification

Cooper-Rand intraoral artificial larynx

coordination
> visual-motor c.

copal
> c. varnish

Copalite cavity varnish

cope

Cophene-B

Cophene XP

coping
> image c.'s
> paralleling c.
> primary c.
> c. retainer
> secondary c.
> telescopic c.
> transfer c.

copolymer
> LactoSorb c.
> c. resin

copolymerization

copper
> c. amalgam
> c. band
> c. band-acrylic splint

> c. cement
> c. dental cement
> electroplated c.
> gold-c. system
> c. nose
> c. phosphate cement
> silver-c. system
> c. sulfate
> c. vapor laser

copperhead snake

copperplated die

copperplating

coprolalia

copula linguae

Co-Pyronil 2 Pulvules

COR
> conditioned orientation reflex
>> COR audiometry

Coral
> C. Plus fluoride paste

coralline hydroxyapatite

coral snake

cord
> condyle c.
> dental c.
> enamel c.
> false vocal c.
> gubernacular c.
> retraction c.
> true vocal c. (TVC)
> vocal c.

cordectomy

cordopexy

cordotomy

Cordran
> C. SP

core
> amalgam c.
> c. build-up
> cast c.
> composite c.
> disappearing c.
> full-coping c.
> laboratory c.
> mesodermal c.
> c. needle biopsy
> pulp c.
> suppurative c.
> c. vocabulary

cored structure

Coreform

Co-Re-Ga denture adhesive powder

CoreVent Implant system

Corex instrument

Corgard

Coricidin
> C. D

corium
> gingival c.

corkscrew esophagus

corn

cornea
> apex c. (acor)

corneal
> c. abrasion
> c. reflex
> c. ulceration

corneoretinal potential

corner-of-the-mouth smile

corner tooth

corneum
> orthokeratotic stratum c.
> stratum c.

corniculate
> c. cartilage
> c. tubercle

cornified
> c. layer

cornmeal

cornu, gen. **cornus**, pl. **cornua**
> c. cutaneum

corolliform papillae of tongue

corona, pl. **coronae, coronas**
> c. clinica
> c. dentis
> tuberculum coronae

coronad

coronal
> c. bleaching
> c. brow lift
> c. cementum
> c. dentin
> c. foreheadplasty
> c. necrosis
> c. oblique projection
> c. odontoma
> c. plane
> c. polishing
> c. pulp
> c. pulp tissue
> c. ring
> c. scaling
> c. synostosis
> c. translucency
> c. trusion
> c. zone

coronalis
> pulpa c.

coronary
> c. artery disease
> café c.
> c. odontoma
> c. thrombosis

coronas (*pl. of* corona)

coronavirus virus

coronion, koronion

coronoid
> c. hyperplasia
> c. process
> c. process of mandible

coronoidectomies
> bilateral c.

coronoidectomy
> transoral c.

coronoplasty

coronoradicular stabilization

cor pulmonale

corpus, pl. **corpora**
> corpora amylacea
> c. callosum
> c. callosum agenesis
> corpora cavernosa
> c. cavernosum
> erectile corpora
> c. spongiosum

corpuscle
> cement c.
> Golgi c.
> Hassall c.
> Krause c.
> Meissner tactile c.
> Merkel c.'s
> Pacini c.
> salivary c.
> Schwalbe c.
> tactile c.'s
> taste c.

correctable impression

correction
> anteroposterior c.
> bat ear c.
> cephalometric c.
> c. of chordee
> notch c.
> occlusal c.
> one-stage esthetic c.
> secondary c.
> skeletal c.
> speech c.

NOTES

C

correction *(continued)*
    Whitlow and Constable alar cartilage c.
correctionist
    speech c.
corrective
    c. feedback
    c. impression
    c. impression wax
    c. orthodontics
    c. therapy (CT)
corrector
    Fränkel III functional c.
    function c.
correlation
    coefficient of c.
    negative c.
    Pearson product-moment coefficient of c.
    positive c.
    product-moment c.
corrodens
    Eikenella c.
corrosion
corrosive
    c. substance
corrugated
    c. forehead retractor
    c. gold foil
corrugator
    c. muscle
    c. muscle resection
    c. resection
    c. supercilii muscle
corset platysmaplasty
Cort
    S-T C.
CortaGel
Cortaid
    C. Maximum Strength
    C. with Aloe
Cortatrigen Otic
Cort-Dome
Cortef
cortex, pl. cortices
    auditory c.
    buccal c.
    cerebral c.
    mastoid c.
Corti
    organ of C.
    C. tunnel
cortical
    c. anchoring screw
    c. auditory evoked response (CAER)
    c. auditory evoked response audiometry

    c. bone
    c. bone graft
    c. bone plate
    c. deafness
    c. lateralization
    c. mastoidectomy
    c. necrosis
    c. oral plate
    c. perforation
    c. respiration
    c. supranuclear paralysis
    c. vein
corticalis
    amaurosis c.
corticalosteotomy
cortices (*pl. of* cortex)
corticocancellous
    c. block graft
    c. bone
cortico-spongeous bone granule
corticosteroid
    c. antibiotic
    c.-antibiotic combination
    17-hydroxy c.
corticotropin
cortilymph
cortisol
cortisone
    c. acetate
Cortisporin
    C. Ophthalmic Ointment
    C. Ophthalmic Suspension
    C. Otic
    C. Topical Cream
    C. Topical Ointment
Cortizone-5
Cortizone-10
Cortone Acetate
Corynebacterium
    C. diphtheriae
    C. fusiforme
    C. hemolyticum
coryza
    allergic c.
    c. caseosa
Coschwitz duct
Cosgrove mitral valve retractor
cosine
    c. angle
    c. wave
CosMedical
    C. AHA marine moisture creme
    C. lipid drops
Cosmegen
cosmesis
    good c.
cosmetic
    camouflage c.

c. dentistry
c. orthodontics
c. surgery
CO_2-snow test
costal
c. cartilage
c. cartilage graft
Costen syndrome
costochondral
c. graft (CCG)
c. graft mandibular ramus construction
c. graft reconstruction
costosternoplasty
Cotrim
C. DS
co-trimoxazole
Cottle
C. columella clamp
C. elevator
C. knife
C. maneuver
C. nasal retractor
C. nasal speculum
cotton
c. linters
c. pellet
c. pledget
c. pliers
c. roll injury
cottonmouth snake
cottonoid
neurosurgical c.
cotton-roll gingivitis
cottonseed
cottonwood
Arizona/Fremont c.
cotton-wool appearance
Cottony-Dacron hollow suture
Cotunnius
nerve of C.
couchgrass
cough
brassy c.
Diphen C.
c. mechanism
nervous c.
privet c.
reflex c.
c. reflex

spasmodic laryngeal c.
weaver's c.
could not test (CNT)
coulomb (Q)
coumadin necrosis
counseling
count
gingival-bone c.
helper T cell c.
salivary *Lactobacillus* c.
T cell c.
word c.
counter
c. conditioning
Geiger-Müller c.
c. incision
c. irritation
joule c.
counterdie
counterincision
counterirritant
counterirritation
counterpart analysis
countersink bur
coup
c. de glotte
c. de sabre
coupler
Ackerman-Proffitt orthogonal analysis acoustic c.
Precise anastomotic c.
coupling
c. fitness test
nasal c.
cover
c. cell
c. dentin
E-Z Flap burr hole c.
c. screw
surface c.
TiMesh burrhole c.
coverage
flap c.
covering
allograft wound c.
Biobrane wound c.
biosynthetic wound c.
fibroelastic c.
fibrous c.
xenograft wound c.
covert response

C

NOTES

cow
 c. dander
 c. milk
Cowden
 C. disease
 C. syndrome
cowhorn
 c. explorer
 c. forceps
Cox
 C. II ocular laser shield
 C. regression analysis of partially
  edentulous jaw
coxsackie virus
CP
 carbamide peroxide
 central pit
 cerebellopontine
 commercially pure
  CP titanium
CPA
 cerebellopontine angle
  CPA collision tumor
CPAC
 Clinical Probes of Articulation
  Consistency
CPAP
 continuous positive airway pressure
  nasal CPAP
  CPAP ventilation
CPDD
 calcium pyrophosphate dihydrate deposit
CPG
 computerized pattern generator
CPLS
 cleft palate and lateral synechia syndrome
CPR
 cardiopulmonary resuscitation
 cochleopalpebral reflex
cps
 cycles per second
CR
 crown
  CR inlay cement
crabgrass
 c. effect
crack
 canal c.
 cemental c.
 intradentin c.
cracked-tooth synergistic syndrome
cracking
 surface c.
crackling
 c. jaw
 ping-pong ball c.

cradle
 neonatal audiometry response c.
 neonatal auditory response c.
cramp
 laryngeal c.
crampbark
Crandall syndrome
Crane
 C. elevator
 C. Vitapulp pulp tester
crane
 c. pick
 c. procedure
Crane-Kaplan marker pocket
crania (*pl. of* cranium)
cranial
 c. anchorage
 c. arteritis
 c. base defect
 c. base landmark
 c. base neoplasm
 c. coronal ring articulation
 c. dysraphism
 c. flap fixation
 c. fossa defect
 c. nerve
 c. polyneuritis
 c. prosthesis
 c. suture joint
 c. suture synostosis
 c. vault suture
cranialization
 sinus c.
craniectomy
 anterior c.
craniocaudal
craniocervical
 c. chordoma
craniodentofacial deformity
craniofacial
 c. anomaly
 c. appliance
 c. complex
 c. deformity
 c. dysjunction
 c. dysjunction fracture
 c. dysmorphism
 c. dysostosis
 c. dysplasia
 c. fixation
 c. instrumentation
 c. microsomia
 c. multidisciplinary team
 c. notch
 c. osteogenic sarcoma
 c. resection
 c. surgery
 c. suspension wiring

craniofaciocervical
craniomandibular dysfunction (CMD)
craniomaxillofacial
    c. callus distraction
    c. surgery
craniomedial
cranio-orbital
    c.-o. neurofibromatosis
craniopharyngioma
cranioplasty
craniostenosis
craniosynostosis, pl. **craniosynostoses**
    kleeblattschädel c.
    nonsyndromic c.
    Saethre-Chotzen c.
craniotabes
craniotomy
    attached c.
    bifrontal c.
    detached c.
    frontal c.
    osteoplastic c.
    posterior fossa c.
    retromastoid c.
cranium, pl. **crania**
    dysmorphic c.
Crataegus
    C. laevigata
    C. oxyacantha
crater
    alveolar process c.
    bone c.
    bony c.
    c. formation
    gingival c.
    interalveolar bone c.
crater-shaped erosion
craze line
crazing
CR/CO
    centric relation-centric occlusion
CRCS
    calcium hydroxide root canal sealer
creak
cream (*See also* creme)
    allantoin vaginal c.
    Aqua Glycolic c.
    AVC C.
    azelaic acid c.
    Azelex c.
    BioMedic MicroEncapsulated
      retinol c.

    Catrix c.
    Cortisporin Topical C.
    Denavir C.
    Eldopaque Forte c.
    Eldoquin Forte c.
    EMLA c.
    Gly Derm c.
    kojic acid c.
    Lamisil C.
    Lotrimin AF C.
    Massé Breast C.
    Maximum Strength Desenex
      Antifungal C.
    M.D. Forté rejuvenating eye c.
    Neosporin C.
    penciclovir c.
    Prevacare moisturizing c.
    Prevacare personal protective c.
    Renova c.
    Retin-A c.
    Sea-Bond denture adhesive c.
    Silvadene c.
    Solaquin Forte c.
    SSD C.
    tretinoin emollient c.
    Viquin Forte c.
    Viractin C.
    Zonalon Topical C.
crease
    alar c.
    helical c.
    inframammary c.
    lateral neck c.
    palmar c.
    preauricular c.
    submammary c.
    vertical glabellar c.
Credo topical gel
creed
    Millard c.
creep
    c. recovery
    skin c.
cremaster muscle
creme (*See also* cream)
    CosMedical AHA marine
      moisture c.
    Fungoid C.
    Gormel C.
    Iamin post laser c.
    Vite E C.

C

NOTES

cremoris
>*Streptococcus c.*

crenation of tongue
crepitation
crepitus
Cresanol root canal dressing
Cresatin
crescent
>sublingual c.
>traumatic c.

crescentic
>c. advancement flap
>c.-shaped skin paddle
>c. ulceration

crest
>alveolar c.
>c. of alveolar ridge
>ampullary c.
>buccinator c.
>dental c.
>endoalveolar c.
>falciform c.
>gingival c.
>iliac c.
>incisor c.
>infrazygomatic c.
>mandibular c.
>marginal c.
>c. of ridge
>superficial temporal c.
>transverse c.
>triangular c.
>turbinal c.
>vertical c.
>vomeropremaxillary c.
>zygomatic c.

crestal
>c. bone
>c. bone loss
>c. bone response
>c. fiber
>c. resorption

Cresylate
Crête-Manche implant
cretinism
Creutzfeldt-Jakob disease
crevice
>gingival c. (GC)

crevicular
>c. epithelium
>c. fluid
>c. fluid flow rate (CFFR)
>c. incision
>c. method of toothbrushing
>c. volume flow

crib
>allogenic c.
>allogenic bone c.
>alloplastic c.
>Jackson c.
>lingual c.
>lip-sucking habit c.
>c. splint
>TiMesh mandibular c.
>tongue c.

Crib-O-Gram
>C.-O.-G. audiometer

cribriform
>c. pattern
>c. plate
>c. plate of alveolar process
>c. plate injury
>c. salivary carcinoma of the excretory duct (CSCED)

cricket
cricoarytenoid
>c. ankylosis
>c. arthrodesis
>c. joint
>c. joint fixation
>c. muscle

cricohyoidoepiglottopexy
>supracricoid laryngectomy with c.
>supracricoid partial laryngectomy with c. (SCPL-CHEP)

cricoid
>c. cartilage
>c. ring
>c. split

cricoidynia
cricopharyngeal myotomy
cricopharyngeus muscle
cricothyroid
>c. angle
>c. artery
>c. joint
>c. ligament
>c. membrane
>c. muscle
>c. paralysis

cricothyroidotomy, cricothyrotomy
cricotomy
cricotracheal anastomosis
cricovocal membrane
cri du chat syndrome
crimping
>emulsion c.

crinion
crinis, pl. **crines**
crinkling effect
Crinone
crippling of oral cavity
crisis, pl. **crises**
>addisonian c.
>laryngeal c.

Crismani
> C. attachment
> C. stress-breaker

crista, pl. **cristae**
> c. ampullaris
> c. buccinatoria
> c. conchalis maxillae
> c. dentalis
> c. ethmoidalis maxillae
> c. falciformis
> c. frontalis
> c. galli
> c. infratemporalis
> c. marginalis
> c. palatina
> c. temporalis
> c. transversalis
> c. triangularis

cristobalite
> c. investment

criterion, pl. **criteria**
> behavioral c.
> Mark May sinus disease criteria
> c.-referenced test
> c. related validity

critical
> c. band
> c. band concept
> c. pH

Criticare
> C. comprehensive vital sign
>   monitor
> C. monitor
> C. 507N noninvasive blood
>   pressure monitor
> C. 507O pulse oximeter/NIBP
>   monitor
> C. POET TE end-tidal CO_2
>   respiration monitor
> C. 503 pulse oximeter
> C. 507S vital sign monitor

CRMO
> chronic recurrent multifocal osteomyelitis

crocodile
> c. tears
> c. tongue

Crocus sativus
Crohn disease
Crolom Ophthalmic Solution
Crombie ulcer
cromolyn sodium

CROS
> contralateral routing of offside signals
> binaural CROS
> criss-CROS
> power CROS

cross
> c. arch bar splint
> c. arch bar splint connector
> c. arch fulcrum line
> c. arch splinting
> c. bite
> c. bridge
> c. flap
> c. hearing
> c. probe
> c. talk

crossbar
crossbite, cross bite
> anterior c.
> buccal c.
> incisor c.
> lingual c.
> c. occlusion
> posterior c.
> scissors-bite c.
> c. teeth
> telescoping c.

cross-consonant injection method
cross-contamination
cross-cut
> c.-c. straight fissure bur
> c.-c. tapered fissure bur

crossed laterality
cross-facial
> c.-f. nerve graft
> c.-f. technique

cross-finger flap
cross-hatch incision
cross-hatching
> c.-h. undermining

cross-head displacement
cross-innervation
cross-leg flap
cross-lid flap
cross-linked polymer
cross-modal
> c.-m. naming paradigm
> c.-m. priming (CMP)

cross-modality perception
crossover
> axon c.
> facial nerve c.

NOTES

C

cross-pin tooth
cross-sectional projection
cross-section technique
cross-talk transmission
crotchless compression garment
croup
    inflammatory c.
    spasmodic c.
    c. tent
croupous
    c. laryngitis
croupy
Crouzon
    C. craniostenotic defect
    C. disease
    C. syndrome
crowded tooth
crowding
    canine c.
    extreme c.
    hereditary c.
    mandibular incisor c.
    molar c.
    premolar c.
    c. of teeth
Crowe-Davis
    C.-D. mouth gag
    C.-D. mouth retractor
crowing inspiration
crown (CR)
    acrylic veneer c.
    adequate c.
    alumina-reinforced porcelain c.
    aluminoceramic c.
    aluminum c.
    C. amalgamator
    anatomic c.
    anatomical c.
    artificial c.
    c. and bar space maintainer
    basket c.
    bell c.
    bell-shaped c.
    Bonwill c.
    c. and bridge prosthodontics
    c. and bridge resin
    c. and bridge type implant
    Carmichael c.
    cast core and c.
    cast glass ceramic c.
    Celay InCeram c.
    celluloid strip c.
    ceramic-metal c.
    clinical c.
    collar c.
    complete c.
    complete veneer c.
    c. and crib space maintainer

Davis c.
dental c.
c. dentin
dowel c.
c. down technique
extra-alveolar clinical c.
faced c.
feldspathic porcelain c.
c. flask
c. fracture
free-standing single c.
full c.
full veneer c.
gold c.
gold shell c.
half-c.
half-cap c.
C. Hylastic gold wire alloy
inadequate c.
c. inclination
Ion c.
jacket c.
C. K inlay
C. Knapp No. 3, No. 9, Supreme, T,T gold
Lang c.
c. ledge
length of c.
Libra III bridge and c.
metal c.
metal-ceramic c.
modified metal c.
C. No. 1 gold
open-face c.
overlay c.
partial c.
partial veneer c.
physiological c.
pinledge c.
platinum-bonded alumina c.
polycarbonate c.
porcelain c.
porcelain-faced dowel c.
porcelain-fused-to-metal c.
porcelain veneer gold c.
post and core c.
preformed c.
c. remover
Renaissance c.
restoration c.
c. restoration
Richmond c.
sheared c.
shell c.
shoulderless jacket c.
stained c.
stainless steel c.
steel c.

tapered c.
telescopic c.
temporary c.
temporary acrylic c.
thimble c.
three-quarter c.
c. of tooth
c. tubercle
veneered c.
veneer metal c.
Weston c.
window c.
Crown-A-Matic
C.-A.-M. crown and bridge remover
crown-contouring method
crowncork tympanoplasty
crown-crimping pliers
crowning
crown-root
c.-r. fracture
c.-r. ratio
crow's
c. feet
c. foot incision
Crozat
C. clasp
C. dental orthopaedics
C. philosophy
C. removable orthodontic appliance
C. therapy
CRR
canal resonance response
C-R syringe
crucial incision
cruciate incision
crucible former
crumpled aluminum foil
crural
c. feet
c. foot reduction
crus, pl. crura
c. commune
helical c.
c. helicis
lateral c.
medial c.
posterior c.
crush injury
crusta, pl. crustae
c. petrosa dentis

cry
birth c.
Cryer
C. elevator
C. forceps
C. root elevator
cryoglobulin
CryoLife light-activated fibrin sealant
cryopreservation
cryostat
Reichert Histo-Stat c.
cryosurgery
cryotherapy
crypt
enamel c.
follicular c.
cryptectomy
cryptococcal
c. meningitis
c. pulmonary infection
cryptococcosis
labyrinthine c.
Cryptococcus neoformans
cryptodontic brachymetacarpia
cryptophthalmus, cryptophthalmos
c. syndrome
cryptopia
cryptotia
crystal
apatite c.
calcium oxalate c.
calcium tungstate c.
cementum c.
cholesterol c.
dentin c.
desiccating c.
dihydrate c.
c. gold
gypsum c.
hemihydrate c.
hydroxyapatite c.
myxoid c.
needle shape c.
rhomboidal c.
silver precipitated c.
tyrosine c.
unaffected c.
unexposed c.
Whitlockite c.
zinc acetate c.
crystalline interface
crystallization

C

NOTES

crystalloid
    c. body
    c. infusion
Crysticillin A.S.
CS
    Poly-Histine CS
CSAR
    conservative subtraction-addition
      rhinoplasty
CSCED
    cribriform salivary carcinoma of the
      excretory duct
CSF
    cerebrospinal fluid
    colony-stimulating factor
      CSF rhinorrhea
C-shaped
    C.-s. canal
    C.-s. tooth
CSI
    Calculus Surface Index
CSL
    computerized speech lab
      CSL software
CSOM
    chronic suppurative otitis media
CSP attachment
CST
    Completing Sentence Test
CT
    computed tomography
    corrective therapy
      3D CT
        three-dimensional computed
          tomography
CTB
    calciotraumatic band
CTCL
    cutaneous T-cell lymphoma
CT-guided balloon inflation
CTR
    carpal tunnel release
C-Trak handheld gamma probe
CTRS
    carpal tunnel release system
      CTRS device
CTS
    carpal tunnel syndrome
C-TUB instrument receptacle
ctx
    cyclophosphamide
CU
    cusp
cubital artery
cubitale
    pterygium c.

cuboidal
    c. cell
    c. epithelium
cucumber
cue
    auditory c.
    kinesthetic c.
    visual c.
cued speech
cuff
    attached gingival c.
    epithelial c.
    gingival c.
    gum c.
    V-Lok disposable blood pressure c.
cuirass ventilation
cul-de-sac
culdoplasty
Culp pyeloplasty
cultivated
    c. barley smut
    c. corn smut
    c. oat smut
    c. rye smut
    c. wheat smut
cultural
    c. biases
    c. norm
Culture
culture
    anaerobic c.
    bacterial c.
    endodontic c.
    endodontic medium c.
    C. Fair Intelligence Test
    negative c.
    positive c.
    c. test
cultured
    c. autograft
    c. autologous keratinocyte
    c. autologous melanocyte
    c. mucosal graft
    c. periosteal cell
culturing
    c. technique
Cummer
    C. classification
    C. guideline
cumulative effect
cumulus cloud effect
cuneiform
    c. cartilage
    c. cartilage of Wrisberg
    c. osteotomy
    c. tubercle
cuniculatum
    carcinoma c.

cup-and-ball osteotomy
cup ear
Cupid
    Arch of C.
    C.'s bow
    C.'s bow peak
cupped forceps
cupula, cupola
cupulolithiasis
cupulometry
Curcuma domestica
curcumin
cure
curettage
    apical c.
    gingival c.
    infrabony pocket c.
    periapical c.
    root c.
    soft tissue c.
    subgingival c.
    ultrasonic c.
curette, curet
    Billeau wax c.
    Buck wax c.
    Columbia c.
    disposable c.
    double-ended c.
    Goldman c.
    Gracey c.
    Hartmann c.
    Lucas alveolar c.
    McCall c.
    Moult c.
    oval c.
    Shapleigh wax c.
    sharp loop c.
    surgical c.
    universal c.
    wax c.
    Younger-Good c.
curing
    dental c.
    denture c.
curled enamel
currant
current
    action c.
    alternating c. (AC)
    direct c. (DC)
Curretab Oral

curse
    Ondine c.
curtain
    lip c.
curvature
    buccolingual c.
    canal c.
    gingival c.
    mesial c.
    occlusal c.
curve
    alignment c.
    anti-Monson c.
    apical c.
    articulation c.
    bayonet c.
    bell-shaped c.
    buccal c.
    catenary c.
    compensating c.
    defalcated c.
    dilacerated c.
    dipper c.
    discrimination c.
    dose-effect c.
    dose-response c.
    elastic c.
    falling c.
    frequency response c.
    gaussian c.
    gradual c.
    Hurter-Driffield c.
    isodose c.
    labial c.
    marked falling c.
    milled-in c.'s
    Monson c.
    nasogram c.
    normal probability c.
    c. of occlusion
    parabolic c.
    Pleasure c.
    probability c.
    reverse c.
    saddle c.
    saucer c.
    sensitometric c.
    shadow c.
    sharply falling c.
    sickle-shaped c.
    ski slope c.
    c. of Spee

C

NOTES

curve (*continued*)
    steep drop c.
    strain-time c.
    strength duration c.
    stress-strain c.
    sudden drop c.
    trough c.
    tuning c.
    U-shaped c.
    von Spee c.
    waterfall c.
    Wilson c.
curved
    c. base Lewis bracket
    c. base twin bracket
    c. canal
    c. cannula
    c. chisel
    c. Kelly hemostat
    c. laryngeal mirror
    c. layer tomography
    c. longitudinal incision
    c. magnifying mirror
    c. mosquito hemostat
    c. turbinate scissors
    c. turbinectomy scissors
curvilinear
    c. incision
Curvularia
    C. geniculata
    C. lunata
CUSA laparoscopic tip
Cushing
    C. forceps
    C. syndrome
    C. ulcer
cushingoid
    c. change
    c. symptom
cushion
    Ezo dental c.
    Passavant c.
    retroarticular c.
    sucking c.
Cu-Sil attachment
cusp (CU)
    accessory c.
    accessory buccal c.
    c. angle
    buccal c. (BC)
    c. of Carabelli
    central c.
    distal c. (DC)
    distobuccal c. (DBC)
    distolingual c. (DLC)
    c. height
    lingual c. (LC)
    mesiobuccal c. (MBC)

    mesiolingual c. (MLC)
    c. plane
    plunger c.
    c. restoration
    c. ridge
    shearing c.
    shoeing c.
    stamp c.
    c. stamp
    supporting c.
    talon c.
    tipping of c.
    c. writer
cuspad
cuspal
    c. inclination
    c. interference
cusp-forming pliers
cusp-fossa relation
cuspid
    c. guidance
    mandibular c.
    maxillary c.
    c. protected occlusion
    c. tooth
cuspidate
    c. tooth
cuspidatus, pl. cuspidati
    dens c.
    dentes cuspidati
cuspides (*pl. of* cuspis)
cuspid-molar position
cuspidor
cuspis, pl. cuspides
    c. dentis
cuspless tooth
Cusp-Lok
    C.-L. bracket
    C.-L. cuspid traction system
custom
    c. matrix
    c. staining
    c. tip
    c. total alloplastic TMJ
      reconstruction prosthesis
custom-made mouth protector
cut
    c. amalgam alloy
    full spectrum low c.
    c. taper needle
cutaneoglandular
cutaneoperiosteal flap
cutaneous
    c. blue nevus
    c. capillary formation
    c. chromophore
    c. circulation
    c. fibrous histiocytoma

c. flap
c. focal mucinosis
c. forearm flap
c. horn
c. melanoma
c. meningioma
c. metastasis
c. nerve of the cervical plexus
c. paddle
c. polly beak
c. proteinaceous coagulation
c. protein coagulation
c. pulse oximetry
c. syringocystadenoma papilliferum
c. T-cell lymphoma (CTCL)
c. tuberculosis
c. vascular abnormality
c. vascular lesion

cutaneum
cornu c.

cuticle
acquired c.
acquired enamel c.
attachment c.
cemental c.
dental c.
enamel c.
Nasmyth c.
posteruption c.
primary c.
primary enamel c.
secondary c.
transposed crevicular c.

cuticula, pl. cuticulae
c. dentis

cuticularization

cutis
c. aplasia congenita
c. graft
primary osteoma c.
retinacula c.

cutisector
Cutivate
Cutler-Beard flap
Cutler-Ederer
C.-E. life-table methodology
C.-E. prediction table

cutter
arch bar c.
bone c.
hollow c.
ligature c.

Lindeman bone c.
pin and ligature c.
wire c.

cutting
c. bur
c. cone
c. disk
c. edge
c. instrument
c. movement
c. tooth

cuttle
cuttlefish disk
CV
collecting vein
consonant-vowel

CVA
cerebrovascular accident

CVC
consonant-vowel-consonant

Cvek-type pulpotomy
CVN
cochleovestibular neurectomy

cyanoacrylate
c. cement
c. resin

Cyano-Dent material
cyanosis
cybernetics
cybernetic theory of stuttering
Cyberware 3030RGB digitizer
cycle
cell c.
chewing c.
citric acid c.
duty c.
glottal c.
c. loading of skin
masticating c.
vibratory c.

cycles per second (cps)
cyclic
c. adenosine monophosphate
c. adenosine 3′,5′-monophosphate (cAMP)
c. adenosine 3′5′-monophosphate
c. neutropenia

cyclin D1 protein
cyclizine
cyclobenzaprine
Cyclocort Topical

NOTES

Cyclogyl
cyclohexylchloroethylnitrosurea (CCNU)
Cyclomydril Ophthalmic
cyclooxygenase
cyclopentolate
    c. and phenylephrine
cyclophosphamide (ctx)
cyclosporin A
cyclosporine
Cycofed Pediatric
Cycrin Oral
Cyfra 21-1 IRMA kit
Cyklokapron
Cylex
cylinder
    blood-free c.
    c. bur
    c. collimator
    gold c.
    gold foil c.
    TPS-coated c.
cylinder-type implant
cylindroma
cylindromatous lesion
cyma (ogee) closure
cymba
    c. conchae
    c. conchal cartilage graft
    midconcha c.
cynodont
Cynosure laser
cypress
    Arizona c.
    bald c.
    Italian c.
    Monterey c.
cyproheptadine
cyproteron acetate
Cyrano nose
cyst
    aneurysmal bone c. (ABC)
    antral mucosal c.
    apical c.
    apical periodontal c.
    apical radicular c.
    arachnoid c.
    Bartholin c.
    Blandin-Nuhn c.
    bone c.
    botryoid odontogenic c.
    Boyer c.
    branchial c.
    branchial cleft c.
    branchial pouch c.
    branchiogenic c.
    bronchogenic c.
    buccal c.
    calcified oil c.

    calcifying c.
    calcifying and keratinizing
     odontogenic c.
    calcifying odontogenic c.
    cervical c.
    cholesterol granuloma c.
    choristomatic c.
    daughter c.
    dental c.
    dental root c.
    dentigerous c.
    dentinal lamina c.
    dentoalveolar c.
    dermoid c.
    dermoid inclusion c.
    duplicative c.
    dysontogenetic c.
    enteric c.
    enterogenous c.
    epidermal inclusion c.
    epidermoid c.
    eruption c.
    extravasation c.
    fissural c.
    follicular c.
    follicular odontogenic c.
    functional parathyroid c.
    ganglion c.
    gingival c.
    glandular odontogenic c.
    globulomaxillary c.
    Gorlin c.
    hemorrhagic c.
    hemorrhagic bone c.
    heterotrophic c.
    heterotrophic oral gastrointestinal c.
    hydatid c.
    incisive canal c.
    inclusion c.
    inflammatory c.
    intraoral c.
    intraosseous c.
    intraosseous ganglion c.
    keratinizing epithelial
     odontogenic c.
    Klestadt c.
    laryngeal saccular c.
    lateral c.
    lateral periodontal c.
    lingual c.
    lymphoepithelial c.
    mandibular c.
    mandibular median c.
    maxillary c.
    maxillary median anterior c.
    maxillary sinus c.
    median alveolar c.
    median anterior maxillary c.

median mandibular c.
median palatal c.
mucosal c.
mucous c.
mucous retention c.
multilocular c.
nasoalveolar c.
nasolabial c.
nasopalatine c.
nasopalatine duct c.
nasopharyngeal c.
nonepithelial bone c.
nonfunctional parathyroid c.
nonodontogenic c.
nonsecreting mucosal c.
odontogenic c.
oil c.
orthokeratinized c.
palatine papilla c.
papillary c.
paradental c.
parakeratinized c.
parathyroid c.
parotid c.
periapical c.
periodontal c.
periosteal c.
pilar c.
preauricular c.
primordial c.
pulpoperiapical c.
radicular c.
raphe c.
residual c.
retention c.
root c.
root end c.
saccular c.
salivary duct c.
salivary gland c.
salivary gland retention c.
sebaceous c.
sialo-odontogenic c.
simple bone c.
sinus tract c.
soft tissue c.
solitary bone c.
sphenoidal c.
Stafne bone c.
static bone c.
sublingual c.
surgical ciliated c.

teratoid c.
thyroglossal duct c.
thyroglossal tract c.
Tornwaldt c.
traumatic c.
traumatic bone c.
true c.
unicameral c.
unicameral bone c.
Valsalva-induced cervical thymic c.

cystadenolymphoma
cystadenoma lymphomatosum
cystic
   c. adenoid epithelioma
   c. fibrosis
   c. hygroma
   c. lesion
   c. lymphangioma
   c. lymphoepithelial AIDS-related
    lesion
   c. odontoma
   c. oncocytic metaplasia
cystica
   spina bifida c.
cysticum
   epithelioma adenoides c.
   hygroma colli c.
cyst-like appearance
cystogenic carcinoma
cystoplasty
Cystospaz-M
cystostomy
   trocar c.
cytochrome oxidase
CytoGam
cytokeratin
   c. filament
   c. marker
cytokine
cytologic atypia
cytology
   aspiration biopsy c.
   exfoliative c.
   fine-needle aspiration c. (FNAC)
   FNA c.
   needle aspiration c.
cytomegalic inclusion disease
cytomegalovirus (CMV)
   c. chorioretinitis
   c. disease
   c. immune globulin intravenous-
   human

C

NOTES

cytometry
> flow c.

cytoplasm
> oxyphilic c.
> perinuclear c.
> Schwann cell c.
> serous cell c.

cytoplasmic
> c. eosinophilia
> c. granule
> c. process

cytosine arabinosyl

cytotoxicity
> antibody-dependent cellular c.
> (ADCC)

Cytovene

Cytoxan
> C. Injection
> C. Oral

Czermak
> globular spaces of C.

Δ (*var. of* delta)
δ (*var. of* delta)
D
  deciduous
  dentin
  deuterium
  dexter
  diopter
  duration
2D
  two-dimensional
    2D flat plate
    2D linear plating system
    2D railed plate
    2D US
3D
  three-dimensional
    3D CT
    3D plate
    3D plating system
    3D railed plate
    3D record
    3D US
3D-flat
    3D-f. Lactosorb plate
DAC
    Guiatuss DAC
    Guiatussin DAC
    Halotussin DAC
    Mytussin DAC
dacarbazine
Dacron
    D. batting
    D. netting
Dacron-backed implant
dacryocystorhinostomy (DCR)
    endonasal d.
    endoscopic d.
    d. procedure
dacryorhinocystostomy
dacryostenosis
dactinomycin
dactyl
    d. speech
dactylology
D.A.D. mattress
DAE complex
DAF
    delayed auditory feedback
D.A.II Tablet
daisy
    oxeye d.
Dakin solution
Dakrina Ophthalmic Solution

Dalalone
    D. D.P.
    D. L.A.
Dalbo
    D. extracoronal attachment
    D. extracoronal unit
    D. stud attachment
    D. stud unit
Dale
    D. abdominal binder
    D. Foley catheter holder
    D. oxygen cannula support
    D. tracheostomy tube holder
    D. ventilator tubing support
Dalgan
Dalla
    D. Bona attachment
    D. Bona ball and socket abutment
Dallergy
    D.-D Syrup
Dall-Miles cable grip system
dam
    post d.
    rubber d.
    rubber punch d.
damage
    actinic d.
    epidermal actinic d.
    left hemisphere brain d. (LHD)
    noise-induced d.
    right hemisphere brain d. (RHD)
Damascus disk
Damason-P
damiana
damped wave
damping
dandelion
dander
dander
    cat d.
    cattle d.
    chicken feather d.
    cockatiel feather d.
    cow d.
    deer hair d.
    dog d.
    duck feather d.
    ferret d.
    French poodle d.
    gerbil d.
    goat d.
    guinea pig d.
    hamster d.
    horse hair d.
    mohair d.

D

dander *(continued)*
    monkey d.
    moth d.
    mouse d.
    rat d.
    sheep d.
    silk d.
    swine d.
    turkey feather d.
Dandy-Walker malformation
danger space
Daniel EndoForehead instrument
Dapacin Cold Capsule
dapiprazole
dappen dish
DAPS
    Differentiation of Auditory Perception Skill
dapsone
Daranide
d'Arcet metal
Dardour flap
Darier-White disease
dark lateral
darkroom
    d. processing
dartos
    d. fascia
    d. fasciocutaneous flap
    d. muscle
    d. musculocutaneous flap
Darvocet-N
    D.-N 100
    D.-N 50
Darvon
    D. compound 65
    D. Compound-65 Pulvules
    D.-N
darwinian
    d. ear
    d. tubercle
DASE
    Denver Articulation Screening Examination
D'Assumpcão clamp
DAT
    dental aptitude test
    Developmental Articulation Test
Datascope pulse oximeter
date
daughter cyst
daunorubicin
David-Baker
    D.-B. clamp
    D.-B. eyelid retractor
    D.-B. lip clamp

Davis
    D. crown
    D. graft
Davis-Crowe mouth gag
Davis-Kitlowski procedure
Davol dermatome
Day
    Actifed Allergy Tablet (D.)
    Acutrim Late D.
Daypro
DB
    distobuccal
dB
    decibel
DBC
    distobuccal cusp
DBCR
    distobuccal cusp ridge
DBDG
    distobuccal developmental groove
DBFF
    distally based fasciocutaneous flap
DBO
    distobucco-occlusal
DBP
    distobuccopulpal
DBR
    distobuccal root
DC
    direct current
    distal cusp
    distocervical
        Bromanate DC
        Myphetane DC
DCP
    dynamic compression plate
DCR
    dacryocystorhinostomy
    distal cusp ridge
3D CT
    three-dimensional computed tomography
DDR
    Direct Digital radiography
DDS
    Doctor of Dental Surgery
DDSc
    Doctor of Dental Science
DE
    Ru-Tuss DE
de
    d. la Plaza transconjunctival retractor
    D. Morgan spot
    d. novo tumor
    d. Quervain granulomatous thyroiditis
    d. Quervain syndrome

dead
    d. nerve
    d. pulp
    d. room
    d. space
    d. tooth
    d. tract
deaf
    d. speech
    telecommunication device for
        the d. (TDD)
deafferentation
    bilateral vestibular d.
    total unilateral vestibular d.
deaffrication
deaf-mute
deafmutism
    endemic d.
deafness
    acoustic trauma d.
    adventitious d.
    Alexander d.
    boilermaker's d.
    catarrhal d.
    central d.
    conductive d.
    congenital d.
    conversion d.
    cortical d.
    familial d.
    functional d.
    gusher-associated d.
    high-frequency d.
    hysterical d.
    industrial d.
    low tone d.
    mixed d.
    Mondini d.
    nerve d.
    noise-induced d.
    nonorganic d.
    occupational d.
    organic d.
    perceptive d.
    postlingual d.
    prelingual d.
    prevocational d.
    psychogenic d.
    pure word d.
    retrocochlear d.
    Scheibe d.
    sensorineural d.

    tone d.
    toxic d.
    word d.
    X-linked d.
deamination
    tryptophane d.
Dean
    D. fluorosis index
    D. periosteal elevator
    D. scissors
    D. tonsil hemostat
death
    pulp d.
    d. rattle
Deaver retractor
debanding
deblocking
debonding
    d. pliers (DP)
debridement
    canal d.
    cavity d.
    epithelial d.
    root canal d.
debris
    canal d.
    d. index
    Malassez d.
    oral d.
Debrisan
Debrox Otic
debulking
    secondary d.
    surgical d.
Decadron
    D.-LA
    D. Phosphate
Decaject
    D.-LA
decalcification
decalcified
    d. cementum
    d. enamel
    d. freeze-dried bone allograft
        (DFDBA)
    d. freeze-dried cortical bone
        (DFDCB)
decannulation
decantation
decarboxylation
    tryptophane d.

D

NOTES

decay
>
> acoustic reflex d.
> baby bottle tooth d.
> dental d.
> free induction d. (FID)
> d. period
> d. rate
> rate of d.
> senile d.
> tone d.
> tooth d.

decayed
>
> d., extracted, and filled
> d., extracted, filled deciduous teeth (def)
> d., extracted, filled permanent teeth (DEF)
> d. and filled deciduous teeth (df)
> d. and filled permanent teeth (DF)
> d. and filled teeth
> d., missing, filled deciduous teeth (dmf)
> d., missing, filled deciduous teeth surfaces (dmfs)
> d., missing, filled permanent teeth (DMF)
> d., missing, filled permanent teeth surfaces (DMFS)
> d., missing, filled surfaces deciduous teeth (dmfs)
> d., missing, filled surfaces permanent teeth (DMFS)

decentration

decibel (dB)
>
> perceived noise d. (PNdB)

deciduous (D)
>
> d. dentition
> d. incisor
> d. molar
> d. tooth

deciduus, pl. decidui
>
> dens d.
> dentes decidui

decision
>
> Bates d.

declarative sentence

decoder

decoding

Decofed Syrup

Decohistine
>
> D. DH
> D. Expectorant

decompression
>
> carpal tunnel d.
> endolymphatic sac d.
> endoscopic orbital d.
> facial nerve d.
> gastric d.

jugular bulb d.
microvascular d. (MVD)
orbital d.
sac-vein d.
subfascial carpal tunnel d.
three-wall orbital d.
transantral orbital d.
transconjunctival endoscopic orbital d.
wide d.

Decon
>
> Par D.

Deconamine
>
> D. SR
> D. Syrup
> D. Tablet

deconditioning

decongestant
>
> New D.
> topical d.

decongestion
>
> local d.

Deconsal
>
> D. II
> D. Sprinkle

decontamination

decorative tattoo

decorticated flap

decruitment

decubitus
>
> d. ulcer

decuspation

decussation

dedentition

dedifferentiated chordoma

Dedo laryngoscope

deduction

deep
>
> d. articulation test
> d. bite
> d. cervical fascia
> d. facial lymph node
> d. hemangioma
> d. inferior epigastric artery
> d. inferior epigastric vein
> d. lateral node
> d. lobectomy
> d. muscular aponeurotic system (DMAS)
> d. overbite
> d. parotid lobe
> d. parotid node
> d. peroneal nerve
> d. petrosal nerve
> d. plantar arch
> d. scaler
> d. scaling
> d. space

d. structure
d. subdermal
d. suspension suture
d. temporal fascia (DTF)
D. Test of Articulation
d. vertical overlap

deepening
    d. pocket
    web space d.

Deepep-Hard
de-epithelialization, de-epithelization
    periareolar d.-e.
    vertical rhomboid d.-e.

de-epithelialize
de-epithelialized
    d.-e. doughnut
    d.-e. local flap
    d.-e. revascularized lateral
      intercostal flap
    d.-e. transverse rectus abdominis
      musculocutaneous pedicle flap

de-epithelization (*var. of* de-epithelialization)
deep-lobe parotid tumor
deeply placed, unerupted maxillary
    third molar
deep-plane
    d.-p. face lift
    d.-p. rhytidectomy

deer
    d. fly
    d. hair dander

Deesix
Deetwo
DEF
    decayed, extracted, filled permanent teeth
    DEF caries index
    DEF rate

def
    decayed, extracted, filled deciduous teeth
    def caries index

defalcated
    d. curve
    d. root canal

defatted
defatting
    internal d.

defect
    acquired d.
    alveolar bone d.
    birth d.
    bone d.

buccal d.
calvarial d.
congenital d.
contour d.
cranial base d.
cranial fossa d.
Crouzon craniostenotic d.
extirpative d.
extraoral d.
full-thickness d.
heminasal d.
intercalated d.
interradicular osseous d.
intrabony d.
intraoral mucosal d.
mandibular d.
Mohs d.
one-buttress d.
orbitomaxillary d.
oromandibular d.
oropharyngeal d.
osteoporotic marrow d.
pars flaccida d.
periodontal d.
periodontal bony d.
periodontal intrabony d.
pharyngoesophageal d.
post-ablation d.
postresection d.
repair of alveolar ridge d.
resorptive d.
sacrococcygeal d.
saddle d.
saddle-nose d.
segmental bone d.
segmental continuity d.
speech d.
suboccipital dural d.
three-buttress d.
through-and-through d.
two-buttress d.

Defen-LA
defense cell
defensive dentin
deferential orthodontic force
deficiency
    acquired immunoglobulin A d.
    arch length d.
    immune d.
    intraoral lining d.
    iron d.
    malar d.

D

NOTES

deficiency (*continued*)
    mandibular d.
    mandibular sagittal d.
    maxillary d.
    premaxilla peripyriform d.
    submalar d.
    vitamin A, B d.
deficit
    receptive d.
    residual expressive language d.
    strength d.
defined
    d. frequency
    d. sterilization
definitive prosthesis
deflation
    implant d.
deflective
    d. malocclusion
    d. occlusal
    d. occlusal contact
defluoridation
deformation
    condylar d.
    dentinoblastic d.
    elastic d.
    permanent d.
deformational frontal plagiocephaly
deformity
    Andy Gump d.
    Bishop collar d.
    boutonniere d.
    Burow triangle d.
    cleft lip d.
    coloboma of iris, heart deformities,
      choanal atresia, retarded growth,
      genital and ear d.'s (CHARGE)
    columellar d.
    complete bilateral d.
    contour d.
    craniodentofacial d.
    craniofacial d.
    dentofacial d.
    dish-face d.
    double-bubble breast d.
    d. of ear lobe
    facial d.
    facial contour d.
    gibbus d.
    gingival d.
    halo d.
    harlequin d.
    hourglass nasal d.
    iatrogenic d.
    lambdoid synostosis d.
    lateral facial cleft d.
    middle vault d.
    Mondini d.

    nasal tip d.
    parrot-beak d.
    Pinocchio tip d.
    Poland chest-wall d.
    polly beak nasal d.
    posterior plagiocephaly d.
    postmaxillectomy d.
    ripple d.
    saddle d.
    saddle-nose d.
    scaphocephalic d.
    soft-tissue d.
    step d.
    supratip d.
    swan neck d.
    Treacher Collins d.
    unaesthetic contour d.
    unilateral cleft lip nose d.
    uni-tip d.
    whistling d.
    witch's chin d.
DEFS
    Detailed Evaluation of Facial Symmetry
degassing
degeneration
    calcific d.
    hyaline d.
    myxomatous d.
    wallerian d.
degenerative
    d. zone
Degest 2 Ophthalmic
deglove
degloved amputation
degloving
    d. injury
    midfacial d.
deglutition
    d. apnea
    d. maneuver
    d. reflex
deglutitory disturbance
degradation
degrees
    hearing impairment d.
degree of voicelessness (DUV)
dehiscence
    alveolar d.
    congenital tympanic plate d.
    intimal d.
    levator d.
    root d.
    soft tissue d.
    wound d.
dehiscent
    d. mandibular canal
dehydrated

dehydration
    d. of gingivae
dehydroepiandrosterone (DHEA)
dehydrogenase
    glucose 6-phosphate d.
    11β-hydroxysteroid d.
    lactic d.
    malic d.
    succinate d.
    succinic d.
dehydrosterone
deictic
Deiters nucleus
DEJ
    dentinoenamel junction
déjà vu
Dejerine syndrome
delay
    expressive language d.
    toddler language d.
delayed
    d. auditory feedback (DAF)
    d. dentition
    d. distally based total sartorius flap
    d. echolalia
    d. eruption
    d. expansion
    d. feedback audiometry (DFA)
    d. graft
    d. hypersensitivity
    d. language
    d. reinforcer
    d. response
    d. speech
Delcort
Delerm and Elbaz technique
deletion
    d. of final consonant
    d. of initial consonant
    stridency d.
    syllable d.
    d. of unstressed syllable
    weak syllable d.
delivery
    d. assistance sleeve
    d. hose
Del-Mycin Topical
delphian node
Del Rio Language Screening Test, English/Spanish

delta, δ, Δ
    apical d.
    d. rhythm
    d. wave
Delta-Cortef Oral
Deltasone
Delta-Tritex
deltopectoral flap
deltoscapular flap
delusion
    somatic d.
demand speech
demarcation
    areolar d.
    d. line
Demarquay symptom
Demazin Syrup
Dembone
    D. demineralized cancellous chips
    D. demineralized cortical chips
    D. demineralized cortical dental block
    D. demineralized cortical granule
    D. demineralized cortical powder
    D. demineralized cortical powder Pastegraft
    D. demineralized cortical powder Pulvograft
    D. demineralized corticocancellous chips
    D. demineralized human bone
    D. freeze dried bone
    D. graft
demecarium
dementia
Demerol
demilune
    serous d.
demineralization
demineralized
    d. bone (DMB)
    d. bone graft
    d. bone matrix
    d. cortical bone powder
    d. flexible laminar bone strip
    d. freeze-dried bone (DFDB)
    d. freeze-dried bone allograft (DFDBA)
Demodex folliculorum
demonstrative
demonstrative-entity
demucosation

D

NOTES

demyelinating disease
demyelination
    segmental d.
Denar articulator
denasal
denasality
denasalization
denaturation
denatured bioburden
Denavir Cream
dendrite
dendritic
    d. cell
denervated muscle
denervation
    chemical d.
Denholz appliance
Denis Browne tonsil forceps
DenLite illuminated hand-held mirror
Denonvilliers aponeurosis
denotation
    lexical d.
Denquel
dens, pl. dentes
    dentes acustici
    dentes acuti
    d. angularis
    dentes bicuspidi
    d. bicuspidus
    dentes canini
    d. caninus
    dentes cuspidati
    d. cuspidatus
    dentes de Chiaie
    dentes decidui
    d. deciduus
    d. in dente
    dentes incisivi
    d. incisivus
    d. invaginatus
    d. invaginatus gestant odontoma
    d. lacteus
    dentes molares
    d. molaris
    d. permanens
    dentes permanentes
    dentes premolares
    d. premolaris
    d. sapientiae
    d. serotinus
    d. succedaneus
densification
Densite
Densitometer
    Victoreen Digital D.
densitometric
    d. analysis
densitometry

density
    alveolar bone d.
    cohesive site d.
    microvessel d. (MVD)
    d. radiograph
    sound power d.
Denstone
DENT
    Dental Exposure Normalization
    Technique
Dentacolor
dentagra
dental
    d. abscess
    d. adhesive
    d. aerosol
    d. alveolus
    d. amalgam
    d. amalgam alloy
    d. amalgam packer
    d. anatomy
    d. anesthesia
    d. ankylosis
    d. anomaly
    d. apparatus
    d. aptitude test (DAT)
    d. arch
    d. arch expansion
    d. artery
    d. articulation
    d. articulator
    d. aspirator
    d. auxiliary
    D. Auxiliary Utilization
    d. base cement
    d. biomechanics
    d. biophysics
    d. bridge
    d. calculus
    d. canal
    d. caries
    d. cast
    d. casting
    d. casting gold
    d. casting gold alloy
    d. cavity
    d. cement
    d. ceramics
    d. chart
    d. compound
    d. cord
    d. crest
    d. crown
    d. curing
    d. cuticle
    d. cyst
    d. decay
    d. disk

d. drill
d. dysfunction
d. dysplasia
d. eburnation
d. elevator
d. enamel
d. engine
d. engineering
d. excavator
D. Exposure Normalization Technique (DENT)
d. fenestration
d. fiber
d. film
d. fistula
d. floss
d. follicle
d. foramen
d. forceps
d. formula
d. furnace
d. galvanism
d. geriatrics
d. germ
d. gold
d. gold alloy
d. granuloma
d. groove
d. hammer
d. headache
d. health care provider (DHCP)
D. H topical fluoride gel
d. hygiene
d. impaction
d. implant
d. implant cover screw
d. impression
d. inclusion
d. index (DI)
d. inlay casting wax
d. inlay wax
d. instrument
d. investment
d. jurisprudence
d. key
d. laboratory lathe
d. laboratory technician
d. laboratory technologist
d. lamina
d. ledge
d. length
d. lever

d. lisp
d. lymph
d. material
d. mercury
d. microbiota
d. mirror
d. model
d. nerve
d. occlusion
d. operculum
d. orthopaedics
d. osteoma
d. papilla
d. pathology
d. perimeter
d. periosteum
d. phenomenon
d. plaque
d. plaster
d. plate
d. polyp
d. porcelain
d. premedication
d. process
d. prognosis
D. Pro II camera
d. prophylaxis
d. prosthesis
d. prosthetic laboratory procedure
d. prosthetics
d. psychosedation
d. pulp
d. pulp extirpation
d. pulp hyperemia
d. pump
d. puncture
d. record
d. resin
d. restoration
d. ridge
d. root abscess
d. root cyst
d. sac
d. sealant
d. senescence
d. shelf
d. shield
d. stain
d. stone
d. surgeon
d. surgery
d. surveyor

D

NOTES

dental *(continued)*
    d. syringe
    d. tape
    d. technician
    d. technologist
    d. tophus
    d. trauma
    d. trepanation
    d. tubercle
    d. ulcer
    d. unit
    d. varnish
    d. wax
    d. wedge
dentalgia
dentalis
    alveolus d.
    Amoeba d.
    crista d.
    odontalgia d.
Dentalvision
dentary center
Dentascan
Dentaseptic
dentate
    d. section
    d. straight fissure bur
    d. suture
    d. tapered fissure bur
Dentatus
    D. articulator
    D. screw
dente
    dens in d.
Dentemp ZOE temporary cement
dentes (*pl. of* dens)
Dent G. No. 1, 2 gold
dentia
    d. praecox
    d. tarda
dentibuccal
DentiCAD system
denticle
    adherent d.
    attached d.
    embedded d.
    false d.
    free d.
    interstitial d.
    pulp d.
    true d.
denticola
    Treponema d.
denticulate
dentification
dentiform
dentifrice
    d. abrasion

accepted d.
fluoride d.
Macleans d.
monofluorophosphate d.
provisionally accepted d.
sodium fluoride d.
stannous fluoride d.
dentigerous
    d. cyst
dentilabial
dentilingual
Dentillium
    D. CB
    D. CB alloy
dentimeter
dentin, dentine (D)
    adventitious d.
    affected d.
    apical d.
    black d.
    d. bonding
    d. bridge
    calcified d.
    carious d.
    d. cell
    circumpulpal d.
    d. cleaner
    d. collagen
    coronal d.
    cover d.
    crown d.
    d. crystal
    defensive d.
    desensitizing d.
    developmental d.
    d. dysplasia
    eburnation of d.
    functional d.
    globular d.
    d. globule
    hereditary opalescent d.
    human radicular d.
    hypersensitive d.
    d. hypersensitivity
    infected d.
    d. innervation
    interglobular d.
    intermediate d.
    intertubular d.
    irregular d.
    irritation d.
    mantle d.
    d. matrix
    mature d.
    d. mud
    opalescent d.
    pericanal d.
    peripheral d.

peritubular d.
d. permeability
postnatal d.
prenatal d.
primary d.
radicular d.
reparative d.
residual carious d.
sclerotic d.
secondary d.
secondary irregular d.
sensitive d.
shaving d.
solid d.
d. substitute
d. surface
tertiary d.
d. thickness
transparent d.
traumatic d.
uncalcified d.
vascular d.
dentinal
d. canal
d. caries
d. cartilage
d. crack syndrome
d. dysplasia
d. fiber
d. fibril
d. fluid
d. intratubular nerve
d. lamina cyst
d. lymph
d. matrix
d. permeability
d. pulp
d. sclerosis
d. sheath
d. system
d. tubule
d. tubules orifice
d. wall
dentinalgia
Dentinbloc dentin desensitizer
dentin-bonded resin composite
dentine (*var. of* dentin)
dentin/enamel bonding resin
dentinification
dentinoblast
columnar d.

dentinoblastic
d. cell
d. deformation
d. injury
d. layer
d. nucleus
d. process
d. zone
dentinoblastic-predentin junction
dentinoblastic-subdentinoblastic junction
dentinocemental
d. junction
dentinocementum
dentinoclast
dentinoenamel
d. junction (DEJ)
d. membrane
dentinogenesis
d. hypoplastica hereditaria
d. imperfecta
radicular d.
dentinogenic
d. fiber
dentinoid
d. formation
dentinoma
immature d.
dentinosteoid
dentin-producing cell
dentinum
dentiparous
Dentipatch
dentis
apex radicis d.
cavitas d.
cavum d.
cervix d.
cingulum d.
collum d.
corona d.
cuticula d.
ebur d.
facies contactus d.
facies distalis d.
facies facialis d.
facies lingualis d.
facies mesialis d.
facies occlusalis d.
facies vestibularis d.
foramen apicis d.
gubernaculum d.
iter d.

D

NOTES

dentis *(continued)*
    pulpa d.
    radix d.
    tuberculum d.
dentist
    Fellow of the American College of D.'s
    Fellow of the International College of D.'s (FICD)
dentistry
    ceramic d.
    community d.
    cosmetic d.
    esthetic d.
    forensic d.
    four-handed d.
    industrial d.
    interceptive restorative d.
    legal d.
    operative d.
    pediatric d.
    preventive d.
    prophylactic d.
    prosthetic d.
    psychosomatic d.
    public health d.
    reconstructive d.
    restorative d.
    seat-down d.
    washed-field d.
dentition
    aplasia of d.
    artificial d.
    deciduous d.
    delayed d.
    diphyodont d.
    first d.
    heterodont d.
    homodont d.
    mandibular d.
    maxillary d.
    mixed d.
    monophyodont d.
    natural d.
    neonatal d.
    permanent d.
    polyphyodont d.
    postpermanent d.
    precocious d.
    predeciduous d.
    premature d.
    primary d.
    prosthetic d.
    retarded d.
    secondary d.
    succedaneous d.
    temporary d.
    terminal d.

    third d.
    transitional d.
dentium
    iter d.
    stridor d.
DentlBright
dentoalveolar
    d. abscess
    d. cyst
    d. dysplasia
    d. fracture
    d. ligament
dentoalveolitis
dentoaural
dentode
dentoepithelial junction
Dentofacial
    D. Planner software
dentofacial
    d. anomaly
    d. complex
    d. deformity
    d. dysplasia
    d. esthetics
    d. orthopaedics
    d. surgery
    d. zone
dentoform
dentogenic
    d. movement
dentogingival
    d. fiber
    d. junction
    d. lamina
dentography
dentoid
dentolabial dysplasia
dentolegal
Dent-O-Lux
    D.-O.-L. Smooth-Flow gutta-percha plug
Dentomat triturator
dentomechanical
dentonomy
dentoperiodontal unit
dentoperiosteal
    d. fiber
dentopulmonary syndrome
dentoskeletal
dentosurgical
dentotropic
Dentsply
    D. FlexoFiles
    D. implant
    D. implant system
dentulism
dentulous
    d. dental arch

denture
    d. abrasion
    acrylic d.
    acrylic resin d.
    d. adherent paste
    d. adherent powder
    d. adhesive
    articulated partial d.
    bar joint d.
    d. basal surface
    basal surface of d.
    d. base
    d. base resin
    d. base saddle
    bilateral partial d.
    d. bolt
    d. border
    broken-stress partial d.
    d. brush
    cantilever fixed partial d.
    cantilever partial d.
    d. characterization
    clasp d.
    d. classification
    d. cleaner
    d. cleanser
    complete d.
    conditioning d.
    continuous gum d.
    d. curing
    design d.
    distal extension d.
    d. edge
    esthetic d.
    d. esthetics
    extension partial d.
    d. finish
    fixed partial d.
    d. flange
    d. flask
    d. foundation
    d. foundation area
    d. foundation surface
    d. frame
    full d.
    heel of d.
    hidden-lock d.
    d. hyperplasia
    immediate insertion d.
    implant d.
    implant-retained d.
    d. implant superstructure

    d. impression surface
    d. injury
    d. injury tumor
    interim d.
    Lee d.
    d. leverage
    d. magnet
    maxillary removable implant-retained d.
    metal base d.
    model wax d.
    mucosa-borne d.
    occlusal surface of d.
    d. occlusal surface
    onlay d.
    overlay d.
    d. packing
    partial d., distal extension
    periphery d.
    d. periphery
    polished surface d.
    porcelain d.
    precision retained d.
    d. processing
    d. prognosis
    d. prosthetics
    provisional d.
    removable d.
    removable partial d.
    d. retention
    retention d.
    sectional partial d.
    d. service
    soft-lined d.
    d. sore mouth
    space d.
    d. space
    d. stability
    d. stomatitis
    swing-lock d.
    d. teeth
    telescopic d.
    temporary partial d.
    Ticonium d.
    Ticonium hidden-lock d.
    tissue-borne partial d.
    tooth-borne d.
    tooth-borne partial d.
    tooth-borne/tissue-borne partial d.
    tooth and mucosa-borne d.
    transitional d.
    treatment partial d.

D

NOTES

denture *(continued)*
    trial d.
    d. ulcer
    unilateral partial d.
    d. vulcanite bur
    wax model d.
denture-bearing area
denture-dislodging force
denture-retaining force
denture-supporting
    d.-s. area
    d.-s. structure
denturism
denturist
Dentvision
    KTD D.
denudation
    interdental d.
denude
denuded
    d. finger
    d. furca
    d. furcation
    d. tissue
Denver Articulation Screening Examination (DASE)
deodorizing mouthwash
deoxidizing
depalatalization
depigmenting skin
deplate
depletion
    end-stage nutritional d.
depolarization
depolymerization
depolymerizing
Depo-Medrol Injection
Depo-Provera Injection
deposit
    calcium d.
    calcium pyrophosphate dihydrate d. (CPDD)
deposition
    bone d.
    collagen d.
depression
    lingual salivary gland d.
    mesial developmental d. (MDD)
    prejowl d.
    tooth d.
    trochanteric d.
depressor
    d. anguli oris muscle
    d. labii inferioris muscle
    d. labii oris muscle
    d. muscle of angle of mouth
    d. septi

    d. septi muscle
    tongue d.
Deproist Expectorant with Codeine
depth
    mandibular d.
    maxillary d.
    oral vestibular d.
    pocket d.
    probing d. (PD)
    vestibular d.
derangement
    alveolar arch d.
    internal d. (ID)
derivation
    sentence d.
derived sentence
Derm
    Gly D.
Derma
    D. K combination laser
    D. 20 laser
dermabrader
    high-speed d.
dermabrasion, dermoabrasion
Dermacort
dermal
    d. analogue tumor
    d. atrophy
    d. brassiere technique
    d. fat free flap
    d. fat free tissue transfer
    d. fat pedicle flap
    d. graft
    d. grafting
    d. melanosis
    d. network
    d. orbicular pennant technique
    d. pedicle technique
    d. pouch
    d. pouch reconstruction
    d. pyramidal flap
    d. vascularized pedicle
    d. vascular plexus
dermal-fat graft
Dermanet wound contact layer
dermaplaning
Dermarest Dricort
Derma-Smoothe/FS
Dermastat dermatology handpiece
dermatan
    d.-4 sulfate
    d. sulfate
dermatitis
    atopic d.
    contact d.
    d. herpetiformis (DH)
    d. medicamentosa
    perioral d.

retinoid d.
seborrheic d.
d. venenata
dermatoalloplasty
dermatoautoplasty
dermatochalasis
true d.
dermatofibroma
d. protuberans
dermatofibrosarcoma protuberans
dermatoheteroplasty
dermatohomoplasty
dermatome
Brown electric d.
Davol d.
drum d.
electric d.
Padgett d.
Rees d.
dermatomyositis
Dermatop
dermatopathologist
Dermatophagoides
D. farinae antigen
D. pteronyssinus
dermatoplastic
dermatoplasty
dermatosis, pl. **dermatoses**
d. papulosa nigra
dermatoxenoplasty
Dermedex
Donell D.
DERMED specialty skin care product
DERMESS specialty skin care product
DermiCort
dermis
activated d.
AlloDerm preserved human d.
d. fascia
fresh autologous de-
epidermalized d.
new d.
dermoabrasion (*var. of* dermabrasion)
dermoadipose
d. flap
d. tissue
dermoepidermal Gillies stitch
dermofasciectomy
dermofat
d. flap
d. graft
d. technique

dermoid
d. cyst
d. inclusion cyst
Dermo-Jet
D.-J. high pressure injector
D.-J. injector
Dermolate
dermolipectomy
abdominal d.
brachial d.
dermoplasty
d. procedure
Dermtex HC with Aloe
descending
d. necrotizing mediastinitis (DNM)
d. palatine artery (DPA)
d. pitch break
d. technique
d. technique audiometry
d. vestibular nucleus
descent
description
thick d.
descriptive
d. linguistics
d. phonetics
Desenex
Prescription Strength D.
desensitization
desensitize
desensitizer
Dentinbloc dentin d.
desensitizing
d. dentin
d. paste
desert ragweed
desiccans
glossitis d.
desiccate
desiccating crystal
desiccation
design
d. denture
radial-landed d.
Design Veronique compression wear
Desitin
desk-type auditory trainer
Desmarres retractor
desmin
d. filament
desmodont
desmoid tumor

D

NOTES

desmolysis
desmolytic stage
desmoplasia
    stromal d.
desmoplastic
    d. ameloblastoma
    d. fibroma
    d. melanoma
desmosome
    modified d.
desonide
DesOwen Topical
desoximetasone
desoxyribonuclease
    fibrinolysin and d.
desquamate
desquamated epithelial cell
desquamating epithelium
desquamation
    erosion d.
desquamativa
    otitis d.
desquamative
    d. gingivitis
destabilization
    postganglionectomy wrist d.
    d. surgery
destruction
    bony d.
Desyrel
detached
    d. cranial section
    d. craniotomy
detachment
    retinal d.
Detachol
Detailed Evaluation of Facial Symmetry
  (DEFS)
detectability threshold
detection
    gap d.
    speech d.
    d. threshold
detector
    TubeCheck esophageal intubation d.
detergent
    Enzol enzymatic d.
deterioration
determinants of occlusal morphology
determination
    exposure d.
    videostroboscopic diagnostic d.
determiner
    regular d.
determinism
    linguistic d.
detorque
detrition

Detussin Expectorant
deuterium (D)
devascularization
devascularized material
developer
    All-Pro automatic film d.
    d. solution
developing time
development
    Bayley Scales of Infant D.
    cognitive d.
    Houston Test for Language D.
    language d.
    Screening Kit of Language D.
    (SKOLD)
    Sequenced Inventory of
    Communication D.
    slow expressive language d.
    (SELD)
    speech d.
    Test of Language D.-Intermediate
    (TOLD-I)
    Test of Language D.-Primary
    (TOLD-P)
    Tests of Early Language D.
    (TELD)
    Utah Test of Language D.
developmental
    d. age
    d. aphasia
    D. Articulation Test (DAT)
    d. articulatory apraxia
    d. assessment
    d. dentin
    d. groove
    d. guidance
    d. hesitation
    d. imbalance
    d. line
    d. nevus
    d. period
    d. phonological process
    d. scale
    D. Sentence Scoring (DSS)
deviant
    d. articulation
    d. language
    d. speech
    d. swallowing
deviated septum
deviation
    mandibular d.
    septal d.
    standard d.
device
    Agee d.
    Algo-1, -2 automated auditory
    brainstem response d.

Algo-2 hearing screening d.
alternative communication d.
Ameflow d.
angled delivery d. (ADD)
assistive listening d. (ALD)
assistive technology d.
augmentative communication d.
behind-the-ear listening d.
blade-form d.
BTE listening d.
carpal tunnel release system d.
central-bearing tracing d.
charge-coupled d. (CCD)
Chick patient transfer d.
CIC listening d.
circumaural hearing protection d.
cohesive d.
completely-in-the-canal listening d.
CTRS d.
distraction d.
Douek-Med ear d.
DRH monitoring d.
EEA stapling d.
Endermologie noninvasive body
  contouring d.
Endo-Bender bending d.
EndoLift d.
esophageal detection d. (EDD)
Flutter therapeutic d.
GSI 60 distortion-product
  otoacoustic emission d.
hearing protection d. (HPD)
Hemovac suction d.
Heyer Schulte implant d.
insert hearing protection d.
Insta-Mold ear protection d.
interrupter d.
in-the-ear listening d.
ion collection monitoring d.
ITE listening d.
language acquisition d. (LAD)
Lewy suspension d.
LySonix 2000 ultrasound d.
Magna-Finder locating d.
magnetic jaw tracking d.
3M CTRS d.
Medicamat ultrasound d.
Medicon ultrasonic liposuction d.
Medicon US liposuction d.
Mentor ultrasound d.
Minnesota thermal disk temperature
  testing d.

3M microvascular anastomotic
  coupling d.
Morwel ultrasound d.
Orthofix lengthening d.
Parascan scanning d.
PhotoDerm PL pulsed light d.
Plastibell clamp-on d.
PLM d.
position indicating d. (PID)
precise lesion measuring d.
Pressurefuse automatic constant
  pressure d.
presyntactic d.
Pron-Pillo head positioning d.
provisionally acceptable d.
rigid internal fixation d.
Rinn XCP radiographic
  paralleling d.
root-form d.
Sebbin ultrasound d.
semiaural hearing protection d.
Senso listening d.
Serena and Serena Mx hand-held
  apnea detection d.
SMEI ultrasound d.
Sonic Air 1500 d.
Sono-stat Plus sound d.
Steri-Oss implant d.
Sure-Closure d.
Surgitron 3000 ultrasound d.
titanium fixation d.
tongue-retaining d. (TRD)
unacceptable d.
Virtual Model 330 distortion-
  product otoacoustic emission d.
Vitallium d.
Widex listening d.

devil's
  d. claw
  d. incision mammaplasty
devitalization
  pulp d.
devitalize
devitalized
  d. pulp
  d. tooth
devitrification
devoicing of final consonant
dewlap
  radiation d.
Dexacidin
Dexacort

D

NOTES

dexamethasone
> neomycin and d.
> neomycin, polymyxin B, and d.
> tobramycin and d.

Dexasone
> D. L.A.

Dexasporin

Dexatrim Pre-Meal

dexbrompheniramine and pseudoephedrine

Dexchlor

dexchlorpheniramine

Dexone
> D. LA

Dexon surgically knitted mesh

Dexotic

dexter (D)
> auris d. (AD)
> D. clear polyester casting resin

dexterity

dextral

dextrality

dextran
> d.-40
> low-molecular-weight d. (LMD)

dextranomer

dextromethorphan
> acetaminophen and d.
> carbinoxamine, pseudoephedrine, and d.
> chlorpheniramine, phenylephrine, and d.
> chlorpheniramine, phenylpropanolamine, and d.
> guaifenesin, phenylpropanolamine, and d.
> guaifenesin, pseudoephedrine, and d.
> pseudoephedrine and d.

Dey-Drop Ophthalmic Solution

dezocine

DF
> decayed and filled permanent teeth
> distal fossa
> DF caries index

df
> decayed and filled deciduous teeth
> df caries index

DFA
> delayed feedback audiometry

DFDB
> demineralized freeze-dried bone

DFDBA
> decalcified freeze-dried bone allograft
> demineralized freeze-dried bone allograft

DFDCB
> decalcified freeze-dried cortical bone

DFNX3
> X-linked progressive mixed deafness with perilymphatic gusher

DG
> distogingival

β-ᴅ-galactosidase

β-ᴅ-glucosidase

DH
> dermatitis herpetiformis
>> Codehist DH
>> Decohistine DH
>> Dihistine DH

DHCP
> dental health care provider

DHC Plus

DHEA
> dehydroepiandrosterone

D.H.E. 45 Injection

DHI
> Dizziness Handicap Inventory

DI
> dental index

diabetes
> d. mellitus

diabetic
> d. coma
> d. gingivitis
> d. neuropathy

diachronic linguistics

diacritic

diacrylate resin

diadochokinesia, diadochokinesis

diadochokinetic rate

diagnosis, pl. diagnoses
> differential d.

diagnosogenic theory

diagnostic
> d. articulation test
> d. audiology
> d. audiometry
> d. cast
> d. excisional biopsy
> d. implant cast
> d. setup
> d. teaching
> d. test
> d. therapy (Dx)
> d. wire

diagram
> branching tree d.
> Lund-Browder burn d.
> tree d.
> Venn d.

diagraph

Diaket sealer

dialdehyde solution

dialect
    regional d.
    d. speech community
diameter
    aerodynamic equivalent d. (AED)
    buccal-lingual alveolar d.
    buccolingual d.
    cervicobregmatic d.
    internal d.
    labiolingual d. of crown
    mesiodistal d. of crown
    temporal d.
diametral tensile strength
Diamine T.D.
diamond
    d. bur
    d. cutting instrument
    d. disk
    d. drill
    d. finishing bur
    d. fraise
    d. rotary instrument
    d. stone
    d. wafering saw
    d. wheel
diamond-edged fingernail file
Diamond-Edge Supercut scissors
Diamond-Jaw needle holder
Diamox
    D. Sequels
diapedesis
diaphanoscopy
diaphragm
    styloid d.
diaphragmatic-abdominal respiration
diaphragmatic hernia
diaphysis
diarthrodial synovial joint
diascopy
Diasonic DRF 1000 sonograph
diastase digestion
diastasis
    d. recti
diastema, pl. **diastemata**
    anterior d.
    closed median d.
    frenum d.
    multiple diastemata
diathermal needle
diathermy knife
diathesis
diatomaceous silicon dioxide abrasive

diatoms
diatoric
    d. teeth
diazepam
diazone
dibasic sodium citrate
Dibbell cartilage strut technique
dibromodulcitol
dichloralphenazone
    acetaminophen, isometheptene, and d.
dichlorodifluoromethane and trichloromonofluoromethane
dichlorotetrafluoroethane
    ethyl chloride and d.
dichlorphenamide
dichotic
    d. consonant-vowel test
    d. digit
    d. listening
    d. messages
dichotomous
dichotomy
diclofenac
dicloxacillin
diction
Didronel
die
    amalgam d.
    copperplated d.
    electroplated d.
    epoxy d.
    gypsum d.
    d. lubricant
    metal-plated d.
    d. plate
    plated d.
    D.-Rock
    silverplated d.
    d. spacer
    D. Stone
    stone d.
    waxing d.
Dieffenbach method
dielectric
diencephalon
diet
    postgastroplasty d.
diethyldithiocarbamate
    sodium d.
difference
    just noticeable d. (JND)

NOTES

D

difference *(continued)*
    language d.
    d. limen (DL)
    masking level d.
    d. tone
differential
    d. diagnosis
    d. eruption
    d. force
    d. force appliance
    d. force technique
    d. function
    d. reinforcement
    d. relaxation
    d. response
    d. retention
    d. threshold
differentiated
    d. cell
    d. thyroid cancer
differentiation
    auditory d.
    D. of Auditory Perception Skill
    (DAPS)
difficulty
    relaxation d.
    word-finding d.
diffracted wave
diffuse
    d. alveolar atrophy
    d. calcification
    d. esophageal spasm
    d. fibroma of gingiva
    d. gingivitis
    d. hyperplasia
    d. idiopathic skeletal hyperostosis
    (DISH)
    d. intravascular coagulopathy
    d. large cell lymphoma
    d. phoneme
    d. pulmonary hypoplasia
    d. pulp calcification
    d. sclerosing osteomyelitis (DSO)
    d. serous labyrinthitis
    d. suppurative labyrinthitis
    d. vocal polyposis
diffusion root canal filling method
diflorasone
Diflucan
diflunisal
digastric
    d. fossa
    d. muscle
    d. muscle flap
    d. ridge
    d. space
    d. triangle

digestion
    diastase d.
digit
    dichotic d.
    d. duplication
digital
    d. caliper
    d. hearing aid
    d. manipulation
    d. sound processing (DSP)
digitale
    pterygium d.
digitized lateral cephalogram
digitizer
    Cyberware 3030RGB d.
    Polhemus 3Space d.
digitopalmar arch
diglossia
digluconate
    chlorhexidine d.
dignathus
dignity
Dihistine
    D. DH
    D. Expectorant
dihydrate
    calcium pyrophosphate d.
    d. crystal
dihydrocodeine compound
dihydroergotamine
diketone
dilacerated
    d. canal
    d. curve
    d. tooth
dilaceration
    sharp d.
Dilantin
dilantin
    d. enlargement
    d. gingival hyperplasia
    d. gingivitis
dilatans
    pneumosinus d.
dilated odontoma
dilation, dilatation
    esophageal d.
dilator
    Anthony quadrisected minigraft d.
    bisected minigraft d.
    hydrostatic d.
    implant site d.
    Jackson triangular brass d.
    Marritt d.
    micrograft d.
    minigraft d.
    d. naris muscle
    Porges Neoflex d.

quadrisected-graft d.
quadrisected minigraft d.
tracheoesophageal puncture d.

Dilaudid
    D.-5
    D.-HP

diluent
    D. Complex V
    glycerin-saponin d.

dilute local anesthesia

Dimacol Caplets

Dimaphen
    D. Elixir
    D. Tablet

dimenhydrinate

dimension
    buccolingual d.
    occlusal vertical d. (OVD)
    postural vertical d. (PVD)
    restoration of vertical d.
    rest vertical d.
    vertical d.

dimensional
    d. change
    d. stability

Dimetabs Oral

Dimetane
    D.-DC
    D. Decongestant Elixir
    D. Extentabs

Dimetapp
    D. Elixir
    D. Extentabs
    D. 4-Hour Liqui-Gel Capsule
    D. Sinus Caplets
    D. Tablet

dimethacrylate
    bisphenol A glycidyl d.
    d. cement
    light-cured d.
    phosphonated d.
    d. polymer
    d. resin
    d. sealant
    urethane d. (UDMA)

dimethyl methacrylate

dimethylsiloxane

dimethyltriazeno-imidazole-carboxamide (DTIC)

diminutive

dimple
    müllerian d.

palatal d.
philtral d.
vaginal d.

dimpling

Dinamap Plus multiparameter monitor

Dinate Injection

dinatriumklodronate

Dine Digital Macro camera

Dingman retractor

dinitrofluorobenzene (DNFB)

diode
    d. pumped Nd:YAG laser

Diolite 532 laser system

diopter (D)

diotic
    d. listening
    d. messages

dioxide
    carbon d. (CO_2)
    chlorine d.
    end-tidal carbon d. ($ETCO_2$)
    sulfur d. (SO_2)

DIP
    distal interphalangeal
    DIP joint

diphallia

diphasic spike

diphemanil methylsulfate

Diphen Cough

Diphenhist

diphenhydramine
    acetaminophen and d.
    d. and pseudoephedrine

diphenidol

diphenylhydantoin
    d. gingivitis

diphtheria

diphtheriae
    Corynebacterium d.

diphtheritica
    angina d.

diphtheroid

diphthong

diphyodont
    d. dentition

dipivefrin

diplacusis
    d. binauralis
    d. dysharmonica
    d. echoica
    d. monauralis

NOTES

D

diplegia
  congenital facial d.
diploë, diploe
diplophonia
diplopia
dipper curve
Diprivan anesthesia
Diprolene
  D. AF
dipropionate
  beclomethasone d.
Diprosone
diprosopus
direct
  d. acrylic restoration
  d. bonding
  d. bone impression
  d. casting
  d. composite resin restoration
  d. conduction theory
  d. current (DC)
  D. Digital radiography (DDR)
  d. filling gold
  d. filling gold compaction
  d. filling resin
  d. flap
  d. gold restoration
  d. immunofluorescence
  d. innervation
  d. labial veneer
  d. laryngoscopy
  d. light reflex
  d. method for making inlay
  d. motor system
  d. neural stimulation
  d. porcelain matrix
  d. pulp capping
  d. puncture intralesional
    embolization
  d. resin filling
  d. resin restoration
  d. retainer
  d. retention
  d. selection communication board
  d. supracillary excision
  d. technique
directed fine-needle aspiration biopsy
direct/indirect technique
direction
  ampullopetal d.
directional
  d. brush stroke discrimination
  d. microphone
  d. preponderance (DP)
directionality
directivity
Directon resin
direct-vision carpal tunnel release

dirithromycin
disability
  learning d. (LD)
  Slingerland Screening Tests for
    Identifying Children with Specific
    Language D.
Disalcid
disappearing
  d. core
  d. mandible
disarticulation
disassimilation, dissimilation
disassociation (*var. of* dissociation)
Disc
  Clear Away D.
disc (*var. of* disk)
discharge
  purulent d.
  serosanguineous d.
discharged granule
discharging sinus
disclosing
  d. agent
  d. solution
discoid
  d. carver
  d. lupus erythematosus
discoid-cleoid
discoloration
  congenital d.
  endodontic d.
  gingival d.
  post-endodontic d.
  tetracycline d.
  traumatic d.
discomfort
  threshold of d. (TD)
discontiguous
discontinuous neck dissection
discourse
  D. Comprehension Test
  d. processing
  structured d.
discrepancy
  anterior-posterior d.
  arch d.
  envelope of d.
  posterior occlusal d.
  tooth size d.
  transverse d.
discrete disease
discrimination
  auditory d.
  auditory figure-ground d.
  d. curve
  directional brush stroke d.
  dynamic two-point d. (D-2PD)

Goldman-Fristoe-Woodcock Test of Auditory D.
d. loss
moving two-point d.
oral sensory d.
Picture Sound D.
Schiefelbush-Lindsey Test of Sound D.
d. score
spacial d.
speech d. (SD)
speech sound d.
static two-point d. (S-2PD)
Testing-Teaching Module of Auditory D. (TTMAD)
Tests of Nonverbal Auditory D. (TENVAD)
d. training
Tree/Bee Test of Auditory D.
two-point d. (2 PD)
visual d.
visual figure-ground d.

disease, pl. **diseases**
acute respiratory d.
Addison d.
Albers-Schönberg d.
Alzheimer d. (AD)
Apert d.
autoallergic d.
autoimmune d.
autoimmune inner ear d.
Barclay-Baron d.
Barlow d.
Basedow d.
Behçet d.
Besnier-Boeck-Schaumann d.
bleeder d.
Bowen d.
Breda d.
Brill-Symmers d.
brittle bone d.
Buerger d.
bullous/erosive d.
Caffey-Silverman d.
calculous d.
cardiovascular d.
catarrhal d.
cat scratch d.
Chagas d.
Chagas-Cruz d.
collagen d.
collagen-vascular d.

d. concept
congenital polycystic d.
coronary artery d.
Cowden d.
Creutzfeldt-Jakob d.
Crohn d.
Crouzon d.
cytomegalic inclusion d.
cytomegalovirus d.
Darier-White d.
demyelinating d.
discrete d.
Dupuytren d.
dysgenetic polycystic d. (DPD)
Engman d.
Fabry d.
Fauchard d.
Feer d.
fibrocystic d.
Fordyce d.
fusospirochetal d.
Gaucher d.
Gilchrist d.
granulomatous d.
Graves d.
hand-foot-and-mouth d.
Hand-Schüller-Christian d.
Hansen d.
Hashimoto d.
Heck d.
Hodgkin d.
human immunodeficiency virus-associated salivary gland d. (HIV-SGD)
hydatid d.
iatrogenic d.
I cell d.
inclusion d.
infectious d.
inflammatory d.
intransit d.
Jod-Basedow d.
Kawasaki d.
Keinböck d.
kissing d.
Korsakoff d.
Letterer-Siwe d.
linear IgA bullous d.
locoregional d.
Lyme d.
Magitot d.
marble bone d.

D

NOTES

165

disease *(continued)*
    Meige d.
    Menetrier d.
    Ménière d.
    Meyenburg d.
    micrometastatic d.
    Mikulicz d.
    Möller d.
    Mondor d.
    mycotic d.
    no evidence of d. (NED)
    nonspecific granulomatous d.
    Norrie d.
    obstructive airway d.
    occlusive artery d.
    occupational d.
    Ollier d.
    Oschler d.
    ototrophic viral d.
    Owren d.
    Paget d.
    parasitic d.
    Parkinson d.
    periodontal d.
    peripheral arterial occlusive d.
    (PAOD)
    Pfaundler-Hurler d.
    pilonidal d.
    Pleasants d.
    Plummer d.
    polycystic d.
    pulmonary d.
    regional d.
    Rendu-Osler-Weber d.
    rheumatic d.
    rheumatic heart d.
    Riga-Fede d.
    Riggs d.
    Romberg d.
    Sainton d.
    salivary gland virus d.
    Schilder d.
    sexually transmitted d. (STD)
    Simmonds d.
    Spira d.
    submandibular gland d.
    Sutton d.
    Takahara d.
    Tornwaldt d.
    van Buchem d.
    vanishing bone d.
    vascular occlusive d.
    vertebral-basilar artery d.
    Vincent d.
    Voltolini d.
    von Meyenburg d.
    von Recklinghausen d.
    Werdnig-Hoffman d.

    Winkler d.
    Wohlfart-Kugelberg-Welander d.
disease-specific functional status
disequilibrium
disfluency *(var. of* dysfluency)
DISH
    diffuse idiopathic skeletal hyperostosis
dish
    dappen d.
    Petri d.
disharmony
    facial d.
    maxillomandibular d.
    midline d.
    occlusal d.
dished-in face
dish-face deformity
dish-shaped erosion
disinfectant
    aqueous synthetic dual phenolic d.
    chlorine dioxide d.
    glutaraldehyde d.
    hydrophilic virus kill d.
    iodophor d.
    phenolic d.
    surface d.
    water-based d.
disinfection
    root canal d.
    spray-wipe-spray d.
    surface d.
disinsertion
    levator d.
disjoined pyeloplasty
disk, disc
    abrasive d.
    aluminum oxide d.
    Amici d.
    articular d.
    articular d.
    Burlew d.
    carborundum d.
    coarse d.
    composite resin finishing d.
    cutting d.
    cuttlefish d.
    Damascus d.
    dental d.
    diamond d.
    Dr Scholl's D.
    emery d.
    fine d.
    d. herniation
    interarticular d. of
    temporomandibular joint
    Jo Dandy d.
    lead d.
    d. mandrel

medium d.
polishing d.
safe-side d.
sandpaper d.
separating d.
silicon carbide d.
superfine d.
transport d.
XX fine d.
Disk-Criminator instrument
dislocation
fracture d.
d. fracture
mandibular d.
temporomandibular joint d.
dislodgement
Disobrom
disocclude
disodium
etidronate d.
Disophrol
D. Chronotabs
D. Tablet
disorder
articulation d.
attention deficit d. (ADD)
attention deficit hyperactivity d. (ADHD)
auditory d.
auditory processing d.
behavior d. (BD)
body dysmorphic d.
body image d.
breathing d.
central auditory d.
central language d. (CLD)
Charcot-Marie-Tooth d.
communication d.
communicative d.
conceptual d.
contiguity d.
endocrine d.
endonasal d.
esophageal motility d.
eye motility d.
false role d.
fluency d.
functional articulation d.
Haws Screening Test for Functional Articulation D.
language d.
lymphoproliferative d.

masticatory muscle d.
motor d.
myofacial pain-dysfunction d.
neuralgic d.
neurogenic language d.
olfactory d.
organic articulation d.
perceptual d.
pervasive developmental d. (PDD)
phonological d.
psychogenic d.
resonance d.
respiratory d.
rheumatic d.
Screening Test for Identifying Central Auditory D. (SCAN)
speech d.
temporomandibular d. (TMD)
temporomandibular pain-dysfunction d.
TMPD d.
vascular d.
vestibular system d.
vestibulospinal d.
voice d.
disordered
d. phonology
d. speech motor control
Dispers
Visio D.
Dispersalloy amalgam
dispersed phase alloy
dispersion
d. alloy
amphotericin B colloidal d.
d. phase alloy
d. system alloy
Dispertab Tablet
displaceability
tissue d.
displaced
d. malar fracture
d. sideburn
d. speech
d. tooth
displacement
anterior d. (AD)
cross-head d.
eye d.
mesial d.
disposable
d. bikini

D

NOTES

disposable (*continued*)
    d. cannula tip
    d. coaxial Endostat
    d. curette
    d. glove
    d. microclamp
    d. needle
    d. sculptured Endostat
    d. styrofoam block
Dispos-A-Cap amalgam alloy
disproportion
    skeletal d.
dissatisfaction
    body image d.
dissecans
    osteochondritis d. (OCD)
dissecta
    lingua d.
dissection
    axillary node d.
    balloon d.
    bilateral neck d.
    blunt d.
    cold d.
    cold-knife d.
    discontinuous neck d.
    elective lymph node d. (ELND)
    elective neck d. (END)
    electrosurgical d.
    ESP d.
    extended supraplatysmal plane d.
    facial nerve d.
    functional neck d. (FND)
    hydraulic d.
    mediastinal d.
    modified neck d. (MND)
    neck d.
    plane of d.
    radical neck d. (RND)
    retrograde d.
    selective neck d. (SND)
    sharp d.
    d. snare
    subgaleal d.
    subperichondrial d.
    subperiosteal d.
    suprahyoid neck d.
    supraomohyoid neck d.
    supra-perichondrial d.
    tongue-jaw-neck d.
    two-team d.
dissector
    #10 d.
    Chajchir d.
    endoscopic d.
    Hurd d.
    Resposable Spacemaker surgical
      balloon d.

    synovial d.
    Toledo d.
disseminated
    d. form Albright syndrome
    d. *Mycobacterium avium* complex
      (DMAC)
dissimilation (*var. of* disassimilation)
dissipation
dissociation, disassociation
    scapholunate d.
dissociative reaction
dissonance
    cognitive d.
distal
    d. angle
    d. based flap
    d. caries
    d. cavity
    d. cusp (DC)
    d. cusp ridge (DCR)
    d. end
    d. extension denture
    d. extension restoration
    d. force
    d. fossa (DF)
    d. interphalangeal (DIP)
    d. marginal ridge (DMR)
    mesial, occlusal, and d. (MOD)
    d. movement
    d. oblique groove (DOG)
    d. oblique molar radiograph
    d. occlusion
    d. pedicle flap
    d. pedicle flap technique
    d. phalanx
    d. pit (DP)
    d. root (DR)
    d. surface
    d. terminal bar
    d. triangular fossa (DTF)
DistaLens
distally based fasciocutaneous flap
  (DBFF)
distal-occlusal
distance
    interalveolar d.
    interarch d.
    interincisal d.
    interocclusal d.
    interridge d.
    large interarch d.
    maximum interincisal d. (MID)
    orbito-temple d.
    reduced interarch d.
    small interarch d.
    tube-patient d.
distancing
    cognitive d.

distant flap
distensae
    striae d.
distinction
    voicing d.
distinctive
    d. feature analysis
    d. features
distoangular
    d. impaction
    d. position
distoaxiogingival
distoaxioincisal
distoaxio-occlusal
distobuccal (DB)
    d. alveolus
    d. cusp (DBC)
    d. cusp ridge (DBCR)
    d. developmental groove (DBDG)
    d. line angle
    d. root (DBR)
distobucco-occlusal (DBO)
    d.-o. point angle
distobuccopulpal (DBP)
distocervical (DC)
distoclination
distoclusal, disto-occlusal (DO)
    d. point angle
distoclusion, disto-occlusion
    bilateral d.
    class II d.
    unilateral d.
distogingival (DG)
distoincisal
distolabial (DLA, DLa)
    d. line angle
distolabioincisal (DLAI, DLaI)
    d. point angle
distolabiopulpal
distolingual
    d. cusp (DLC)
    d. cusp ridge (DLCR)
    d. developmental groove
    d. fossa (DLF)
    d. groove (DLG)
    d. line angle
distolinguoincisal (DLI)
    d. point angle
distolinguo-occlusal (DLO)
    d.-o. point angle
distolinguopulpal (DLP)

distomolar
disto-occlusal (*var. of* distoclusal) (DO)
disto-occlusion (*var. of* distoclusion)
distoplacement
distopulpal (DP)
distopulpolabial
distopulpolingual (DPL)
distorted tragus
distortion
    amplitude d.
    figure-ground d.
    harmonic d.
    intermodulary d.
    nonlinear d.
    perceptual d.
    positional d.
    speech d.
    transient d.
    waveform d.
distortional bone conduction
distortion-product
    d.-p. masquerade of emission
    d.-p. otoacoustic emission (DPOAE)
distoversion
distractibility
distraction
    craniomaxillofacial callus d.
    d. device
    forward mandibular d.
    d. lengthening
    d. osteogenesis (DO)
    d. osteosynthesis
    d. pin
    rigid external d. (RED)
    simple mandibular d.
    skeletal d.
    d. TRAM
distractor
    Molina mandibular d.
    multidirectional d.
    MULTIGUIDE mandibular d.
    RED system rigid external d.
distress
    respiratory d.
distributed force
distribution
    capelike d.
    complementary d.
    contrastive d.
    gaussian d.
    noncontrastive d.
    normal d.

D

NOTES

distribution *(continued)*
    parallel d.
    V2 nerve d.
disturbance
    Appraisal of Language D. (ALD)
    architectural d.
    body image d.
    deglutitory d.
    emotional d.
    occlusal d.
    perceptual d.
disturbed voice quality
disyllable
ditched filling
ditching
ditransitive verb type
diuretic
diutinum
    eosinophilicum d.
dive
    HBO d.
    hyperbaric oxygen therapy d.
divergence
    anterior d.
    d. circuit
    posterior d.
diversion
    laryngeal d.
    laryngotracheal d.
diver's position
diverticulum, pl. **diverticula**
    cervical d.
    esophageal d.
    hypopharyngeal d.
    pharyngoesophageal d.
    pulsion d.
    tracheal d.
    traction d.
    Zenker d.
divider
    stress d.
division
    maxillary d.
    T12 nerve d.
divot
    liposuction d.
Dix-Hallpike maneuver
Dizmiss
dizziness
    D. Handicap Inventory (DHI)
DL
    difference limen
DLA, DLa
    distolabial
DLAI, DLaI
    distolabioincisal
DLC
    distolingual cusp

DLCR
    distolingual cusp ridge
DLF
    distolingual fossa
DLG
    distolingual groove
DLI
    distolinguoincisal
DLO
    distolinguo-occlusal
DLP
    distolinguopulpal
DLS
    ductlike structure
DM
    Anatuss DM
    Carbodec DM
    Cardec DM
    Humibid DM
    Profen II DM
    Pseudo-Car DM
DMAC
    disseminated *Mycobacterium avium*
    complex
DMAS
    deep muscular aponeurotic system
DMB
    demineralized bone
DMD
    Doctor of Dental Medicine
DMEM
    Dulbecco modified Eagle medium
DMF
    decayed, missing, filled permanent teeth
    DMF caries index
    DMF rate
dmf
    decayed, missing, filled deciduous teeth
    dmf caries index
DMFS
    decayed, missing, filled permanent teeth
    surfaces
    decayed, missing, filled surfaces
    permanent teeth
    DMFS caries index
dmfs
    decayed, missing, filled deciduous teeth
    surfaces
    decayed, missing, filled surfaces
    deciduous teeth
    dmfs caries index
DMR
    distal marginal ridge
DNFB
    dinitrofluorobenzene
DNM
    descending necrotizing mediastinitis

DO
distoclusal
disto-occlusal
distraction osteogenesis
DO cavity
Doan's
Extra Strength D.
D. Original
dock
bitter d.
sour d.
tall d.
yellow d.
Doctor
D. of Dental Medicine (DMD)
D. of Dental Science (DDSc)
D. of Dental Surgery (DDS)
doctorate of audiology (AuD)
doctrine
Godrina d.
usage d.
Doerfler-Stewart (D-S)
D.-S. test
DOG
distal oblique groove
dog
d. dander
d. ear of anastomosis
d. epithelium antigen
d. fennel
d. nose
dog-ear
d.-e. repair
Dolacet
Dolder
D. bar
D. bar joint attachment
D. bar unit
Dolene
dolichocheilia
dolichouranic, dolichuranic
Dolobid
Dolophine
dolor
domain
abdominal d.
amplitude d.
time/frequency d.
dome
nasal d.

Domeboro
Otic D.
D. solution
dome-sectioning technique
dominance
cerebral d.
lateral d.
dominant
d. hue
d. language
Donaldson tube
Donders
space of D.
Donell Dermedex
dong quai
donkey breathing
Donnamar
donor
autologous d.
d. bone marrow engraftment
d. incision
d. nipple
d. site
Dontrix gauge
Doppler
D. audiometry
color flow D. (CDF)
D. effect
D. flowmeter
Hadeco MiniDop D.
D. phenomenon
D. shift
Smartdop D.
D. ultrasonic probe
Dopram Injection
Dorello canal
Dormarex 2 Oral
Dormin Oral
Dorrance
D. closure
D. palatal pushback
dorsa (*pl. of* dorsum)
dorsal
d. antebrachial cutaneous nerve
d. back roll
d. cross-finger flap
d. lingual artery
d. lingual mucosa
d. thoracic fascia free flap
dorsalis
d. pedis artery
d. pedis-FDMA system

D

NOTES

dorsalis *(continued)*
    d. pedis flap
    tabes d.
dorsum, pl. **dorsa**
    nasal d.
    d. sella
Doryx
    D. Oral
dorzolamide
Dos Amigos Verbal Language Scale
dose
    maximum accumulated d. (MAD)
    maximum permissible d. (MPD)
    d. perturbation
    roentgen absorbed d. (rad)
    threshold d.
    tumoricidal d.
dose-effect curve
Dosepak
    Medrol D.
dose-response curve
dosimeter
dosimetry
    thermoluminescent d.
dotted tongue
Double
    D. D needle
double
    d. assimilation
    d. club elevator
    d. consonant
    d. cord retraction
    d. cross-lip flap
    d. emulsion film
    d. exposure
    d. gloving
    d. jaw surgery
    d. keyhole loop archwire
    d. keyhole loop wire
    d. lingual bar
    d. lip
    d. lumen implant
    d. opposing Z-plasty
    d. papilla graft
    d. papilla pedicle graft
    d. pedicle flap
    d. pedicle technique
    d. pendulum flap
    d. protrusion
    d. rectus harvest
    d. seal
    d. skin paddle fibular flap
    d. tunnel
    d. V-Y flap
    d. V-Y plasty with paired inverted
    Burow triangle excisions
double-barreled fibular bone graft
double-bubble breast deformity

double-cannula tracheostomy tube
double-cross-plasty
double-ended
    d.-e. curette
    d.-e. instrument
    d.-e. scaler
double-eyelid plasty
double-lumen suction irrigation tube
double-paddle
    d.-p. flap
    d.-p. island flap
double-pedicle transverse rectus
    abdominis musculocutaneous flap
double-plane instrument
double-sealant technique
double-sided instrument
double-spoon biopsy forceps
double-walled audiometric test booth
doubling
Douek-Med ear device
doughnut
    de-epithelialized d.
doughy
    d. consistency
Douglas
    D. fir
    D. graft
douloureux
    tic d.
dovetail
    lingual d.
    occlusal d.
    d. stress broken abutment
dowel
    d. crown
    d. rest attachment
    Thompson d.
dowel-core placement
Downes nasal speculum
downgrafting
    maxillary d.
Downs
    D. analysis
    D. cephalometric analysis
Down syndrome
doxapram
doxepin
doxorubicin
Doxy-Caps
Doxychel
    D. Injection
    D. Oral
doxycycline
    d. hyclate
Doxy Oral
Doyle
    D. bi-valved airway splint
    D. II silicone stent

DP
  debonding pliers
  directional preponderance
  distal pit
  distopulpal
  driving pressure
D.P.
  Dalalone D.P.
DPA
  descending palatine artery
DPD
  dysgenetic polycystic disease
D-2PD
  dynamic two-point discrimination
DPL
  distopulpolingual
DPM
  dual-pedicle dermoparenchymal
    mastopexy
DPOAE
  distortion-product otoacoustic emission
DR
  distal root
Dr.
  D. Scholl's Athlete's Foot
  D. Scholl's Disk
  D. Scholl's Maximum Strength
    Tritin
  D. Scholl's Wart Remover
drag
drain
  Axiom d.
  Blake d.
  Blake silicone d.
  H d.
  Hemovac d.
  Jackson-Pratt d.
  pencil d.
  Penrose d.
  TLS surgical d.
  tube d.
drainage
  fluctuant d.
  incision and d. (I&D)
  lumbar d.
  lymphatic d.
  one-way d.
  retrograde venous d.
  submandibular d.
  suction d.
  d. system
  through-and-through d.

draining lymph node
Dramamine
  D. II
  D. Oral
Drechlsera
Dremel Moto-tool
dressing
  Abdopatch Gel Z adhesive d.
  Alldress multilayered wound d.
  Alvogyl surgical d.
  Aquaplast d.
  Biobrane d.
  Chloro-Thymonol root canal d.
  ClearSite wound d.
  CollaCote wound d.
  CollaPlug wound d.
  CollaTape wound d.
  Cresanol root canal d.
  DuoDerm d.
  Elastoplast tension d.
  Flexzan d.
  Flexzan Extra d.
  Flexzan topical wound d.
  fluffs d.
  FyBron d.
  GraftCyte moist d.
  hydrocolloid d.
  Hypergel wound d.
  Iamin Hydrating Gel wound d.
  Kalginate calcium alginate
    wound d.
  Kirkland cement d.
  LaserSite wound d.
  Mammopatch gel self adhesive d.
  Medipatch Gel Z adhesive d.
  Mepitel d.
  Mepitel nonadherent silicone d.
  Mesalt sodium chloride
    impregnated d.
  Micropore d.
  moustache d.
  Normlgel protective wound d.
  occlusive d.
  occlusive semipermeable d.
  Omniderm d.
  OsmoCyte island wound care d.
  OsmoCyte pillow wound d.
  periodontal d.
  Pillo Pro d.
  PolyMem d.
  Reston foam d.
  Rhino Rocket d.

NOTES

D

dressing *(continued)*
 semiocclusive d.
 SignaDRESS d.
 Silastic foam d.
 Silon-TSR wound d.
 super-absorptive polymer d.
 Tegaderm d.
 Telfa d.
 tie-over d.
 Vigilon d.
 wet-to-dry d.
DRH monitoring device
Dri-Angles obstructor
Dricort
 Dermarest D.
drift
 mesial d.
 physiologic d.
drifting
 d. tooth
drill
 bibeveled d.
 bur d.
 Calcitek d.
 Canal Master d.'s
 centering d.
 cobra-head d.
 dental d.
 diamond d.
 Feldman d.
 Gates-Glidden d.
 Hall surgical d.
 high-speed d.
 IMCOR d.
 intraosseous d.
 lentula spiral d.
 MicroMax speed d.
 Osteon d.
 Peeso d.
 Shannon d.
 spear-point d.
 Spirec d.
 Stryker d.
 twist d.
 Zimmer Micro-E fixation d.
drill-induced hearing loss
drilling
drip
 postnasal d.
 succinylcholine d.
Dristan
 D. Cold Caplets
 D. Long Lasting Nasal Solution
 D. Sinus Caplets
driver
 UAM universal fixation d.
driving pressure (DP)
Drixomed

Drixoral
 D. Cough & Congestion Liquid Caps
 D. Cough & Sore Throat Liquid Caps
 D. Non-Drowsy
 D. Syrup
drool
drooling
drop
 Afrin Children's Nose D.'s
 Allerest Eye D.'s
 Allergan Ear D.'s
 Americaine Otic ear d.'s
 Auro Ear D.'s
 Coly-Mycin S Otic D.'s
 CosMedical lipid d.'s
 ear d.'s
 enamel d.
 Luride D.'s
 Mallazine Eye D.'s
 Moisture Ophthalmic D.'s
 Murine Ear D.'s
 N'ice Vitamin C D.'s
 Pearl D.'s
 Rondamine-DM D.'s
 Rondec D.'s
 saline d.'s
 Triaminic Oral Infant D.'s
 Tussafed D.'s
droperidol plus fentanyl
droplet
 lipid d.
 d. nucleus
 d. spread
droppings
 pigeon d.
Drowsiness
 Allerest No D.
 Ornex No D.
 Sinarest, No D.
 Sinutab Without D.
 Tylenol Cold No D.
drug
 anticonvulsive d.
 antituberculous d.
 endodontic d.
 non-S-phase specific d.
 nonsteroidal anti-inflammatory d. (NSAID)
 ototoxic d.
 parasympathetic d.
 parasympatholytic d.
 parasympathomimetic d.
 prophylactic d.
 radiosensitizing d.
 S-phase specific d.

d. therapy
vestibulotoxic d.
drug-induced immunosuppression
drum
    d. dermatome
    d. membrane
drumhead
Drummond
    artery of D.
dry
    D. Eyes Solution
    D. Eye Therapy Solution
    d. felt wheel
    d. field technique
    d. heat oven sterilization
    d. heat sterilizer
    d. hoarseness
    d. mouth
    d. socket
    d. socket syndrome
    d. strength
    d. vermilion
dryer
    L&R X-ray film d.
dry-eye syndrome
Drysol
DS
    Bactrim DS
    Cotrim DS
    Septra DS
    Tolectin DS
D-S
    Doerfler-Stewart
    D-S test
DSC
    Parafon Forte D.
D-shaped implant
DSO
    diffuse sclerosing osteomyelitis
DSP
    digital sound processing
D-speed film
DSS
    Developmental Sentence Scoring
DTF
    deep temporal fascia
    distal triangular fossa
DTIC
    dimethyltriazeno-imidazole-carboxamide
DTIC-Dome
DTPA
    gadolinium D.

D-TRAM pedicle flap
D-tubocurarine
D-type reamer
Duadacin Capsule
dual
    d. bite
    d. impression
    d. impression technique
    d. wavelength spectrophotometry
dual-chambered
    d.-c. implant
    d.-c. prosthesis
dual-cured luting composite resin
dual-cure resin
dual-meaning idiomatic phrase
dual-pedicle dermoparenchymal mastopexy (DPM)
dual-port
    d.-p. arthroscopy
    d.-p. lavage
duboid cell
Dubreuil-Chambardel syndrome
duck
    d. feather dander
    d. lips exercise
duckbill
    d. voice prosthesis
duct
    Bartholin d.
    d. cannulation
    cochlear d.
    Coschwitz d.
    endolymphatic d.
    excretory d.
    frontonasal d.
    intercalated d.
    interlobular d.
    intralobular d.
    lacrimal d.
    lingual d.
    müllerian d.
    nasofrontal d.
    nasolacrimal d.
    nasopalatine d.
    parotid d.
    perilymphatic d.
    periotic d.
    pharyngoinfraglottic d.
    Rivinus d.
    saccular d.
    salivary d.
    secretory d.

D

NOTES

duct (continued)
    semicircular d.
    Stensen d.
    striated d.
    sublingual d.
    submandibular d.
    submaxillary d.
    thoracic d.
    thyroglossal d.
    utricular d.
    utriculosaccular d.
    vestibulo-infraglottic d.
    Wharton d.
ductal
    d. carcinoma
    d. obstruction
    d. stricture
ductile material
ductility
ductless
ductlike structure (DLS)
ductule
ductus reuniens
Dulbecco modified Eagle medium (DMEM)
Dulguerov T stage
Dull-C
Dumbach
    D. mandibular reconstruction system
    D. mini mesh
    D. regular mesh
    D. titanium mesh
dummy
Dumon-Harrell bronchoscope
Dumon silicone stent
Duncan multiple range test
Dunlap cold compression wrap system
Dunning-Leach index
DuoCet
duodenal
    d. adenoma
    d. ulcer
DuoDerm
    D. dressing
DuoFilm
Duoloid impression system
DuoPlant Gel
duplex ultrasound
duplicating
    d. impression
    d. radiograph
duplication
    digit d.
    d. of the face
    limb d.
    nasal d.
    syllable d.
duplicative cyst

duplicator
    radiographic d.
Dupuy-Dutemps operation
Dupuytren disease
dura
    lamina d.
    lyophilized d.
    d. mater
    d. mater venous sinus
Duracell Activair hearing aid battery
Duract
Durafill
    D. adhesive
    D. bonding resin
    D. dental restorative material
    D. VS
Duraflor sodium fluoride varnish
Duragesic Transdermal
Dura-Gest
dural
    d. grafting
    d. venous sinus injury
Duralay inlay resin
Duralone Injection
Duramist Plus
Duramorph Injection
Duranest
duraplasty
Durascope endoscope
Dur-A-Sil
    D.-A.-S. ear impression material
    D.-A.-S. silicone impression system
duration (D)
Duration Nasal Solution
Dura-Vent
    D.-V./DA
Durelon cement
Durette
    D. dental shield
    D. external laser shield
    D. system
Durham tube
Duricef
dust
    barn d.
    grain d.
    house d.
Dutch strain
duty cycle
DUV
    degree of voicelessness
DUX system
dwarf
    pituitary d.
dwarfed enamel
Dwelle Ophthalmic Solution
Dx
    diagnostic therapy

dyad
> parent-child d.

Dyazide

Dycal
> D. cement

Dycill

Dyclone

dyclonine

dye
> fluorescein d.
> fluorescent d.
> d. injection
> isosulfan blue d.
> occlusal registration d.
> radiopaque d.
> rhodamine B fluorescent d.

Dymenate Injection

Dynabac
> D. tablet

Dynabond resin

Dynacin Oral

Dynafed
> D. IB
> D., Maximum Strength

Dynaflex prosthesis

DynaGraft
> D. bioimplant
> D. gel
> D. granule
> D. putty

Dyna-Hex Topical

Dynamic
> D. Bridging plate
> D. Mesh craniomaxillofacial pre-angled connecting bar

dynamic
> d. anchorage
> d. aphasia
> d. bite opener
> d. compression plate (DCP)
> d. computed tomography
> d. fascial transfer procedure
> d. graciloplasty
> d. modulus
> d. muscle transfer procedure
> d. platform posturography
> d. posturography
> d. range
> d. relation
> d. resilience
> d. sling

> d. stress
> d. two-point discrimination (D-2PD)

dynamometer
> Lido Multi Joint II isokinetic d.

Dynapen

DynaSurg electric handpiece

DynaTorq wrench

Dynatrak handpiece

dyne

dynein arm

dysacusia, dysacousia, dysacusis

dysallilognathia

dysarthria
> ataxic d.
> ataxic and spastic d.
> flaccid d.
> hyperkinetic d.
> hypokinetic d.
> d. literalis
> neurogenic d.
> parkinsonian d.
> peripheral d.
> somesthetic d.
> spastic d.
> d. syllabaris spasmodica

dysarthric

dysarthrosis

dysaudia

dyscalculia

dyscephaly
> mandibulo-oculofacial d.

dyschromia

dyscinesia (*var. of* dyskinesia)

dysconjugate gaze

dyscrasia
> hematologic d.

dysesthesia
> palmar d.

dysfluency, disfluency

dysfunction
> baroreflex d. (BRD)
> brain d. (BD)
> craniomandibular d. (CMD)
> dental d.
> eustachian tube d. (ETD)
> facial neuromuscular d.
> minimal brain d. (MBD)
> myofacial pain-d. (MPD)
> neurological d.
> temporomandibular joint d. (TMD, TMJ)
> temporomandibular pain d. (TMPD)

D

NOTES

dysfunction *(continued)*
    vestibular d.
    voice d.
dysfunctional nasal valve
dysgenesis
    d. iridodentalis
dysgenetic polycystic disease (DPD)
dysgeusia
dysglossia
dysgnathia
dysgnathic
    d. anomaly
dysgraphia
dysharmonica
    diplacusis d.
dysjunction
    craniofacial d.
    Le Fort III craniofacial d.
    pterygomaxillary d.
dyskeratoma
    warty d.
dyskeratosis
    benign intraepithelial d.
    d. congenita
    hereditary benign intraepithelial d.
      (HBID)
    intraepithelial d.
    malignant d.
dyskeratotic leukoplakia
dyskinesia, dyscinesia
    primary ciliary d. (PCD)
dyslalia
    functional d.
    organic d.
dyslexia
dyslexic
dyslogia
dyslogomathia
dysmasesis
dysmathia
dysmetria
    ocular d.
dysmorphic cranium
dysmorphism
    craniofacial d.
dysmorphology
    orbital d.
dysmorphophobia
dysnomia
dysodontiasis
dysontogenetic cyst
dysosmia
    congenital d.
dysostosis
    cleidocranial d.
    craniofacial d.
    faciomandibular d.
    mandibulofacial d.

    maxillonasal d.
    multiplex d.
    d. multiplex
    Nager acrofacial d.
    orodigitofacial d.
    otomandibular d.
dysphagia
    d. lusoria
    d. nervosa
    neurogenic d.
    sideropenic d.
    vallecular d.
dysphasia
dysphemia
    d. and biochemical theory
dysphonia
    adductor spasmodic d.
    hyperkinetic d.
    pediatric hyperfunctional d.
    d. plicae ventricularis
    spasmodic d.
    spastic d.
    d. spastica
    ventricular d.
    ventricular fold d.
dysphrasia
dyspigmentation
dysplasia
    anteroposterior d.
    anteroposterior facial d.
    brachycephalofrontonasal d.
    cemental d. (*var. of* florid
      osseous d.)
    chondroectodermal d.
    cleidocranial d.
    condylar d.
    craniofacial d.
    dental d.
    dentin d.
    dentinal d.
    dentoalveolar d.
    dentofacial d.
    d. dentofacialis
    dentolabial d.
    ectodermal d.
    enamel d.
    familial fibrous d.
    familial white folded d.
    fibromuscular d.
    fibro-osseous d.
    fibrous d. of jaws
    florid osseous d., cemental d.
    focal cementoosseous d. (FCOD)
    focal osseous d.
    frontonasal d.
    hereditary ectodermal d.
    hypohidrotic ectodermal d.
    iridodental d.

maxillomandibular d.
Mondini d.
monostotic fibrous d.
nasal d.
nasomaxillary d.
oculodento-osseous d.
odontogenic d.
osseous d.
otodental d.
periapical cemental d.
peripheral cemental d.
polyostotic fibrous d.
vertical d.

dysplastic
d. nevi
d. nevus

dyspnea
dyspraxia
dysprosody
dysraphism
cranial d.

dysrhythmia

dysrhythmic phonation
dyssyllabia
dystocia
shoulder d.

dystomia
dystonia
oromandibular d.

dystopia
globe d.
orbital d.

dystrophic
d. calcification
d. mineralization
d. myotonia

dystrophica
epidermolysis bullosa d.

dystrophy
facioscapulohumeral muscular d.
fibrous pulp d.
mucopolysaccharide keratin d.
muscular d.
reflex sympathetic d. (RSD)

NOTES

D

E

enamel
  E space

E₂

prostaglandin E_2

E/200 contra-angle 1:5 press-button chuck

EA

educational age
  EA surgical contra-angle 10:1
    press-button chuck

EAAS

electrothermal atomic absorption
  spectrophotometry

EAC

external auditory canal

Eagle

E. MEM
E. syndrome

eagle's beak pliers

EAL

electronic apex locator

Eames technique

EAP

endoscopic access port
Guyuron EAP

E-A-R

E-A-R Hi-Fi earplugs
E-A-R LINK eartips
E-A-R TONE earphones

ear

artificial e.
aviator's e.
Aztec e.
Blainville e.'s
e. bowl
bowl of e.
boxer's e.
Cagot e.
e. canal
cauliflower e.
cockleshell e.
constricted e.
cup e.
darwinian e.
e. drops
ERO E.
external e.
glue e.
helix of e.
inner e.
internal e.
e. lobule
lop e.
middle e.

Morel e.
Mozart e.
Otocalm E.
outer e.
outstanding e.
persistent lop e.
Pneumocystis carinii in middle e.
prominent e.
protruding e.
question mark e.
scroll e.
e. shape
e. speculum
Stahl e.
e. surgery
swimmer's e.
telephone e.
tin e.
e. training
e. wax
Wildermuth e.

earache

eardrum

earlobe

e. adipose tissue
cleft e.
e. composite graft
incomplete cleft of e.
e. keloid

early

e. hard palate closure
e. intervention service
e. obstetric brachial plexus palsy
e. tooth

earmold

e. lab
nonoccluding e.
open e.
perimeter e.
shell e.
skeleton e.
standard e.
vented e.

earmuffs

earphones

E-A-R TONE e.

EarPlanes

earplugs

E-A-R Hi-Fi e.

EARR

external apical root resorption

earring

pressure e.
pressure-producing e.

ears, nose, and throat (ENT)

E

earth wax
eartips
> E-A-R LINK e.

earwax
EASIC
> Evaluating Acquired Skills in
> Communication

Easprin
Easy Introduction system (EIS)
Eaton-Lambert syndrome
EBA cement
EBER
> Epstein-Barr virus-encoded ribonucleic
> acid
> EBER in situ hybridization

EBL
> endemic Burkitt lymphoma
> endoscopic band ligation

E-BM
> evidence-based medicine

Ebner, von Ebner
> E. glands
> imbrication lines of von E.
> incremental lines of von E.

ebonics
eboris
> membrana e.

ébranlement
EBSL
> external branch of the superior laryngeal
> EBSL nerve

ebur
> e. dentis

eburnation
> dental e.
> e. of dentin

eburnea
> substantia e.

eburnitis
EBV
> Epstein-Barr virus
> EBV-encoded RNA

ECA
> external carotid artery

eccentric
> e. checkbite
> e. dynamic compression plating
> (EDCP)
> e. interocclusal record
> e. jaw position
> e. jaw relation
> e. maxillomandibular record
> e. occlusion
> e. relation
> e. slide

ecchymosis

Eccovision
> E. acoustic reflection imaging
> system
> E. acoustic rhinometry system

eccrine
> e. acrospiroma
> e. hidrocystoma
> e. poroma
> e. spiradenoma

ECF-A
> eosinophil chemotactic factor of
> anaphylaxis

Echinacea angustifolia
Echinococcus granulosus
ECHO
> enterocytopathogenic human orphan
> ECHO virus

echo
> e. chamber
> cochlear e.
> e. reaction
> e. speech
> e. time

echoacousia
echogenic
> e. interface

echoica
> diplacusis e.

echoic operant
echolalia
> delayed e.
> immediate e.
> mitigated e.
> unmitigated e.

echoless
echologia
echophasia
echophrasia
echothiophate iodide
eclabium
eclecticism
ECM
> extracellular matrix
> ECM contraction

ECoG
> electrocochleography

ecological theory
E-Complex-600
econazole
Econopred Plus Ophthalmic
Ecotrin
> E. Low Adult Strength

ECS
> extracapsular spread
> extracellular space

ectatic
> e. capillary channels
> e. vertebral artery

ecthyma
ectocanthus
ectocranial
ectocyst
ectoderm
ectodermal
    e. dysplasia
    e. tumor
ectomesenchymal origin
ectomesenchyme
ectopia
    primary cerebellar e.
ectopic
    e. adenoma
    e. eruption
    e. synapse
ECTR
    endoscopic carpal tunnel release
    single-portal ECTR
ectrodactyly
ectropion
    paralytic e.
    posttraumatic e.
    residual senile e.
eczematoid external otitis
EDA
    electrodermal audiometry
Ed A-Hist Liquid
EDB
    extensor digitorum brevis
EDCP
    eccentric dynamic compression plating
EDD
    esophageal detection device
EDDA
    expanded duty dental auxiliary
eddying
edema
    angioneurotic e.
    brawny e.
    cerebral e.
    facial e.
    e. glottidis
    inflammatory e.
    labial e.
    laryngeal e.
    palatal e.
    penoscrotal e.
    purulent e.
    Reinke e.
    retropharyngeal e.
edentate

edentia
    compensated e.
edentics
edentulate
edentulism
edentulous
    e. dental arch
    lower completely e. (LCE)
    lower partially e. (LPE)
    e. patient
    e. ridge
    e. space
    upper completely e. (UCE)
    upper partially e. (UPE)
EDGE
    E. coated blade
    E. coated needle electrode
edge
    cartilage e.
    cutting e.
    denture e.
    feathered e.
    incisal e.
    labioincisal e. (LIE)
    linguoincisal e. (LIE)
    shearing e.
    e. strength
edge-strength
edge-to-edge
    e.-t.-e. bite
    e.-t.-e. occlusion
edgewise
    e. attachment
    e. bracket
    e. buccal tube
    e. fixed orthodontic appliance
    e. slot
    e. technique
    e. torque
Edinger-Westphal nucleus
Edlan-Mejchar operation
Edlan vestibulotomy
EDMA
    euclidean distance matrix analysis
EDRA
    electrodermal response test audiometry
edrophonium
    e. chloride
    e. chloride test
ED-SPAZ
EDTA
    ethylenediaminetetraacetic acid

E

NOTES

183

EDTAC
ethylenediaminetetraacetic acid Cetavlon
educable mentally retarded (EMR)
educational
e. age (EA)
e. audiology
e. quotient (EQ)
educationally mentally handicapped (EMH)
EDXA
energy dispersed x-ray analysis
EEA
electroencephalic audiometry
end-to-end anastomosis
EEA stapling device
EEG
electroencephalogram
eel cobra tip
EEM
Test for Examining Expressive Morphology
EEMG
evoked electromyography
EENT
eye, ear, nose, and throat
EEP
end expiratory pressure
E.E.S.
E. Oral
EF
eosinophilic fasciitis
EFDA
extended function dental assistant
effect
adaptation e.
arcading e.
Bauschinger e.
Bernoulli e.
body baffle e.
cascading e.
check-rein e.
consistency e.
crabgrass e.
crinkling e.
cumulative e.
cumulus cloud e.
Doppler e.
electrophonic e.
Féré e.
halo e.
head shadow e.
Karolyi e.
lysing e.
neurotoxic e.
occlusion e.
off e.
on e.
placebo e.

spiral e.
tethering e.
truncated cone e.
vestibulotoxic e.
wedging e.
Wever-Bray e.
Z-plasty e.
effective
e. amplitude
e. masking
e. setting expansion
effector
e. operation
e. organ
efferent
e. motor aphasia
e. nerve
Effersyl
efficiency
masking e.
masticatory e.
vocal e.
effort
e. level
paradoxic respiratory e.
vocal e.
effusion
chronic otitis media with e. (COME)
endotoxin-mediated otitis media with e.
extradural e.
middle ear e. (MEE)
mucopurulent hemorrhagic e.
otitis media with e. (OME)
Efidac/24
Efodine
Efudex
EGF
epidermal growth factor
egg
e. white
e. yolk
eggplant
eggshell appearance
egobronchophony
egocentric
e. language
e. speech
egophonic
egophony
egress
Eicken method
5,8,11,14-eicosatetraynoic acid (ETYA)
eidetic
e. imagery
EIE
E. 150F operating microscope

E. MiniEndo piezoelectric ultrasonic
unit
eighth
  e. cranial nerve
  e. nerve action potential (8NAP)
  e. nerve tumor
Eikenella corrodens
EIS
  Easy Introduction system
ejector
  apical fragment e.
  hygroformic saliva e.
  saliva e.
E/KM surgical contra-angle 40:1 press-button chuck
EL
  elastic limit
ELAFF
  extended lateral arm free flap
Elase
  E.-Chloromycetin Topical
  E. Topical
elastase
elastic
  e. band fixation
  e. curve
  e. deformation
  e. fiber
  e. hook
  e. impression
  e. impression material
  intermaxillary e.
  intramaxillary e.
  e. ligature
  e. limit (EL)
  maxillomandibular e.
  e. modulus
  e. plastic splint
  e. recoil
  rubber dam e.
  e. stain
  e. thread
  e. traction
  vertical e.
elasticity
elasticus
  conus e.
  nodulus e.
elastomer
  e. shell
  silicone e.

elastomeric
  e. impression
  e. impression material
elastometric tie
Elastoplast tension dressing
elastosis
Elavil
elbow
  e. zip
Elbrecht splint
Eldecort
elder
  marsh e.
  rough marsh e.
Elderly
  Hearing Handicap Inventory for
  the E. (HHIE)
Eldopaque
  E. Forte
  E. Forte cream
Eldoquin
  E. Forte
  E. Forte cream
elecampane
elected mutism
elective
  e. lymph node dissection (ELND)
  e. mutism
  e. neck dissection (END)
  e. neck irradiation (ENI)
Electraloy alloy
electric
  e. casting machine
  e. current shunting
  e. dermatome
  e. field
  e. irritability
  e. nerve stimulator
  e. pulp test
  e. pulp tester
  e. pulp testing
  e. response audiometry (ERA)
  e. shock
  e. toothbrush
electrical
  e. artificial larynx
  e. measurement of speech
  production
  e. potential
electrically stimulated anal neosphincter
electroacoustic
electroactivation

E

NOTES

electrocauterization
electrocautery
    needle-point e.
electrocoagulation
electrocoagulator
electrocochleogram
electrocochleography (ECoG)
electrode
    e. array
    Cardiff e.
    Clark polarographic oxygen e.
    Colorado MicroNeedle needle e.
    EDGE coated needle e.
    E-Z Clean laparoscopic e.
    Iomed Phoresor e.
    LLETZ/LEEP loop e.
    MegaDyne arthroscopic hook e.
    Neotrode II neonatal e.
electrodeposition
electrodermal
    e. audiometry (EDA)
    e. response test audiometry
    (EDRA)
electrodermatome
electrodesiccation
electrodiagnostic
    e. study
    e. testing
electroencephalic
    e. audiometry (EEA)
    e. response audiometry (ERA)
electroencephalogram (EEG)
electroencephalograph
electroencephalography
electroetched
electroetching
electroformer
electroforming
electroglottograph
electroglottographic
electroglottography
electrogustometer
electrogustometry
electrohydraulic extracorporeal
    lithotripsy
electrolarynx
electrolyte
electrolytic
    e. gold
    e. solution
electrolyzer
electromagnetic
    e. induction
    e. lithotriptor
    e. radiation
    e. spectrum
    e. wave

electromallet
    e. condenser
    McShirley e.
electrometric testing
electromotive force (EMF)
electromyograph
    Viking II EMG system e.
electromyographic relaxation biofeedback
electromyography (EMG)
    evoked e. (EEMG)
electron
    e. beam
    e. micrograph
    e. microscope
electroneurography
electroneurography/nerve conduction
    study
electroneuronography (ENog, ENoG)
electronic
    e. apex locator (EAL)
    e. artificial larynx
    e. knife
    e. speckle pattern interferometry
    (ESPI)
electronystagmogram
electronystagmography (ENG)
electro-oculography (EOG)
electrophonic effect
electrophoresis
    polyacrylamide gel e.
    sodium dodecyl sulfate-
    polyacrylamide gel e. (SDS-
    PAGE)
electrophysiologic
    e. audiometry
    e. mapping
electrophysiology
electroplated
    e. copper
    e. die
    e. silver
electroplating
electropolishing
electroresection
electrosalivogram
electroscission
electrosection
electrosterilization
    root canal e.
electrosterilizer
electrosurgery
electrosurgical
    e. current intensity
    e. dissection
    e. scaling
    e. scalpel
Electro-Surgical instrument (ESI)
electrotherapy

electrothermal atomic absorption
  spectrophotometry (EAAS)
element
    morphological e.
    neural e.
    syntactic e.
elements of performance objective
elephantiasis
    filarial e.
    e. gingivae
    scrotal e.
Eleutherococcus senticosus
elevate
elevation
    FAME midface e.
    flap e.
    medial e.
    mucoperichondrial e.
    periosteal e.
    philtral column e.
    pitch e.
    sinus e.
    subgaleal e.
    subperiosteal e.
    transblepharoplasty subperiosteal
      midface e.
  elevator
    46, 190, 191, 301 e.
    angled e.
    angular e.
    apical e.
    Cameron e.
    Cottle e.
    Crane e.
    Cryer e.
    Cryer root e.
    Dean periosteal e.
    dental e.
    double club e.
    ESI lighted suction e.
    e. esophagus
    e. extraction
    fine periosteal e.
    Freer e.
    Freer septal e.
    e. grain dust mite
    Hajek e.
    Howarth e.
    Hu-Friedy e.
    Joseph periosteal e.
    lip e.
    MacKenty septal e.

malar e.
Miller Apexo e.
Molt No. 4 e.
Ohl e.
periosteal e.
Pollock-Dingman e.
Potts e.
Pritchard e.
Ramirez periosteal e.
root apex e.
root-tip e.
screw e.
Seldin e.
sharp e.
straight inclined plane e.
subperiosteal e.
suction e.
T-bar e.
Tenzel e.
tooth e.
wedge e.
Woodson No. 1 e.
eleventh cranial nerve
Elgiloy archwire
ELI
    Environmental Language Inventory
elicit
elicited imitation
elimination
    e. pocket
    wax e.
    e. wax
elinguation
ELISA
    enzyme-linked immunosorbent assay
    ELISA test
elision
Elite cement
elixir
    Brofed E.
    Bromaline E.
    Bromanate E.
    Cold & Allergy E.
    Dimaphen E.
    Dimetane Decongestant E.
    Dimetapp E.
    Genatap E.
Elliott flap
Ellipse compact spacer
ellipsis, pl. ellipses
elliptical
    e. excision technique

NOTES

E

elliptical *(continued)*
    e. flap
    e. incision
    e. plication of Grazer
    e. recess
Ellis-van Creveld syndrome
Ellman press-form system
elm
    American e.
    Chinese e.
    fall e.
    slippery e.
    e. tree antigen
Elmex Protector
ELND
    elective lymph node dissection
Elocon Topical
Elon
elongation
    tooth e.
ELS
    endolymphatic sac surgery
Elysee Lasercare
EMA
    epithelial membrane antigen
embarrassment
    neurologic e.
embed
embedded
    e. cementicle
    e. denticle
    e. sentence
    e. sound
    e. tooth
embolectomy
    Fogarty catheter e.
embolism
    air e.
    endovascular e.
    pulmonary e.
embolization
    e. coil
    direct puncture intralesional e.
    transarterial e.
embolus
    air e.
embrasure
    buccal e.
    e. clasp
    gingival e.
    e. hook
    incisal e.
    interdental e.
    labial e.
    lingual e.
    occlusal e.
    e. space
embryo

embryogenesis
embryological
    e. approach
embryology
embryonic
    e. bone
embryoplastic odontoma
Emdogain
    E. gel
    E. treatment
EME
    epithelial-myoepithelial
    EME carcinoma
emergence
Emergence Profile implant system
emergent
    e. language
emery
    e. disk
EMF
    electromotive force
EMG
    electromyography
Emgel Topical
EMH
    educationally mentally handicapped
eminence
    arcuate e.
    articular e.
    canine e.
    hypobranchial e.
    hypopharyngeal e.
    hypophysial e.
    hypothenar e.
    malar e.
    pyramidal e.
    retromylohyoid e.
    temporomandibular joint articular e.
    thenar e.
    triangular e.
eminectomy
eminentia
    e. arcuata
    e. triangularis
emissary vein
emission
    click-evoked otoacoustic e.
    context-specific nasal e.
    distortion-product masquerade of e.
    distortion-product otoacoustic e.
    (DPOAE)
    evoked otoacoustic e.
    nasal e.
    otoacoustic e. (OAE)
    Otodynamics model ILO-92
    distortion-product otoacoustic e.
    spontaneous e.
    stimulated e.

transient evoked otoacoustic e.
(TEOAE)
EMLA
eutectic mixture of local anesthetics
EMLA cream
Emory EndoPlastic retractor
emotion
anticipatory e.
negative e.
positive e.
emotional
e. disturbance
e. voice handicap score
emphysema
orbital e.
subcutaneous e.
subgaleal e.
empiric
empiricist theory
Empirin
E. With Codeine
empty movement
empyema
mastoid e.
recurrent e.
EMR
educable mentally retarded
EMS
eosinophilia-myalgia syndrome
emulsification
fat e.
emulsifier
emulsion
e. crimping
E-Mycin
E.-M. Delayed-Release Tablet
E.-M. Oral
en
e. bloc
e. bloc resection
e. plaque tumor
ENAC
ENAC II
ENAC ultrasonic instrument system
enactment
enamel (E)
e. aplasia
aprismatic e.
e. bonding
e. cap
e. caries
ceramic e.

cervical e.
e. chisel
e. cleaner
e. cleavage
e. cleaver
e. cord
e. crypt
curled e.
e. cuticle
decalcified e.
dental e.
e. and dental aplasia
e. and dentin hypocalcification
e. drop
dwarfed e.
e. dysplasia
e. epithelium
erupted e.
e. excrescence
e. fiber
e. fissure
e. fracture
e. germ
gnarled e.
e. hatchet
human e.
e. hypocalcification
e. hypomaturation
e. hypomineralization
e. hypoplasia
hypoplastic e.
e. knot
e. lamella
e. ledge
e. margin
e. matrix
e. maturation
e. membrane
mottled e.
nanoid e.
e. navel
e. niche
e. nodule
opaque e.
e. organ
e. organ remnant
e. pearl
e. pellicle
porcelain e.
postnatal e.
prenatal e.
e. prism

E

NOTES

enamel *(continued)*
    e. projection
    e. pulp
    e. ridge
    e. rod
    e. rod inclination
    e. sac
    e. spike
    e. spindle
    e. spur
    straight e.
    subsurface e.
    e. surface index (ESI)
    e. tearout
    e. tongue
    e. tuft
    e. wall
    white e.
    whorled e.
enamel-bonding agent
enamel-dentin bonding
enamelin
Enamelite 500 adhesive
enamelogenesis
    e. imperfecta
enameloma
enameloplasty
enamelum
enanthem, pl. **enanthema**
ENB
    esthesioneuroblastoma
encapsulate
encapsulated powdered gold
encapsulation
encapsulization
encatarrhaphy
encephalitis, pl. **encephalitides**
    granulomatous amebic e.
    mumps e.
    varicella-zoster e.
encephalocele
    sphenoorbital e.
    tegmental e.
encephaloma
encephalomeningocele
enchondroma
encoder
encoding
    e. communication board
END
    elective neck dissection
end
    e. cell
    distal e.
    e. expiratory pressure (EEP)
    e. organ
    e. tube
    two open e.'s

Endal
endaural
    e. mastoid incision
    e. retractor
end-biting
    e.-b. blunt nosed rongeur
    e.-b. rongeur
end-cutting
    e.-c. bur
    e.-c. fissure bur
endemic
    e. Burkitt lymphoma (EBL)
    e. deafmutism
    e. fluorosis
Endermologie
    E. adipose destruction system
    E. noninvasive body contouring
        device
ENDEX
    E. apex locator
    E. apex sensor
ending
    inflectional e.
    nerve e.
    vesiculated e.
endoalveolar crest
Endo-Bender bending device
EndoCaddy
endocamera
    Olympus e.
endocarditis
    bacterial e.
    infective e.
    subacute bacterial e. (SBE)
endocentric construction
endochondral
    e. bone
endochondroma
endocochlear potential
endocranial
endocrine
    e. disorder
    e. neoplasia
    e. system
endocyst
endodontalis
    Bacteroides e.
    Porphyromonas e.
endodontia
endodontic
    e. armamentarium
    e. broach
    e. bur
    e. cavity
    e. cement
    e. culture
    e. discoloration
    e. drug

e. endosseous implant
e. endosteal implant
e. file
e. instrument
e. irrigating syringe
e. irrigation
e. medium culture
E. Meter SII
e. pin
e. plugger
e. reamer
e. sealer
e. stabilizer
e. surgery
e. technique
e. therapy
e. timetable
e. treatment
endodontics
   one-sitting e.
   pedodontic e.
   surgical e.
endodontist
endodontium
endodontologist
endodontology
endodontoma
endoesophagitis
endoforehead
   e. lift
endoforehead-endomidface lift
endoforehead-periorbital-cheek lift
endoforeheadplasty
   laser e.
endogauge
endogenous
   e. algogenic agent
Endo-grasper
   Babcock E.-g.
   E.-g. by Babcock
Endo-Gripper endodontic handpiece
EndoLift device
endolith
endolymph
endolymphatic
   e. decompression surgery
   e. duct
   e. hydrops
   e. sac
   e. sac decompression
   e. sac/shunt surgery
   e. sac surgery (ELS)

endolymphatic-subarachnoid shunt
EndoMax endoscopic instrumentation
endomethasone
endometriosis
endomidface
   e. lift
endomolare
endomysium
endonasal
   e. approach
   e. dacryocystorhinostomy
   e. disorder
   e. fenestration
   e. incision
   e. rhinoplasty
endonerve stripper
endoneurial
   e. tube
   e. tubule
endoneurium
Endo-Otoprobe
endophytic
Endoplan workstation
endoplasm
endoplasmic
   e. reticulum (ER)
   e. retinaculum
Endopore
   E. dental implant system
   E. implant
Endopost
   Kerr E.
end-organ of hearing
endoscope
   Circon/ACMI e.
   Durascope e.
   Padgett e.
   Sine-U-View e.
   Storz 30- and 70-degree e.
   Storz Sine-U-View e.
endoscope-assisted
   e.-a. rectus abdominis muscle flap
      harvest
   e.-a. suction extraction
endoscopic
   e. access port (EAP)
   e. band ligation (EBL)
   e. brow lift
   e. brow lift with simultaneous
      carbon dioxide laser resurfacing
   e. carpal tunnel release (ECTR)
   e. cholangiopancreatography

E

NOTES

endoscopic *(continued)*
  e. dacryocystorhinostomy
  e. dissector
  e. ethmoidectomy
  e. face lift
  e. face-lifting
  e. forceps
  e. forehead-brow rhytidoplasty
  e. forehead lift
  e. guidance
  e. harvest
  e. intranasal frontal sinusotomy
  e. medial maxillectomy
  e. muscle plication
  e. orbital decompression
  e. procedure
  e. sinus surgery (ESS)
  e. sphenoethmoidectomy with
    septoplasty
  e. subperiosteal forehead lift
  e. subperiosteal forehead and
    midface lift
  e. subperiosteal midface lift
  subperiosteal minimally invasive
    laser e. (SMILE)
  e. transaxillary submuscular
    augmentation mammaplasty
  e. variceal ligation (EVL)
endoscopically
  e. assisted abdominoplasty
  e. harvested tissue
**endoscopic-assisted facial implant
  insertion**
endoscopy
  e. brow pexy
  flexible fiberoptic e.
  fluorescein e.
  nasal e.
  peroral e.
endosonic file
endosonics
endosseous
  e. blade implant
  e. dental implant placement for
    replacement of missing teeth
  e. HA implant
  e. hydroxyapatite implant
  e. implant needle mandrel
  e. stress
  e. vent implant
Endostat
  disposable coaxial E.
  disposable sculptured E.
  E. disposable sterile fiber
endosteal
  e. implant
  e. implant anchor

  e. implant arm
  e. implant blade
  e. implant system
endosteum
Endo stop
Endotec spreader
endotemporal-endomidface lift
endotemporal lift
endothelial
  e. cell
  e. sarcoma
endothelin-1
endothelioma
endothelium
  vascular e.
endothermic
endotherm knife
endotoxin
**endotoxin-mediated otitis media with
  effusion**
**Endotrac endoscopic carpal tunnel
  release system**
endotracheal
  e. intubation
  e. stylet
  e. tube (ETT)
Endotron-Lipectron ultrasonic scalpel
Endovage syringe
endovascular
  e. balloon
  e. embolism
  e. management
endovenous antibiotic
Endowel
endplate
  motor e.
end-stage nutritional depletion
end-tidal carbon dioxide (ETCO$_2$)
end-to-end
  e.-t.-e. anastomosis (EEA)
  e.-t.-e. bite
  e.-t.-e. microvascular anastomosis
  e.-t.-e. occlusion
  e.-t.-e. venous anastomosis
end-to-side
  e.-t.-s. anastomosis
  e.-t.-s. venous anastomosis
Endur
  E. adhesive
  E. resin
end-Z file
energy
  acoustic e.
  e. dispersed x-ray analysis (EDXA)
  kinetic e.
  pneumoballistic e.
  potential e.

ENG
    electronystagmography
      Nystar Plus ENG
Engerix-B
engine
    Acrotorque hand e.
    e. arm
    dental e.
    e. H-file
    e. reamer
    Robbins Acrotorque hand e.
    e. S-file
    e. T-file
engine-driven
    e.-d. instrument
    e.-d. reamer
engineering
    dental e.
    tissue e.
English
    Black E.
    manual E.
    pidgin Sign E. (PSE)
    E. plantain
    E. plantain antigen
    E. rhinoplasty
    Seeing Essential E. (SEE$_1$)
    signed E.
    Signing Exact E. (SEE$_2$)
English/Spanish
    Del Rio Language Screening
      Test, E.
    Toronto Tests of Receptive
      Vocabulary, E.
Engman disease
engorgement
engraftment
    donor bone marrow e.
engram
enhancement
    gadolinium-diethylenetriamine
      pentaacetic acid e.
    e. gun
    lip e.
    V-LACE real-time digital video e.
enhancer
    Aerosol Cloud e. (ACE)
ENI
    elective neck irradiation
enlarged frenum
enlargement
    dilantin e.

gingival e.
gingival hormonal e.
idiopathic e.
salivary gland e.
tumor-like gingival e.
ENog, ENoG
    electroneuronography
enolase
    neuron-specific e.
Enomine
enophthalmos, enophthalmia
    posttraumatic e.
enosseous implant
enostosis
ENT
    ears, nose, and throat
Entamoeba
    E. gingivalis
enteral feeding
enteric cyst
Enterobacter
enterocutaneous fistula
**enterocytopathogenic human orphan
(ECHO)**
**enterocytopathogenic human orphan
virus**
enterogenous cyst
enteropathy
    gluten-sensitive e.
enteroplasty
Entex
    E. LA
    E. PSE
enthesis
enthetic
entity
entocone
entoconid
entomophthoramycosis
    e. conidiobolae
    rhinofacial e.
entrapment
Entrease variable depth punch
**Entree disposable CO_2 insufflation
needle**
entropion
    temporary e.
entubulization
enucleation
    orbital e.
enunciate

E

NOTES

envelope
    e. of discrepancy
    e. flap
    nuclear e.
    shriveled skin e.
envenomation
environment
    neurotropic e.
    oral e.
environmental
    E. Language Inventory (ELI)
    e. noise
    E. Pre-language Battery
environs
ENZA laser skin care program
Enzol enzymatic detergent
enzyme
    e. activity
    angiotensin-converting e. (ACE)
    mitochondrial oxidative e.
    peroxidative e.
    proteolytic e.
    transferring e.
enzyme-linked immunosorbent assay (ELISA)
EOG
    electro-oculography
EOS
    Extra Oral System
eosin
    hematoxylin and e. (H&E)
eosinophil
    e. chemotactic factor of
        anaphylaxis (ECF-A)
eosinophilia
    cytoplasmic e.
eosinophilia-myalgia syndrome (EMS)
eosinophilic
    e. fasciitis (EF)
    e. granuloma
    e. hyperplasia
    e. nucleus
    e. proteinaceous material
    e. proteinaceous secretions
    e. ulcer
    e. ulcer of oral cavity
eosinophilicum diutinum
epaulet flap
ephaptic transmission
ephedrine
ephelis, pl. ephelides
epicanthal fold
epicanthus
Epicoccum
epicranium
epicranius
    e. muscle

epidemic
    e. hiccup
    e. parotiditis
epidemiology
epidermal
    e. actinic damage
    e. growth factor (EGF)
    e. growth factor receptor
    e. inclusion cyst
    e. necrosis
    e. nevus
    e. sliding
epidermatoplasty
epidermic graft
epidermidis
    Staphylococcus e.
epidermization
epidermodysplasia verruciformis
epidermoid
    e. carcinoma
    e. cyst
    e. resection
    e. tumor
epidermolysis
    e. bullosa
    e. bullosa dystrophica
Epidermophyton
Epi-Derm silicone gel sheeting
epididymoplasty
epidural abscess
Epifrin
epigastric
    e. artery
    e. flap
    e. voice
epiglottic
    e. hematoma
    e. reconstruction
    e. tubercle
epiglottidectomy
epiglottiditis
epiglottis
    absent e.
    bifid e.
    suprahyoid e.
    e. swing
epiglottitis
epignathus
EpiLaser
    E. hair removal laser
    E. system
epilate
epilepsy
    laryngeal e.
    temporal lobe e.
EpiLight hair removal system
epiloia
E-Pilo-x Ophthalmic

epimyoepithelial island
epimyoepithelium
epimysium
Epinal
epinephrine
    pilocarpine and e.
    racemic e.
epinephryl borate
epineural window
epineurial
    e. repair
    e. suture
epineurium
epiperineurial suture
epiphora
epirubicin
episioplasty
episode
    aphonic e.
episodic
    e. variation
    e. vertigo
epistaxis
epistropheus
    odontoid process of e.
epithelia (*pl. of* epithelium)
epithelial
    e. adaptation
    e. attachment
    e. atypia
    e. cell
    e. cicatrization
    e. cuff
    e. debridement
    e. granuloma
    e. inlay
    e. invagination
    e. marker
    e. membrane antigen (EMA)
    e. migration
    e.-myoepithelial carcinoma
    e. neoplasm
    e. pearl
    e. peg
    e. proliferation
    e. rest
    e. rete peg
    e. ridge
    e. sarcoma (ES)
    e. seam
    e. sheath
    e. strand

epithelialization, epithelization
    e. technique
    vaginal e.
epithelial-myoepithelial (EME)
epithelioid
    e. cell
    e. sarcoma
epithelioid-cell sialadenitis
epithelioma
    e. adenoides cysticum
    cystic adenoid e.
    e. of Malherbe
epithelium, pl. epithelia
    attachment e.
    autologous-cultured e. (ACE)
    buccal e.
    crevicular e.
    cuboidal e.
    desquamating e.
    enamel e.
    external dental e.
    external enamel e.
    follicular e.
    gingival e.
    hornified e.
    inner dental e.
    inner enamel e.
    junctional e.
    keratinized e.
    noncornified e.
    nonhornified e.
    nonkeratinized e.
    olfactory e.
    oral e.
    outer enamel e.
    parakeratinized e.
    pocket e.
    reduced enamel e.
    respiratory e.
    squamous e.
    stratified squamous e.
    sulcal e.
    sulcular e.
    supporting cell of olfactory e.
    urethral e.
    vestibular e.
epithelization (*var. of* epithelialization)
epitope
EpiTouch
    E. Alex laser hair removal system
    E. Ruby SilkLaser

E

NOTES

EpiTouch (*continued*)
    E. ruby SilkLaser hair removal system
epitympanic air cell
epitympanum
epoxy
    e. die
    E. Die material
    E. Die resin
    e. resin
    e. resin sealer
Epoxydent
Epoxylite 9070, 9075
Epstein-Barr
    E.-B. virus (EBV)
    E.-B. virus-encoded ribonucleic acid (EBER)
Epstein pearl
ePTFE
    expanded polytetrafluoroethylene
    ePTFE augmentation membrane
    ePTFE implant
    ePTFE membrane
epulis
    congenital e. of newborn
    e. fibromatosa
    fibrous e.
    e. fissuratum
    giant cell e.
    e. gigantocellularis
    e. granulomatosa
    e. gravidarum
    e. of newborn
    pigmented e.
epulis-like lesion
epulofibroma
epuloid
EQ
    educational quotient
equal
    e. loudness contour
equalization
    pressure e. (PE)
equalizer
    stress e.
Equanil
equation
    Larmor e.
equidistant
equilibration
    mandibular e.
    occlusal e.
equilibrium
equina
    cauda e.
equipment
    American Medical Source laparoscopic e.

    containment e.
    Luxar Silhouette noninvasive body appearance e.
    Storz e.
    Wolf e.
Equisetum arvense
EquiTest
    E. motor coordination test
    E. sensory organization test
equivalent
    grammatical e.
    migraine e.
    e. speech reception threshold
E-R
    Indochron E-R
ER
    endoplasmic reticulum
ERA
    electric response audiometry
    electroencephalic response audiometry
    evoked response audiometry
Erb
    E. palsy
    E. score
Erb-Duchenne-Klumpke palsy
Erb-Duchenne palsy
Erbium
    E. CrystaLase laser
    2.5 joule E. resurfacing laser
erbium:YAG laser system
Ercaf
erectile corpora
erg
Ergomar
ergometer
    bicycle e.
ergonovine maleate
ergotamine
    e. tartrate
Erich
    E. alar cartilage relocation
    E. dental arch bar
eriodictylol glycoside
Erkoflex plastic
eroded incus
ERO Ear
erosion
    crater-shaped e.
    e. desquamation
    dish-shaped e.
    notch-shaped e.
    saucer-shaped e.
    V-shaped e.
    wedge-shaped e.
erosive lichen planus
errant approach
error
    articulation e.

inborn e. of metabolism
noise-induced e.
phonemic articulation e.
phonetic articulation e.
phonological e.
vowel e.
erupted enamel
eruption
accelerated e.
active e.
altered passive e.
clinical e.
continuous e.
e. cyst
delayed e.
differential e.
ectopic e.
febrile-associated vesicular e.
forced e.
functional phase of tooth e.
guided e.
Kaposi varicelliform e.
nonfebrile-associated vesicular e.
passive e.
prefunctional phase of tooth e.
premature e.
e. sequestrum
surgical e.
tooth e.
eruptive
e. blue nevus
e. gingivitis
e. phase
e. stage
e. tooth movement
ERV
expiratory reserve volume
ERx Avulsed Tooth kit
Eryc Oral
Eryderm Topical
Erygel Topical
Erymax Topical
EryPed Oral
erysipelas
Ery-Tab Oral
erythema
e. migrans
e. migrans linguae
e. multiforme
e. nodosum
erythematosus
discoid lupus e.

lupus e.
systemic lupus e.
erythroblastosis fetalis
erythrocephalgia
Erythrocin
E. Oral
erythrodontia
erythromycin
e. and sulfisoxazole
e., topical
erythroplakia
precancerous e.
erythroplakic lesion
erythroplasia
e. of Queyrat
erythropoietin
recombinant e.
erythroprosopalgia
Eryzole
ES
epithelial sarcoma
Vicodin ES
escape
e. learning
nasal e.
e. reaction
escapement spaces
Escat phlegmon
eschar
black e.
escharotomy
Escherichia
E. coli
E. vulneris
ESI
Electro-Surgical instrument
enamel surface index
ESI fiberoptic light source
ESI lighted suction elevator
ESI light-weight, narrow
mammaplasty retractor
ESI Lite-Pipe fiberoptic cable
ESI Lite-Pipe fiberoptic instrument
ESI Lite-Pipe plastic surgery
instrument
ESI long, narrow mammaplasty
retractor
ESI mammary retractor
Esmarch bandage
E-Solve-2 Topical
esophageal
e. atresia

E

NOTES

esophageal *(continued)*
   e. balloon tamponade
   e. candidiasis
   e. compression
   e. detection device (EDD)
   e. dilation
   e. diverticulum
   e. hemangioma
   e. hiatus
   e. manometry
   e. motility disorder
   e. spasm
   e. speech
   e. sphincter
   e. stricture
   e. varix
   e. voice
   e. web
esophagectomy
   Lewis-Tanner e.
esophagism
esophagitis
   herpetic e.
   infectious e.
   peptic e.
esophagocardioplasty
esophagocutaneous fistula
esophagogastric hypothermia
esophagography
esophagoplasty
esophagoscope
   Jackson e.
   Jesberg e.
esophagoscopy
esophagostomy
   cervical e.
esophagotrachea
esophagus
   cervical e.
   corkscrew e.
   elevator e.
esorubicin
Esoterica
   E. Facial
   E. Regular
   E. Sensitive Skin Formula
   E. Sunscreen
esotropia
ESP
   extended supraplatysmal plane
   ESP dissection
   ESP face lift technique
Espe
   E. Ketac-Bond Aplicap
   E. Ketac-Endo sealer
   E. Photac-Bond Aplicap
E-speed intraoral film

ESPI
   electronic speckle pattern interferometry
espundia
esquinancea
ESS
   endoscopic sinus surgery
Essar handle
essential
   e. blepharospasm
   e. tremor
Esser
   E. graft
   E. operation
Essig
   Essig-type E.
   E. splint
esterase
esthesioneuroblastoma (ENB)
esthetic, aesthetic
   e. appearance
   e. breast reconstruction
   e. CO_2 laser
   e. dentistry
   e. denture
   e. laser system
   e. restoration
   e. rhinoplasty
   e. septorhinoplasty
   e. surgery
   e. Taylor mandibular angle implant
esthetics, aesthetics
   dentofacial e.
   denture e.
   facial e.
   gingival tissue e.
   profile e.
Estilux
   E. C
   E. resin
Estivin II Ophthalmic
Estlander
   E. flap
   E. operation
Estlander-Abbe flap
17β-estradiol
estriol
estrogen
estrone
etch
   phosphoric acid gel e.
   e. system
etchant
   acid e.
etched
   e. cast resin bonded bridge
   e. tooth
etching
   acid e.

ETCO$_2$
    end-tidal carbon dioxide
ETD
    eustachian tube dysfunction
ethambutol
ethanol
Ethibloc
Ethibond extra polyester suture
Ethicon
    E. SAS
    E. ST-4 straight taper-point needle
    E. suture
ethics
Ethilon suture
ethinamate
ethmoid
    e. air cells
    anterior e.
    e. bone
    e. plate
    posterior e.
    e. punch forceps
    e. registration point
    supraorbital e.
ethmoidal
    e. artery
    e. bulla
    e. cells
    e. fissure
    e. infundibular system
    e. infundibulum
    e. infundibulum
    e. labyrinth
    e. labyrinth cell
    e. mucosa
    e. nerve
    e. notch
    e. ostium
    e. periostitis
    e. prechamber
    e. sinus
    e. sinusitis
ethmoidale
ethmoidalis
    bulla e.
    fovea e.
ethmoid-Blakesley forceps
ethmoidectomy
    anterior e.
    endoscopic e.
    external e.

    internal e.
    intranasal e.
    partial e.
    total e.
    transantral e.
ethmoiditis
    chronic e.
ethmoidomaxillary
    e. plate
    e. suture
ethnographer
ethnographic method
ethyl
    e. alcohol
    e. chloride
    e. chloride and
        dichlorotetrafluoroethane
    e. methacrylate
ethylene
    e. glycol
    e. oxide
    e. oxide sterilization
ethylenediaminetetraacetic
    e. acid (EDTA)
    e. acid Cetavlon (EDTAC)
etidocaine
    e. HCl
etidronate disodium
etiology
etodolac
etoposide
ETS-2% Topical
ETT
    endotracheal tube
ETYA
    5,8,11,14-eicosatetraynoic acid
etymology
Eubacterium lentum
eucalyptol
    oil of e.
eucalyptus
eucapercha
Eucerin Plus
euclidean distance matrix analysis (EDMA)
Eudal-SR
eugenol
    e. pack
    zinc oxide-e. (ZOE, ZnOE)
eugenolate
    zinc e.

E

NOTES

eugnathia
eugnathic
    e. anomaly
eunuchoid voice
euophthalmus
euosmia
euphemism
Euphrasia officinalis
eupnea
Eupolin ointment
Euro-Collins solution
eurygnathic
eurygnathism
eurygnathous
eustachian
    e. catheter
    e. tube
    e. tube dysfunction (ETD)
    e. tube orifice
eustachitis
eutectic
    e. alloy
    e. mixture of local anesthetics
    (EMLA)
euthymol
euthyroid
evacuation
    laser smoke e.
evacuator
    hatchet e.
    high volume e. (HVE)
    oral e.
    Surgilase ECS.01 smoke e.
evagination
Evaluating
    E. Acquired Skills in
    Communication (EASIC)
    E. Communicative Competence
evaluation
    audiological e.
    Békésy Ascending-Descending
    Gap E. (BADGE)
    Compton Speech and Language
    Screening E.
    hearing aid e. (HAE)
    Orzeck Aphasia E.
    Post-Exposure E.
Evans articulator
evaporation
event
    antecedent e.
Everbest
    E. Prosonic
    E. Prosonic cleaner
Eve reconstructive procedure
eversion
everted
evidence-based medicine (E-BM)

E-Vista
E-Vitamin
EVL
    endoscopic variceal ligation
evoked
    e. electromyography (EEMG)
    e. otoacoustic emission
    e. potential
    e. response
    e. response audiometry (ERA)
    e. visual potential test
evolution
evolutionary phonetics
evulsed
    e. tooth
evulsion
    nerve e.
    tooth e.
Ewart procedure
Ewing
    E. sarcoma
    E. sign
E.X.
    Extra Strength Dynafed E.X.
exaggerated
    e. feminine tooth
    e. masculine tooth
EXAKT
    E. cutting/grinding system
    E. cutting/grinding unit
examination
    Body Dysmorphic Disorder E.
    Boston Diagnostic Aphasia E.
    Denver Articulation Screening E.
    (DASE)
    Mini-Mental State E. (MMSE)
    neurotologic e.
    oral peripheral e.
exanthematous
    e. rhinitis
Excaliber handpiece
excavating bur
excavation
excavator
    dental e.
    hatchet e.
    hoe e.
    spoon e.
Excedrin
    E., Extra Strength
    E. P.M.
Exceltech
    E. imaging
    E. patient imaging software
excementosis, pl. excementoses
    extension e.
    intraepithelial e.

pronglike e.
ultraterminal e.

excess
mandibular e.
marginal e.
maxillary e.
e. overhang
e. sealer
vertical maxillary e. (VME)

excessive
e. lip support
e. nasality
e. overbite
e. spacing

exchange
saline implant e.

exchanger
HumidFilter heat and moisture e.

excimer ultraviolet laser

excision
alar rim e.
alar wedge e.
anterior port scalp e.
direct supracillary e.
double V-Y plasty with paired
inverted Burow triangle e.'s
Feldman e.
flared-W e.
interdental e.
inverted T skin e.
local e.
L-shaped skin e.
lunate e.
Mohs e.
mucosal e.
neuroma e.
osteocartilaginous e.
radical e.
serial scar e.
tangential e.
through-and-through buttonhole
fashion e.
U-shaped skin e.
vertical skin e.
V-shaped skin e.
wide e.
wound e.

excisional biopsy
excitatory synapse
exclamatory sentence
excrescence
enamel e.

excretory duct
excursion
eyelid e.
lateral e.
left lateral e.
protrusive e.
retrusive e.
right lateral e.

executive aphasia
Exelderm Topical
exenterate
exenterated orbit
exenteration
radical e.
total pelvic e.

exercise
cat sneer e.
duck lips e.
rabbit sniffing e.

exeresis
exfoliated
exfoliation
exfoliativa
glossitis areata e.

exfoliative
e. cytology
e. peri-implantoclasia

exfoliator
Bi-Phasic e.

exhalation
exhaust
automobile e.

Exidine Scrub
exit tip
exocentric construction
exocranial orifice
exocytosis
exodontia
exodontics
exodontist
exodontology
exogenous
exognathia
exognathion
exolever
exomphalos
exoneurolysis
exophoric
e. pronoun

exophthalmia

E

NOTES

exophthalmometer
    Hertel e.
    Naugle e.
exophthalmometry
    Hertel e.
exophthalmos
    pulsatile e.
    tumoral e.
exophytic mass
exorbitism
    posttraumatic e.
    traumatic e.
exostosis, pl. exostoses
    osteocartilaginous e.
exothermic
exotoxin
exotropia
Expandacell sponge
expanded
    e. duty dental auxiliary (EDDA)
    e. polytetrafluoroethylene (ePTFE)
    e. polytetrafluoroethylene implant
expander
    AccuSpan tissue e.
    Biospan anatomical tissue e.
    Integra tissue e.
    e. pocket
    saline-filled e.
    slow palatal e.
    subperiosteal tissue e. (STE)
    tissue e.
expansible
    e. infrastructure endosteal implant
    e. osseous neoplasm
expansile
    e. forceps
    e. Mercedes incision
expansion
    e. and activator therapy
    e. of the arch
    e. arch
    balloon e.
    delayed e.
    dental arch e.
    effective setting e.
    hygroscopic e.
    intraoperative skin e.
    investment e.
    linear thermal e.
    maxillary e.
    mercuroscopic e.
    palatal e.
    e. plate
    e. plate appliance
    postexcision skin e.
    preexcision skin e.
    rapid maxillary e. (RME)
    scalp e.

    e. screw
    secondary e.
    setting e.
    slow maxillary e.
    surgical assisted-rapid palatal e.
      (SA-RPE)
    thermal coefficient e.
    tissue e.
    wax e.
expectorant
    Codafed E.
    Decohistine E.
    Detussin E.
    Dihistine E.
    Fedahist E.
    Genamin E.
    Isoclor E.
    Myminic E.
    Nucofed Pediatric E.
    Phenhist E.
    Ru-Tuss E.
    Silaminic E.
    SRC E.
    Theramin E.
    Triaminic E.
    Tri-Clear E.
    Triphenyl E.
    Tussafin E.
expectorate
expectoration
experiment
    hertzian e.
experimental
    e. audiology
    e. delayed auditory feedback
    e. phonetics
expiration
expiratory
    e. reserve volume (ERV)
    e. stridor
explantation
    mammary prosthesis e.
expletive
exploding head syndrome
exploratory stroke
explorer
    cowhorn e.
explosive
    e. speech
    e. tinnitus
expose
exposed
    e. intraoral film
    e. pulp
exposure
    accidental pulp e.
    carious pulp e.
    E. Control Plan

e. determination
double e.
fast film e.
e. guideline
incident e.
industrial e.
e. keratitis
log relative e.
mechanical pulp e.
Nissenbaum surgical e.
noise e.
occupational e.
e. period
surgical pulp e.
e. time
e. timer
e. unit

expression
facial e.
nonvolitional facial e.

expressive
e. aphasia
e. language
e. language delay
E. One-Word Picture Vocabulary Test
E. One-Word Picture Vocabulary Test-Upper Extension
e. vocabulary

expressive-receptive aphasia
Exprin DQ1 biopsy instrument
Exserohilum
extended
e. anatomical chin
e. clasp
e. frontal approach
e. function dental assistant (EFDA)
e. jargon paraphasia
e. lateral arm free flap (ELAFF)
e. lateral arm free flap for head/neck reconstruction
e. liposuction
e. mesh technique
e. multiplanar multivector face-lift
e. open-tip rhinoplasty
e. posterior rhytidectomy
e. shoulder flap
e. sub-SMAS face-lift
e. supraplatysmal plane (ESP)
e. supraplatysmal plane dissection
e. supraplatysmal plane face lift technique

Extendryl SR
extension
attached gingiva e.
e. base
e. bridge
e. excementosis
Expressive One-Word Picture Vocabulary Test-Upper E.
extraosseous e.
fascial e.
e. form
groove e.
e. partial denture
partial denture, distal e.
e. for prevention
ridge e.
e. ridge
e. semantics

extensive blue nevus
extensor
e. carpi radialis brevis muscle
e. carpi radialis longus muscle
e. carpi ulnaris muscle
e. digiti minimi muscle
e. digiti minimi tendon
e. digitorum brevis (EDB)
e. digitorum communis tendon
e. digitorum longus muscle
e. digitorum muscle
e. hallucis longus muscle
e. indicis muscle
e. indicis proprius tendon
e. pollicis brevis muscle
e. pollicis longus muscle

Extentabs
Dimetane E.
Dimetapp E.

exterior bolster fixation
exteriorized
e. stuttering

externa
benign necrotizing otitis e. (BNOE)
malignant necrotizing otitis e. (MNOE)
otitis e.

external
e. apical root resorption (EARR)
e. auditory canal (EAC)
e. auditory meatus
e. bevel incision
e. branch of the superior laryngeal (EBSL)

E

NOTES

external *(continued)*
    e. branch of the superior laryngeal nerve
    e. carotid artery (ECA)
    e. dental epithelium
    e. ear
    e. enamel epithelium
    e. ethmoidectomy
    e. fixator
    e. frame function
    e. jugular vein
    e. ligament of mandibular articulation
    e. ligament of temporomandibular articulation
    e. mouth protector
    e. nasal nerve
    e. nose
    e. oblique aponeurosis
    e. oblique line
    e. oblique ridge
    e. otitis
    e. paralateronasal skin incision
    e. pharyngotomy approach
    e. pin fixation
    e. pin fixation, biphase
    e. root resorption
    e. tooth resorption
    e. traction
externalization
exteroception
    tactile e.
exteroceptor
extinction
extirpate
extirpation
    dental pulp e.
    e. of ganglion
    pulp e.
    surgical e.
extirpative defect
Extra
    E. Oral System (EOS)
    E. Strength Adprin-B
    E. Strength Bayer Enteric 500 Aspirin
    E. Strength Bayer Plus
    E. Strength Doan's
    E. Strength Dynafed E.X.
extra-alveolar
    e.-a. clinical crown
extra-articular
extra-axial
    e.-a. injury
    e.-a. tumor
extrabuccal
extracanalicular resorption

extracapsular
    e. rupture
    e. spread (ECS)
    e. tissue
extracellular
    e. matrix (ECM)
    e. matrix contraction
    e. space (ECS)
extracoronal
    e. attachment
    e. retainer
    e. retention
    e. splint
    e. splinting
extracranial
    e. meningioma
    e. pneumatocele
    e. pneumocele
extract
extracted tooth
extracting forceps
extraction
    elevator e.
    endoscope-assisted suction e.
    forceps e.
    e. forceps
    progressive e.
    rubber-band e.
    serial e.
    e. space
    suction e.
    tooth e.
    e. trap
extractor
    buccal fat e.
    e. injector
    Luxator e.
    Thomas post e.
extradental
    e. intraoral radiography
    e. projection
extradural
    e. abscess
    e. effusion
extrafollicular
extraglandular lithiasis
extralabyrinthine symptom
extralaryngeal
    e. approach
    e. muscle
    e. skeleton
extraluminal silicone
extramaxillary anchorage
extramedullary plasmacytoma
extraneous
    e. movement
    e. noise

extranodal
- e. malignant lymphoma
- e. non-Hodgkin lymphoma

extraocular muscle

extraoral
- e. anchorage
- e. appliance
- e. approach
- e. defect
- e. film
- e. force
- e. fracture appliance
- e. orthodontic appliance
- e. prosthesis
- e. radiograph
- e. radiographic examination profile
- e. radiography
- e. Rison neck incision
- e. sigmoid notch retractor
- e. tracing

extraosseous
- e. chondrosarcoma
- e. extension
- e. plasma cell tumor

extraperitoneal fat

extrapolation

extrapyramidal
- e. pathway
- e. system
- e. tract

extrasellar

extraskeletal
- e. chondrosarcoma
- e. osseous tumor

extravasate

extravasation
- e. cyst
- e. of mouse urine
- e. phenomenon

extravelar muscle bundle

extraversion

extreme
- e. crowding
- e. hearing loss

extremis
- in e.

extrinsic
- e. color
- e. coloring
- e. environmental staining
- e. feedback
- e. mechanism

- e. muscles of larynx
- e. muscle of tongue

extroversion

extrovert

extrude

extruded teeth

extrudoclusion

extrusion
- sealer e.
- e. of a tooth
- tube e.

extubate

extubation

exudate
- gingival e.
- purulent e.
- sanguineous e.
- serous e.
- suppurative e.

exudation
- gingival e.
- purulent e.

exudative
- e. zone

exuviation

eye
- e. aperture
- Clear E.'s
- e. displacement
- e. exposure guideline
- e. motility disorder
- e. strain
- e. tooth

eyeball
- rectus muscle of e.

eyebright

eyebrow
- e. height
- high e.
- e. lift
- e. ptosis

eyebrowpexy

eyedrops
- fluorometholone and neomycin sulfate e.
- FML-Neo e.

eye, ear, nose, and throat (EENT)

eye-ear plane

eyeglasses
- protective e.

eyelid
- e. crease suture

E.

NOTES

eyelid *(continued)*
    e. excursion
    gray line of upper e.
    inelastic lower e.
    e. ptosis
    e. redundancy
    e. sphincter
    e. sulcus placement
    e. tightening
Eye-Lube-A Solution

Eyesine Ophthalmic
eyewear
    protective e.
E-Z
    E-Z Clean laparoscopic electrode
    E-Z Flap burr hole cover
    E-Z Flap cranial flap fixation
      system
Ezo dental cushion

F
Fahrenheit
F_0
fundamental frequency
fabricate
fabricated implant
fabricating post
fabrication
fabric covered tubing
Fabricius ship
Fabry disease
face
acromegalic f.
bird f.
contralateral f.
dished-in f.
duplication of the f.
frog f.
f. lift
f. lifting
sunken-in f.
f. validity
volume deficient f.
face-bow
adjustable axis f.
Asher high-pull f.
f. fork
Hanau modular articulator f.
kinematic f.
Kloehn f.
Rampton f.
f. record
root high-pull f.
faced crown
face-lift, face lift, facelift (*See also* lift)
conventional SMAS f.-l.
extended multiplanar multivector f.-l.
extended sub-SMAS f.-l.
FAME f.-l.
f.-l. scissors
SMAS imbrication f.-l.
SMAS plication f.-l.
SMILE f.-l.
subperiosteal minimally invasive laser endoscopic f.-l.
vertical f.-l.
face-lifting
endoscopic f.-l.
faceometer
facer
root f.
facet, facette
occlusal f., facette
facial
f. analysis
f. angle
f. animation
f. artery
f. artery musculomucosal (FAMM)
f. asymmetry
f. bevel
f. bipartition procedure
f. bone
f. bone reconstruction with bioactive glass
f. butt joint preparation
f. canal
f. causalgia
f. and cervical cellulitis
f. cleft
f. clefting
f. compression finger closure
f. compression skull cap closure
f. contour deformity
f. contouring
f. deformity
F. Disability Index (FDI)
F. Disability Index Physical (FDIP)
F. Disability Index Social (FDIS)
f. disharmony
f. edema
Esoterica F.
f. esthetics
f. excursion measurement
f. expression
f. fascial layer
f. fracture
f. gesture
F. Grading System (FGS)
F. Grading System Resting symmetry (FGSR)
F. Grading System Synkinesis (FGSS)
F. Grading System voluntary Movement (FGSM)
f. growth
f. hamartoma
f. harmony
f. height
f. hemihypertrophy
F. Impairment Scales for Clefts
f. implant
f. landmark
f. lipodystrophy
f. mimetic muscle
f. mimic
f. motor nucleus
f. moulage

facial *(continued)*
  f. muscle
  f. nerve (FN)
  f. nerve branches
  f. nerve crossover
  f. nerve decompression
  f. nerve dissection
  f. nerve latency
  f. nerve misdirection
  f. nerve paralysis
  f. nerve paresis
  f. nerve-preserving parotidectomy
  f. nerve rerouting
  f. nerve root
  f. neuralgia
  f. neurinoma
  f. neuromuscular dysfunction
  f. node
  f. palsy
  f. paralysis
  f. paralysis reconstruction with
    rectus abdominis muscle
  f. plane
  f. plane angle
  f. plaque
  f. plastic surgery scissors
  f. profile
  f. prosthesis
  f. prosthetics
  f. reanimation
  f. recess
  f. regions
  f. rejuvenation
  f. restoration
  f. root
  f. sling
  f. spasm
  f. subcutaneous lift
  f. support
  f. surface
  f. surface of maxilla
  f. symmetry
  f. synkinesis
  f. tic
  f. translocation
  f. traumagram
  f. triangle
  f. vein
facially aging patient
facies, pl. **facies**
  adenoid f.
  f. contactus dentis
  f. distalis dentis
  f. distalis dentis
  f. facialis dentis
  Greek helmet f.
  f. labialis
  leonine f.

  f. lingualis dentis
  masklike f.
  f. masticatoria
  f. maxillaris alae majoris
  f. maxillaris ossis palatini
  f. mesialis dentis
  f. occlusalis dentis
  permanent smile f.
  f. vestibularis dentis
facilitated communication
facilitating restoration
facilitation
  f. of resonance
facing
  acrylic veneer f.
  interchangeable f.
  Steele f.
  Thom f.
faciolingual
faciomandibular dysostosis
facioplasty
facioscapulohumeral muscular dystrophy
facioversion
FACT-HN
  functional assessment of cancer
    therapy–head and neck
factitious wound
factor-β
factor-α
  tumor necrosis f. (TNF-α)
factor
  angiogenic f.
  basic fibroblastic growth f. (bFGF)
  chemotactic f.
  colony-stimulating f. (CSF)
  epidermal growth f. (EGF)
  force f.
  granulocyte colony-stimulant f.
  Green f.
  growth f.
  Hageman f.
  hematopoietic growth f.
  hybridoma growth f.
  f.-I
  insulin-like growth f.
  insulin-like growth f.-I (IGF)
  f. IX complex human
  Klebanoff f.
  lymphocyte activation f.
  macrophage-activating f. (MAF)
  macrophage-inhibiting f. (MIF)
  migration-inhibiting f. (MIF)
  mitogenic f. (MF)
  nerve f.
  nerve growth f. (NGF)
  neurogenic f.
  osteoclast-activating f. (OAF)
  perpetuating f.

platelet-activating f. (PAF)
platelet-derived growth f. (PDGF)
precipitating f.
predisposing f.
squamous cell carcinoma
  inhibitory f. (SSCIF)
tissue injury f.
transforming growth f.-β (TGF-β)
tumor necrosis f. (TNF)
vascular endothelial growth f.
  (VEGF)

faecalis
  Streptococcus f.

FAHI
functional assessment of human
immunodeficiency virus
FAHI scale

Fahrenheit (F)

failure
cohesive f.
f. of fixation suppression (FFS)
flap f.
mixed f.
porcelain-metal f.

faking
falciform crest
falciformis
crista f.
fall elm
faller
falling
f. curve
f. palate
fallopian
f. bridge technique
f. canal
false
f. aneurysm
f. denticle
f. fluency
f. muscle contraction
f. paracusis
f. ragweed
f. role disorder
f. threshold
f. unicorn root
f. vocal cord
f. vocal fold
false-negative response
false-positive response
falsetto
f. voice

falx cerebri
famciclovir
FAME
F. face-lift
F. midface elevation
F. midface lift
familial
f. deafness
f. fibrous dysplasia
f. hearing loss
f. neurilemmomatosis
f. polythelia
f. white folded dysplasia
family
multicultural f.
family-centered
f.-c. practice
f.-c. service
FAMM
facial artery musculomucosal
FAMM flap
famotidine
fan flap
fang
fan-shaped flap
farad
farcy
Fargin-Fayolle syndrome
Farrior graft augmentation
Fasanella Servat procedure
fascia, gen. and pl. **fasciae**
alar f.
aryepiglottic f.
brachial f.
Buck f.
Buck deep penile f.
capsulopalpebral f.
cervical f.
Colles f.
dartos f.
deep cervical f.
deep temporal f. (DTF)
dermis f.
f. graft
innominate f.
intermediate f.
interposing f.
f. lata
f. lata strip
f. lata transfer
parotid f.
parotidomasseteric f.

F

NOTES

209

fascia *(continued)*
    f. penis superficialis
    pharyngeal f.
    pharyngobasilar f.
    preparotid f.
    pretracheal f.
    prevertebral f.
    rectus f.
    Scarpa f.
    f. sling
    sternocleidomastoid f.
    subgaleal f.
    superficial temporal f. (STF)
    suprasternal f.
    temporalis f.
    temporalis superficialis f.
    temporoparietal f.
    temporoparietalis f.
    tensor fasciae latae
    transversalis f.
    visceral f.

fascial
    f. extension
    f. grafting
    f. plane
    f. plication
    f. sept
    f. sling
    f. space
    f. staple technique
    f. strip
    f. turnover flap

fascicle
    inferior alveolar nerve f.
    nerve f.

fascicular graft
fasciculation
fasciculus, pl. fasciculi
    arcuate f.

fasciectomy
fasciitis, fascitis
    eosinophilic f. (EF)
    infiltrative f.
    necrotizing f. (NF)
    nodular f.
    odontogenic cervical necrotizing f.
    pseudosarcomatous f.

fasciocutaneous
    f. free flap
    f. island flap
    f. vessel

fascioplasty
fasciotomy
fasciovascular pedicle
fascitis *(var. of* fasciitis)
FAST
    Fein Articulation Screening Test
    Flowers Auditory Screening Test

fast
    f. exposure technique
    f. film
    f. film exposure

fastener
    NG strip nasal tube f.

fast-imaging steady precession sequence three-dimensional magnetic resonance imaging (FISP-3D MRI)
Fastrac lighting
fast-setting acrylic
fast-twitch fatigable skeletal muscle
fat
    autologous f.
    buccal f.
    f. cell graft
    f. cell space
    f. embolus syndrome
    f. emulsification
    extraperitoneal f.
    f. fillant
    f. flap
    f. fracture
    f. graft
    f. injection
    jowl f.
    laminar f.
    macroinjection of autologous f.
    f. necrosis
    orbital f.
    parapharyngeal f.
    periorbital f.
    preplatysmal f.
    pseudoherniated f.
    reserve f.
    residual f.
    suborbicularis oculi f. (SOOF)
    subplatysmal f.

fatigue
    auditory f.
    functional vocal f.
    olfactory f.
    perstimulatory f.
    f. striation
    vocal f.
    voice f.

fatty
    f. ball of Bichat
    f. hypertrophy
    f. marrow
    f. zone

fauces
    isthmus of f.

Fauchard disease
faucial
    f. paralysis
    f. reflex
    f. tonsil

faulty
>f. centric occlusion
>f. contact
>f. contact point
>f. interproximal contact
>f. restoration

Fay sign
FBS
>fetal bovine serum

FCG
>fifth cusp groove

FCOD
>focal cementoosseous dysplasia

FDA
>Food and Drug Administration

FDC
>follicular dendritic cell

FDDB
>freeze-dried demineralized bone

FDI
>Facial Disability Index

FDIP
>Facial Disability Index Physical

FDIS
>Facial Disability Index Social

FDMA
>first dorsal metatarsal artery

feared word
feather
>chicken f.'s
>goose f.
>mixed f.'s
>parakeet f.
>parrot f.
>pigeon f.

feathered edge
featheredge
feather-edged proximal finishing line
FeatherTouch SilkLaser
featural surgery
feature
>coarse facial f.
>f. contrasts process
>distinctive f.'s
>junctural f.
>nondistinctive f.
>phonetic f.
>semantic f.

febrile-associated vesicular eruption
fecal fistula
Fedahist
>F. Expectorant

>F. Expectorant Pediatric
>F. Tablet

feedback
>acoustic f.
>afferent f.
>auditory f.
>augmented f.
>corrective f.
>delayed auditory f. (DAF)
>experimental delayed auditory f.
>extrinsic f.
>haptic f.
>intrinsic f.
>inverse f.
>kinesthetic f.
>negative f.
>proprioceptive f.
>f. reduction circuit (FRC)
>simultaneous auditory f.
>tactile f.

feedforward
feeding
>2° f. arteriole
>enteral f.
>oral f.
>parenteral f.
>f. prosthesis
>f. tube

feeling-of-knowing
feeling threshold
Feer disease
feet
>crow's f.
>crural f.

Fein Articulation Screening Test (FAST)
Feldene
Feldman
>F. bur
>F. drill
>F. excision

feldspar
>orthoclase ceramic f.

feldspathic
>f. porcelain
>f. porcelain crown

Fellow
>F. of the American College of Dentists
>F. of the American College of Prosthodontists

F

NOTES

Fellow *(continued)*
F. of the International College of Dentists (FICD)
felon
felt wheel
FEM
finite element method
female-to-male transsexual
Femizole-7
Femizol-M
femoral
f. artery-saphenous bulb region
f. cutaneous nerve
fence
ligamentous facial f.
fenestra, pl. **fenestrae**
f. cochlea
f. nov-ovalis
f. ovalis
f. rotunda
stapes f.
f. vestibuli
fenestram
fissula ante f.
fissula post f.
fenestrated
f. forceps
f. splint
fenestration
alveolar plate f.
f. of alveolar process
apical f.
dental f.
endonasal f.
intercellular f.
labyrinthine f.
f. operation
f. procedure
size of f.
f. technique
tracheal f.
fennel
dog f.
fenoprofen
fentanyl
droperidol plus f.
Fentanyl Oralet
FEP
fluorinated ethylene propylene
Féré effect
Fergusson incision
ferment
proteolytic f.
Fermit-N
F.-N. occlusal hole blockage material
ferret dander
ferric hydroxide

Ferrier
F. 212 gingival clamp
F. separator
ferrule
Ferula
Fer-Will Object Kit
FES
functional endoscopic sinus
FES stent
fescue
meadow f.
FESS
functional endoscopic sinus surgery
festoon
gingival f.
McCall f.
festooning
periocular f.
fetal
f. alcohol syndrome
f. bovine serum (FBS)
f. head constraint
f. valproate syndrome
fetalis
erythroblastosis f.
fetor
f. exore
f. oris
Feulgen reaction
FEV
forced expiratory volume
fever
hay f.
laurel f.
Malta f.
Mediterranean f.
pharyngoconjunctival f.
picket fence f.
rheumatic f.
undulant f.
uveoparotid f.
Feverall
Infants F.
F. Sprinkle Caps
feverfew
fexofenadine
f. HCl
FF
FF abrasive
FFF
FFF abrasive
2-[F-18]-fluoro-2-deoxy-D-glucose
positron emission tomography with -f.-d.-D.-g. (PET-FDG)
FFR
fixed frequency response
FFS
failure of fixation suppression

FGG
  free gingival groove
FGS
  Facial Grading System
FGSM
  Facial Grading System voluntary
    Movement
FGSR
  Facial Grading System Resting symmetry
FGSS
  Facial Grading System Synkinesis
fiber
    A f.
    A-α f.
    A-β f.
    A-δ f.
    A-γ f.
    algogenic pain f.
    alpha f.'s
    alveolar f.
    alveolar crest f.
    alveologingival f.
    apical f.
    argyrophilic collagen f.
    B f.
    f. bundle
    bundle f.
    C f.
    cemental f.
    circular f.
    collagen f.
    collagenous f.
    complex predentinal nerve f.
    crestal f.
    dental f.
    dentinal f.
    dentinogenic f.
    dentogingival f.
    dentoperiosteal f.
    elastic f.
    enamel f.
    Endostat disposable sterile f.
    FiberLase flexible f.
    free gingival f.
    gingival f.
    gingivodental f.
    horizontal f.
    intermediate f.
    interradicular f.
    intervascular smooth muscle f.
      (IMF)
    Korff f.

    lattice f.
    medullated nerve f.
    Micro Link endoscope f.
    myelinated nerve f.
    myelinated sensory nerve f.
    nerve f.
    nonmedullated nerve f.
    oblique f.
    odontogenic f.
    oxytalan f.
    pain f.
    perforating f.
    periodontal ligament f.
    polyester f.
    precollagenous f.
    predentinal nerve f.
    principal f.
    pulpal f.
    f.'s of Rasmussen
    reticular collagen f.
    reticulum f.
    secretomotor f.
    Sharpey f.
    simple marginal pulpal f.
    simple predentinal nerve f.
    striated muscle f.
    supraalveolar f.
    Tomes f.
    tooth attachment f.
    transseptal f.
    UltraLine Nd:YAG laser f.
    unmyelinated nerve f.
FiberLase flexible fiber
fiberoptic
    flexible f.
    f. light (FOL)
    f. lighted mirror
    f. light source
    f. tip
    f. unit
fiberotomy
fiberscope
Fibrel collagen
fibril
    anchoring f.
    aperiodic f.
    argyrophilic f.
    beta f.
    collagen f.
    dentinal f.
    interodontoblastic collagen f.
    sublamina densa f.'s

NOTES

F

fibrilloblast
fibrillogenesis
fibrin
    f. gel
    f. glue
    f. matrix gel (FMG)
    f. sealant
fibrinogen
fibrinolysin and desoxyribonuclease
fibrinolytic system
fibrinopeptide
fibrinous inflammation
fibroadenoma
fibroblast
    f. process
    scar f.
    spindle-cell f.
    wound f.
fibroblastic
    f. cell
    f. reaction
fibroblastoma
    perineural f.
fibrocartilage
    f. plate
fibrocementoma
fibrocystic disease
fibrocyte
fibrodentinoma
    ameloblastic f.
fibroelastic
    f. covering
    f. membrane
fibroepithelioma
fibrofat
fibrofatty
    f. tissue
    f. tumor
fibrogenic sarcoma
fibrogranuloma
    sublingual f.
fibrohemangioma
    gingival f.
fibrolipoma
fibroma
    ameloblastic f.
    benign periapical f.
    cementifying f.
    central f.
    central cementifying f.
    central cementifying/ossifying f.
    central odontogenic f.
    central ossifying f.
    desmoplastic f.
    giant cell f.
    irritation f.
    juvenile ossifying f.
    malignant f.

    nasopharyngeal f.
    f. of nerve
    nonosteogenic f.
    odontogenic f.
    ossifying f.
    osteogenic f.
    periapical f.
    peripheral ameloblastic f.
    peripheral odontogenic f.
    peripheral ossifying f.
    psammomatoid ossifying f.
    psammoosteoid f.
    f. sarcomatosum
    traumatic f.
fibromatosis
    central f.
    f. colli
    gingival f.
    hereditary gingival f.
    idiopathic f.
    pseudosarcomatous f.
fibromuscular dysplasia
fibromxyomatous connective tissue
fibromyalgia
fibromyoma
fibromyxoma
fibromyxomatous lesion
fibromyxosarcoma
fibronectin
fibro-odontoma
    ameloblastic f.-o.
fibro-osseous
    f.-o. ankylosis
    f.-o. dysplasia
    f.-o. lesion
    f.-o. process
    f.-o. pseudotumor (FOPT)
fibro-ossification
fibro-osteogenic myxoma
fibro-osteoma
fibropapilloma
fibrosa
    rarefying pericementitis f.
fibrosarcoma
    ameloblastic f.
    infantile f.
    odontogenic f.
fibrosed hematoma
fibrosis
    cystic f.
    oral submucous f.
    productive f.
    pulp f.
    submucous f.
fibrositis
Fibrostat
fibrotomy

fibrous
    f. adhesion
    f. ankylosis
    f. band
    f. capsular contracture
    f. capsule
    f. connective septa
    f. covering
    f. dysplasia of jaws
    f. epulis
    f. foil
    f. gold
    f. histiocytic cell
    f. histiocytoma
    f. nonunion
    f. odontoma
    f. polly beak
    f. pulp dystrophy
    f. shell
    f. tissue
fibrovascular
    f. aponeurosis
    f. ingrowth
fibroxanthoma
fibula
    f. free flap
    f. osteoseptocutaneous flap
fibular
    f. onlay strut graft
    f. osteocutaneous free flap
FICD
    Fellow of the International College of Dentists
FID
    free induction decay
fiducial marker
field
    auditory f.
    f. cancerization
    electric f.
    free f.
    minimum acceptable f. (MAF)
    minimum audible f. (MAF)
    operating f.
    sound f.
    sterile f.
fifth
    f. cranial nerve
    f. cusp groove (FCG)
fig
    weeping f.
figurative language

figure
    mitotic f.
    f. of speech
figure-eight
    f.-e. preparation
    f.-e. reverse filling
figure-ground
    auditory f.-g.
    f.-g. distortion
    visual f.-g.
figure-of-eight stitch
filaggrin
filament
    cytokeratin f.
    desmin f.
    intracytoplasmic intermediate f.
    keratin f.
    neural f.
    Semmes-Weinstein pressure aesthesiometer f.
    thin f.
    vimentin f.
fila olfactoria
filarial elephantiasis
filariasis
Filatov
    F. flap
    F. spot
Filatov-Gillies
    F.-G. flap
    F.-G. tubed pedicle
file
    Antaeos C f.
    bone f.
    diamond-edged fingernail f.
    endodontic f.
    endosonic f.
    end-Z f.
    fingernail f.
    finishing f.
    Flexicut f.
    Flex-R-File f.
    gold f.
    Greater Taper F.
    GT F.'s
    Hedström f.
    Hirschfeld f.
    Hirschfeld-Dunlop f.
    H-type f.
    initial f.
    Kerr K-Flex f.
    K-type f.

F

NOTES

file *(continued)*
    Lightspeed f.
    master apical f. (MAF)
    McXIM f.
    Mity Gates Glidden f.
    Mity Hedström f.
    Mity Turbo File f.
    nickel-titanium f.
    NiTi nickel-titanium endodontic f.'s
    Onyx-R NiTi f.
    Orban f.
    periodontal f.
    precurved f.
    precurving f.
    ProFile f.
    Quantec Series 2000 micro f.'s
    rat-tail f.
    root canal f.
    rubber f.
    S-f.
    scaler f.
    Schwed Flexicut f.
    Star root canal f.
    SureFlex nickel-titanium f.
    taper hand f.
    temporary master apical f. (TMAF)
    triangular blank f.
    turbo f.
    vulcanite f.

filet *(var. of* filet)
filiform papilla
filing
    anticurvature f.
    circumferential f.
fill
    Prisma F.
fillant
    fat f.
filled
    decayed, extracted, and f.
filler
    BIO-OSS maxillofacial bone f.
    bovine-derived bone f.
    f. graft
    lentula root canal f.
    omental f.
    f. paste
    resin f.
fillet, filet
    f. flap procedure
    f. of foot free flap
filling
    bead technique f.
    brush technique f.
    f. canal
    complex f.
    composite f.
    compound f.

    direct resin f.
    ditched f.
    figure-eight reverse f.
    f. first technique
    flow technique f.
    four-canaled f.
    indirect f.
    f. material
    f. material condensation
    Mosetig-Moorhof f.
    nature's root canal f.
    permanent f.
    postresection f.
    pressure technique f.
    retrograde f.
    Retroplast f.
    reverse f.
    root canal f.
    root-end f.
    temporary f.
    treatment f.

film
    Agfa Dentus M2 comfort intraoral radiograph f.
    Agfa Dentus RP 6 blue-sensitive extraoral radiograph f.
    Agfa Dentus ST8 G green-sensitive extraoral radiograph f.
    autoradiographic f.
    f. badge
    bent f.
    bitewing f.
    dental f.
    double emulsion f.
    D-speed f.
    E-speed intraoral f.
    exposed intraoral f.
    f. exposure technique
    extraoral f.
    fast f.
    f. fog
    f. holder
    f. identification
    interproximal f.
    intrafilling f.
    intraoral f.
    intraoral occlusal f.
    latent image f.
    lateral jaw f.
    measurement f.
    f. mount
    f. mounting
    occlusal f.
    panoramic x-ray f.
    periapical f.
    f. processing
    Salactic f.
    scout f.

screen f.
Softopac intraoral f.
unexposed intraoral f.
x-ray f.

Filmtab
Rondec F.

filopodium

filter
ACE autografter bone f.
active f.
aluminum f.
bacterial f.
band-pass f.
GBX f.
high-pass f.
labial f.
low-pass f.
notch f.
octave-band f.
pass-band f.
power peak f.
third octave f.
tunable notch f.
wave f.

filtered speech

filtral
f. arch
f. ridge

filtration

fimbriated fold

final
f. cementation
f. cone position
f. consonant position
f. impression

Finapec APC root canal filling material

finasteride

finding
Test of Word f (TWF)

fine
f. disk
f. line
f. motor
f. particle composite
f. periosteal elevator
f. pinch

fine-bore catheter

fine-needle
f.-n. aspiration (FNA)
f.-n. aspiration biopsy (FNAB)
f.-n. aspiration cytology (FNAC)
f.-n. biopsy

fineness

fine-tipped mosquito hemostat

finger
f. agnosia
avulsion of portion of f.
denuded f.
f. grasp
mallet f.
f. ruler
f. spreader
f. spring

fingernail file

fingerspelling

finger-sucking re-education appliance

fingertip

finish
denture f.
f. line
satin f.

finishing
f. appliance
f. archwire
f. bur
f. file
f. knife

finite
f. element method (FEM)
f. grammar

Fiorinal
F. With Codeine

fir
Douglas f.

fire
f. ant
St. Anthony f.

firebush

fired porcelain

fireweed

firing
air f.
high biscuit f.
high bisque f.
low biscuit f.
medium biscuit f.
medium bisque f.

first
f. branchial cleft sinus
f. cone position
f. cranial nerve
f. deciduous molar tooth
f. dentition
f. dorsal metatarsal artery (FDMA)

F

NOTES

first *(continued)*
    f. molar
    f. order bend
    f. permanent molar
    f. premolar
    f. premolar alveolus
    f. premolar tooth
    f. sentence
    f. teeth
    f. word
first-state cementoma
Fischer
    F. aspirative lipoplasty
    F. curette technique
    F. nasal rasp
fish
    tuna f.
Fisher exact test
Fisher-Logemann Test of Articulation Competence
fishtail burnisher
FISP-3D MRI
fissula
    f. ante fenestram
    f. post fenestram
fissum
    palatum f.
fissura, pl. **fissurae**
fissural
    f. cyst
fissurata
    lingua f.
fissuratum
    epulis f.
fissure
    f.'s antitragohelicina
    f. bur
    f. burnisher
    f. caries
    f. cavity
    enamel f.
    ethmoidal f.
    gingival f.
    glaserian f.
    globulomaxillary f.
    inferior orbital f.
    infraorbital f.
    lateral f.
    linguogingival f.
    longitudinal cerebral f.
    mandibular f.
    maxillary f.
    medial canthal f.
    oral f.
    orbital f.
    palpebral f.
    petrotympanic f.
    pharyngomaxillary f.

    pterygomaxillary f.
    pterygopalatine f.
    retrocuticular f.
    f. of Rolando
    Santorini f.'s
    f. sealant
    superior orbital f.
    sylvian f.
    f. of Sylvius
    tympanomastoid f.
    zygomatic f.
fissured
    f. fracture
    f. tongue
fistula, pl. **fistulae**
    alveolar f.
    arteriovenous f. (AVF)
    f. auris congenita
    AV f.
    branchial f.
    carotid-cavernous sinus f. (CCSF)
    chyle f.
    f. colli congenita
    dental f.
    enterocutaneous f.
    esophagocutaneous f.
    fecal f.
    gingival f.
    high-flow arteriovenous f.
    intralabyrinthine f.
    labyrinthine f.
    locoregional treatment oral f.
    lymphatic f.
    oroantral f.
    orocutaneous f.
    orofacial f.
    oronasal f.
    oval window f.
    palatoalveolar f.
    perilymph f. (PLF)
    pharyngeal f.
    pharyngocutaneous f.
    preauricular f.
    salivary f.
    f. sign
    speech f.
    spontaneous perilymph f.
    submental f.
    f. takedown
    f. test
    thrombosed renal dialysis f.
    thyroglossal f.
    tracheal f.
    tracheocutaneous f.
    tracheoesophageal f. (TEF)
    traumatic carotid-cavernous sinus f.
fistulation, fistulization
    artificial f.

fistulogram
fistulous
FIT
  fusion-inferred threshold
    FIT test
fit
Fit-Checker
fitting
  Luer lock f.
Fitzgerald Key
five-pin staple
five-position turret
Five Slate System
fixable-removable cross arch bar
fixation
  AO rigid f.
  biphase pin f.
  circumalveolar f.
  circummandibular f.
  circumzygomatic f.
  condylar process fracture axial
    anchor screw f.
  cranial flap f.
  craniofacial f.
  cricoarytenoid joint f.
  elastic band f.
  exterior bolster f.
  external pin f.
  external pin f., biphase
  intermaxillary f. (IMF)
  internal f.
  intramedullary f.
  intraosseous f.
  LactoSorb resorbable
    craniomaxillofacial f.
  lag screw f.
  mandibulomaxillary f.
  maxillomandibular f. (MMF)
  McIndoe and Reese alar cartilage
    suture f.
  medullary f.
  microplate f.
  miniplate f.
  nasomandibular f.
  open reduction internal f. (ORIF)
  osseous f.
  f. pinning
  plate f.
  repeat open reduction internal f.
  resorbable rigid f.
  restorative f.
  rigid internal f. (RIF)

  rigid lag screw f.
  rigid plate f.
  Roger-Anderson pin f.
  f. screw
  semi-rigid f.
  skeletal pin f.
  tension-free scalp f.
  three-point f.
  titanium rigid f.
  transcalvarial suture f.
  wire f.
fixative
fixator
  external f.
  Hoffman external f.
  Joe Hall-Morris external f.
fixed
  f. bridge
  f. bridge prosthesis
  f. bridge prosthodontics
  f. bridgework
  f. expansion prosthesis
  f. forceplate posturography
  f. frequency response (FFR)
  f. interval reinforcement schedule
  f. maintainer space
  f. malleus
  f. mandibular implant (FMI)
  f. orthodontic appliance
  f. partial denture
  f. partial denture splint
  f. prosthodontics
  f. ratio reinforcement schedule
  f. space maintainer
  f. support
fixed-fixed bridge
fixed-movable bridge
fixed-removable space maintainer
fixed-tissue technique
fixer
  f. solution
fixing
  f. process
  f. time
fixture
  implant f.
  osseointegrated f.
FK-506
flaccid
  f. dysarthria
  f. paralysis
  f. skin

F

NOTES

flaccida
pars f. (PF)
flaccidity
abdominal f.
flag flap
Flagyl
flame
f. bur
manometric f.
flammeus
nevus f.
flange
buccal f.
f. contour
denture f.
f. guide appliance
labial f.
lingual f.
mandibular lingual f.
flank
male f.
f. roll
flap
Abbe f.
Abbe-Estlander f.
abdominal axial subcutaneous
pedicle f.
adenoadipose f.
adipofascial f.
adipofascial axial pattern cross-
finger f.
adipofascial turnover f.
advancement f.
allogenically vascularized
prefabricated f.
angiosomal f.
antegrade island f.
anterior helical rim free f.
anterolateral thigh f.
apron f.
arterial f.
arterialized f.
axial f.
axial-based f.
axial pattern vascularized skin f.
axial temporoparietal fascial f.
Bakamjian f.
Banner f.
base of f.
BELL f., bell flap
Berlin tulip f.
bicoronal scalp f.
bilateral inferior epigastric artery f.
(BIEF)
bilobed transposition f.
bipedicle f.
bipedicled delay f.
bipedicled TRAM f.

bone f.
boomerang rectus abdominis
musculocutaneous free f.
buccal envelope f.
buccal mucosal f.
buccal musculomucosal f.
buccinator myomucosal f.
buried de-epithelialized local f.
caterpillar f.
cellulocutaneous f.
cervical f.
cervicopectoral f.
cheek advancement f.
cheek-lip f.
cheek mucous-muscle f.
cheek rotation f.
chest f.
Chinese f.
circular subcutaneous island f.
circumflex scapular f.
cleft margin f.
columellar f.
composite chondrocutaneous f.
composite osteomyocutaneous
preformed f.
compound f.
conical f.
conjoint extensor digitorum brevis
muscle and dorsalis pedis
osteocutaneous island f.
f. consonant
Converse f.
f. coverage
crescentic advancement f.
cross f.
cross-finger f.
cross-leg f.
cross-lid f.
cutaneoperiosteal f.
cutaneous f.
cutaneous forearm f.
Cutler-Beard f.
Dardour f.
dartos fasciocutaneous f.
dartos musculocutaneous f.
decorticated f.
de-epithelialized local f.
de-epithelialized revascularized
lateral intercostal f.
de-epithelialized transverse rectus
abdominis musculocutaneous
pedicle f.
delayed distally based total
sartorius f.
deltopectoral f.
deltoscapular f.
dermal fat free f.
dermal fat pedicle f.

dermal pyramidal f.
dermoadipose f.
dermofat f.
digastric muscle f.
direct f.
distal based f.
distally based fasciocutaneous f.
  (DBFF)
distal pedicle f.
distant f.
dorsal cross-finger f.
dorsalis pedis f.
dorsal thoracic fascia free f.
double cross-lip f.
double-paddle f.
double-paddle island f.
double pedicle f.
double-pedicle transverse rectus
  abdominis musculocutaneous f.
double pendulum f.
double skin paddle fibular f.
double V-Y f.
D-TRAM pedicle f.
f. elevation
Elliott f.
elliptical f.
envelope f.
epaulet f.
epigastric f.
Estlander f.
Estlander-Abbe f.
extended lateral arm free f.
  (ELAFF)
extended shoulder f.
f. failure
FAMM f.
fan f.
fan-shaped f.
fascial turnover f.
fasciocutaneous free f.
fasciocutaneous island f.
fat f.
fibula free f.
fibula osteoseptocutaneous f.
fibular osteocutaneous free f.
Filatov f.
Filatov-Gillies f.
fillet of foot free f.
flag f.
flat f.
forehead f.
forked f.

free arterialized venous forearm f.
free bone f.
free forearm f.
free jejunal f.
free medial plantar fasciocutaneous
  sensory f.
free microvascular f.
free posterior interosseous f.
free temporal fascial f.
free temporoparietal fascial f.
free toe-to-finger hemipulp f.
free toe-to-fingertip neurovascular f.
free transverse rectus abdominis
  musculocutaneous f.
free vascularized bone f.
French f.
Fricke f.
full-thickness periodontal f.
fusiform f.
fusiform island f.
galea-frontalis f.
galea-occipital f.
galea-periosteal f.
gate f.
geometric nasal f.
Gillies fan f.
Gillies up and down f.
gingival f.
glabellar bilobed f.
glabellar rotation f.
gluteal f.
gluteus maximus
  musculocutaneous f.
gracilis muscle f.
gracilis musculocutaneous f.
groin f.
hemiback f.
hemitongue f.
hinged f.
homodigital island f.
horizontal preputial vascularized f.
Hughes f.
hypogastric f.
ideal f.
iliac crest free f.
iliac crest osseous f.
iliac crest osteocutaneous f.
iliac crest osteomuscular f.
immediate f.
inchworm f.
Indian f.
innervated platysma f.

F

NOTES

flap (*continued*)
  insensate f.
  instep island f.
  interdigitated muscle f.
  interdigitating zigzag skin f.
  internal oblique osteomuscular f.
  interpolated f.
  interpolation f.
  intraoral f.
  island fasciocutaneous f.
  Italian f.
  jejunal free f.
  jump f.
  Juri f.
  Karapandzic f.
  Koerner f.
  lateral cutaneous thigh f.
  lateral distally based
    fasciocutaneous f.
  lateral intercostal f.
  lateral supramalleolar f.
  lateral thigh free f.
  lateral trapezius f.
  lateral upper arm f.
  latissimus dorsi muscle f.
  latissimus dorsi musculocutaneous f.
  latissimus dorsi myocutaneous f.
    (LDMCF)
  latissimus dorsi/scapular bone f.
  latissimus fasciocutaneous
    turnover f.
  latissimus muscle f.
  Leibinger E-Z f.
  lifeboat f.
  Limberg f.
  Limberg-type cutaneous f.
  lined f.
  lingual mucoperiosteal f.
  lingual tongue f.
  lip-lip f.
  lip switch f.
  Littler neurovascular island f.
  local rotation f.
  lower trapezius f.
  lumbar periosteal turnover f.
  Malaga f.
  masseter muscle f.
  mastectomy skin f.
  medial cutaneous thigh f.
  medial distally based
    fasciocutaneous f.
  medial plantar sensory f.
  medial upper arm f.
  median forehead f.
  melolabial f.
  mental V-Y island advancement
    island f.
  mesiolabial bilobed transposition f.

  microsurgical free pulp f.
  microvascular free posterior
    interosseous f.
  midface avulsion f.
  midline forehead f.
  modified Singapore f.
  monitor muscle f.
  moustache-like f.
  mucochondrocutaneous f.
  mucoperichondrial f.
  mucoperiosteal periodontal f.
  mucoperiosteal sliding f.
  mucosal periodontal f.
  mucosal prelaminated f.
  muscle-periosteal f.
  musculocutaneous f.
  musculofascial f.
  Mustardé lateral cheek rotation f.
  Mustardé rotation-advancement f.
  myocutaneous f.
  myodermal f.
  myofascial f.
  myomucosal f.
  nape of neck f.
  nasolabial rotation f.
  Nataf lateral f.
  neck f.
  f. necrosis
  neurocutaneous f.
  neurosensorial free medial
    plantar f.
  neurosensory f.
  neurovascular free f.
  Ochsenbein-Luebke f.
  omental transposition f.
  omocervical f.
  open f.
  opening f.
  f. operation
  osteocutaneous filet f.
  osteocutaneous scapular f.
  osteomusculocutaneous f.
  osteomyocutaneous f.
  palatal mucoperiosteal f.
  palmar f.
  palmaris longus composite f.
  parabiotic f.
  paramedian forehead f.
  PARAS f.
  parascapular f.
  parasitic f.
  parieto-occipital f.
  partial-thickness f.
  pectoralis major f.
  pectoralis major myocutaneous f.
  pectoralis myofascial f.
  pedicle f.

pedicled compound rib-latissimus dorsi osteomusculocutaneous f.
pedicled galeal frontalis f.
pedicled groin f.
pedicled latissimus f.
pedicled mucosa f.
pedicled myocutaneous f.
pedicled pericranial f.
pedicled tibial bone f.
peg f.
penile f.
peninsula f.
peno-preputial vascularized f.
perforator-based f.
f. perfusion
perialar crescentic advancement f.
pericoronal f.
pericranial f.
perineal artery axial f.
perineoscrotal f.
periodontal f.
periosteal f.
permanent pedicle f.
pharyngeal f.
platysma myocutaneous f.
Ponten-type fasciocutaneous f.
posterior thigh fasciocutaneous f.
postpharyngeal f.
prefabricated temporoparietal fascial f.
prefabricated thin f.
f. prefabrication
preputial island f.
proximally based medial gastrocnemius f.
quadrapod f.
quadri-lobed f.
radial forearm f.
RAM f.
random fasciocutaneous f.
random pattern f.
random temporoparietal fascial f.
rectus abdominis free f. (RAFF)
rectus abdominis muscle f.
rectus abdominis myocutaneous f. (RAMCF)
rectus turnover f.
regional f.
retroauricular free f.
reversal pedicle f.
reversed digital artery f.
reversed fasciosubcutaneous f.

reverse digital artery f.
reverse digital artery island f.
reverse dorsal digital island f.
reverse flow island f.
reverse Karapandzic f.
reverse medial arm f.
rhomboid transposition f.
rope f.
rotation f.
Rubens f.
Rybka myocutaneous f.
sandwich epicranial f.
scalping f.
scalp sickle f.
scapula free f.
scapular island f.
scapular osteocutaneous f.
Scarpa adipofascial f.
scored alar mucocartilaginous f.
second-toe wraparound f.
semilunar f.
sensate f.
sensate medial plantar free f.
serratus anterior muscle f.
shaped glandular f.
shaped random pattern f.
shutter f.
sickle f.
simple periodontal f.
single-pedicle f.
skin f.
sliding f.
SMAS-platysma f.
split-thickness periodontal f.
steeple f.
subcutaneous laterodigital reverse f.
subcutaneous pedicled f.
subcutaneous turnover f.
subgaleal f.
submental artery f.
submental island f.
submentonian dermo-fatty f.
subscapular system free f.
superficial brachial f.
superiorly based Dardour lateral f.
superiorly based Nataf lateral f.
supraperiosteal f.
switch f.
temporalis f.
temporal island pedicle scalp f.
temporalis muscle f.
temporoparietal fascial f. (TPFF)

F

NOTES

flap *(continued)*
  temporoparietalis fascia f.
  temporoparieto-occipital Juri f.
  Tennison-Randall triangular f.
  Tennison triangular f.
  tensor fasciae latae f.
  thenar f.
  thoracoacromial f.
  thoracodorsal fascia f.
  three-paddle tensor fasciae latae
    free f.
  f. tip
  tongue f.
  TRAM f.
  TRAMP f.
  transposition f.
  transverse pedicled f.
  transverse rectus abdominis
    muscle f.
  transversus and rectus abdominis
    musculoperitoneal f.
  trapezius f.
  trapezoidal f.
  f. tray
  triangular skin f.
  trilobed f.
  Tripier bipedicle skin and
    muscle f.
  triple-paddle f.
  tubed f.
  tubed pedicle f.
  tunnelized dermic f.
  turned down forearm f.
  turnover f.
  tympanomeatal f.
  type C fasciocutaneous f.
  unipedicle f.
  unpedicled f.
  unrepositioned f.
  upper trapezius f.
  U-shaped interdigitated muscle f.
  V f.
  f. vascularity
  vascularized calvarial f.
  vascularized island bone f.
  vascularized preputial f.
  vascularized tibial bone f.
  venous f.
  vermilion Abbe f.
  versatile f.
  vertical preputial vascularized f.
  visor f.
  volar tissue f.
  vomer f.
  von Langenbeck bipedicle
    mucoperiosteal f.
  von Langenbeck palatal f.
  von Langenbeck pedicle f.

  V-Y mucosal f.
  V-Y transposition f.
  waltzed f.
  Washio f.
  web space f.
  Widman f.
  Wookey f.
  wrap-around f.
  Y f.
  Y-V f.
  Z f.
  Zimany bilobed f.
  Zitelli bilobed nasal f.

flare
  red f.
flared-W excision
Flarex
flaring
  f. apex
  labial f.
  overzealous f.
  reverse f.
flash
flashlamp
  f. pulse-dye laser (FLPD)
  f. pumped pulsed dye laser
    (FPPDL)
flask
  casting f.
  f. closure
  crown f.
  denture f.
  injection f.
  refractory f.
flasking
flat
  f. burnisher
  f. flap
  f. fluctuating hearing loss
  f. stone
  f. tongue
flat-bladed nasal speculum
flatness
  malar f.
flava
  macula f.
***Flavobacterium* group II-b**
flavor
Flavorcee
flavus
  Aspergillus f.
flaw
  perioral f.
Flaxedil
flaxseed
flea venom
Fleck cement
Fleischmann hygroma

fleur-de-lis shape
fleur-de-lis-shaped skin paddle
Flexaphen
Flexblock
Flexeril
flexibility
    f. clasp
flexible
    f. fiberoptic
    f. fiberoptic bronchoscopy
    f. fiberoptic endoscopy
    f. fiberoptic laryngoscopy
    f. finishing appliance
    f. laminar bone strip
    f. spiral wire (FSW)
    f. spiral wire retainer
Flexicon material
Flexicut file
flexion
    f. contracture
    f. reflex
flexion-extension reflex
Flexipost
Flexisensor sensor
Flexlite
    Zelco F.
FlexoFile
    Dentsply F.'s
flexoplasty
    Steindler f.
flexor
    f. carpi radialis tendon
    f. carpi ulnaris muscle
    f. carpi ulnaris tendon
    f. digitorum brevis muscle
    f. digitorum longus muscle
    f. digitorum profundus muscle
    f. digitorum superficialis muscle
    f. hallucis longus muscle
    f. pollicis longus muscle
Flexoreamer Batt tip
Flex-R-File file
flexure
    f. clasp
Flexzan
    F. dressing
    F. Extra dressing
    F. topical wound dressing
flint abrasive
floating
    f. premaxilla
    f. tooth

flocculonodular lobe
flocculus of cerebellum
Flonase
floor
    f. of mouth (FOM)
    nasal f.
    pulpal f.
floor-of-mouth
    f.-o.-m. closure
    f.-o.-m. lesion
flora
    bacterial f.
    fusospirochetal f.
    mouth f.
    oral f.
florid
    f. osseous dysplasia
    f. reactive periositis
Florocid fluoride
Florone
    F. E
Floropryl Ophthalmic
floss
    dental f.
    Quik f.
    Reach Easy Slide shred-resistant f.
    Reach Floss Gentle Gum Care
      dental f.
    f. silk
    f. tape
    unwaxed regular dental f.
flottant
    pouce f.
Flovent
flow
    air f.
    antegrade blood f.
    crevicular volume f.
    f. cytometry
    gingival blood f. (GBF)
    f. loop
    mucociliary f.
    parabolic f.
    salivary f.
    speech sound f.
    f. technique
    f. technique filling
flower
    F. dental index
    purple cone f.
Flowers
    F. Auditory Screening Test (FAST)

NOTES

F

Flowers *(continued)*
    F. implant
    F. mandibular glove
    F. Test of Auditory Selective
      Attention
Flowers-Costello Test of Central
  Auditory Abilities
flowmeter
    Assess peak f.
    Doppler f.
    laser Doppler f.
    transit-time f.
    Transonic f.
flowmetry
    laser Doppler f.
flowprobe
Floxin
    F. Otic
Floxite
    F. mirror light
    F. mirror lite
floxuridine (5-FUdR)
FLPD
    flashlamp pulse-dye laser
fluconazole
fluctuance
fluctuant drainage
fluctuating hearing loss
flucytosine
fluence
    f. initiating gesture
fluency
    basal f.
    f. disorder
    false f.
    verbal f.
fluent
    f. aphasia
fluffs dressing
FLUFTEX gauze roll
Fluharty Speech and Language
  Screening Test
fluid
    cerebrospinal f. (CSF)
    f. colloidal system
    crevicular f.
    dentinal f.
    gingival f.
    gingival crevicular f. (GCF)
    intercellular f.
    oral f.
    periciliary f.
    periprosthetic f.
    proteinaceous f.
    Rossman f.
    serous f.
    silicone f.
    sulcular f.

    temporomandibular joint synovial f.
     (TMJ-SF)
    f. wax
    f. wax impression
Fluid-Air Plus bed
flumazicon
flunisolide
fluocinolone
fluocinonide
Fluonid
Fluor-A-Day Supplements
fluorescein
    f. dye
    f. endoscopy
fluorescence
fluorescent dye
fluoridate
fluoridated teeth
fluoridation
fluoride
    acidulated f.
    acidulated phosphate f.
    f. dentifrice
    Florocid f.
    Fluoristan f.
    Fluoritab f.
    f. hypocalcification
    Karidium f.
    Lemoflur f.
    Listermint with F.
    Ossalin f.
    Ossin f.
    Pro-Dentx Home F.
    silver f.
    sodium f.
    f. solution
    Stanide stannous f.
    stannous f.
    Villaumite sodium f.
    Zymafluor f.
Fluorident liquid
fluoridization
Fluorigard
    F. mouthrinse
Fluori-Methane Topical Spray
fluorinated ethylene propylene (FEP)
fluorine
Fluorinse
    Pacemaker F.
Fluoristan fluoride
Fluoritab
    F. fluoride
    F. liquid
fluoroandrolinide
fluoroapatite
FluoroCore resin composite
Fluoro-Ethyl topical anesthetic
Fluor-O-Kote topical fluoride gel

fluorometholone
>f. and neomycin sulfate eyedrops
>sulfacetamide sodium and f.

fluorometric study

Fluor-Op

Fluoroplex

fluoroquinolone

fluoroscopy

fluorosis
>chronic endemic f.
>chronic endemic dental f.
>endemic f.

Fluoro-Thin cement

fluorouracil
>5-f. (5-FU)

Fluothane

Flura-Drops

Flura-Gel

Flura-Loz
>F.-L. lozenge

flurandrenolide

flurbiprofen

Fluro-Ethyl Aerosol

Flurosyn

flute

fluted
>f. finishing bur
>f. tongue

Flutex

fluticasone
>f. propionate

flutter
>alar f.
>auditory f.

Flutter therapeutic device

flux

fluxed wax

fly
>black f.
>deer f.

FM
>frequency modulation

FMA
>Frankfort mandibular angle

FMG
>fibrin matrix gel

FMI
>fixed mandibular implant

FMIA
>Frankfort mandibular incisor angle

FML
>F. Forte

>F.-Neo eyedrops
>F.-S Ophthalmic Suspension

FN
>facial nerve

FNA
>fine-needle aspiration
>FNA biopsy
>FNA cytology

FNAB
>fine-needle aspiration biopsy

FNAC
>fine-needle aspiration cytology

FND
>functional neck dissection

Fo
>phonation

foam
>f. and dome method
>Laclede Fluoride F.
>open cell f.
>Oral-B Minute F.
>polyurethane f. (PUF)
>f. posturography
>Reston polyurethane f.

focal
>f. calcific regression of pulp
>f. cementoosseous dysplasia (FCOD)
>f. condensing osteitis
>f. dermal hypoplasia
>f. epithelial hyperplasia
>f. keratosis
>f. (oral) keratosis
>f. osseous dysplasia
>f. palmoplantar and marginal gingival hyperkeratosis
>f. spot condition
>f. trough

focus, pl. foci
>hilar foci
>tone f.
>vocal f.
>voice tone f.

Foeniculum vulgare

fog
>film f.
>radiation f.

Fogarty
>F. adherent clot catheter
>F. catheter
>F. catheter embolectomy

F

NOTES

foil

adhesive f.
aluminum f.
f. carrier
cohesive gold f.
f. condenser
corrugated gold f.
crumpled aluminum f.
fibrous f.
gold f.
laminated gold f.
mat f.
noncohesive gold f.
f. passer
platinum f.
f. plugger
f. rope
semicohesive gold f.
tin f.

foil-carrying pliers
FOL

fiberoptic light

fold

anterior mallear f.
antihelical f.
aryepiglottic f.
bowed vocal f.
epicanthal f.
false vocal f.
fimbriated f.
glossoepiglottic f.
Herb f.
incudal f.
inframammary f. (IMF)
intercartilaginous f.
interossicular f.
labiomental f.
laryngeal f.
lateral glossoepiglottic f.
lateral incudal f.
lateral mallear f.
mallear f.
medial incudal f.
median glossoepiglottic f.
median thyrohyoid f.
mucobuccal f.
mucolabial f.
mucosobuccal f.
nail f.
nasojugal f.
nasolabial f. (NLF)
obturatoria stapedis f.
palatine f.
palatopharyngeal f.
pharyngoepiglottic f.
polypoid degeneration of the
   true f.

pretarsal f.
pterygomandibular f.
salpingopalatine f.
semilunar f.
stapedial f.
sublingual f.
superior incudal f.
superior mallear f.
tensor f.
thyrohyoid f.
triangular f.
true vocal f.
tympanic f.
ventricular f.
vestibular f.
vocal f.
white dural f.

folded aluminum ear splint
folding technique
Folex PFS
Foley

F. catheter
F. operation
F. Y-plasty pyeloplasty

foliate

f. papilla
f. papillitis

folic acid
folk healer
follicle

dental f.
lingual f.
lingual lymph f.
lymphatic f.

follicular

f. adenoiditis
f. carcinoma
f. crypt
f. cyst
f. dendritic cell (FDC)
f. epithelium
f. formation
f. lymphoid hyperplasia
f. lymphoma
f. odontogenic cyst
f. pattern
f. thyroid carcinoma
f. tonsillitis

follicularis

keratosis f.

folliculitis

f. nares perforans

folliculorum

Demodex f.

FOM

floor of mouth

Fome-Cuf tracheostomy tube

Fomon
    F. face lift scissors
    F. graft augmentation
Fones
    F. method
    F. method of toothbrushing
    F. technique
Fonix 6500-CX hearing aid test system
Fontana-Masson staining
fontanel, fontanelle
    posterior f.
food
    F. and Drug Administration (FDA)
    f. impaction
foot
    Aftate for Athlete's F.
    f. condenser
    Dr Scholl's Athlete's F.
    f. plugger
footplate
    stapes f.
foot-pound
FOPT
    fibro-osseous pseudotumor
foramen, pl. foramina
    alveolar foramina
    anterior ethmoidal f.
    apical f. (AF)
    f. apicis dentis
    f. cecum
    f. cecum of tongue
    dental f.
    greater palatine f.
    histologic f.
    f. of Huschke
    incisive f.
    inferior orbital f.
    infraorbital f.
    jugular f.
    f. lacerum
    lingual f.
    f. magnum
    f. mandibulae
    mandibular f.
    mastoid f.
    maxillary f.
    mental f.
    multiple foramina
    nasopalatine f.
    optic f.
    f. ovale
    palatine f.

    posterior ethmoidal f.
    pulpal f.
    f. radicis dentis
    root f.
    f. rotundum
    Scarpa f.
    f. singulare
    sphenopalatine f.
    f. spinosum
    stylomastoid f.
    superior maxillary f.
    teardrop f.
    zip f.
    zygomatic f.
force
    anchorage f.
    anterior f.
    anterior component of f.
    F. 9 arch
    bite f.
    biting f.
    chewing f.
    component of f.
    compressive f.
    concentrated f.
    condensing f.
    constant f.
    deferential orthodontic f.
    denture-dislodging f.
    denture-retaining f.
    differential f.
    distal f.
    distributed f.
    electromotive f. (EMF)
    extraoral f.
    f. factor
    gravitational f.
    headgear f.
    incisal f.
    intermittent f.
    interrupted f.
    light wire torque f.
    f. of mastication
    masticatory f.
    maximum bite f.
    nerve f.
    occlusal bite f.
    optimal f.
    optimum orthodontic f.
    orthodontic f.
    orthopaedic f.
    f. platform

F

NOTES

force *(continued)*
    reciprocal f.
    f. and stress
    strong f.
    tensile f.
    threshold f.
    tooth-moving f.
    unilateral isometric bite f.
    f. vector
    F. wire

forced
    f. duction test
    f. eruption
    f. expiratory volume (FEV)
    f. vibration
    f. whisper

forceps
    Adson f.
    Adson-Brown f.
    alligator f.
    Allison f.
    Allis tissue f.
    American style f.
    antrum punch f.
    apical fragment f.
    Ash f.
    ASSI f.
    backbiting f.
    ball f.
    bayonet root tip f.
    biopsy f.
    bipolar f.
    Blakesley f.
    Blakesley-Weil upturned ethmoid f.
    Blakesley-Wilde f.
    bone f.
    Brigham 1x2 teeth f.
    Brown-Adson side-grasping f.
    Castroviejo f.
    center-action f.
    chalazion f.
    clamp f.
    C. L. Jackson head-holding f.
    C. L. Jackson pin-bending
     costophrenic f.
    continuous clip f.
    cowhorn f.
    Cryer f.
    cupped f.
    Cushing f.
    Denis Browne tonsil f.
    dental f.
    double-spoon biopsy f.
    endoscopic f.
    ethmoid-Blakesley f.
    ethmoid punch f.
    expansile f.
    extracting f.

    extraction f.
    f. extraction
    fenestrated f.
    foreign body f.
    giraffe biopsy f.
    Gordon bead f.
    Griffith-Brown f.
    Halsted mosquito f.
    hemostatic f.
    horn beak f.
    iris f.
    ivory rubber dam clamp f.
    Jackson approximation f.
    Jackson broad staple f.
    Jackson button f.
    Jackson conventional foreign
     body f.
    Jackson cross-action f.
    Jackson cylindrical object f.
    Jackson double-prong f.
    Jackson dull rotation f.
    Jackson flexible upper lobe
     bronchus f.
    Jackson globular object f.
    Jackson papilloma f.
    Jackson ring jaw globular object f.
    Jackson sharp-pointed rotation f.
    Jansen-Middleton punch f.
    jeweler's f.
    Kahler f.
    Kazanjian f.
    Kelly f.
    Kerrison f.
    Kinder Design pedo f.
    Kleinert-Kutz bone-cutting f.
    Lalonde extra fine skin hook f.
    Lalonde skin hook f.
    LaRoe undermining f.
    Löwenberg f.
    lower anterior f.
    lower universal f.
    mandibular f.
    Matthew f.
    maxillary f.
    McGivney f.
    Mead f.
    mosquito f.
    O'Brien fixation f.
    O'Brien tissue f.
    optical biopsy f.
    oval f.
    papilloma f.
    Peet f.
    Pierse tip f.
    point f.
    Potts-Smith tissue f.
    R f.
    Radial Jaw biopsy f.

right-angle f.
Rochester oral tissue f.
Rochester Russian tissue f.
rongeur f.
root-tip f.
round f.
Rowe disimpaction f.
rubber dam clamp f.
Semken f.
Semken-Taylor f.
side-biting Stammberger punch f.
side-lip f.
silver point f.
sister-hook f.
small cup biopsy f.
Smith & Nephew Richards
  bipolar f.
splinter f.
sponge f.
Stammberger punch f.
S&T Lalonde hook f.
straight f.
suction f.
suture f.
Takahashi f.
tenaculum f.
thumb f.
tissue f.
tissue-spreading f.
tongue f.
tonsil f.
Tucker staple f.
Tucker tack and pin f.
universal f.
University of Washington rubber
  dam clamp f.
upbiting f.
upper universal f.
upturned f.
upward bent f.
Vickers ring tip f.
Watson duckbill f.
wedge and post f.
Wilde ethmoid f.

Fordyce
  F. disease
  F. granules
  F. spot

forefoot
fore-glide
forehead
  f. asymmetry

broad f.
convex f.
f. flap
f. lag
f. positioner
f. wrinkling

forehead-brow complex
forehead-nose position
foreheadplasty
  coronal f.
  open f.

foreign
  f. accent
  f. body
  f. body aspiration
  f. body forceps
  f. body giant cell reaction
  f. body granuloma
  f. body magnet
  f. body removal
  f. body remover
  f. body sensation

forelock
forensic
  f. dentistry
  f. odontology

foreshortening
fork
  banking the f.
  bite f.
  face-bow f.
  transfer f.
  tuning f.

forked
  f. flap
  f. tongue
  f. uvula

form
  access f.
  anatomic f.
  arch f.
  cavity preparation f.
  convenience f.
  disseminated f. Albright syndrome
  extension f.
  free f.
  ion crown f.
  language f.
  occlusal f.
  oral-like language f.
  outline f.
  posterior tooth f.

F

NOTES

form *(continued)*
    preextirpative f.
    resistance f.
    retention f.
    spherical f.
    tooth f.
    wax f.
    f. word
    written-like language f.
formal
    f. method
    f. universals
formaldehyde
formalin
formant
    f. frequency
    singer's f.
formation
    aortoenteric fistula f.
    crater f.
    cutaneous capillary f.
    dentinoid f.
    follicular f.
    keloid f.
    root f.
    twin f.
    zip f.
formative stage
formed clasp
forme fruste
former
    angle f.
    base f.
    crucible f.
    manual t. f.
    sprue f.
    vacuum type f.
formocresol
    Buckley f.
    f. pulpotomy
formula, pl. **formulas, formulae**
    Bayer Select Pain Relief F.
    Black f.
    dental f.
    Esoterica Sensitive Skin F.
    Grossman f.
    Kligman f.
    Mollifene Ear Wax Removing F.
    F. Q
    Rickert f.
    Sine-Off Maximum Strength No
      Drowsiness F.
    Triaminic AM Decongestant F.
formulation
fornix
    vestibular f.
    f. vestibuli
Foroblique bronchoscopic telescope

forsythus
    Bacteroides f.
Fortaz
Forte
    Aristocort F.
    Eldopaque F.
    Eldoquin F.
    FML F.
    Lignospan F.
    M.D. F.
    Norgesic F.
    Robinul F.
    Solaquin F.
    Triam F.
Forticast alloy
fortis consonant
fortuitum
    Mycobacterium f.
forward
    f. coarticulation
    f. mandibular distraction
    f. masking
    f. protrusion
Fosamax
foscarnet
Foscavir Injection
Fosdick-Hansen-Epple test
fossa, pl. **fossae**
    antecubital f.
    anterior cranial f.
    articular surface of mandibular f.
    Bichat f.
    buccal groove of central f.
      (BGCF)
    canine f.
    central f. (CF)
    central groove of central f.
      (CGCF)
    digastric f.
    distal f. (DF)
    distal triangular f. (DTF)
    distolingual f. (DLF)
    glenoid f.
    incisive f.
    infratemporal f.
    jugular f.
    lacrimal f.
    lateral bulbar f.
    lingual f. (LF)
    mandibular f.
    f. mandibularis
    maxillary f.
    mesial triangular f. (MTF)
    mesiolingual f. (MLF)
    middle cranial f.
    nasal f.
    oral f.
    piriform f.

posterior f.
posterior cranial f. (PCF)
pterygomaxillary f.
f. pterygopalatina
pterygopalatine f.
retromandibular f.
f. retromandibularis
retromolar f.
f. of Rosenmüller
saccular f.
scaphoid f.
subarcuate f., f. subarcuata
sublingual f.
submandibular f.
submaxillary f.
supratonsillar f.
temporal f.
temporal-pterygomaxillary f.
temporomandibular joint f.
tonsillar f.
triangular f.
f. triangularis
vestibular f.

Foster bed frame
Fotofil adhesive
foul odor
foundation
    denture f.
    f. surface
four-canaled filling
four-flap Webster-Bernard technique
four-handed dentistry
Fourier
    F. analysis
    F. law
Fournier
    F. gangrene
    F. glossitis
    F. teeth
    F. tip
four-pronged liposuction cannula
four-stage light wire appliance
four-tailed bandage
fourteen-and-six Hertz positive spike
fourth
    f. branchial anomaly
    f. cranial nerve
    f. molar
4-Way Long Acting Nasal Solution
fovea
    f. ethmoidalis

fowleri
    Naegleria f.
Fox scissors
foxtail
    meadow f.
Fox-Williams probe
FPPDL
    flashlamp pumped pulsed dye laser
fracture
    alveolar process f.
    alveolar socket wall f.
    anterior f.
    blow-in f.
    blow-out f.
    cemental f.
    cementum f.
    Colles f.
    compound f.
    condylar process f.
    craniofacial dysjunction f.
    crown f.
    crown-root f.
    dentoalveolar f.
    dislocation f.
    f. dislocation
    displaced malar f.
    enamel f.
    facial f.
    fat f.
    fissured f.
    frontal sinus f.
    greenstick f.
    Guérin f.
    horizontal f.
    horizontal maxillary f.
    hyoid bone f.
    impacted f.
    incomplete vertical root f. (IVRF)
    intracapsular f.
    laryngeal cartilage f.
    Le Fort I, II, III f.
    malar f.
    mandibular body f.
    mandibular condyle f.
    mandibular ramus f.
    mandibular symphysis f.
    marginal ridge f.
    maxillary f.
    maxillofacial f.
    f. medialization
    mesiodistal f.
    midface f.

F

NOTES

fracture *(continued)*
    midfacial f.
    nasal f.
    nasal-septal f.
    nasoethmoidal f.
    naso-ethmoid-orbital f.
    naso-orbito-ethmoid f.
    NOE f.
    open f.
    orbital blow-in f.
    orbital blow-out f.
    pancraniomaxillofacial f.
    panfacial f.
    petrous pyramid f.
    porcelain f.
    posterior f.
    pyramidal f.
    root f.
    single f.
    f. splint
    spontaneous f.
    symphysial f.
    temporal bone f.
    tooth f.
    transverse facial f.
    transverse maxillary f.
    traumatic f.
    trimalar f.
    tripod f.
    undisplaced f.
    vertical f.
    vertical tooth f.
    ZMC f.
    zygomatic arch f.
    zygomatic complex f.
    zygomatic maxillary complex f.
fractured
    f. tooth
    f. tuberosity
fragile X syndrome
fragilitas ossium
fragment
fraise
    diamond f.
frame
    CircOlectric bed f.
    denture f.
    Foster bed f.
    halo head f.
    implant f.
    implant superstructure f.
    f. implant superstructure
    Nygaard-Otsby f.
    occluding f.
    Otsby f.
    Otsby dam f.
    radiolucent f.
    ramus f.

    rubber dam f.
    Stryker bed f.
    subperiosteal f.
    superstructure f.
    Wizard f.
    Young f.
framework
    implant f.
    osteocartilagenous f.
Franceschetti syndrome
Francisella tularensis
Fränkel
    F. III functional corrector
    F. removable orthodontic appliance
Frankfort
    F. horizontal light line
    F. horizontal plane
    F. mandibular angle (FMA)
    F. mandibular incisor angle
    (FMIA)
    F. mandibular plane
    F. mandibular plane angle
franklinic taste
Frank technique
Fraser syndrome
Frazier
    F. aspirator
    F. incision
    F. suction tip aspirator
FRC
    feedback reduction circuit
    functional residual capacity
freckle
    Hutchinson f.
free
    f. arterialized venous forearm flap
    Arthritis Foundation Pain Reliever,
      Aspirin F.
    f. autogenous corticocancellous iliac
      bone graft
    f. autogenous pearl fat graft
    f. bone flap
    f. bone reconstruction
    f. cementicle
    f. colon transfer
    f. composite graft
    f. composite lip-switch procedure
    f. cutaneous nerve graft
    f. denticle
    f. fat graft
    f. field
    f. field room
    f. flap procedure
    f. flap vaginoplasty
    f. forearm flap
    f. form
    f. gingiva
    f. gingival fiber

f. gingival graft
f. gingival groove (FGG)
f. gingival margin
f. graft from urinary bladder mucosa
f. groove
f. gum
f. gum margin
f. induction decay (FID)
f. jejunal flap
f. jejunal graft procedure
f. mandibular movement
f. medial plantar fasciocutaneous sensory flap
f. microvascular flap
f. morpheme
f. muscle graft
f. muscle transfer
f. posterior interosseous flap
f. skin graft
f. support
f. temporal fascial flap
f. temporoparietal fascial flap
f. thyroxin index (FTI)
f. tissue transfer
f. toe-to-finger hemipulp flap
f. toe-to-fingertip neurovascular flap
f. transverse rectus abdominis musculocutaneous flap
f. variation
f. vascularized bone flap
f. vibration

free-end
f.-e. base
f.-e. saddle
f.-e. spring
free-flap reconstruction
free-hand knife
Freer
F. elevator
F. septal elevator
free-standing
f.-s. implant
f.-s. single crown
free-tissue transfer reconstruction
freeway space
freeze-dried demineralized bone (FDDB)
freeze trim
Freezone Solution
frena (*pl. of* frenum)
frenata
lingua f.

French
F. flap
F. method
F. plane
F. poodle dander
French-line
F.-l. abdominoplasty
F.-l. method
frenectomy
frenoplasty
frenotomy
frenulum, pl. **frenula**
f. linguae
lingual f.
f. of superior lip
f. of tongue
frenum, pl. **frena, frenums**
buccal f.
f. diastema
enlarged f.
labial f.
lingual f.
f. pull
f. of tongue
Frenzel maneuver
Freon solution
frequency
band f.
defined f.
formant f.
fundamental f. (F_0)
high f. (HF)
infrasonic f.
f. jitter
Larmor f.
low f. (LF)
modal f.
f. modulation (FM)
f. modulation auditory trainer
natural f.
octave f.
primary peak f.
f. range
range of f.'s
resonant f.
respiratory f.
f. response
f. response curve
speech f.
f. theory
ultrasonic f.
frequency-place theory

NOTES

F

fresh autologous de-epidermalized dermis
Frey, von Frey
    F. hairs
    F. syndrome
friable
    f. vessel
FRIALITE-2 dental implant system
fricative
    gliding of f.
    groove f.
    slit f.
    stopping of f.
Fricke flap
friction
    f. attachment
frictional wall retention
frictionless
friction-retained pin
friction/trauma-associated leukoplakia
Friedman splint
Friedreich ataxia
Frigiderm topical anesthetic
frit
frog
    f. face
    f. in the throat
Froment sign
front
    f. consonant
    f. phoneme
    f. recess drainage system
    f. routing of signals (FROS)
    f. vowel
frontal
    f. artery
    f. bone
    f. bone resorption
    f. bossing
    f. branch
    f. bulla
    f. craniotomy
    f. furrow
    f. gyri
    f. irrigation
    f. lisp
    f. lobe
    f. margin
    f. mirror
    f. nerve
    f. ostium
    f. plagiocephaly
    f. plane
    f. process
    f. projection
    f. recess
    f. region
    f. resorption

    f. sinus
    f. sinus fracture
    f. sinusitis
    f. sinus mucocele
    f. sinus septoplasty
    f. sulcus
    f. suture
    f. view
frontalis
    f. hypertactivity
    f. muscle
    f. muscle paralysis
    f. sling procedure
    f. suspension
fronting
    palatal f.
    velar f.
frontocaudal
frontoethmoidal
    f. cell
    f. meningoencephalocele
frontoethmoidectomy
frontoglabella wrinkle
frontolateral laryngectomy
frontomalar suture
frontomaxillary suture
frontonasal
    f. duct
    f. dysplasia
fronto-orbital rim
frontoparietal region
frontotemporal
frontotemporale
frontozygomatic (FZ)
    f. suture
FROS
    front routing of signals
frostbite
Frosted Flex earmold material
frosting
    light white f.
Frost stitch
frowning
    oral f.
frozen
    f. knee joint
    f. section
fruste
    forme f.
frustration tolerance
fry
    glottal f.
    vocal f.
FSW
    flexible spiral wire
FTI
    free thyroxin index

5-FU
>5-fluorouracil

fucci
>*Bacteroides f.*

Fuchs position
Fucus vesiculosus
5-FUdR
>floxuridine

fugax
>amaurosis f.

Fuji Dentacam EDC 2
fulcrum
>f. line
>f. of tooth
>f. tooth

fulguration
full
>f. arch bridge implant
>f. cast restoration
>f. crown
>f. denture
>f. denture prosthetics
>f. face laser resurfacing
>f. flap in mucogingival surgery
>f. mouth series
>f. shoulder preparation
>f. spectrum low cut
>f. veneer crown

full-coping core
full-denture smile
Fullerton Language Test for Adolescents
full-face peel
full-jacketed
>f.-j. bullet wound
>f.-j. military round

fullness
>aural f.
>supratip f.
>upper pole f.

full-thickness
>f.-t. defect
>f.-t. periodontal flap
>f.-t. periodontal graft
>f.-t. skin graft

fulminans
>purpura f.

fulminant
>f. invasive infection
>f. mediastinitis
>f. tenosynovitis

Fulvicin P/G

Fulvicin-U/F
Fu Manchu pattern
fumigatus
>*Aspergillus f.*

functio laesa
function
>affective f.
>articulation-gain f.
>auditory f.
>central auditory f.
>Clinical Evaluation of Language F.'s (CELF)
>Clinical Evaluation of Language F.-Preschool (CLEF-P)
>cochlear outer hair cell f.
>f. corrector
>differential f.
>external frame f.
>gap f.
>Gilbert classification of shoulder f.
>language f.
>liver f.
>occlusal f.
>performance-intensity f.
>referential f.
>semi-autonomous systems concept of brain f.
>speech-motor f.
>velopharyngeal f.
>visual-motor f.
>f. word

functional
>f. activator
>f. aphonia
>f. appliance
>f. articulation disorder
>f. assessment of cancer therapy–head and neck (FACT-HN)
>f. assessment of human immunodeficiency virus (FAHI)
>f. chew-in record
>F. Communication Profile
>f. deafness
>f. dentin
>f. dyslalia
>f. endoscopic sinus (FES)
>f. endoscopic sinus stent
>f. endoscopic sinus surgery (FESS)
>f. form of supporting structure
>f. hearing
>f. hearing loss

F

NOTES

functional *(continued)*
- f. hypertrophy
- f. impression
- f. jaw orthopaedics
- f. lift
- f. malposition
- f. mandibular movement
- f. neck dissection (FND)
- f. occlusal harmony
- f. occlusal registration
- f. occlusion
- f. orthodontic therapy
- f. parathyroid cyst
- f. phase
- f. phase of tooth eruption
- f. repair
- f. residual capacity (FRC)
- f. ridge
- f. splint
- f. veloplasty
- f. vocal fatigue

function corrector
functioning
- general intellectual f.

functor
fundamental
- f. frequency (F_0)
- f. tone

fundoplication
- Nissen f.

fundus, pl. fundi
funduscopy
fungal
- f. antigen
- f. infection

fungal-specific IgE
fungi (*pl. of* fungus)
fungiform papilla
Fungizone
- F. oral suspension

Fungoid
- F. Creme
- F. Solution
- F. Tincture

fungoides
- mycosis f.

fungus, pl. fungi
- ray f.

funicular graft
funnelform
- f. preparation
- f. taper

funnel shaped
fur
Furacin Topical
furca, pl. furcae
- denuded f.
- invaded f.
- f. invasion
- f. involvement

furcal
- f. nerve

furcation
- f. canal
- f. caries
- denuded f.
- invaded f.
- f. perforation
- root f.

Furlow
- F. closure
- F. double opposing Z-plasty
- F. double opposing Z-plasty palatoplasty
- F. double reversing Z-plasty
- F. procedure

furnace
- annealing f.
- dental f.
- inlay f.
- muffle f.
- porcelain f.
- f. pyrometer

furoate
- mometasone f.

furred tongue
furrow
- frontal f.
- nasal-labial f.
- orbital-palpebral f.
- sagittal f.
- shoulder of f.

furrowed tongue
Furstenberg regimen
furuncle
furunculosis
Fusarium
fused teeth
fusiform
- f. flap
- f. island flap
- f. plication
- f. scar

fusiforme
- *Corynebacterium f.*
- *Fusobacterium f.*

fusiformis
- *Bacillus f.*
- *Sphaerophorus f.*

fusing point
fusion
- auditory flutter f.
- binaural f.
- root f.
- STT f.
- f. temperature wire method

temporal line of f.
    f. welding
fusion-inferred
    f.-i. threshold (FIT)
    f.-i. threshold test
Fusobacterium
    F. fusiforme
    F. necrophorum
    F. nucleatum
    F. plauti-vincenti
fusospirillary
    f. marginal gingivitis

fusospirillosis
fusospirochetal
    f. disease
    f. flora
    f. gingivitis
    f. stomatitis
fuzzy coat
FyBron dressing
FZ
    frontozygomatic

NOTES

F

γ (*var. of* gamma)
G
  gingiva
  gingival
G₁
    G₁ block
    G₁ checkpoint
G5 Neocussor percussor
GA
  gingivoaxial
GABHS
  group A β-hemolytic streptococcus
gadolinium
    g. diethylamine triamine penta-
      acetic acid (Gd-DPTA)
    g. DTPA
**gadolinium-diethylenetriamine pentaacetic
acid enhancement**
GAEL
  Grammatical Analysis of Elicited
    Language
Gaerny bar
GAG
  glycosaminoglycan
gag
    Crowe-Davis mouth g.
    Davis-Crowe mouth g.
    Millard mouth g.
    Molt mouth g.
    mouth g.
    g. reflex
gagging
gain
    acoustic g.
    g. control
    HAIC g.
    HF average full-on g.
    peak acoustic g.
    g. potentiometer
    primary g.
    secondary g.
gait
    lurching g.
galactorrhea
galea
    aponeurotic g.
    g. aponeurotica
    lateral g. aponeurotica
galea-aponeurotic plication
galea-frontalis
    g.-f. advancement
    g.-f. flap
galea-frontalis-occipitalis release
galea-occipital flap
galea-periosteal flap

Galen
    G. anastomosis
    G. nerve
    G. ventricle
galeni
    ansa g.
galeoperiosteum
Galilean loupe
gallamine triethiodide
galli
    cleft crista g.
    crista g.
Gallium aparine
gallstone
galoche chin
Galton whistle
galvanic
    g. skin resistance
    g. skin response (GSR)
    g. skin response audiometry
      (GSRA)
galvanism
    dental g.
galvanometer
Gambel oak
Gamimune N
gamma, γ
    g. camera
    g. knife
    g. locking nail
    g. probe radiolocalization (GPRL)
    g. ray
gammacism
Gammagard
    G. S/D
Gammar-P I.V.
ganciclovir
ganglion, pl. ganglia
    basal g.
    Blandin g.
    cervical g.
    ciliary g.
    g. cyst
    extirpation of g.
    gasserian g.
    geniculate g.
    Meckel g.
    motor roots of submandibular g.
    otic g.
    parasympathetic root of
      submandibular g.
    pterygopalatine g.
    recurrent g.
    Scarpa g.
    sphenopalatine g.

G

ganglion *(continued)*
    spiral g.
    submandibular g.
    submaxillary g.
    superior cervical g.
    sympathetic root of
      submandibular g.
    vestibular g.
ganglionectomy
    wrist g.
ganglioneuroblastoma
ganglioneuroma
ganglionic
    g. blocker
    g. blocking agent
    g. nerve cell
    g. saliva
gangosa
gangrene
    clostridia g.
    Fournier g.
    gas g.
    hospital g.
    mammary g.
    pulp g.
gangrenosum
    pyoderma g.
gangrenous
    g. periosteitis
    g. pharyngitis
    g. pulp necrosis
    g. rhinitis
    g. stomatitis
Gantanol
Gantrisin
GAP
    general all purpose
    GAP verb
gap
    air-bone g.
    comprehension-production g.
    contraction g.
    g. detection
    g. function
    interocclusal g.
    g. junction
    mean residual g. (MRG)
    nerve g.
    receptive-expressive g.
Garamycin
    G. Injection
    G. Ophthalmic
    G. Topical
Gardner
    G. needle holder
    G. syndrome
gargle
gargoylism

Gariot articulator
garlic
garment
    Canfield facial plastics g.
    compression g.
    crotchless compression g.
    Marena by LySonix compression g.
    surgical compression g.
garnet
    g. abrasive
Garré
    G. osteomyelitis
    G. periostitis
gas
    argon g.
    g. gangrene
    g. welding
gas-air blowtorch
Gasparotti bevel tip
gasserian ganglion
gastric
    g. decompression
    g. mucosa
    g. outlet obstruction
gastritis
gastrocnemius
Gastrocrom Oral
gastroepiploic artery
gastroesophageal reflux
Gastrografin
gastrointestinal
    g. adenocarcinoma
    g. bleeding
    g. carcinoma
    g. licorice
gastroplasty
    vertical banded g. (VBG)
gastroschisis
gastroscope
gastroscopy
Gastrosed
gastrostomy
    g. feeding tube
gate
    g. control theory
    g. flap
    locking g.
Gates-Glidden
    G.-G. bur
    G.-G. drill
Gaucher disease
gauge
    bite g.
    Boley g.
    Dontrix g.
    leaf g.
    machinist's g.
    Starret wire g.

strain g.
Synthes mini-depth g.
test file g.
Tycos g.
g. undercut
undercut g.

gaussian
g. curve
g. distribution
g. noise

gauze
Adaptic g.
Kling g.
g. pack
g. pad
petrolatum g.
Telfa g.
Vaseline-coated g.
Xeroform g.

gay bowel syndrome

gaze
dysconjugate g.
g. nystagmus
g. paresis
g. stability
g. test

GBA
gingivobuccoaxial

GBF
gingival blood flow

GBI
gingival bleeding index

GBR
guided bone regeneration

GBR-200
REGENTEX GBR-200

GBX filter

GC
gingival crevice

GCF
gingival crevicular fluid

GCS
Glasgow Coma Scale

GCT
giant cell tumor
granular cell tumor

Gd-DPTA
gadolinium diethylamine triamine pentaacetic acid

Geiger-Müller counter

gel
acidulated phosphate-fluoride g.

APF g.
bioexcretable g.
calcium alginate g.
Cavi-Trol acidulated phosphate
fluoride topical g.
Codesco topical fluoride phosphate
anticaries g.
Credo topical g.
Dental H topical fluoride g.
DuoPlant G.
DynaGraft G.
Emdogain g.
fibrin g.
fibrin matrix g. (FMG)
Fluor-O-Kote topical fluoride g.
Gel-Kam Home Care G.
Healthco topical fluoride g.
H.P. Acthar G.
Hurricaine g.
hydrofluoric acid etching g.
hydrophilic g.
hydrophobic g.
hydroquinone g.
Karidium phosphate fluoride
topical g.
Kerr Topical Flura-Gel g.
Luride topical g.
Nufluor g.
Oral-B Minute G.
orthophosphoric acid etch g.
Pacemaker topical fluoride g.
phosphoric acid g.
pigment g.
platelet g.
polymer g.
Predent topical fluoride
treatment g.
PreviDent Brush-On G.
Rafluor topical g.
Regranex g.
Rescue Squad topical g.
Sal-Plant G.
g. sheeting
silicone g.
silver-stained polyacrylamide g.
sodium fluoride-orthophosphoric
acid g.
So-Flo phosphate topical g.
Solaquin Forte g.
g. state
Sultan Topex 00:60 second topical
fluoride g.

NOTES

G

gel *(continued)*
>   Super-Dent topical fluoride g.
>   T-4 G.
>   g. technique
>   thixotropic fluoride g.

gelatin
>   absorbable g.
>   g., pectin, and methylcellulose
>   g. sponge

gelatinosa
>   substantia g.

Gel-Drops
>   Thera-Flur G.-D.
>   Thera-Flur-N G.-D.

gel-filled bladder

Gelfilm
>   G. Ophthalmic

Gelfoam
>   G. Topical

Gel-Kam
>   G.-K. FluoroCare dual rinse kit
>   G.-K. Home Care Gel

Gell classification

Gellé test

Gelpirin

GelShapes scar management system

Gel-Tin

Gemella morbillorum

geminate

geminated teeth

gemination

Gemini alloy

Gemini II

Genac Tablet

Genagesic

Genahist Oral

Genamin
>   G. Cold Syrup
>   G. Expectorant

Genapap

Genaspor

Genatap Elixir

gender dysphoria syndrome

gene
>   p53 tumor suppressor g.

general
>   g. all purpose (GAP)
>   g. all purpose verb
>   g. anesthesia
>   G. Aspirator Q
>   g. intellectual functioning
>   g. linguistics
>   g. oral inaccuracy
>   g. phonetics
>   g. semantics

generalization
>   g. response
>   stimulus g.

generalized
>   g. chondromalacia
>   g. cortical hyperostosis
>   g. diffuse gingivitis
>   g. intellectual impairment
>   g. mastoid hypocellularity
>   g. osteoarthritis (GOA)
>   g. pulpitis
>   g. reinforcer
>   g. spacing

generated occlusal path

generation

generative
>   g. grammar
>   g. semantics
>   g. transformational grammar

generator
>   artificial sound g.
>   ballistic energy g.
>   computerized pattern g. (CPG)
>   Lithoclast ballistic energy g.
>   noise g.
>   Scan Pattern g.
>   ultrasound g.

genetics

Geneye Ophthalmic

genial
>   g. advancement plate
>   g. hypertrophy
>   g. tubercle

geniculate
>   g. ganglion
>   g. ganglion neuralgia
>   medial g.
>   g. neuralgia
>   g. otalgia
>   g. zoster

Genie resin

genioglossus muscle

geniohyoglossus
>   g. muscle

geniohyoid
>   g. muscle
>   g. space
>   g. tubercle

genioid tubercle

genioplasty
>   advancement g.
>   augmentation g.
>   centering g.
>   jumping g.
>   lengthening g.
>   lengthening/advancing g.
>   g. procedure
>   reduction g.
>   reduction/advancement g.
>   sliding g.

staged g.
two-tiered g.
genital branch
genitofemoral
g. causalgia
g. nerve
g. neuralgia
genitoplasty
Genius 4/Digoxigenin RNA labeling kit
genodermatosis
genokeratosis
Genoptic S.O.P. Ophthalmic
Genpril
Gentacidin Ophthalmic
Gentak Ophthalmic
gentamicin
intratympanic g.
prednisolone and g.
Gentian violet
gentle onset
genu
carotid g.
Geocillin
geographica
lingua g.
geographic tongue
geometric nasal flap
geophagia
Georgiade rasp
Gerber
G. attachment
G. hinge
G. space maintainer
gerbil dander
Gerhardt-Semon law
Gerhardt sign
geriatric
g. audiology
geriatrics
dental g.
Geristore
G. repair material
G. restoration
Gerlach tonsil
germ
dental g.
enamel g.
reserve tooth g.
tooth g.
German
G. cockroach

G. measles
G. method
germicidal
germicide
germinal
g. cap
g. center
g. layer
germination
Germ-X
gerodontic
gerodontics
gerodontist
gerodontology
gerontologist
gerontology
Gerow-Harrington retractor, heart-shaped distal end
Gerstmann syndrome
gestant
g. anomaly
g. odontoma
gesture
communicative g.
complementary g.
facial g.
fluence initiating g.
g. language
representational g.
speech g.
supplementary g.
ghost
g. pain
g. tooth
GI
Gingival Index
Giampapa technique
giant
g. cell
g. cell arteritis
g. cell epulis
g. cell fibroma
g. cell hyaline angiopathy
g. cell lesion
g. cell reparative granuloma
g. cell tumor (GCT)
g. follicle lymphoma
g. nevus
g. ragweed
g. word
Gianturco expanding metallic stent
gibberish

G

NOTES

gibbus deformity
Gibson
    G. bandage
    G. inner ear shunt
gigantic benign facial tumor
gigantiform
    g. cementoma
    g. monstrous cementoma
gigantism
gigantomastia
Gigli wire saw
Gilbert
    G. classification of shoulder
      function
    G. stage shoulder abduction
Gilchrist disease
Gilles de la Tourette syndrome
Gillies
    G. cocked hat procedure
    G. fan flap
    G. operation
    G. up and down flap
Gillmore needle
Gilmer
    G. splint
    G. wire
    G. wiring
Gilmore probe
Gilson fixable-removable bar
ginger
gingiva, gen. and pl. **gingivae (G)**
    alveolar g.
    areolar g.
    attached g.
    buccal g.
    cemental g.
    cemented g.
    dehydration of gingivae
    diffuse fibroma of g.
    elephantiasis gingivae
    free g.
    g. index
    interdental g.
    interproximal g.
    labial g.
    lingual g.
    marginal g.
    papillary g.
    prosthetic g.
    septal g.
    stippling g.
    unattached g.
gingiva-bone count index
gingival (G)
    g. abrasion
    g. abscess
    g. anatomy
    g. architecture

    g. asymmetry
    g. atrophy
    g. attachment
    g. augmentation
    g. blanching
    g. bleeding
    g. bleeding index (GBI)
    g. blood flow (GBF)
    g. blood supply
    g. buccal sulcus incision
    g. cartilage
    g. cavity
    g. cavity wall
    g. clamp
    g. cleft
    g. collar
    g. color
    g. consistency
    g. contour
    g. corium
    g. crater
    g. crest
    g. crevice (GC)
    g. crevicular fluid (GCF)
    g. cuff
    g. curettage
    g. curvature
    g. cyst
    g. deformity
    g. denture contour
    g. discoloration
    g. embrasure
    g. enlargement
    g. epithelium
    g. exudate
    g. exudation
    g. festoon
    g. fiber
    g. fibrohemangioma
    g. fibromatosis
    g. finishing line
    g. fissure
    g. fistula
    g. flap
    g. fluid
    g. gland
    g. groove
    g. hemorrhage
    g. hormonal enlargement
    g. hyperplasia
    g. hypertrophy
    G. Index (GI)
    g. inflammation
    g. lancet
    g. ligament
    g. line
    g. margin (GM)
    g. margin trimmer (GMT)

g. massage
g. mat
g. mucosa
g. necrosis
g. nerve
g. onlay graft
g. papilla
G.-Periodontal Index (GPI)
g. physiology
g. pigmentation
g. plasmocytosis
g. pocket
g. point
g. position
g. proliferation
g. radiography
g. recession
g. recession index
g. recontouring
g. relief
g. repositioning
g. resorption
g. retraction
g. septum
g. shrinkage
g. slot
g. space
g. stimulation
g. stippling
g. sulcus
g. surface
g. surface texture
g. third
g. tissue
g. tissue esthetics
g. tissue pack
g. topography
g. trough
g. tumefaction
g. unit
g. zone
gingival-bone
g.-b. count
g.-b. index
gingivalgia
gingivalis
Bacteroides g.
Entamoeba g.
Porphyromonas g.
sulcus g.

gingivectomy
chemosurgical g.
Ochsenbein g.
gingivitis
acute necrotizing g.
acute necrotizing ulcerative g. (ANUG)
acute ulcerating g.
acute ulceromembranous g.
allergic g.
atrophic senile g.
atypical g.
bismuth g.
catarrhal g.
chronic atrophic senile g.
chronic desquamative g.
combined g.
cotton-roll g.
desquamative g.
diabetic g.
diffuse g.
dilantin g.
diphenylhydantoin g.
eruptive g.
g. expulsiva
fusospirillary marginal g.
fusospirochetal g.
generalized diffuse g.
g. gravidarum
hemorrhagic g.
herpetic g.
hormonal g.
human immunodeficiency virus g. (HIV-G)
hyperplastic g.
g. hypertrophica
idiopathic g.
leukemic hyperplastic g.
localized g.
marginal g.
g. marginalis suppurativa
menstruation g.
necrotizing g.
necrotizing ulcerative g. (NUG)
nephritic g.
nonspecific g.
papillary g.
phagedenic g.
plasma cell g.
pregnancy g.
proliferative g.
pseudomembranous g.

NOTES

G

gingivitis *(continued)*
    puberty g.
    recurrent g.
    scorbutic g.
    senile atrophic g.
    streptococcal g.
    suppurative g.
    tuberculous g.
    ulcerative g.
    ulceromembranous g.
    uremic g.
    Vincent g.
gingivoaxial (GA)
gingivobuccal
    g. region
    g. sulcus
gingivobuccoaxial (GBA)
gingivodental
    g. fiber
    g. ligament
gingivoglossitis
gingivolabial
    g. sulcus
gingivolinguoaxial (GLA)
gingivo-osseous
gingivoperiosteoplasty
gingivoplasty
gingivosis
gingivostomatitis
    acute herpetic g.
    acute infectious g.
    acute primary keratotic g. (APKG)
    allergic g.
    atypical g.
    bismuth g.
    herpetic g.
    idiopathic g.
    membranous g.
    menopausal g.
    necrotizing ulcerative g.
    plasma cell g.
    g. syndrome
    white folded g.
ginglymus
ginseng
    American g.
    Asian g.
    Siberian g.
giraffe biopsy forceps
girdle
    compression g.
    Lipo-Medi g.
    Lipopanty g.
    male compression g.
Giromatic handpiece
GLA
    gingivolinguoaxial
glabella

glabellar
    g. bilobed flap
    g. frown line
    g. line
    g. rotation flap
    g. wrinkle
glabrous
    g. skin
glacial
    g. phosphoric acid
glairy
    g. mucus
    g. secretion
gland
    accessory salivary g.
    apocrine g.
    Bauhin g.
    Blandin g.
    Blandin and Nuhn g.'s
    Bowman g.'s
    buccal g.
    buccal mucous g.
    cardiac g.
    Ebner g.'s
    gingival g.
    glossopalatine g.
    intramuscular g. of tongue
    labial g.
    labial minor salivary g.
    lacrimal g.
    lingual g.
    malar g.
    mandibular g.
    meibomian g.
    minor salivary g.
    mixed tumor of salivary g.
    molar g.
    mucous g.
    nasal sebaceous g.
    Nuhn g.
    palatal g.
    palatine g.
    parathyroid g.
    parotid g.
    pituitary g.
    Rivinus g.
    salivary g. (SG)
    sebaceous g.
    seromucous g.
    serous g.
    sublingual g.
    sublingual salivary g.
    submandibular g.
    submaxillary salivary g.
    Suzanne g.
    thyroid g.
    g. of tongue
    Weber g.

glanders
glandular
    g. atrophy
    g. hypertrophy
    g. massage
    g. neoplasm
    g. odontogenic cyst
    g. stroma
    g. zone
glandularis
    cheilitis g.
glans
    reduced g.
glanular triangular flap technique
glanulopasty
    meatoplasty and g. (MAGPI)
glaserian fissure
Glasgow Coma Scale (GCS)
glass
    g. bead sterilizer
    bioactive g.
    g. ceramic
    facial bone reconstruction with
      bioactive g.
    g. ionomer
    g. ionomer cement
    g. ionomer cement light-cured
    g. ionomer cement self-cured
    g. ionomer restorative material
Glastone
glaucoma
Glaucon
GlaucTabs
glaze
    high g.
    low g.
glazing
glenoid fossa
glial tumor
Glick instrument
Glickman periodontal probe
glide
    acentric g.
    mandibular g.
    occlusal g.
    vocalic g.
gliding
    g. of fricative
    g. of liquids
    g. movement
    g. occlusion
Gliocladium

gliofibrosarcoma
glioma
    heterotopic g.
    nasal g.
    peripheral g.
Glisson capsule
global
    g. aphasia
globe
    g. dystopia
    proptotic g.
    g. retropulsion
globular
    g. abdomen
    g. collection
    g. dentin
    g. spaces of Czermak
globule
    dentin g.
globulin
    immune g.
    lymphocyte immune g.
    thyroxine-binding g. (TBG)
globulomaxillary
    g. cyst
    g. fissure
glomerulus, pl. glomeruli
    olfactory glomeruli
glomus
    g. jugulare
    g. jugulare tumor
    g. tympanicum tumor
    g. vagale
    g. vagale tumor
gloss
    loss of g.
glossagra
glossal
glossalgia
glossanthrax
glossectomy
    partial g.
    subtotal g.
    total g.
glossitis
    g. areata exfoliativa
    atrophic g.
    benign migratory g.
    Clarke-Fournier g.
    g. desiccans
    Fournier g.
    glossodynia exfoliativa g.

G

NOTES

glossitis *(continued)*
    Hunter g.
    idiopathic g.
    median rhomboid g.
    g. migrans
    Moeller g.
    parenchymatous g.
    pellagrous g.
    unilateral g.
glossocele
glossocinesthetic *(var. of*
  glossokinesthetic)
glossodontotropism
glossodynia
    g. exfoliativa glossitis
glossodyniotropism
glossoepiglottic
    g. fold
glossograph
glossokinesthetic, glossocinesthetic
glossolalia
glossolaryngeal anastomosis
glossology
glossolysis
glossomantia
glossoncus
glossopalatine
    g. ankylosis
    g. arch
    g. gland
    g. muscle
glossopalatinus
    arcus g.
glossopathy
glossopexy
glossopharyngeal
    g. breathing
    g. nerve
    g. neuralgia
    g. press
    g. tic
glossophytia
glossoplasty
glossoplegia
glossoptosis
glossopyrosis
glossorrhaphy
glossoschisis
glossoscopy
glossospasm
glossosteresis
glossotomy
    labiomandibular g.
    median labiomandibular g.
glossotrichia
glottal
    g. area
    g. attack

    g. catch
    g. chink
    g. click
    g. consonant
    g. cycle
    g. fry
    g. pulse
    g. region
    g. replacement
    g. stop
    g. stroke
    g. tone
    g. vibration
    g. waveform
glottalization
glotte
    coup de g.
glottic
    g. cancer
    g. carcinoma
    g. chink
    g. closure
    g. larynx
    g. prosthesis
    g. spasm
    g. squamous cell carcinoma
    g. stenosis
glottic-subglottic squamous cell
  carcinoma
glottidospasm
glottis, gen. glottidis, pl. glottides
    edema glottidis
    rima glottidis
    spasmus glottidis
glottitis
glottograph
glottology
glove
    Biogel Sensor surgical g.
    Biogel surgeons' g.'s
    disposable g.
    Flowers mandibular g.
    latex g.
    neoprene g.
    nitrile latex utility g.
    Nouvisage Deep Hydration g.
    polynitrile g.
    utility g.
gloving
    double g.
glucagon
glucocorticoid
gluconate
    chlorhexidine g. (CHX)
glucose
    g. 6-phosphate dehydrogenase
glucosteroid
β-glucuronidase

β-D-glucuronidase
glue
 g. ear
 fibrin g.
 histacryl g.
 hydroxyapatite fibrin g.
 Tisseel fibrin g.
 tissue g.
glued-on ear appearance
Gluma
 G. dentin bonding agent
Glutall
glutamate
glutaraldehyde
 acid g.
 g. disinfectant
 g. solution
 g. sterilization
glutaraldehyde/HEMA
Glutarex
glutathione
 oxidized g.
 reduced g.
gluteal
 g. cleft
 g. flap
 g. infarction
gluten-sensitive enteropathy
gluteus
 g. maximus
 g. maximus musculocutaneous flap
Gly
 G. Derm
 G. Derm alphahydroxy acid
 G. Derm cream
 G. Derm glycolic acid
glycerin
 g., lanolin, and peanut oil
 g.-saponin diluent
glycerol
 iodinated g.
 g. test
Glycofed
glycogen
glycol
 ethylene g.
glycolic
 g. acid
 g. acid peeling
 g. skin peel
**glycolide trimethylene carbonate
material**

glycoprotein
glycopyrrolate
glycosaminoglycan (GAG)
 g. chain
glycosialorrhea
glycoside
 eriodictylol g.
Glycyrrhiza
 G. glabra
 G. uralensis
GlyMed
 G. Camouflage System
 G. Plus post-surgical skin care system
 G. Plus skin care product
Gly-Oxide
 G.-O. Oral
GM
 gingival margin
GMT
 gingival margin trimmer
G-myticin Topical
gnarled enamel
gnashing
gnathalgia
gnathic
 g. index
 g. replicator
gnathion
gnathode
gnathodynamics
gnathodynamometer
 bimeter g.
gnathodynia
gnathograph
gnathography
Gnatholator
gnathologic
 g. instrument
 g. orthopaedics
gnathological
gnathology
gnathopalatoschisis
gnathoplasty
gnathoschisis
gnathoscope
Gnathosimulator
gnathostat
gnathostatic cast
gnathostatics
GOA
 generalized osteoarthritis

G

NOTES

goat
 g. dander
 g. milk
goblet cell
Goddio disposable cannula
Godrina doctrine
goiter
 adenomatous g.
 multinodular g.
gold
 Aderer No. 3 Bridge g.
 g. alloy
 g. amalgam
 g. burnisher
 24 carat g.
 g. casting
 cohesive g.
 g. condenser
 g. crown
 Crown Knapp No. 3, No. 9,
  Supreme, T,T g.
 Crown No. 1 g.
 g. and crown scissors
 crystal g.
 g. cylinder
 dental g.
 dental casting g.
 Dent G. No. 1, 2 g.
 direct filling g.
 electrolytic g.
 encapsulated powdered g.
 g. eyelid implant
 fibrous g.
 g. file
 g. foil
 g. foil compaction
 g. foil condensation
 g. foil cylinder
 g. foil pellet
 g. foil rope
 inlay g.
 g. inlay
 Knapp No. 2 g.
 g. knife
 Leff "C" g.
 Leff hard g.
 Leff medium soft g.
 Libra IV extra hard g.
 g. lid load
 mat g.
 MF-Y g.
 Mowrey g.
 noncohesive g.
 g. plate technique
 g. plugger
 25 G. portable CO_2 laser
 powdered g.
 Rx Jeneric dental casting g.

 g. saw
 G. Series bone drilling system
 g. shell crown
 g. shrinkage
 g. sodium thiomalate
 g. solder
 sponge g.
 g. tempering
 white g.
gold-based alloy
gold-copper
 g.-c. alloy
 g.-c. system
Goldenberg implant system
Goldenhar syndrome
goldenrod
goldenseal
Goldent
golden tooth
Goldman
 G. curette
 G. Fox probe
 G. nasal tip reconstruction
Goldman-Fox
 G.-F. knife
 G.-F. scissors
Goldman-Fristoe Test of Articulation
Goldman-Fristoe-Woodcock
 G.-F.-W. Auditory Skills Battery
 G.-F.-W. Test of Auditory
  Discrimination
Goldman-Ponti technique
Goldner modification
gold-palladium
 g.-p. alloy
 g.-p. sputter
Goldscheider syndrome
Goldsmith I inlay
gold-weight procedure
golf tee hollow titanium cannula
Golgi
 G. apparatus
 G. complex
 G. corpuscle
 G. membranes
 G. saccule
 G. system
Goltz syndrome
Gomco
 G. clamp
 G. pump
Gomori methenamine silver stain
gomphosis
gonadal
 g. exposure guideline
 g. shield
Gonak

gondii
>   *Toxoplasma g.*

gonial angle
goniometer
gonion
Goniosol
gonococcal stomatitis
gonorrhoeae
>   *Neisseria g.*

Gonzalez specialized dissecting cannula
good
>   g. cosmesis
>   g. take

Goodenough draw-a-man test
Goody Headache Powders
gooseberry
goose feather
Gordofilm Liquid
Gordon bead forceps
gordonii
>   *Streptococcus g.*

Gore
>   G. Resolut regenerative tissue
>   membrane
>   G. subcutaneous augmentation
>   material

Gore-Tex
>   G.-T. alloplastic material
>   G.-T. augmentation material
>   (GTAM)
>   G.-T. augmentation membrane
>   (GTAM)
>   G.-T. closure
>   G.-T. graft
>   G.-T. lip augmentation
>   G.-T. membrane
>   G.-T. mesh
>   G.-T. periodontal material
>   G.-T. regenerative material
>   G.-T. soft-tissue patch
>   G.-T. tag

Gorlin
>   G. cyst
>   G. syndrome

Gormel Creme
Gorney face lift scissors
gorondou
Goshgarian transpalatal bar
Goslee tooth
Gothic
>   G. arch
>   G. arch tracer

G. arch tracing
G. palate

Gottlieb epithelial attachment
gouge
>   U X-Acto g.
>   X-Acto g.

Gougerot-Sjögren syndrome
Goulian knife
goundou
gout
gouty pearl
GPI
>   Gingival-Periodontal Index

GPRL
>   gamma probe radiolocalization

GPX
>   G. bur
>   G. rotary instrument

Gracey curette
gracilis
>   g. muscle
>   g. muscle flap
>   g. musculocutaneous flap
>   g. myocutaneous vaginal
>   reconstruction

graciloplasty
>   dynamic g.
>   stimulated g.

grade
>   Baker g.
>   Brackman g.
>   House-Brackman g. I–VI
>   g. I–IV breast ptosis
>   Kaplan-Feinstein comorbidity g.
>   lymphedema g. II, III
>   Meurmann external ear anomaly g.

Gradenigo syndrome
gradient
>   g. echo technique
>   g. recalled acquisition in the
>   steady state (GRASS)

grading
>   insufficient jaw g.
>   jaw g.
>   mean rejection g. (MRG)

gradual
>   g. curve
>   g. tooth separation
>   g. topic shift

graft
>   accordion g.
>   adipodermal g.

NOTES

G

graft *(continued)*
　　alar batten g.
　　AlloDerm acellular dermal g.
　　AlloDerm cellular dermal g.
　　allogenic g.
　　allogenic keratinocyte g.
　　alloplastic g.
　　alveolar bone g.
　　alveolar cleft g.
　　amnion g.
　　anastomosed g.
　　animal g.
　　aortofemoral bypass g.
　　augmentation g.
　　auricular cartilage g.
　　auricular composite g.
　　autodermic g.
　　autogeneic g.
　　autogenous bone g.
　　autogenous cartilage g.
　　autogenous corticocancellous g.
　　autogenous fat g.
　　autogenous nerve g.
　　autologous fat g.
　　autologous iliac crest bone g.
　　autologous rib bone g.
　　autoplastic g.
　　Baker composite g.
　　BioGran resorbable synthetic
　　　bone g.
　　BioGran synthetic g.
　　Blair-Brown g.
　　bone g.
　　brephoplastic g.
　　buccal mucosa g.
　　cable g.
　　calvarial bone g.
　　cancellous cellular bone g.
　　cantilever g.
　　cantilevered bone g.
　　cartilage g.
　　cartilaginous g.
　　cartilaginous autologous thin
　　　septal g.
　　CATS g.
　　cavum conchal cartilage g.
　　CCB g.
　　chessboard g.
　　chip g.
　　chondromucosal g.
　　composite inlay antral and nasal
　　　bone g.
　　conchal cartilage g.
　　connective tissue g.
　　cortical bone g.
　　corticocancellous block g.
　　costal cartilage g.
　　costochondral g. (CCG)

　　cross-facial nerve g.
　　cultured mucosal g.
　　cutis g.
　　cymba conchal cartilage g.
　　Davis g.
　　delayed g.
　　Dembone g.
　　demineralized bone g.
　　dermal g.
　　dermal-fat g.
　　dermofat g.
　　double-barreled fibular bone g.
　　double papilla g.
　　double papilla pedicle g.
　　Douglas g.
　　earlobe composite g.
　　epidermic g.
　　Esser g.
　　fascia g.
　　fascicular g.
　　fat g.
　　fat cell g.
　　fibular onlay strut g.
　　filler g.
　　free autogenous corticocancellous
　　　iliac bone g.
　　free autogenous pearl fat g.
　　free composite g.
　　free cutaneous nerve g.
　　free fat g.
　　free gingival g.
　　free muscle g.
　　free skin g.
　　full-thickness periodontal g.
　　full-thickness skin g.
　　funicular g.
　　gingival onlay g.
　　Gore-Tex g.
　　g. harvest
　　heterologous g.
　　heteroplastic g.
　　heterospecific g.
　　heterotopic g.
　　heterotrophic bone g.
　　homologous g.
　　homoplastic g.
　　hydroxyapatite block g.
　　hyperplastic g.
　　hypod interposition g.
　　iliac crest bone g.
　　implantation g.
　　infusion g.
　　inlay g.
　　interspecific g.
　　isogeneic g.
　　isologous g.
　　isoplastic g.
　　Kiel g.

Kimura cartilage g.
Krause g.
Krause-Wolfe g.
lateral pedicle g.
LifeCell AlloDerm acellular
  dermal g.
linear g.
lyophilized dura g.
mattressed onlay g.
McIndoe inlay g.
McIndoe skin g.
mesh g.
meshed split-thickness skin g.
metatarsal free vascularized g.
microvascular g.
mucoperiosteal periodontal g.
mucosal periodontal g.
muscular g.
nerve g.
neuromuscular pedicle g.
nonvascularized bone g. (NVBG)
nonvascularized fibular strut g.
Ollier g.
Ollier-Thiersch g.
omental skin g.
onlay bone g.
onlay tip g.
orthotopic g.
orthotropic bone g.
OsteoGen bone g.
osteoperiosteal g.
overlay cantilever bone g.
papilla g.
papillary pedicle g.
partial-thickness periodontal g.
pedicle g.
pedicled cartilage g.
pedicled skin g.
pelvic peritoneal g.
perichondrocutaneous g.
PerioGlas synthetic bone g.
periosteal g.
Phemister g.
pinch g.
polytetrafluoroethylene membrane g.
porcine skin g.
postage stamp g.
primary skin g.
punch g.
revascularized bone g.
Reverdin g.
Robinson vein g.

saphenous vein interposition g.
scapula crest pedicled bone g.
septal chondromucosal g.
shield-type g.
sieve g.
skin g.
sleeve g.
split calvarial g.
split-skin g.
split-thickness periodontal g.
split-thickness skin g. (STSG)
spreader g.
Stent g.
subepithelial connective tissue g.
substernal colon interposition g.
sural nerve cable g.
sutured in place, shield-shaped
  tip g.
swaging g.
syngeneic g.
synthetic bone g.
temporalis fascia g.
tendon g.
Thiersch skin g.
transposition of g.
T-shaped g.
twin-barreled fibular g.
umbrella g.
undemineralized bone g.
underlayer cantilever bone g.
unmeshed split-thickness skin g.
vascularized bone g. (VBG)
vascularized tendon g.
white g.
Wolfe g.
Wolfe-Krause g.
zooplastic g.

Graftac absorbable skin tack
Graftac-S skin stapler
GraftCyte
  G. hydrating mist
  G. moist dressing
  G. system for wound care
grafting
  alveolar g.
  aortofemoral bypass g.
  areolar g.
  autogenous g.
  bone g.
  dermal g.
  dural g.
  fascial g.

NOTES

G

grafting (*continued*)
  mucosal g.
  onlay bone g.
  osseous g.
  preprosthetic g.
  skin g.
graft-versus-host-disease (GVHD)
grain dust
gramicidin
  neomycin, polymyxin B, and g.
gramma grass
grammar
  case g.
  finite g.
  generative g.
  generative transformational g.
  particular g.
  pedagogical g.
  phrase structure g.
  pivot g.
  prescriptive g.
  scientific g.
  traditional g.
  transformational g.
  transformational generative g.
  universal g.
grammatic
  g. closure
  g. method
grammatical
  g. analysis
  G. Analysis of Elicited Language
    (GAEL)
  g. category
  g. component
  g. equivalent
  g. meaning
  g. morpheme
  g. structure
gram-negative microorganism
gram-positive
  g.-p. bacteria
  g.-p. microorganism
gram-rad
Gram stain
grand mal
Granger articulator
granular
  g. bacteriosis
  g. bed
  g. cell
  g. cell myeloblastoma
  g. cell myoblastoma
  g. cell tumor (GCT)
  g. layer
  g. reticulum

granulation
  g. polyp
  g. tissue
granule
  Birbeck g.
  Bollinger g.
  cortico-spongeous bone g.
  cytoplasmic g.
  Dembone demineralized cortical g.
  discharged g.
  DynaGraft g.
  Fordyce g.'s
  immature g.
  keratohyalin g.
  lamellar g.
  mucigen g.
  mucin g.
  secretory g.
  serous g.
  sulfur g.
  Zymogen g.
Granulex
granulocyte colony-stimulant factor
granulocytic phagocyte
granulocytopenia
granuloma
  g. annulare
  apical g.
  central giant cell g.
  central giant cell reparative g.
  cholesterol g.
  contact g.
  dental g.
  eosinophilic g.
  epithelial g.
  g. fissuratum
  foreign body g.
  giant cell reparative g.
  g. gravidarum
  histiocytic g.
  histocytic g.
  infectious g.
  internal pulp g.
  intracordal g.
  Langerhans cell eosinophilic g.
  laryngeal g.
  lethal midline g.
  lipophagic g.
  midline lethal g.
  midline malignant reticulosis g.
  necrotizing g.
  oil g.
  ointment g.
  paraffin g.
  periapical g.
  peripheral giant cell reparative g.
  peripheral reparative g.
  pulpal g.

pulse g.
purulent apical g.
pyogenic g.
g. pyogenicum
reparative giant cell g.
root end g.
silicone g.
specific g.
Teflon g.
g. telangiectaticum
traumatic g.
traumatic eosinophilic g.
traumatic ulcerative g.
tuberculoid g.
ulcerated g.
ulcerative eosinophilic g.

granulomatic reaction
granulomatosa
cheilitis g.
granulomatosis
Langerhans cell g.
Wegener g.
granulomatous
g. amebic encephalitis
g. cheilitis
g. disease
g. inflammation
g. sialadenitis
g. tenosynovitis
g. tissue
g. zone
granulosum
stratum g.
granulosus
Echinococcus g.
grape
grapefruit
graph
logarithmic g.
grapheme
graphite tattoo
grasp
finger g.
modified pen g.
palm-and-thumb g.
pen g.
grasper
Blakesley g.
GRASS
gradient recalled acquisition in the steady
state

grass
Bahia g.
Bermuda g.
canary g.
gramma g.
Johnson g.
June g.
oat g.
orchard g.
perennial rye g.
redtop A g.
reed canary g.
rye g.
salt g.
sorghum g.
sweet vernal g.
timothy g.
velvet g.
wild rye g.
Zoysia g.
grasses antigen
grass-line ligature
gravel voice
grave phoneme
Graves
G. disease
G. ophthalmopathy
gravidarum
epulis g.
granuloma g.
striae g.
gravis
myasthenia g.
gravitational
g. force
g. problem
gravity
center of g. (COG)
gray (Gy)
g. appearance
G. flexible intramedullary reamer
g. green stone
g. line of upper eyelid
g. stone
Grazer
G. abdominoplasty
elliptical plication of G.
great auricular nerve
greater
g. horn
g. palatine artery
g. palatine canal

G

NOTES

greater *(continued)*
    g. palatine foramen
    g. palatine sulcus of maxilla
    g. petrosal nerve
    g. superficial petrosal nerve
    G. Taper File
    g. wing of sphenoid
Greco cutting block
Greek helmet facies
Green
    G. Endo-Ice pulp tester
    G. factor
green
    g. amaranth
    g. ash
    g. bean
    g. coffee bean
    g. pepper
    g. stain
    g. stone
    g. tooth
greenstick
    g. fracture
    g. medialization
greffotome
Greig syndrome
gression
Grice suture needle
Griesinger
    G. sign
    G. symptom
Griffin appliance
Griffith-Brown forceps
Grifulvin V
grimace
grinding
    habitual g.
    g. movement
    nonfunctional g.
    selective g.
    spot g.
    g. surface
    g. tooth
    g. wheel
grinding-in
Grip
    G. cement
grip strength
Grisactin Ultra
Grisel syndrome
griseofulvin
Gris-PEG
Gritman No. 6. carver
gritty
groin flap
grommet
Groningen button

groove
    abutment g.
    ala-facial g.
    alar facial g.
    alveolingual g.
    anterior palatine g.
    buccal g. (BG)
    buccal developmental g. (BDG)
    central developmental g. (CDG)
    dental g.
    developmental g.
    distal oblique g. (DOG)
    distobuccal developmental g. (DBDG)
    distolingual g. (DLG)
    distolingual developmental g.
    g. extension
    fifth cusp g. (FCG)
    free g.
    free gingival g. (FGG)
    g. fricative
    gingival g.
    interdental g. (IDG)
    intermandibular g.
    intertubercular g.
    labiomental g.
    lingual g. (LG)
    lingual developmental g. (LDG)
    mesial marginal developmental g. (MMDG)
    mesiobuccal developmental g. (MBDG)
    mesiolingual g. (MLG)
    mesiolingual developmental g. (MLDG)
    nasofacial g.
    palatine g.
    palatomaxillary g.
    retention g.
    supplemental g. (SG)
grooved
    g. hemostat
    g. tongue
grooving
gross
    g. lesion
    g. motor
    g. sound
Grossan
    G. nasal irrigator tip with Water Pik
    G. nasal irrigator tip with Water Pik and saline
Grosse & Kempf locking nail
Grossman
    G. formula
    G. formula root canal sealer

ground
  g. lamella
  g. substance
ground-glass lesion
groundsel
group
  g. A β-hemolytic streptococcus
    (GABHS)
  g. audiometer
  g. audiometry
  control g.
grouping
  tumor stage g.
growth
  asymmetric maxillomandibular g.
  basicranial sagittal g.
  chondromatous g.
  facial g.
  g. factor
  hamartomatous g.
Gruber method
GSI
  GSI 16 audiometer
  GSI 60 distortion-product
    otoacoustic emission device
GSR
  galvanic skin response
GSRA
  galvanic skin response audiometry
GSW
  gunshot wound
GTAM
  Gore-Tex augmentation material
  Gore-Tex augmentation membrane
GT Files
GTR
  guided tissue regeneration
G-type reamer
Guaifed
  G.-PD
guaifenesin
  hydrocodone, pseudoephedrine,
    and g.
  g. and phenylephrine
  g. and phenylpropanolamine
  g., phenylpropanolamine, and
    dextromethorphan
  g., phenylpropanolamine, and
    phenylephrine
  g. and pseudoephedrine
  g., pseudoephedrine, and codeine

  g., pseudoephedrine, and
    dextromethorphan
Guaifenex
  G. PPA 75
  G. PSE
GuaiMAX-D
Guaipax
Guaitab
Guaivent
Guai-Vent/PSE
guard
  Ad-hear cerumen g.
  bite g.
  mouth g.
  occlusal g.
Guberina
  system universal verbotonol
    audition G. (SUVAG)
gubernacular
  g. canal
  g. cord
gubernaculum
  gubernaculum dentis
Guérin fracture
Guiatex
Guiatuss
  G. CF
  G. DAC
  G. PE
Guiatussin DAC
guidance
  condylar g.
  cuspid g.
  developmental g.
  endoscopic g.
  incisal g.
guide
  adjustable anterior g.
  anterior g.
  condylar g.
  incisal g.
  microdrilling g.
  mold g.
  g. plane
  shade g.
  Slick stylette endotracheal tube g.
  V-tunnel g.
guided
  g. bone regeneration (GBR)
  g. eruption
  g. tissue regeneration (GTR)

NOTES

guideline
>bone marrow exposure g.
>clasp g.
>Cummer g.
>exposure g.
>eye exposure g.
>gonadal exposure g.
>operator's x-ray exposure g.
>parotid gland exposure g.
>patient exposure g.
>thyroid exposure g.
>x-ray exposure g.

guiding
>g. incline
>g. plane

Guillain-Barré syndrome
guillotine
>tonsil g.

guinea pig dander
gullwing
>g. incision
>g. pattern

gum
>g. contour
>g. cuff
>free g.
>Karaya g.
>g. lancet
>g. line
>g. massage
>g. pad
>g. polyp
>g. resection
>g. septum
>sterculia g.
>trench g.

gumboil
gumma
gummatous necrosis
gummy smile
gun
>B-D g.
>enhancement g.
>Messing g.
>Messing root canal g.
>root canal g.

Gunderson conjunctival flap procedure
Gunning
>G. one-piece splint
>G. two-piece splint

gunshot wound (GSW)
gusher
>labyrinthine g.
>perilymph g.
>perilymphatic g.
>X-linked progressive mixed
>deafness with perilymphatic g.
>(DFNX3)

gusher-associated deafness
gustatory
>g. bud
>g. center
>g. lacrimation
>g. pore
>g. reflex
>g. rhinorrhea
>g. sweating
>g. tearing

Gustilo soft tissue classification
gutta-percha
>g.-p. baseplate
>cold g.-p.
>compacted g.-p.
>condensed g.-p.
>g.-p. cone
>partially dissolved g.-p.
>g.-p. point
>g.-p. spreader
>thermoplastic g.-p.
>warm g.-p.

guttural
>g. voice

gutturophonia
gutturotetany
Guyon
>G. canal
>G. canal release

Guyuron EAP
GVHD
>graft-versus-host-disease

Gy
>gray

gynecomastia
>g. vest

Gyne-Lotrimin
gynoplasty
gypoglossal nerve
gypsum
>g. crystal
>g. die
>g. hardener
>g. hemihydrate
>g. retarder

Gyroscan
>Philips G.

gyrus, pl. gyri
>angular g.
>frontal gyri
>Heschl gyri
>postcentral g.
>precentral g.
>supramarginal g.
>supramarginal angular gyri
>temporal g.
>transverse temporal gyri

Gysi articulator

HA
 hydroxyapatite
 hydroxylapatite
  Osteograf/N HA
habenula perforata
habilitation
 audiologic h.
habit
 normal swallowing h.
habit-breaking appliance
Habitrol
habitual
 h. centric
 h. grinding
 h. occlusion
 h. pitch
 h. temporomandibular joint luxation
habituation
 h. therapy
hackberry
HA-coated
 H.-c. root-form dental implant
Hadeco MiniDop Doppler
Hader
 H. bar clip
 H. bar pattern
 H. implant bar
Hade-ring attachment
HAE
 hearing aid evaluation
Haemogram blood loss monitor
Haemophilus influenzae
Hageman factor
hag teeth
HAIC
 H. gain
 H. output
hair
 h. bulb
 h. cell
 h. collar sign
 Frey h.'s
 h. step
 h. tooth
 h. transplantation
 h. transplant punch
hairline
hair-on-end appearance
hairpin clasp
hairy
 h. leukoplakia (HL)
 h. nevus
 h. tongue

Hajek
 H. elevator
 H. incision
halcinonide
Halcion
Halenol Childrens
half-and-half clasp
half-cap crown
half-mouth technique
Halfprin 81
half-seated recumbent dorsal position
half-value
 h.-v. layer (HVL)
 h.-v. thickness
halisteresis
halitosis
Hall
 H. surgical drill
Haller
 H. cell
 H. plexus
Hallermann-Streiff syndrome
Hallgren syndrome
Hall-Morris biphase
Hallpike
 H. maneuver
 H. position
 H. test
hallucination
hallux valgus
halo
 h. blue nevus
 h. deformity
 h. effect
 h. head frame
 h. test for CSF leak
 h. test for CSF rhinorrhea
halobetasol
Halog
 H.-E
halogen
 h. dual lightsource
 h. lamp
 h. light source
halothane
Halotussin
 H. DAC
 H. PE
Halstead
 H. radical mastectomy
 H. radical mastectomy procedure
Halsted
 H. mosquito forceps
 H. mosquito hemostat
Haltran

H

halzoun
hamartoma
    angiomatous lymphoid h.
    h. of dental lamina
    facial h.
    neuromuscular h.
    odontogenic gingival epithelial h.
hamartomatous
    h. growth
Hamas and Rohrich technique
hammer
    dental h.
    h. nose
    sledge h.
hammock ligament
Hammond splint
hamster dander
hamular
    h. notch
    h. process
hamuloglossus
hamulus
    pterygoid h.
Hamy plane
Hanau
    H. 130-21 articulator
    H. modular articulator face-bow
hand
    h. condenser
    h. ischemia
    h. mechanical spatulator
    h. scaling
    h. sensibility
    h. skeleton
    spoon-shaped h.
    h. spreader
    ulnar club h.
handcutting instrument
handedness
    left-h.
    right-h.
hand-foot-and-mouth disease
hand-held probe
handicap
    International Classification of
    Impairments, Disabilities, and H.'s
    (ICIDH)
    voice h.
handicapped
    educationally mentally h. (EMH)
    multiply h.
    perceptually h.
    trainable mentally h. (TMH)
Handi-Liner cavity varnish
handle
    Bard-Parker h.
    Essar h.
    Klein Delrin Luer lock h.

    knurled h.
    love h.'s
    h. of malleus
    measurement control h.
    test h.
    Unigauge h.
handler
    intermediate h.
handpiece
    air-bearing turbine h.
    contra-angle h.
    Dermastat dermatology h.
    DynaSurg electric h.
    Dynatrak h.
    Endo-Gripper endodontic h.
    Excaliber h.
    Giromatic h.
    hexascan computerized
     dermatology h.
    high-speed h.
    Kerr M4 safety h.
    low-speed h.
    Micro oral surgery h.
    micropigmentation h.
    Microstat h.
    M4 safety h.
    oral surgery h. (OSH)
    Racer h.
    right-angle h.
    h. round bur
    straight h.
    SureScan scanning h.
    Surgitek h.
    Titan slow-speed h.
    h. tubing
    ultra-high-speed h.
    ultrasonic h.
    water-turbine h.
    W&H h.
Hand-Schüller-Christian disease
handwashing
hanging
    h. chain method
    h. columella
hangnail
Hanhart syndrome
Hank Balanced Salt Solution
Hannover Polytrauma Score
Hansen
    cells of H.
    H. disease
Hanson speed bracket
Hapex bioactive material
haplology
Hapsburg
    H. jaw
    H. lip
Hapset bone graft plaster

haptic
   h. feedback
   h. perception
   h. system
hard
   American Gold "C" partial
      extra h.
   American Gold "T" bridge h.
   h. biscuit
   h. bisque
   h. bristle
   h. calculus
   h. cleft palate
   h. glottal attack
   h. of hearing
   h. mallet
   h. palate
   h. percussion
   h. set alginate
   h. and soft tissue
   h. solder
   h. tissue
   h. tissue replacement (HTR)
   h. x-ray
hardener
   gypsum h.
hardening
   h. heat treatment
   h. solution
hardness
   Brinell h.
   indentation h.
   Knoop h.
   Mohs h.
   h. resistance
hard-soft palate junction
hard-wire auditory trainer
Hardy retractor
harelip
   h. suture
Har-el pharyngeal tube
harlequin
   h. deformity
   h. orbit
harmonic
   h. distortion
harmony
   facial h.
   functional occlusal h.
   occlusal h.
   h. process
harnessing extra skin

Harpagophytum procumbens
harshness
   phonation type h.
Hart-Dunn attachment
Hartmann curette
Hartman solution
harvest
   double rectus h.
   endoscope-assisted rectus abdominis
      muscle flap h.
   endoscopic h.
   graft h.
harvesting
   h. pistol
Harvey vapor sterilizer
HAS
   high-amplitude sucking
   HAS technique
Hashimoto disease
Hassall corpuscle
Hassan-type port
Hasson laparoscopic trocar
Hatch
   H. clamp
   H. gingival clamp
hatchet
   black h.
   California h.
   enamel h.
   h. evacuator
   h. excavator
HA-threaded hexlock implant
HAV
   hepatitis A virus
haversian
   h. bone
   h. canal
   h. system
hawk-bill incisor
Hawley
   H. bite plate
   H. chart
   H. retainer
   H. retaining orthodontic appliance
Haws
   H. Screening Test for Functional
      Articulation Disorder
   H. type brachydactyly
hawthorn berry
hay
   h. fever
   h. rake fixed orthodontic appliance

NOTES

H

Hayfebrol Liquid
Hayflick limit of fibroblast replication
hazardous waste
hazelnut
HB
    Tagamet HB
HBcAg
    hepatitis B core antigen
HBeAg
    hepatitis B e antigen
HBGS
    House-Brackman Grading Scale
HBID
    hereditary benign intraepithelial
      dyskeratosis
HBIG
    hepatitis B immunoglobulin
HBO
    hyperbaric oxygen
      HBO dive
      HBO therapy
HBO-induced angiogenesis
HBsAg
    hepatitis B surface antigen
HBV
    hepatitis B virus
HC
    Bancap HC
HCl
    azelastine HCl
    cetirizine HCl
    Cleocin HCl
    etidocaine HCl
    fexofenadine HCl
    hydromorphine HCl
    minocycline HCl
    oxymetazoline HCl
    pentazocine HCl
    propoxyphene HCl
    pseudoephedrine HCl
    ranitidine HCl
HCl/hydrocortisone
    ciprofloxacin HCl/h.
H-conformation
HCV
    hepatitis C virus
HDP
    high definition power
H drain
HDV
    hepatitis delta virus
H&E
    hematoxylin and eosin
      H&E staining
head
    cold in the h.
    condyle h.
    contra-angle h.

    malleus h.
    h. of malleus
    mandibular h.
    h. mirror
    h. and neck cancer
    h. and neck squamous cell
      carcinoma (HNSCC)
    h. shadow effect
    h. turn technique
headache
    cluster h.
    dental h.
    migraine h.
    muscle contraction h.
    muscle tension h.
    ocular h.
    tension h.
    traction h.
    vascular h.
headcap
    plaster h.
    h. plaster
headgear
    h. force
    high-pull h.
    horizontal pull h.
    Kloehn h.
headlamp
    Keeler fiberoptic h.
headlight
    Clip-Lite clip-on h.
    Heine UBL 100 h.
    Welch Allyn Solarc h.
head-neck replacement (HNR)
headpiece
    Novascan scanning h.
healed dental caries
healer
    folk h.
healing screw
Healthco
    H. topical fluoride gel
    H. VLC
hear
hearing
    h. aid
    h. aid evaluation (HAE)
    central h.
    color h.
    h. conservation
    cross h.
    end-organ of h.
    functional h.
    H. Handicap Inventory for the
      Elderly (HHIE)
    Helmholtz theory of h.
    h. impairment
    h. impairment degrees

h. level (HL)
h. loss
mean h.
normal h.
h. protection device (HPD)
h. protector
resonance theory of h.
h. science
h. threshold level (HTL)
H. Threshold Level scale
visual h.
Weber test for h.
Hear Now research project
Heartline
Heart pillow infusor
heat
h. shock proteins
steam h.
h. temperature vulcanized (HTV)
h. treatment
heat-curing
h.-c. plastic
h.-c. resin
heated plugger
heater
compound h.
heat-seal pouch
heat-sear technique
Heat-Treated
Profilnine H.-T.
heat-up period
heavy
h. body impression material
h. condensation
h. skin
heavy-bodied material
Hecht-Beals-Wilson syndrome
Heck disease
Hedström file
heel
h. of denture
Heerfordt syndrome
Heft-Parker pain scale
height
alveolar h.
anterior facial h. (AFH)
buccopalatal h.
h. of contour
cusp h.
eyebrow h.
facial h.
lower anterior dental h.

h. of mandibular ramus
mental h.
nasal h.
h. of occlusion
orbital h.
h. of palate
philtral h.
sural h.
tongue h.
vertical bony h.
Heimlich
H. maneuver
H. tube
Heine UBL 100 headlight
helcoplasty
helical
h. coil
h. crease
h. crus
h. loop archwire
h. rim
h. spring
h. surgery
helicis (*gen. and pl. of* helix)
helicoid
h. endosseous implant
h. endosteal implant
helicotrema
Heliomolar system
Helio Progress
Heliosit resin
Helistat
helium
h. neon beam
h. speech
helium-neon laser
helix, gen. and pl. **helicis**
cauda helicis
crus helicis
h. of ear
spina helicis
sulcus cruris helicis
Helmholtz
H. place theory
H. theory of hearing
Helminthosporium halodes **antigen**
Helonias dioica
helper T cell count
helping verb
Helweg-Larssen syndrome
HEMA
2-hydroxyethyl methacrylate

NOTES

H

hemagluttination
hemangioameloblastoma
hemangioendothelioma
    spindle cell h.
hemangiofibroma
    juvenile h.
hemangioma
    arteriovenous h.
    capillary h.
    cavernous h.
    central h.
    cherry h.
    congenital subglottic h.
    deep h.
    esophageal h.
    hypertrophic h.
    intramuscular h.
    laryngeal h.
    mixed h.
    sclerosing h.
    scrotal h.
    senile h.
    strawberry h.
    subglottic h.
    superficial h.
hemangiomatosis
hemangiomatous
hemangiopericytoma
    malignant h.
hemangiosarcoma
hematogenetic calculus
hematogenous
    h. metastasis
hematologic dyscrasia
hematoma
    calcific h.
    epiglottic h.
    fibrosed h.
    orbital h.
    subcutaneous h.
    subungual h.
hematopoietic growth factor
hematotympanum
hematoxylin
    h. and eosin (H&E)
    iron h.
    periodic acid-Schiff h.
hemiageusia, hemiageustia, hemigeusia
hemianosmia
hemiatrophy
    lingual h.
    h. of the tongue
hemiback flap
hemiclavicular line
hemidesmosome
hemiface
hemifacial
    h. atrophy

    h. hypertrophy
    h. microsomia (HFM, HM)
    h. microsomia anomaly
    h. spasm
hemigeusia (*var. of* hemiageusia)
hemiglossal
hemiglossectomy
hemiglossitis
hemignathia
hemihydrate
    α-calcium sulfate h.
    β-calcium sulfate h.
    h. crystal
    gypsum h.
    sulfate h.
hemihypertrophy
    facial h.
    h. of the tongue
hemilaryngectomy
hemilingual
hemimacroglossia
hemimandible
    h. reconstruction
hemimandibular hyperplasia
hemimandibulectomy
hemimaxillae
hemimaxillectomy
    radical h.
hemin
heminasal defect
hemiplegia
hemisect
hemisection
    tooth h.
hemisectomy
hemiseptum of interalveolar bone
hemisphere
hemistransfixion
hemistrumectomy
hemitongue flap
hemitransfixion incision
hemochromatosis
hemoconcentration
hemocyanin
    keyhole limpet h. (KLH)
Hemodent
hemodialysis
    continuous arteriovenous h.
    (CAVHD)
hemolytic streptococcus
α-hemolytic streptococcus
β-hemolytic streptococcus
hemolyticum
    Corynebacterium h.
hemophilia
hemophiliac
hemoptysis
    massive h.

hemorrhage
adenotonsillar h.
alveolar h.
arterial h.
gingival h.
laryngeal h.
nasal h.
petechial h.
postextraction h.
subarachnoid h.
subconjunctival h.
venous h.
hemorrhagic
h. bone cyst
h. cyst
h. gingivitis
h. laryngitis
h. pansinusitis
h. telangiectasia
hemosiderin
h. staining of the skin
hemosiderosis
hemostasis
hemostat
Allis h.
Carmault h.
curved Kelly h.
curved mosquito h.
Dean tonsil h.
h. film holder
fine-tipped mosquito h.
grooved h.
Halsted mosquito h.
Instat collagen absorbable h.
Instat MCH microfibrillar
collagen h.
Kelly h.
microfibrillar collagen h.
mosquito h.
straight mosquito h.
h. technique
hemostatic forceps
Hemotene
hemotympanum
Hemovac
H. drain
H. suction device
hen-cluck stertor
HeNe beam
Henke-Ject intraligamental syringe
Henle
H. spine

Hennebert sign
henpuye
HEPA
high-efficiency particulate air
heparan sulfate
heparin
h. irrigation
hepatitis
h. A virus (HAV)
h. B core antigen (HBcAg)
h. B e antigen (HBeAg)
h. B immunoglobulin (HBIG)
h. B surface antigen (HBsAg)
h. B transmission
h. B virus (HBV)
chronic active h.
h. C virus (HCV)
h. delta
h. delta virus (HDV)
infectious h.
non-A h.
non-B h.
serum h.
viral h.
Heptavax-B
Herb fold
Herbst appliance
Herculite
H. XRV Lab system
hereditary
h. benign intraepithelial dyskeratosis
(HBID)
h. brown opalescent teeth
h. crowding
h. dark teeth
h. ectodermal dysplasia
h. enamel hypocalcification
h. gingival fibromatosis
h. hemorrhagic telangiectasis
h. opalescent dentin
h. opalescent teeth
heredity
Hering-Breuer reflex
hermaphrodite
hermetic seal
hernia
diaphragmatic h.
hiatal h.
muscle h.
planned ventral h.
herniation
disk h.

NOTES

H

267

hernioplasty
herpangina
herpes
    h. labialis
    h. simplex
    h. simplex virus antibody
    h. simplex virus, type 1, 2
    h. stomatitis
    h. virus
    h. zoster
    h. zoster cephalicus
    h. zoster ophthalmicus
    h. zoster oticus
herpesvirus
    human h.
Herpesvirus hominis
herpetic
    h. esophagitis
    h. gingivitis
    h. gingivostomatitis
    h. stomatitis
    h. ulcer
    h. whitlow
herpetiform
    h. aphthae
herpetiformis
    dermatitis h. (DH)
Herplex Ophthalmic
herringbone pattern
Herrmann syndrome
Hertel
    H. exophthalmometer
    H. exophthalmometry
    H. eye position evaluation system
    H. ophthalmometer
    H. value
Hertwig
    H. epithelial root sheath
    root sheath of H.
    H. sheath
hertz (Hz)
hertzian experiment
Herxheimer reaction
Herying sign
HES
    hypereosinophilic syndrome
Heschl gyri
hesitation
    developmental h.
    h. phenomenon
heterodermic
heterodont
    h. dentition
heterogeneous
    h. word
heterogenous
heterograft
heterolalia

heteroliteral
heterologous
    h. graft
    h. material
hetero-osteoplasty
heterophemy
heterophile antibody test
heterophonia
heterophthongia
heteroplastic graft
heteroplasty
heterosexual
heterospecific
    h. graft
heterotopia, heterotropy
heterotopic
    h. glioma
    h. graft
heterotransplantation
heterotrophic
    h. bone graft
    h. cyst
    h. gastrointestinal mucosa of oral
      cavity
    h. oral gastrointestinal cyst
heterotropy (*var. of* heterotopia)
Hetter pyramid tip
hexachlorophene
Hexadrol
    H. Phosphate
hexahydrate
    aluminum chloride h.
hexamethylmelamine
hexascan
    h. computerized dermatology
      handpiece
    tunable laser with h.
hex implant
hexlock implant
hexokinase
hexosediphosphatase
hexose phosphate
hexylresorcinol
Heyer Schulte implant device
HF
    high frequency
      HF average full-on gain
      HF average SSPL 90
H-file
    engine H.-f.
    Mity engine H.-f.
HFJV
    high-frequency jet ventilation
H-flap incision
HFM
    hemifacial microsomia
HGM Spectrum K1 krypton yellow &
green laser

HHIE
  Hearing Handicap Inventory for the Elderly
hiatal hernia
hiatotomy
hiatus
  esophageal h.
  h. semilunaris
  h. semilunaris posterior
Hibiclens Topical
Hibistat Topical
hiccup
  epidemic h.
Hickman catheter
hickory
  shagbark h.
Hi-Cor 1.0, 2.5
HICROS
  high-frequency contralateral routing of offside signals
hidden-lock denture
hidradenitis
  axillary h.
  h. suppurativa
hidradenoma
  clear cell h.
hidrocystoma
  apocrine h.
  eccrine h.
hierarchy
  response h.
high
  h. biscuit
  h. biscuit firing
  h. bisque firing
  h. definition power (HDP)
  h. density polyethylene
  h. eyebrow
  h. frenum attachment
  h. frequency (HF)
  h. glaze
  h. heat casting technique
  h. labial arch
  H. Level SISI
  h. lip line
  h. oxygen pressure (HOP)
  h. smile line
  h. volume evacuator (HVE)
  h. vowel
high-amplitude
  h.-a. sucking (HAS)
  h.-a. sucking technique

high-copper alloy
high-efficiency particulate air (HEPA)
high-energy gunshot wound
high-flow
  h.-f. arteriovenous fistula
  h.-f. arteriovenous malformation
  h.-f. lesion
high-frequency
  h.-f. audiometry
  h.-f. contralateral routing of offside signals (HICROS)
  h.-f. deafness
  h.-f. jet ventilation (HFJV)
  h.-f. pulp tester
  h.-f. response
high-fusing porcelain
high-gold alloy
high-lateral-tension abdominoplasty
high-molecular weight network polymer
Highmore antrum
high-noble alloy
high-palladium alloy
high-pass filter
high-performance liquid chromatography (HPLC)
high-pressure pulsatile lavage
high-pull headgear
high-resolution
  h.-r. computed tomography (HRCT)
  h.-r. ultrasound
high-speed
  h.-s. dermabrader
  h.-s. diamond three-tiered depth cutting bur
  h.-s. diamond wheel bur
  h.-s. drill
  h.-s. handpiece
  h.-s. tungsten carbide bur
  h.-s. two-grit bir
high-stimulus speech
high-strength
  h.-s. base
  h.-s. stone
high-velocity gunshot wound
high volume evacuator (HVE)
highway
  ciliary h.
hila (*pl. of* hilum)
hilar
  h. foci
  h. sign
Hilger facial nerve stimulator

NOTES

H

Hill stopping
Hilton
    laryngeal saccule of H.
hilum, pl. hila
himantosis
Hinderer lower nasal base implant
hindfoot
hinge
    Ancorvis h.
    h. area
    h. articulator
    h. axis
    h. axis point
    h. bow
    Gerber h.
    h. movement
    h. osteotomy
    h. position
    h. stress breaker
    h. stress-breaker
hinged flap
Hinsberg operation
hip
    h. rotationplasty
    h. strategy
hirci
    barbula h.
Hirschfeld
    H. canals
    H. file
    H. method
    H. silver point
Hirschfeld-Dunlop file
hirsutism
Hirudo medicinalis
His
    H. line
    H. plane
Hiskey-Nebraska Test of Learning
    Aptitude
Hismanal
histacryl glue
Histalet
    H. Forte Tablet
    H. Syrup
    H. X
histamine
    h. cephalgia
Histatab Plus Tablet
Hista-Vadrin Tablet
histiocyte
histiocytic granuloma
histiocytoma
    aneurysmal benign fibrous h.
    aneurysmal fibrous h.
    angiomatoid fibrous h. (AFH)
    benign fibrous h.
    cutaneous fibrous h.

    fibrous h.
    malignant fibrous h. (MFH)
histiocytosis
    acute disseminated h. X
    Langerhans cell h.
    h. X, Y
histoacryl sealer
histochemical technique
histochemistry
histoclasia implant
histocompatibility
histocompatible
histocytic granuloma
histodifferentiation
histogenesis
histogram
    poststimulus time h.
histoincompatibility
    h. barrier
histologic
    h. foramen
    h. tooth repair
histopathology
histophotomicrograph
histophysiology
Histoplasma capsulatum
histoplasmosis
Histor-D
    H.-D. Syrup
    H.-D. Timecelles
historical
    h. linguistics
    h. phonetics
history (Hx)
HIV
    human immunodeficiency virus
    HIV transmission
HIV-associated periodontitis
HIV-G
    human immunodeficiency virus gingivitis
HIV-P
    human immunodeficiency virus-
        associated periodontitis
HIV-SGD
    human immunodeficiency virus-
        associated salivary gland disease
Hixon-Oldfather prediction table
HL
    hairy leukoplakia
    hearing level
HLA
    human lymphocyte antigens
HM
    hemifacial microsomia
HMS Liquifilm
HNR
    head-neck replacement

HNSCC
head and neck squamous cell carcinoma
hoarse
hoarseness
dry h.
rough h.
wet h.
hobnail tongue
hockey-stick incision
Hodgkin
H. disease
H. lymphoma
hoe
h. excavator
monangle h.
h. scaler
surgical h.
Hoefflin suture passer
Hoffman
H. external fixation system
H. external fixator
Hogan and Converse graft augmentation
Holdaway
H. line
H. ratio
holder
Baumgartner needle h.
beam aligning h.
blade-type h.
broach h.
clamp h.
Dale Foley catheter h.
Dale tracheostomy tube h.
Diamond-Jaw needle h.
film h.
Gardner needle h.
hemostat film h.
Lewy laryngoscope h.
lion jaw bone h.
Margraf beam aligning film h.
needle h.
pinion head h.
Rinn XCP film h.
rubber dam clamp h.
speculum h.
Webster needle h.
Young rubber dam h.
holding appliance
hole
bur h.

pilot h.
pour h.
Holinger
H. anterior commissure laryngoscope
H. bronchoscope
Hollenback
H. carver
H. condenser
hollow
h. bulb
h. cutter
h. sunken orbit
hollow-jawed pliers
Hollywood bridge
Holman-Miller sign
holmium:YAG laser
Holmstrom technique
holodontography
hologram
holography
laser h.
holophrastic utterance
holoprosencephaly
Holz phlegmon
homatropine
h. hydrobromide
home
h. language
Leech Mobile H.
home-based smooth speech
homeostasis
hominis
Herpesvirus h.
Mycoplasma h.
homodigital
h. island flap
homodont
h. dentition
homogeneous
h. radiation
homogenizing heat treatment
homogenous
h. tooth transplantation
h. word
homograft
h. reaction
tympanic h.
homograph
homologation
homologous graft
homologue

NOTES

H

271

homonym
homophenes
homophone
homoplastic graft
homoplasty
homorganics
homotransplantation
honeybee
honeycomb appearance
honk
hood
    H. Laboratories Eccovision acoustic
      rhinometer
    preputial h.
    H. technique
    tooth h.
hook
    elastic h.
    embrasure h.
    incisal h.
    intermaxillary h.
    molar h.
    palate h.
    skin h.
    sliding h.
    tracheotomy h.
Hooke law
HOP
    high oxygen pressure
Hope processor
Hopkins
    H. angle-view 30-degree optical
      system
    H. rod lens system
    H. straight-view optical system
Hopmann
    H. papilloma
    H. polyp
hops
hordeolum
    acute h.
Horizon nasal CPAP system
horizontal
    h. angulation
    h. atrophy
    h. canal
    h. fiber
    h. fracture
    h. impaction
    h. incision
    h. lid laxity ,
    h. limb
    h. mattress suture
    h. maxillary fracture
    h. nystagmus
    h. osteotomy
    h. overbite
    h. overlap

    h. plane
    h. plate
    h. plate of palatine bone
    h. preputial vascularized flap
    h. projection
    h. pull headgear
    h. raphe
    h. resorption
    h. resorptive process
    h. tube
horizontal-gaze nystagmus
horizontal-shaped skin paddle
horizontovertical laryngectomy
Hormigueros
Hormodendrum
hormonal
    h. gingivitis
    h. rhinitis
hormone
    adrenocorticotropic h. (ACTH)
    melanocyte-stimulating h.
    osteotropic h.
    parathyroid h.
    thyroid h.
    thyroid-stimulating h. (TSH)
    thyrotropin-releasing h. (TRH)
horn
    h. beak forceps
    cutaneous h.
    greater h.
    lesser h.
    mucosal h.
    pulp h. (PH)
    h. of pulp
Horner
    H. sign
    H. syndrome
    H. teeth
hornet
    white-faced h.
    yellow h.
hornified epithelium
horse
    charley h.
    h. chestnut
    h. hair dander
horsefly
horseshoe
    h. bar
    h. Le Fort I osteotomy
horseshoe-shaped arch
horsetail
Horsley bone wax
Horton histamine cephalgia
hose
    delivery h.
    suction h.
hospital gangrene

host
    h. resistance
    h. response
hot
    h. node
    h. oil sterilizer
    h. potato speech
    h. potato voice
    h. potato voice quality
    h. salt sterilizer
    h. test
    h. tooth
hottentotism
Hounsfield unit
Hour
    Acutrim 16 H.'s
    Claritin-D 24-H.
    Sudafed 12 H.
hourglass nasal deformity
house
    H. classification
    h. dust
    h. dust mite
    h. dust mite antigen
    h. dust mite F
    h. dust mite P
    H. grade facial palsy
    H. wire
    H. wire and Gelfoam technique
House-Brackman
    H.-B. classification
    H.-B. grade I–VI
    H.-B. Grading Scale (HBGS)
Houston Test for Language Development
Howarth elevator
Howe
    H. color scale
    H. silver precipitation method
Howmedica
    H. hip fracture stem
    H. HNR system
Howship lacuna
HP
    hydrogen peroxide
    Vicodin HP
H.P. Acthar Gel
HPD
    hearing protection device
H-plasty
H-plate

HPLC
    high-performance liquid chromatography
HPV
    human papillomavirus
HRCT
    high-resolution computed tomography
Hruska attachment
5-HT
    5-hydroxytryptamine
HTL
    hearing threshold level
HTLV
    human T cell lymphotrophic virus
HTR
    hard tissue replacement
HTR-MFI implant
HT/TCP
    hydroxyapatite/tricalciumphosphate
HTV
    heat temperature vulcanized
H-type file
hue
    bluish h.
    complementary h.
    dominant h.
    primary h.
    secondary h.
Hueston flap procedure
Hueter maneuver
Hu-Friedy
    H.-F. elevator
    H.-F. PermaSharp suture
    H.-F. suction tip aspirator
Hughes flap
Huguier
    H. canal
hum
    sixty-cycle h.
human
    h. amnion
    h. enamel
    factor IX complex h.
    h. herpesvirus
    h. immunodeficiency virus (HIV)
    h. immunodeficiency virus-associated periodontitis (HIV-P)
    h. immunodeficiency virus-associated salivary gland disease (HIV-SGD)
    h. immunodeficiency virus gingivitis (HIV-G)
    h. lymphocyte antigens (HLA)

NOTES

H

human *(continued)*
    h. papillomavirus (HPV)
    h. radicular dentin
    recombinant h. (rHu, rH)
    h. T cell lymphotrophic virus (HTLV)
    tetanus immune globulin h.
Humatrix Microclysmic skin care product
Humby
    H. alar cartilage relocation
    H. knife
Humibid
    H. DM
    H. LA
HumidFilter heat and moisture exchanger
Hummer
    H. microdebrider
    H. V Sputter coater
humor
    aqueous h.
humoral
    h. control
    h. immunity
    h. mediated immune response
Humorsol Ophthalmic
hump
    nasal h.
    h. removal
Hunsaker Mon-Jet tube anesthesia system
Hunstad
    H. Handle flow control
    H. infusion needle
    H. system for tumescent anesthesia
Hunt
    H. neuralgia
    H. syndrome
Hunter
    H. canal
    H. glossitis
    mucopolysaccharidosis type II H. (MPS-II)
    H. syndrome
Hunter-Schreger
    H.-S. bands
    H.-S. line
Hurd
    H. dissector
    H. pillar retractor
Hurler
    mucopolysaccharidosis type I H. (MPS-IH)
    H. syndrome

Hurler-Scheie
    mucopolysaccharidosis type I H.-S. (MPS-IHS)
    H.-S. syndrome
Hurricaine
    H. gel
    H. liquid
    H. spray
    H. swab
Hurst bougie
Hurter-Driffield curve
Hürthle
    H. cell
    H. cell carcinoma
Huschke
    H. auditory teeth
    foramen of H.
huskiness
Hutchinson
    H. crescentic notch
    H. freckle
    H. incisor
    H. sign
    H. teeth
    H. triad
Hutchinson-Gilford syndrome
Hutchison syndrome
Huxley plane
HVE
    high volume evacuator
HVL
    half-value layer
Hx
    history
hyaline
    h. cartilage
    h. cell
    h. degeneration
hyalinization
hyalinized zone
hyalinosis cutis et mucosae
hyaluronic
    h. acid
    h. acid based oil
hyaluronidase
hybrid
    h. based composite
    h. composite resin
    Petrac h.
    h. prosthesis
    h. type implant
hybridization
    EBER in situ h.
hybridoma growth factor
hyclate
    doxycycline h.
Hycodan

Hycomine
    H. Pediatric
Hycort
hyCURE hydrolyzed protein powder and exudate absorber
hydantoin/EDTA
hydatid
    h. cyst
    h. disease
Hydrastis canadensis
hydrate
    chloral h.
    H. Injection
    silver amine sulfate amide h.
hydration
hydraulic dissection
Hydrea
hydrobromide
    homatropine h.
hydrobulbia
Hydrocal cast material
hydrocalcium calcium hydroxide paste
hydrocarbon wax
Hydro-Cast
    H.-C. denture reliner
hydrocele
    cervical h.
    h. colli
hydrocephalus
    otitic h.
Hydrocet
hydrochloric acid
hydrochloride
    meperidine h.
    oxymetazoline h.
    phenylephrine h.
    pilocarpine h.
    ranitidine h.
hydrochlorothiazide
hydrocodone
    h. and acetaminophen
    h. and aspirin
    h. bitartrate and acetaminophen 10/325
    h. bitartrate and ibuprofen
    h. and ibuprofen
    h. PA Syrup
    h., phenylephrine, pyrilamine, phenindamine, chlorpheniramine, and ammonium
    h. and phenylpropanolamine

    h., pseudoephedrine, and guaifenesin
hydrocolloid
    agar h.
    alginate h.
    h. dressing
    h. impression
    h. impression material
    irreversible h.
    reversible h.
Hydrocort
hydrocortisone
    acetic acid, propylene glycol diacetate, and h.
    bacitracin, neomycin, polymyxin B, and h.
    chloramphenicol, polymyxin B, and h.
    colistin, neomycin, and h.
    iodoquinol and h.
    lidocaine and h.
    neomycin and h.
    neomycin, polymyxin B, and h.
    oxytetracycline and h.
    polymyxin B and h.
    urea and h.
    h. valerate
Hydrocortone
    H. Acetate
    H. Phosphate
hydrodynamic
    h. mechanism
    h. shear stress
    h. system
hydrodynamics
    h. theory
Hydrofloss electronic oral irrigator
hydroflow technique
hydrofluoric
    h. acid
    h. acid etching gel
hydrogen
    h. peroxide (HP)
    h. sulfide
Hydrogesic
Hydro-Jel alginate
hydrolytic agent
hydromorphine HCl
hydromorphone
hydromyelia
Hydron
hydroperoxyeicosanoic acid

NOTES

H

hydrophilic
    h. acrylic resin
    h. gel
    h. ground substance
    h. virus
    h. virus kill disinfectant
hydrophobic
    h. gel
    h. monomer
hydrophosphate cement
hydropolymer
    h. beads
    h. pad
hydrops
    cochlear h.
    endolymphatic h.
    labyrinthine h.
    vestibular h.
hydroquinone
    h. gel
    h. USP 4%
hydrostatic
    h. dilator
    h. sialography
HydroStat IR
HydroTex
hydrotherapy
hydrotomy
hydroxide
    calcium h. (CH)
    ferric h.
    iron h.
    lactic acid with ammonium h.
    lanthanum h.
hydroxyamphetamine
    h. and tropicamide
hydroxyapatite, hydroxylapatite (HA)
    h.-40, -300
    h. block graft
    h. coated implant
    coralline h.
    h. crystal
    h. fibrin glue
    Interpore 200 porous h.
    nonresorbable h.
    Osteograf/N natural h.
    porous block h. (PBHA)
    h. ridge augmentation
hydroxyapatite/tricalciumphosphate (HT/TCP)
17-hydroxy corticosteroid
hydroxyeicosanoic acid
hydroxyethyl
    h. cellulose
    h. methacrylate
hydroxylapatite (*var. of* hydroxyapatite) **(HA)**

hydroxylase
    arylhydrocarbon h. (AHH)
Hydroxyline cavity liner
hydroxyprogesterone caproate
hydroxyproline
hydroxypropionic acid
hydroxypropyl
    h. cellulose
    h. methylcellulose
11β-hydroxysteroid dehydrogenase
5-hydroxytryptamine (5-HT)
hydroxyurea
hydroxyzine
hygiene
    dental h.
    mouth h.
    oral h.
Hygienist
    Registered Dental H. (RDH)
hygroformic saliva ejector
hygroma
    cervical h.
    h. colli cysticum
    cystic h.
    Fleischmann h.
hygroscopic
    h. expansion
    h. technique
hygrostomia
Hylutin Injection
Hymed therapeutic skin care
Hymenopterous vespid
Hynes pharyngoplasty
hyoglossal
    h. membrane
    h. muscle
hyoglossus muscle
hyoid
    h. advancement
    h. bar
    h. bone
    h. bone fracture
    h. branchial arch
    h. cartilage
    mandibular plane to h. (MPH)
    h. myotomy
    h. syndrome
hyoscyamine
hypacusis, hypacusia, hypoacusis
Hypaque contrast media
hyperactive
    h. muscle
    h. pulp
hyperactivity
hyperacusis, hyperacusia
hyperalgesia
hyperbaric
    h. oxygen (HBO)

h. oxygen-induced angiogenesis
h. oxygen therapy
h. oxygen therapy dive
hyperbilirubinemia
hyperbole
hyperbolic
hypercalcemia
hypercapnia
hypercemented root
hypercementosis
hypercoagulability
hypercoagulable state
hypercorrect language
hyperdivergent
h. facial pattern
hyperdontia
hyperemia
capillary h.
dental pulp h.
periapical h.
rebound h.
reverse h.
hypereosinophilic syndrome (HES)
hyperesthesia
h. acoustica
cervical h.
laryngeal h.
hypereuryprosopic
hypereversion
hyperextension
hyperflexion
Hyperflex tracheostomy tube
hyperfunction
hyperfunctional
h. facial line
h. glabellar line
h. occlusion
h. voice
Hypergel wound dressing
hyperglycemia
hyperhidrosis
Hypericum peforatum
hyperintense mass
hyperkeratosis
h. complex
h. excentrica
focal palmoplantar and marginal
gingival h.
h. linguae
oral h.
hyperkinesis, hyperkinesia
mimetic h.

hyperkinetic
h. dysarthria
h. dysphonia
h. syndrome
hypermastia
hypermobile mucosa
hypermobility
temporomandibular joint h.
hypernasality
hypernasal speech
hypernephroma
hyperocclusion
hyperosmia
hyperostosis
diffuse idiopathic skeletal h.
(DISH)
generalized cortical h.
infantile cortical h.
reactive h.
subpontic h.
hyperparathyroidism
hyperpermeability
vascular h.
hyperphalangism
hyperphonia
hyperpigmentation
postsclerotherapy h.
hyperplasia
adenomatous h.
angiofollicular lymph node h.
cementum h.
chronic perforating pulp h.
condylar h.
coronoid h.
denture h.
diffuse h.
dilantin gingival h.
eosinophilic h.
focal epithelial h.
follicular lymphoid h.
gingival h.
hemimandibular h.
idiopathic gingival h.
inflammatory fibrous h.
inflammatory papillary h.
lymphoid h.
medication-induced h.
noninflammatory h.
papillary h.
parotid lymph node h.
polypoid h.
primary pseudoepitheliomatous h.

NOTES

H

hyperplasia *(continued)*
    pseudocarcinomatous h.
    pseudoepitheliomatous h.
    pulp h.
    reactive h.
    reactive lymphoid h.
    sebaceous gland h. (SGH)
    tissue h.
    verrucous h.
hyperplastic
    h. adenoiditis
    h. cementum
    h. epithelial lesion
    h. gingivitis
    h. graft
    h. laryngitis
    h. lesion
    h. mucosa
    h. pulpitis
    h. **pulposus**
    h. rhinosinusitis
    h. tissue
    h. tonsillitis
hyperprognathous
hyperptyalism
hyperreactive pulpalgia
hyperreactivity
    vestibular h. (VH)
hyperrecruitment
hyperresonance
hyperrhinolalia
hyperrhinophonia
hypersalivation
hypersecretion
hypersensitive
    h. dentin
    h. pulp
    h. pulpalgia
    h. tooth
hypersensitivity
    anaphylactic h.
    contact h.
    delayed h.
    dentin h.
    immediate h.
    pulp h.
    tooth h.
hypersplenism
hypertactivity
    frontalis h.
hypertaurodontism
hypertelorism
    isolated orbital h.
    orbital h.
hypertension
    benign intracranial h.
    portal h.
    pulmonary artery h. (PAH)

Hyper-Tet
hyperthermia
hyperthyroidism
hypertonia
    lip h.
hypertonic
    h. muscle
hypertrichosis
hypertrophic
    h. adenoiditis
    h. cementum
    h. hemangioma
    h. laryngitis
    h. port wine stain
    h. pulpitis
    h. rhinitis
    h. rosacea
    h. scar
    h. scarring
    h. tonsillitis
hypertrophied papilla
hypertrophy
    bilateral masseteric h.
    breast h.
    cementum h.
    fatty h.
    functional h.
    genial h.
    gingival h.
    glandular h.
    hemifacial h.
    labial h.
    limb h.
    masseteric h.
    masseter muscle h.
    mixed h.
    pseudomuscular h.
    unilateral facial h.
hypervalvular phonation
hypervariable region
hyperventilation
    alveolar h.
hypesthesia, hypoesthesia
    bilateral h.
    olfactory h.
    trigeminal h.
hyphema
    anterior chamber h.
Hy-Phen
hypnodontics
hypnosis
hypnotherapy
hypnotic
hypoactivity
hypoacusis *(var. of* hypacusis)
hypoalbuminemia
hypobranchial eminence
Hypo-Cal cavity liner

hypocalcemia
hypocalcification
    enamel h.
    enamel and dentin h.
    fluoride h.
    hereditary enamel h.
hypocalcified
    h. enamel rod
hypocellularity
    generalized mastoid h.
hypocementogenesis
hypochlorite
    alkaline h.
    sodium h.
hypochondriac
hypochondriasis
hypocone
hypoconid
hypoconule
hypoconulid
hypodermic
    h. needle
    h. syringes
hypodevelopment of vestibular aqueduct
hypod interposition graft
hypodivergence
hypodivergent
hypodontia
hypoechoic
hypoepiglottic ligament
hypoesthesia (*var. of* hypesthesia)
hypoestrogenism
hypofunction
hypogammaglobulinemia
hypogastric flap
hypogastrium
hypogenia
hypogeusia
hypoglobus
hypoglossal
    h. canal
    h. nerve
    h. nerve stimulation
    h. paralysis
hypoglossal-to-facial nerve transfer
hypoglossi
    ansa h.
    nucleus prepositus h.
hypoglossia-hypodactylia syndrome
hypoglottic
hypoglycemia
hypognathous

hypogonadism
hypohidrotic ectodermal dysplasia
hypoinsulinism
hypokinesia, hypokinesis
hypokinetic
    h. dysarthria
hypolarynx
hypologia
hypomagnesemia
hypomastia
hypomaturation
    enamel h.
hypomineralization
    enamel h.
hypomineralized
hypomobile stapes
hyponasal
    h. speech
hyponasality
hypoparathyroidism
hypopharyngeal
    h. diverticulum
    h. eminence
    h. lipoma
    h. squamous cell carcinoma
    h. stenosis
hypopharyngoscope
hypopharynx
hypophonia
hypophosphatasia
hypophosphatemia
hypophrasia
hypophysial, hypophyseal
    h. eminence
hypophysis
hypopigmentation
hypopituitarism
hypoplasia
    condylar h.
    diffuse pulmonary h.
    enamel h.
    focal dermal h.
    lingual h.
    malar h.
    mandibular h.
    mandibular condylar h.
    maxillary-zygomatic h.
    midface h.
    midfacial h.
    soft-tissue h.
    h. of tooth

NOTES

H

hypoplasia *(continued)*
    Turner h.
    zygomaticomaxillary h.
hypoplastic
    h. enamel
    h. mandible
    h. mandibular body
    h. tuberous breast
hypopnea
hypoprosody
hypoproteinemia
hypoptyalism
hyporhinolalia
hyporhinophonia
hyposalivation
hyposialorrhea
hyposmia
hyposmic
hypospadias
    balanic h.
    mid-penile h.
    h. one-stage repair
    penile h.
    proximal h.
    subcoronal h.
hyposphresia
HypoTears PF Solution
hypotelorism
hypotension
hypotensive agent
hypothalamus
hypothenar eminence
hypothermia
    esophagogastric h.
hypothesis
    network h.

    Starling h.
    Whorf h.
    whorfian h.
hypothyroidism
    iatrogenic h.
hypotonic
    h. muscle
hypotympanotomy
hypotympanum
hypoventilation
    alveolar h.
hypovitaminosis
hypoxemia
hypoxia
hypoxic
Hyprogest 250 Injection
hypsodont
Hyrax appliance
Hyrexin-50 Injection
Hyrtl
    H. anastomosis
    H. loop
hysteria
    conversion h.
hysterical
    h. aphonia
    h. deafness
    h. stuttering
hysteroplasty
hysterotracheloplasty
Hy-Tape
    H.-T. surgical tape
Hytone
Hyzine-50
Hz
    hertz

I
>I bar
>I cell disease
>I marker
>I tracing

^{131}I
>iodine ^{131}I

3i
>3i implant
>3i Implant Innovations implant system
>3i wide-diameter abutment
>3i wide-diameter dental implant system

IAC
>internal auditory canal

IAM
>internal auditory meatus

iambic stress

Iamin
>I. Hydrating Gel wound dressing
>I. post laser creme

IAN
>inferior alveolar nerve

iatrogenic
>i. cholesteatoma
>i. deformity
>i. disease
>i. hearing loss
>i. hypothyroidism
>i. immunosuppression
>i. nasal stenosis
>i. perforation
>i. trauma

IBSL
>internal branch of the superior laryngeal
>IBSL nerve

IBU

Ibuprin

ibuprofen
>hydrocodone and i.
>hydrocodone bitartrate and i.
>pseudoephedrine and i.

Ibuprohm

IC
>inspiratory capacity

ICA
>internal carotid artery

ice
>i. stick
>i. test

ICIDH
>International Classification of Impairments, Disabilities, and Handicaps

icons

ICS
>intercellular space

ictus laryngis

ID
>internal derangement
>Ortho ID

I&D
>incision and drainage

IDC
>interdigitating dendritic cell

IDEA
>Individuals with Disabilities Employment Act

ideal
>i. flap
>i. occlusion

ideation

ideational apraxia

identification
>i. audiometry
>film i.
>Word Intelligibility by Picture I. (WIPI)

identifying canal

ideographs

ideomotor apraxia

IDG
>interdental groove

IdI
>interdentale inferius
>point IdI

idioglossia

idioglottic

idiolalia

idiolect

idiom

idiopathic
>i. bone cavity
>i. enlargement
>i. facial paralysis
>i. fibromatosis
>i. gingival hyperplasia
>i. gingivitis
>i. gingivostomatitis
>i. glossitis
>i. incontinence
>i. internal resorption
>i. language retardation
>i. multiple hemorrhagic sarcoma

idiopathic/tobacco-associated leukoplakia

idiosyncratic
>i. allergic reaction
>i. meaning

idiotope

idiotype
IDL
    Index to Dental Literature
idling path
idoxuridine
IdS
    interdentale superius
       point IdS
IFROS
    ipsilateral frontal routing of signals
IFSP
    Individualized Family Service Plan
IgA
    immunoglobulin A
IgE
    immunoglobulin E
       fungal-specific IgE
IgE-mediated immune response
IGF
    insulin-like growth factor-I
IL-1α
    interleukin-1α
IL-1β
    interleukin-1β
IL-6
    interleukin-6
IL-8
    interleukin-8
ileocystoplasty
ileus
iliac
    i. crest
    i. crest bone graft
    i. crest free flap
    i. crest osseous flap
    i. crest osteocutaneous flap
    i. crest osteomuscular flap
iliocostalis
    i. dorsi muscle
    i. lumborum muscle
iliohypogastric
    i. nerve
    i. neuralgia
ilioinguinal
    i. nerve
    i. neuralgia
iliotibial
    i. band
    i. tract
ilium microvascular transfer
Ilizarov
    I. procedure
    I. technique
Illinois
    I. Children's Language Assessment
    Test
    I. Test of Psycholinguistic Abilities
    (ITPA)

illocution
Illouz
    I. aspirative lipoplasty
    I. cannula
    I. liposuction technique
    I. modified tip
    reserve fat of I.
    I. standard tip
illumination
illusion
I.L.MED
    I. instrument
    I. laser
Ilosone Oral
Ilotycin Ophthalmic
ILP
    intralesional laser photocoagulation
ILSA
    Interpersonal Language Skills and
    Assessment
ILVEN
    inflammatory linear verrucous epidermal
    nevus
image
    arthrotomographic i.
    body i.
    i. copings
    latent i.
    radiolucent i.
    radiopaque i.
    radiovisiography i.
    i. sharpness
    x-ray i.
imagery
    eidetic i.
imaging
    computer i.
    Exceltech i.
    fast-imaging steady precession
      sequence three-dimensional
      magnetic resonance i. (FISP-3D
      MRI)
    magnetic resonance i. (MRI)
    magnetic source i. (MSI)
    MedMorph III patient video i.
    Niamtu video i.
    radionuclide i.
    radionuclide-labeled red blood
      cell i.
    surgical prediction i.
    thallium i.
    thermal i.
    time-of-flight i.
    tumor i.
    UniPlast video i.
    vagus nerve i.
imbalance
    central language i.

developmental i.
occlusal i.
orofacial muscle i.
imbibition
plasma i.
imbricate
imbrication
i. lines of von Ebner
platysmal i.
IMCOR
I. drill
I. implant
I. No-Touch implant placement
system
IMF
inframammary fold
intermaxillary fixation
intervascular smooth muscle fiber
IMF wedge excision mastopexy
imipenem and cilastatin
imitation
elicited i.
spontaneous i.
Imitrex
immature
i. bone
i. dentinoma
i. granule
immaturity
perceptual i.
immediate
i. echolalia
i. extension technique
i. flap
i. hypersensitivity
I. Implant Impression system
i. insertion denture
I. Load implant
i. sentence constituent
immersible video camera
immittance
i. test
immobility
ciliary i.
immobilization
tooth i.
immotile cilia syndrome
immune
i. adherence
i. complex
i. deficiency
i. globulin

i. globulin, intramuscular
i. globulin, intravenous
i. modulation
i. response
i. system
immunity
active i.
adaptive i.
cell-mediated i.
humoral i.
innate i.
passive i.
tumor-specific transplantation i.
(TSTI)
immunization
immunobiology
immunocompetent
i. cell
i. site
i. squamous cell cancer model
immunocytochemical
immunocytochemistry
immunodeficiency
severe combined i. (SCID)
immunoelectrophoresis
immunofluorescence
direct i.
immunogenicity
immunoglobulin
i. A (IgA)
i. E (IgE)
hepatitis B i. (HBIG)
salivary i.
secretory i.
immunohistochemical study
immunohistochemistry
immunologic memory
immunology
immunomodulation
immunoperoxidase
i. stain
immunoprophylaxis
immunoradiometric analysis (IRMA)
immunoreactivity
immunosuppressant
immunosuppression
drug-induced i.
iatrogenic i.
immunosuppressive
i. agent
i. therapy
immunosurveillance

NOTES

immunotherapy
IMPA
    incisal mandibular plane angle
impact
    i. injury
    i. sound
impacted
    i. cerumen
    i. fracture
    i. molar
    i. tooth
impaction
    bony i.
    dental i.
    distoangular i.
    food i.
    horizontal i.
    Le Fort I i.
    mesioangular i.
    i. point
    i. tray
    vertical i.
impaired
    language-learning i.
    mentally i. (MI)
impairment
    aphasic phonological i.
    apraxic i.
    auditory comprehension i.
    cognitive i.
    generalized intellectual i.
    hearing i.
    language i. (LI)
    mild hearing i.
    moderate hearing i.
    moderately severe hearing i.
    motor i.
    nonsyndromic hereditary hearing i.
    profound hearing i.
    sensory i.
    severe hearing i.
    slight hearing i.
    smell i.
    specific expressive language i. (SELI)
    specific language i. (SLI)
    speech i.
    visual-spatial i.
impalement injury
impar
    plexus thyroideus i.
impedance
    acoustic i.
    i. audiometry
    i. bridge
    i. matching
    mechanical i.

    static acoustic i.
    i. transfer
impediment
    speech i.
imperative
    i. mood
    i. sentence
imperception
    auditory i.
imperfecta
    amelogenesis i.
    dentinogenesis i.
    enamelogenesis i.
    odontogenesis i.
    osteogenesis i. (OI)
imperforate anus
impermeable junction
impetigo
impingement
ImplaMed
    I.-M. gold screw
    I.-M. implant system
implant
    i. abutment
    adjustable saline breast i.
    AllHear cochlear i.
    alloplastic i.
    anatomical Tobin malar prosthetic i.
    i. anchor
    anterior subperiosteal i.
    arthroplastic i.
    Astra Tech dental i.
    auditory brainstem i. (ABI)
    autologous i.
    bag-gel i.
    Becker i.
    Bicon dental i.
    bilumen i.
    Binder i.
    Biocell anatomical reconstructive mammary i.
    Biocell texture i.
    BioDIMENSIONAL saline-filled i.
    Bio-Vent i.
    Biovert ceramic i.
    bivalve nasal splint i.
    blade endosteal i.
    blade-form i.
    Brånemark i.
    breast i.
    Brink PeriPyriform i.
    i. button
    calcification of breast i.
    Calcitek Integral ThreadLoc i.
    calcium phosphate ceramic i.
    i. cast
    ceramic endosseous i.

ceramic endosteal i.
CeraOne abutment i.
i. cervix
cheek i.
Clarion cochlear i.
cochlear i.
collagen i.
Combi-40 cochlear i.
complete-arch blade endosteal i.
complete subperiosteal i.
i. contouring
Contour Profile Natural saline
  breast i.
Crête-Manche i.
crown and bridge type i.
cylinder-type i.
Dacron-backed i.
i. deflation
dental i.
Dentsply i.
i. denture
i. denture substructure
i. denture superstructure
double lumen i.
D-shaped i.
dual-chambered i.
i. elastomer shell
endodontic endosseous i.
endodontic endosteal i.
Endopore i.
endosseous blade i.
endosseous HA i.
endosseous hydroxyapatite i.
endosseous vent i.
endosteal i.
enosseous i.
ePTFE i.
esthetic Taylor mandibular angle i.
expanded polytetrafluoroethylene i.
expansible infrastructure endosteal i.
fabricated i.
facial i.
fixed mandibular i. (FMI)
i. fixture
Flowers i.
i. frame
i. framework
free-standing i.
full arch bridge i.
i. gingival sulcus
gold eyelid i.
HA-coated root-form dental i.

HA-threaded hexlock i.
helicoid endosseous i.
helicoid endosteal i.
hex i.
hexlock i.
Hinderer lower nasal base i.
histoclasia i.
HTR-MFI i.
hybrid type i.
hydroxyapatite coated i.
3i i.
IMCOR i.
Immediate Load i.
Implantech Binder i.
Implantech facial i.
Implantech Flowers i.
Implantech Mittelman i.
Implantech Terino i.
Imtec premounted threaded i.
IMZ i.
inflatable i.
i. infrastructure
I. Innovations titanium screw
integral i.
intracochlear i.
intramuscular gluteal i.
intraosseous i.
intraperiosteal i.
ITI-Benefit endosseous i.
ITI dental i.
ITI type-F endosseous i.
LaminOss i.
large-pore polyethylene i.
Linkow blade i.
liposuction fat fillant i.
Luhr i.
Maestro i.
magnetic i.
i. malposition
mammary i.
468 McGhan Biocel anatomical
  breast i.
MedDev gold eyelid i.
Medpor facial i.
Medpor malar i.
Medpor reconstructive i.
Medpor surgical i.
Meme i.
Mentor 1600 i.
Mentor breast i.
Mentor H/S Siltex i.
i. mesostructure

NOTES

implant *(continued)*
mesostructure i.
i. metal
metallic i.
Mettelman pre jowl chin i.
Micro-Lok i.
Micro-Vent i.
Micro-Vent^2 i.
Mini-Matic i.
Mittelman i.
i. model
monostructure i.
mucosal i.
multichannel cochlear i.
i. neck
needle endosseous i.
needle endosteal i.
Nobelpharma i.
nonautologous i.
Novagold mammary i.
Nucleus 22 cochlear i.
Nucleus multichannel cochlear i.
Octa-Hex i.
oral i.
osseointegrated cylinder i.
osseointegrated oral i.
Osseotite dental i.
Osseotite two-stage procedure i.
Osteo i.
osteointegrated dental i.
Osteoplate i.
Paragon i.
pergingival i.
Periotest i.
permucosal endosteal i.
pin i.
pin endosseous i.
platinum eyelid i.
polymer tooth replica i.
polytetrafluoroethylene i.
polyurethane-coated silicone
  breast i.
Porex i.
porous polyethylene i.
i. post
post i.
Proplast i.
Proplast-Teflon disk i.
prosthetic i.
PTFE-containing i.
ramus blade i.
ramus endosteal i.
RBM i.
i. related complications (IRC)
Replace system tapered i.
i. restoration
Restore bone i.
Restore RBM i.

root-form dental i.
saline breast i.
SAM facial i.
Sargon i.
i. screw
screw-type i.
Screw-Vent i.
self-tapping screw-type i.
i. shell
Silastic i.
silicone-filled i.
silicone-filled mammary i.
silicone-gel i.
silicone-gel breast i.
silicone gel-filled breast i. (SGBI)
silicone gel-filled mammary i.
  (SGMI)
silicone textured mammary i.
single-chambered saline i.
single-channel cochlear i.
single-stage screw i.
single-tooth root form i.
single-tooth subperiosteal i.
i. site dilator
solid silicone buttock i.
Spectra-System i.
spiral endosseous i.
spiral endosteal i.
Spline Twist dental i.
Spline Twist MTX i.
Spline Twist Ti i.
STAR*LOCK multi-purpose
  submergible threaded i.
STAR*LOCK Press-Fit cylinder i.
Star/Vent one-stage dental screw i.
Star/Vent screw i.
Steri-Oss dental i.
Steri-Oss Hexlock i.
stock i.
i. structure
subdermal i.
submucosal i.
submuscular i.
subpectoral i.
subperiosteal i.
subperiosteal i. one-phase technique
i. substructure interspace
i. substructure strut
i. superstructure attachment
i. superstructure connector
i. superstructure frame
i. superstructure neck
I. Support Systems titanium screw
supraperiosteal i.
i. surgical splint
i. surgical splint superstructure
Sustain HA-coated screw i.
Swede-Vent TL i.

Swede-Vent TL self-tapping
external hex i.
synthetic i.
Synthodont dental i.
i. system
i. template
Terino i.
textured saline breast i.
TG Osseotite single-stage
procedure i.
thick-walled Dacron-backed i.
ThreadLoc i.
TiMesh patient configured titanium
craniomaxillofacial i.
titanium plasma sprayed dental i.
titanium-sprayed IMZ i.
TMI i.
TPS dental i.
transmandibular i. (TMI)
transosseous i.
transosteal i.
triplant i.
triple lumen i.
Twist MTX i.
Twist Ti i.
two-piece i.
Unipost i.
universal subperiosteal i.
vent i.
vent-plate i.
Vitek interpositional i.
Zest i.
zipper amalgam i.
implantation
i. graft
muscle i.
subcutaneous i.
vascular bundle i.
implant-bearing surface
implant-bone interface
implant-borne prosthesis
Implantech
I. Binder implant
I. facial implant
I. Flowers implant
I. Mittelman implant
I. SE-100 smoke aspiration tip
I. Terino implant
implant/flap reconstruction
implantodontics
implantodontist
implantodontology

implantologist
implantology
oral i.
implant-retained denture
Implatome dental tomography system
implication
semantic i.
implicit
i. language
i. stuttering
implosion
implosive
impregnate
impression
agar i.
agar-alginate i.
alginate i.
anatomic i.
i. area
basilar i.
bridge i.
cleft palate i.
closed mouth i.
Coltoflax polysiloxane i.
complete denture i.
composite i.
i. compound
correctable i.
corrective i.
dental i.
direct bone i.
dual i.
duplicating i.
elastic i.
elastomeric i.
final i.
fluid wax i.
functional i.
hydrocolloid i.
indirect i.
intraoral i.
irreversible hydrocolloid i.
lower i.
mandibular i.
i. material
maxillary i.
mercaptan i.
modeling plastic i.
partial denture i.
i. paste
pickup i.
i. plaster

NOTES

impression *(continued)*
  plaster i.
  polyether rubber i.
  polysiloxane i.
  polysulfide rubber base i.
  preliminary i.
  prepared cavity i.
  presurgical i.
  primary i.
  reversible hydrocolloid i.
  rubber i.
  rubber-based i.
  secondary i.
  sectional i.
  silicone i.
  silicone rubber i.
  snap i.
  stone cast i.
  subperiosteal pickup i.
  surface i.
  i. surface
  surgical bone i.
  i. technique
  Thiokol rubber i.
  i. tray
  trigeminal i. of temporal bone
  upper i.
  wash i.
  wax i.
  i. wax
  welded inlay i.
impressioning
impressionistic phonetics
improved stone
improvement
  speech i.
impulse
  nerve i.
  neural i.
  pain i.
  return i.
  sensory and vasomotor i.
Imtec
  I. BioBarrier membrane
  I. premounted threaded implant
Imuran
IMZ
  I. implant
  I. implant system
  I. type restoration
in
  in extremis
  in phase
  in situ
  in vitro grown palatal mucosa
  sheet

inaccuracy
  general oral i.
  oral i.
inactivity
  oral i.
inadequate
  i. crown
  i. planification
I-Naphline Ophthalmic
inarticulate
inborn error of metabolism
incandescence
inchworm flap
incident
  i. exposure
  i. wave
incipient
  i. dental caries
  i. pulpitis
  i. stuttering
incisal
  i. angle
  i. band
  i. canal
  i. cavity
  i. edge
  i. embrasure
  i. force
  i. guidance
  i. guidance angle
  i. guide
  i. guide adjustment
  i. guide pin
  i. hook
  i. mandibular plane angle (IMPA)
  i. margin
  i. path
  i. point
  i. preparation
  i. quadrant view
  i. rest
  i. ridge (IR)
  i. surface
  i. wall
incisalis
  margo i.
incision
  access i.
  angular i.
  anterior hairline i.
  back cut i.
  bicoronal i.
  bikini i.
  Caldwell-Luc i.
  chevron i.
  collar i.
  Conley i.
  counter i.

crevicular i.
cross-hatch i.
crow's foot i.
crucial i.
cruciate i.
curved longitudinal i.
curvilinear i.
donor i.
i. and drainage (I&D)
elliptical i.
endaural mastoid i.
endonasal i.
expansile Mercedes i.
external bevel i.
external paralateronasal skin i.
extraoral Rison neck i.
Fergusson i.
Frazier i.
gingival buccal sulcus i.
gullwing i.
Hajek i.
hemitransfixion i.
H-flap i.
hockey-stick i.
horizontal i.
inferior-conjunctival fornix i.
i. inferius
inner bevel i.
intercartilaginous i.
internal bevel i.
intraoral i.
inverse bevel i.
inverted bevel i.
inverted-U i.
Killian i.
Kocher i.
labicolumellar crease i.
lip-splitting i.
lower lip-splitting i.
low-flying bird i.
MacFee i.
marginal i.
Martin i.
Meisterschnitt i.
Mercedes i.
modified Weber-Ferguson i.
palmar i.
Pfannenstiel i.
postauricular i.
preauricular i.
relief i.
relieving i.

Rethi i.
retromandibular/submandibular i.
reverse bevel i.
right subcostal i.
rim +/-transcolumella i.
Risdon pretragal i.
Rosen i.
Rotterdam extended L i.
Schobinger i.
stepladder i.
sublabial i.
submental i.
i. superius
three-armed stellate i.
transcartilaginous i.
transfixation i.
transmeatal tympanoplasty i.
transverse mid abdominal i.
trapezoid i.
unaesthetic i.
U-shaped i.
Weber-Ferguson i.
Y i.
zigzag i.
incisional
   i. biopsy
   i. pain
incision-halving technique
incisionless otoplasty
incisiva
   papilla i.
incisive
   i. canal
   i. canal cyst
   i. foramen
   i. fossa
   i. fossa of mandible
   i. fossa of maxilla
   i. muscle
   i. muscle of lower lip
   i. muscle of upper lip
   i. nerve
   i. papilla
   i. suture
   i. tooth
incisivus, pl. **incisivi**
   dens i.
   dentes incisivi
incisolabial
incisolingual
incisoproximal

NOTES

incisor
  i. bite position
  central i.
  i. crest
  i. crossbite
  deciduous i.
  hawk-bill i.
  Hutchinson i.
  i. intrusion
  lateral i.
  lower i.
  mandibular i.
  maxillary i.
  medial i.
  i. overjet
  i. path
  peg lateral i.
  point i.
  i. point
  proclination of i.
  second i.
  shovel-shaped i.
  i. tooth
  winged i.
incisura (*See also* incisure)
  i. tensoris
  i. terminalis auris
  i. tympanica
incisure (*See also* incisura)
  Rivinus i.
  sagittal i.
inclination
  axial i.
  condylar guidance i.
  condylar guide i.
  crown i.
  cuspal i.
  enamel rod i.
  lateral condylar i.
  lingual i.
  i. of tooth
incline
  guiding i.
inclusion
  i. cyst
  dental i.
  i. disease
incoherence
incompatible behavior
incompetence, incompetency
  lip i.
  palatal i.
  velopharyngeal i. (VPI)
incompetent upper lip
incomplete
  i. cleft
  i. cleft of earlobe
  i. cleft palate

  i. facial paralysis
  i. medialization
  i. paralysis
  i. recruitment
  i. syndactyly
  i. vertical root fracture (IVRF)
Inconel tube
inconsistent velopharyngeal closure
incontinence
  idiopathic i.
  neuropathic i.
  traumatic i.
incontinentia pigmenti
incoordination
incorporated tissue
increment
  practice i.
incremental
  i. appositional pattern
  i. instrumentation
  i. line
  i. lines of cementum
  i. lines of von Ebner
  i. therapy
incrementally
incudal
  i. fold
  i. ligament
incudectomy
incudomalleolar mass
incudostapedial joint
incus
  eroded i.
  i. interposition
indefinite vowel
indentation
  i. hardness
indenter
Inderal
index, gen. **indicis**, pl. **indexes, indices**
  alveolar i.
  apnea-hypopnea i. (AHI)
  articulation i.
  basilar i.
  bleeding i.
  Bödecker i.
  Borg dizziness i.
  Calculus I., Simplified (CI-S)
  Calculus Surface I. (CSI)
  cephalic i.
  Dean fluorosis i.
  debris i.
  DEF caries i.
  def caries i.
  dental i. (DI)
  I. to Dental Literature (IDL)
  DF caries i.
  df caries i.

DMF caries i.
dmf caries i.
DMFS caries i.
dmfs caries i.
Dunning-Leach i.
enamel surface i. (ESI)
Facial Disability I. (FDI)
i. finger polydactyly
Flower dental i.
free thyroxin i. (FTI)
gingiva i.
gingiva-bone count i.
Gingival I. (GI)
gingival bleeding i. (GBI)
gingival-bone i.
Gingival-Periodontal I. (GPI)
gingival recession i.
gnathic i.
interdental papilla, marginal gingiva and attached gingiva i.
irritation i.
Löe and Silness i.
malocclusion i.
Marginal Line Calculus I. (MLC)
maxilloalveolar i.
Miller i.
Miller mobility i.
Mohs i.
moiré topography i.
nasal i.
Oral Hygiene I. (OHI)
Oral Hygiene I., Simplified (OHI-S)
palatal i.
palatal height i.
palatine i.
palatomaxillary i.
Periodontal I. (PI)
Periodontal Disease I. (PDI)
Plaque I.
PMA i.
Pont i.
Ramfjord i.
respiratory distress i. (RDI)
respiratory disturbance i.
retention i.
root caries i.
Russell Periodontal I.
salivary *Lactobacillus* i.
Schour-Massler i.
Sciatic Function I.
Simplified Oral Hygiene I. (OHI-S)

small increment sensitivity i. (SISI)
Social Adequacy I. (SAI)
Speech with Alternating Masking I. (SWAMI)
Treatment Priority I. (TPI)
Voice Handicap I. (VHI)
Volpe-Manhold I. (V-MI)
Zeiss i.

indexed splint

Indian
    I. flap
    I. method
    I. operation
    I. rhinoplasty

Indican

indicative mood

indicator
    thyration i.

indices (*pl. of* index)

indicis (*gen. of* index)

indirect
    i. axial anchor screw osteosynthesis
    i. bonding
    i. contact
    i. filling
    i. impression
    i. laryngoscopy
    i. method for making inlay
    i. motor system
    i. object
    i. pulpal therapy
    i. pulp capping
    i. restorative method
    i. retainer
    i. retention
    i. technique

indium
    i. 111-diethyltriaminepentaacetic acid-D-Phe-1 (^{111}In-DTPA-D-Phe 1)
    i. 111-diethyltriaminepentaacetic acid-D-Phe-1 octreotide

Individualized Family Service Plan (IFSP)

Individuals with Disabilities Employment Act (IDEA)

Indochron E-R

Indocin
    I. SR

indole

indolent
    i. invasive infection

indomethacin

NOTES

¹¹¹In-DTPA-D-Phe 1
indium 111-diethyltriaminepentaacetic
acid-D-Phe-1
¹¹¹In-DTPA-D-Phe 1 octreotide
inductance
induction
i. coil
electromagnetic i.
i. loop
inductive reactance
inductor
induration
brawny i.
industrial
i. audiometry
i. deafness
i. dentistry
i. exposure
ineffective intrusion
inelastic
i. impression material
i. lower eyelid
inertia
inertial bone conduction
inertness
infancy
melanotic neuroectodermal tumor
of i.
SCM tumor of i.
sternocleidomastoid tumor of i.
infantile
i. apertognathia
i. aphasia
i. autism
i. cortical hyperostosis
i. fibrosarcoma
i. perseveration
i. speech
i. swallowing
Infants Feverall
Infants' Silapap
infarction
gluteal i.
myocardial i.
infected
i. dentin
i. socket
infection
amebic i.
apical i.
bacterial i.
cryptococcal pulmonary i.
fulminant invasive i.
fungal i.
indolent invasive i.
invasive *Aspergillus* i.
invasive fungal i.
late i.

middle ear i.
mycobacterial i.
mycobacterial nodal i.
necrotizing myofascial fungal i.
necrotizing soft tissue i. (NSTI)
noninvasive *Aspergillus* i.
nonopportunistic i.
nosocomial i.
opportunistic i.
oral i.
orbital i.
periapical i.
periimplant i.
periorbital i.
pneumococcal i.
polymicrobial i.
recurrent i.
respiratory tract i.
tuberculous i.
upper respiratory i. (URI)
upper respiratory tract i.
Vincent i.
viral i.
wound i.
infectious
i. agent
i. disease
i. esophagitis
i. granuloma
i. hepatitis
i. lymphadenopathy
i. mononucleosis
i. waste
infective endocarditis
inferential ambiguity
inferior
i. alveolar nerve (IAN)
i. alveolar nerve block
i. alveolar nerve fascicle
i. alveolar neurovascular bundle
arcus dentalis i.
i. cantholysis
chorditis vocalis i.
i. colliculus
i. concha
i. constrictor pharyngeal muscle
i. crus of lateral canthal tendon
i. deep cervical node
i. dental arch
i. dental vessel thrombosis
i. extensor retinaculum
i. laryngeal artery
i. laryngeal nerve
i. laryngotomy
i. lip
i. lip of pons
i. longitudinal muscle of tongue
i. malposition

i. marginotomy
i. maxillary bone
i. meatal antrostomy
i. meatus
i. nasal concha
i. nasal nerve
i. oblique muscle
i. orbital fissure
i. orbital foramen
i. pedicle
i. petrosal sinus
i. pharyngeal constrictor
i. pole peritonsillar abscess
i. rectus muscle
i. retinacular lateral canthoplasty
i. retrognathia
i. surface
i. surface of tongue
i. teeth
i. thyroid artery
i. thyroid vein
i. turbinate
i. turbinated bone
i. tympanic artery
i. vestibular nucleus

inferior-conjunctival fornix incision
inferior-superior zygomatic arch
radiograph
inferius
interdentale i. (IdI)
labrale i.
orbitale i. (oi)
inferomedial
i. aspect
infiltrate
multifocal lymphocytic i.
infiltrating carcinoma
infiltration
leukocytic i.
superwet preoperative
subcutaneous i.
infiltrative
i. fasciitis
i. local anesthesia
infiltrator
Klein i.
Inflamase
I. Forte Ophthalmic
I. Mild Ophthalmic
inflammation
acute i.
central zone i.

chronic i.
fibrinous i.
gingival i.
granulomatous i.
periodontal i.
purulent i.
sanguineous i.
serous i.
subacute i.
suppurative i.
ulcerative i.
inflammatory
i. cell
i. croup
i. cyst
i. disease
i. edema
i. fibrous hyperplasia
i. lesion
i. linear verrucous epidermal nevus
(ILVEN)
i. oncotaxis
i. papillary hyperplasia
i. papillomatosis
i. process
i. response
i. zone
inflatable implant
inflation
CT-guided balloon i.
inflection
inflectional ending
influenza A and B, A, A2 virus
influenzae
Haemophilus i.
infolded
infolding
basal i.
informal method
informed consent
infra
vide i.
infra-areolar scar
infra-auricular mass
infrabony
i. pocket
i. pocket curettage
infrabrow scar
infrabulge
i. clasp
infracartilaginous
infraciliary line

NOTES

infraclusion, infraocclusion
infracrestal pocket
infraction
infracture
infradentale
infraeruption
infraglottic
    i. squamous cell carcinoma
infrahyoid
    i. artery
    i. muscle
    i. strap muscle
infralabyrinthine
    i. air cell
    i. approach
inframammary
    i. crease
    i. fold (IMF)
inframandibular
inframaxillary
inframaxillism
infraocclusion (var. of infraclusion)
infraorbital
    i. artery
    i. block
    i. fissure
    i. foramen
    i. margin
    i. nerve
    i. plate
    i. region
    i. ridge of maxilla
    i. rim
    i. space
    i. space abscess
    i. sulcus of maxilla
    i. tear trough
infrasellar
infrasonic
    i. frequency
infraspinatus muscle
infrastructure
    implant i.
infratemporal
    i. fossa
    i. fossa approach
    i. space
    i. surface of maxilla
    i. wall
infratentorial neoplasm
infratrochlear nerve
infraversion
infrazygomatic crest
Infumorph Injection
infundibular cell
infundibulotomy

infundibulum
    ethmoidal i.
    ethmoidal i.
InfuO.R. drug delivery pump
infuser
    BP Cuff pressure i.
infusion
    colloid i.
    crystalloid i.
    i. graft
infusion/infiltration cannula
infusor
    Alton Deal pressure i.
    Heart pillow i.
ingate
ingestion
    bismuth i.
    caustic i.
    warfarin i.
Ingle classification of pulpoperiapical
  pathosis
ingrowth
    fibrovascular i.
    squamous epithelial i.
inhalant
    ammonia i.
inhalation
    i. method
    solvent i.
inhaler
    AeroBid-M Oral Aerosol I.
    AeroBid Oral Aerosol I.
    Beconase AQ Nasal I.
    budesonide nasal i.
    Intal Oral I.
    Nasacort nasal i.
    Rhinocort nasal i.
    Spiral Mark V portable ultrasonic
      drug i.
    Vancenase AQ I.
    Vancenase Nasal I.
    Vanceril Oral I.
inherent extensibility of skin
inhibition
    commissural i.
    presynaptic i.
    residual i.
inhibitor
    arachidonic acid cascade i. (AACI)
    calculus i.
    plaque i.
    residual i.
inhibitory-excitatory mechanism
inhibitory synapse
initial
    i. consonant position
    i. contact
    i. file

i. lag
i. masking
i. occlusive contact
i. preparation
i. string
i. teaching alphabet
initiation
initiator
initio
ab i.
injectable
Zyderm I, II injectable collagen
injection
Abelcet I.
Adlone I.
air i.
Alfenta I.
A-methaPred I.
Amikin I.
AquaMEPHYTON I.
Articulose-50 I.
Astramorph PF I.
autologous fat i.
Benadryl I.
Ben-Allergin-50 I.
Bicillin C-R 900/300 I.
block i.
Calcimar I.
Cibacalcin I.
Cipro I.
collagen i.
concomitant i.
contralateral frontalis i.
Cytoxan I.
Depo-Medrol I.
Depo-Provera I.
D.H.E. 45 I.
Dinate I.
Dopram I.
Doxychel I.
Duralone I.
Duramorph I.
dye i.
Dymenate I.
fat i.
i. flask
Foscavir I.
Garamycin I.
Hydrate I.
Hylutin I.
Hyprogest 250 I.
Hyrexin-50 I.

Infumorph I.
intramuscular i.
intraosseous i.
intraperiapical i.
intrapulpal i.
Jenamicin I.
Kefurox I.
Key-Pred-SP I.
Konakion I.
mental block i.
mepivacaine HCl i.
i. method
Metro I.V. I.
Miacalcin I.
Microfil i.
Minocin IV I.
i. molding
Monistat i.v. I.
M-Prednisol I.
Nafcil I.
Nallpen I.
nasopalatine i.
Nebcin I.
Neosar I.
Netromycin I.
Osmitrol I.
Osteocalcin I.
periodontal ligament i.
Pitressin I.
Predalone I.
Predcor-TBA I.
Rifadin I.
Salmonine I.
Sandimmune I.
i. sialography
silicone i.
Solu-Medrol I.
Sotradecol I.
Sublimaze I.
Sufenta I.
Teflon i.
Terramycin I.M. I.
Toradol I.
Unipen I.
Ureaphil I.
Vibramycin I.
vocal cord i.
Vumon I.
Wydase I.
Zinacef I.
injection-molded method

NOTES

injector
 Dermo-Jet i.
 Dermo-Jet high pressure i.
 extractor i.
injury
 avulsion i.
 axonotmetic i.
 basement membrane zone i.
 blunt carotid i. (BCI)
 closed degloving i.
 closed head i. (CHI)
 clothesline i.
 cotton roll i.
 cribriform plate i.
 crush i.
 degloving i.
 dentinoblastic i.
 denture i.
 dural venous sinus i.
 extra-axial i.
 impact i.
 impalement i.
 maxillofacial i.
 Mini Inventory of Right Brain I. (MIRBI)
 nerve crush i.
 neurotmetic i.
 obstetric brachial plexus i.
 pulp i.
 reperfusion i.
 ring avulsion i.
 Sunderland type V degree i.
 thermal i.
 traumatic i.
 traumatic brain i.
 zone of i.
^{111}In-labeled octreotide
inlay
 American Gold "M" i.
 American Gold "M-H" i.
 Baker i.
 i. burnout
 cast gold i.
 i. casting wax
 ceramic i.
 Clearfill CR i.
 composite i.
 Crown K i.
 direct method for making i.'s
 epithelial i.
 i. furnace
 i. gold
 gold i.
 Goldsmith I i.
 i. graft
 i. IIB
 indirect method for making i.'s
 Jelenko special i.

 Kulzer i.
 Leff light i.
 Libra II crown and i.
 i. mold
 Mowrey B i.
 i. pattern wax
 porcelain i.
 posterior i.
 i. restoration
 setting i.
 i. splint
 Sterngold i.
 Sterngold Bridgette i.
 Veribest 22 K i.
inlay/onlay
 Coltene i.
in-line trap
innate
 i. immunity
innateness theory
inner
 i. bevel incision
 i. dental epithelium
 i. ear
 i. ear tack procedure
 i. enamel epithelium
 i. fibrous layer
 i. language
 i. speech
innervated platysma flap
innervation
 dentin i.
 direct i.
 reciprocal i.
innominate
 i. artery
 i. fascia
 i. line
Innovar
Innovation implant system
inoculation
inoperable
 i. canal
inorganic
 i. dental cement
 i. pigment
inosculation
input
 i. signal processor (ISP)
inscription
 tendinous i.
insensate flap
insensibility
insert
 i. hearing protection device
 intramucosal i.
 mucosal i.

inserter
  ventilation tube i.
insertion
  endoscopic-assisted facial implant i.
  i. loss
  myringotomy and grommet i.
  path of i.
inset
inside-job protocol
insoluble
inspiration
  crowing i.
inspiratory
  i. capacity (IC)
  i. laryngeal collapse
  i. reserve volume (IRV)
  i. stridor
  i. voice
inspissate
inspissatum
  cerumen i.
instability
  atlantoaxial i.
  scapholunate i.
installation (*var. of* instillation)
Insta-Mold
  I.-M. ear protection device
  I.-M. silicone ear impression
    material
instantaneous power
Insta-Putty silicone ear plug
Instat
  I. collagen absorbable hemostat
  I. MCH microfibrillar collagen
    hemostat
InstaTrak System image-guided surgery
instep island flap
instillation, installation
  intravesical i.
institute
instruction
  oral hygiene i.
instructional objective
instrument
  Accurate Surgical & Scientific I.'s
    (ASSI)
  ASSI nasal and sinus i.'s
  bibeveled cutting i.
  Canal Master rotary i.
  cone-socket i.
  Corex i.
  cutting i.

Daniel EndoForehead i.
dental i.
diamond cutting i.
diamond rotary i.
Disk-Criminator i.
double-ended i.
double-plane i.
double-sided i.
Electro-Surgical i. (ESI)
endodontic i.
engine-driven i.
ESI Lite-Pipe fiberoptic i.
ESI Lite-Pipe plastic surgery i.
Exprin DQ1 biopsy i.
Glick i.
gnathologic i.
GPX rotary i.
handcutting i.
I.L.MED i.
intracanal i.
Isse endo brow i.
Johnson endo-bam i.
Kapp surgical i.
Kirkland i.
Krueger i. stop
Ladmore plastic filling i.
Lightspeed rotary root canal i.
long-handled i.
McCall i.
Mity Roto 360 i.
Mity Roto rotary i.
M4 Kerr Safety Hedstrom i.
i. nib
NOVA DPM 9003 skin testing i.
Obwegeser orthognathic surgery i.
occlusal adjustment i.
orthodontic i.
paralleling i.
periodontal i.
plastic i.
plugging i.
Preschool Language Assessment I.
  (PLAI)
ProFile Variable Taper Rotary I.'s
i. recirculation
I. Recirculation Center (IRC)
root canal i.
Rosenberg gynecomastia
  dissection i.
rotary i.
rotary cutting i.
screwdriver i.

NOTES

instrument *(continued)*
    Semmes-Weinstein monofilament i.
    Sensonic plaque removal i.
    single-beveled cutting i.
    single-plane i.
    standardized i.
    i. stop
    Sutcliffe laser shield and
      retracting i.
    Tessier craniofacial i.
    test handle i.
    the Treaser surgical i.
    Unitech I.'s
    Vilex plastic surgery i.
    XP peritympanic hearing i.
instrumental
    i. avoidance act theory
    i. conditioning
instrumentation
    Baxter V. Mueller laparoscopic i.
    craniofacial i.
    EndoMax endoscopic i.
    incremental i.
    insufficient i.
    Midas Rex i.
    minimal i.
insufficiency
    abdominal wall i.
    adrenal i.
    palatal i.
    pulmonary i.
    respiratory i.
    velar i.
    velopharyngeal i. (VPI)
insufficient
    i. instrumentation
    i. jaw grading
    i. lip support
insufflation
    i. test set
insulin
insulin-induced lipohypertrophy
insulin-like
    i.-l. growth factor
    i.-l. growth factor-I (IGF)
intact canal wall technique
intaglio view
Intal
    I. Inhalation Capsule
    I. Nebulizer Solution
    I. Oral Inhaler
integral
    i. implant
    i. intraoral bilateral posterior
    mesostructure
integrale
integral-total procedure

integration
    binaural i.
    competing messages i.
    prosthetic i.
    semantic i.
    sensory i. (SI)
Integra tissue expander
integrative
    i. language
    i. learning
    i. mastoplasty
integrity
    marginal i. of amalgam
integument
intelligence
    Pictorial Test of I.
    i. quotient (IQ)
    Test of Nonverbal I. (TONI)
    Wechsler Preschool and Primary
    Scale of I. (WPPSI)
intelligibility
    speech i.
    i. threshold
intelligible
intensifying screen
intensity
    electrosurgical current i.
    sound i.
intensive smooth speech
intent
    communicative i.
intentional
    i. marker
    i. replantation
    i. tooth reimplantation
    i. tremor
intention semantics
interaction
    communicative i.
    social i.
interalveolar
    i. bone crater
    i. distance
    i. space
interameloblast
interarch
    i. distance
interarticular disk of
   temporomandibular joint
interarytenoid
    i. muscle
    i. notch
interaural attenuation
interbracket span
intercalated
    i. defect
    i. duct

I

i. duct lumen
i. joint
intercalation
intercanine
intercartilaginous
i. fold
i. incision
intercellular
i. bridge
i. canaliculus
i. fenestration
i. fluid
i. layer
i. matrix process
i. space (ICS)
i. substance
interceptive
i. occlusal
i. occlusal contact
i. orthodontic manipulation
i. orthodontics
i. restorative dentistry
interchangeable facing
interconsonantal vowel
intercostal
i. artery
i. nerve
i. vessel
intercostalis
i. externus muscle
i. internus muscle
intercricothyrotomy
intercuspal
i. position
intercuspation
maximum i.
intercusping
interdent
interdental
i. artery
i. canals
i. caries
i. cleansing
i. cleft
i. denudation
i. embrasure
i. excision
i. gingiva
i. groove (IDG)
i. knife
i. ligament
i. ligation

i. lisp
i. papilla
i. papilla, marginal gingiva and
attached gingiva index
i. resection
i. septum
i. space
i. spacing
i. spillway
i. splint
i. stimulator
i. tip
i. tissue
i. wire
interdentale
i. inferius (IdI)
i. superius (IdS)
interdental papilla, marginal gingiva
and attached gingiva (PMA)
interdentium
interdigitate
interdigitated muscle flap
interdigitating
i. dendritic cell (IDC)
i. zigzag skin flap
interdigitation
buccal i.
interendognathic suture
interface
crystalline i.
echogenic i.
implant-bone i.
metal i.
structural i.
interfacial
i. surface tension
interfascicular guide suture
interference
cuspal i.
i. modification
occlusal i.
interferometry
electronic speckle pattern i. (ESPI)
interferon
i.-α2a
i.-α2b
i.-β
i.-γ
i. gamma
natural human i.-β (nHuIFN-β)
natural human i.-γ (nHuIFN-γ)
interforaminal

NOTES

interfrontal
  i. septum
interglobular
  i. dentin
  i. space
  i. space of Owen
  i. stage
interglobulare
  spatium i.
intergluteal
  i. cleft
  i. sulcus
intergonial
  i. angle
interim denture
interincisal
  i. angle
  i. distance
  i. opening
interiorized stuttering
interjection
interlandmark
interleukin
  i.-1
  i.-1α (IL-1α)
  i.-1β (IL-1β)
  i.-2
  i.-6 (IL-6)
  i.-8 (IL-8)
interlobular duct
intermandibular groove
intermaxillary
  i. anchorage
  i. elastic
  i. fixation (IMF)
  i. hook
  i. relation
  i. suture
  i. traction
intermedia
  Prevotella i.
  thalassemia i.
intermediary
  i. base
  i. movement
  i. nerve
intermediate
  i. abutment
  i. cementum
  i. dentin
  i. fascia
  i. fiber
  i. handler
  i. junction
  i. layer
  i. nerve
  i. plexus
  i. restoration

  i. restorative material (IRM)
  i. string
  i. structure
  i. tendon
  i. zone
intermedium
  stratum i.
intermedius
  Bacteroides i.
  nervus i.
  Streptococcus i.
intermetatarsal ligament
intermittent
  i. aphonia
  i. force
  i. reinforcement schedule
intermodal transfer
intermodulary distortion
intermodulation
interna
  nares i.
  otitis i.
internal
  i. acoustic meatus
  i. attachment
  i. auditory artery
  i. auditory canal (IAC)
  i. auditory meatus (IAM)
  i. auditory vein
  i. bevel incision
  i. branch of the superior laryngeal (IBSL)
  i. branch of the superior laryngeal nerve
  i. caries
  i. carotid artery (ICA)
  i. defatting
  i. derangement (ID)
  i. diameter
  i. ear
  i. elastic membrane
  i. ethmoidectomy
  i. fill reservoir
  i. fixation
  i. hex-thread connection
  i. jugular vein
  i. juncture
  i. mastopexy
  i. maxillary artery
  i. mouth protector
  i. oblique aponeurosis
  i. oblique osteomuscular flap
  i. oblique ridge
  i. occipital protuberance
  i. pterygoid muscle
  i. pulp granuloma
  i. rest
  i. root resorption

i. spiral sulcus
i. tooth resorption
i. traction
international
    I. Acoustic Company audiologic
       assessment room
    I. Classification of Impairments,
       Disabilities, and Handicaps
       (ICIDH)
    I. Organization for Standardization
    I. Phonetic Alphabet (IPA)
    I. Standard Manual Alphabet
    I. Standard Organization (ISO)
    I. System of Units (SI)
    I. Test for Aphasia
    i. two-digit tooth-recording system
interneurosensory learning
internum
    ostium i.
internus
    porus acusticus i.
interocclusal
    i. clearance
    i. distance
    i. gap
    i. record
    i. rest space
interoceptor
interocular
interodontoblastic collagen fibril
interoral speech aid
interorbital space
interosseous
    i. wire
    i. wiring
interossicular fold
interpeak latency
Interpersonal Language Skills and
  Assessment (ILSA)
interphalangeal (IP)
    distal i. (DIP)
interplacodal area
interpolated flap
interpolation flap
Interpore
    I. IMZ implant system
    I. IMZ restoration
    I. 200 porous hydroxyapatite
interposing fascia
interposition
    colonic i.
    incus i.

jejunal i.
temporoparietal fascial flap i.
interpositional gap arthroplasty
interprismatic
    i. space
    i. substance
interprobe system
interproximal
    i. bone
    i. brush
    i. caries
    i. film
    i. gingiva
    i. papilla
    i. radiograph
    i. reduction
    i. space
    i. toothbrush
    i. wear
interproximate space
interradicular
    i. abscess
    i. alveoloplasty
    i. artery
    i. fiber
    i. lesion
    i. osseous defect
    i. septum
    i. space
interridge distance
interrogative sentence
interrupted
    i. force
    i. suture
    i. tracing
interrupter device
intersection
    tendinous i.
intersensory transfer
interseptal osteoclasia
intersinus septum
interspace
    implant substructure i.
    i. implant substructure
interspecific graft
intersphenoid septum
interstitial
    i. cementicle
    i. collagenase
    i. denticle
    i. lamella
    i. radiation therapy

NOTES

interstitial *(continued)*
- i. space
- i. tissue
- i. ulitis
- i. word

intertragic notch
intertriginous area
intertubercular groove
intertubular
- i. dentin
- i. nerve
- i. substance
- i. zone

interval
- scapholunate i.
- i. timer

intervascular smooth muscle fiber (IMF)
intervention
- lexical i.
- second-look i.

interverbal acceleration
intervocalic
intestinal vaginoplasty
in-the-ear (ITE)
- i.-t.-e. hearing aid
- i.-t.-e. listening device

intima
- tunica i.

intimal dehiscence
intolerance
- cold i.

intonation
- i. contour

intoneme
INTRA
- I. angled surgical handpiece, 1:1 speed reduction
- I. angled surgical handpiece, 1:2 speed reduction
- I. straight surgical handpiece, 1:1 speed reduction
- I. surgical handpiece, 4:1 speed reduction
- I. surgical shank 1:1 speed reduction
- I. surgical shank 30:1 speed reduction

intra-alveolar
- i.-a. pocket
- i.-a. root

intra-arterial
- i.-a. chemotherapy
- i.-a. urokinase

intra-aural
- i.-a. muscle reflex

intrabasilar bulla

intrabony
- i. defect
- i. lesion
- i. pocket

intrabuccal
intracanal
- i. instrument
- i. irrigant

intracanalicular resorption
intracapsular
- i. fracture
- i. rupture
- i. temporomandibular joint arthroplasty
- i. tumor removal

intracartilaginous
intracavitary anesthesia
intracellulare
- *Mycobacterium i.*
- *Mycobacterium avium-i.* (MAI)

intracellular keratinization
intracochlear implant
intracordal granuloma
intracoronal
- i. attachment
- i. rest
- i. retainer
- i. retention
- i. splinting

intracoronal-extracoronal retention
intracorporeal lithotripsy
intracranial
- i. tumor

intracuticular running suture
intracytoplasmic
- i. intermediate filament
- i. vacuole

intradentin crack
intradermal
- i. nevus
- i. suture

intraepithelial
- i. carcinoma
- i. dyskeratosis
- i. excementosis

intrafascicular suture
intrafilling film
intraglandular stone
intrajugular
- i. process of temporal bone

intralabyrinthine fistula
intralaminar
- i. thalamic nucleus

intralesional
- i. laser photocoagulation (ILP)
- i. triamcinolone

intraligamentary anesthesia

intralingual
   i. cyst of foregut origin
intralobular duct
intraluminal antibiotic
intramastoid abscess
intramaxillary
   i. anchorage
   i. elastic
intramedullary
   i. fixation
   i. pin
intramembranous
intramucosal
   i. insert
   i. insert base-preparing bur
intramuscular
   i. gland of tongue
   i. gluteal implant
   i. hemangioma
   immune globulin, i.
   i. injection
   i. streptomycin titration therapy
intranasal
   i. ethmoidectomy
   i. polypectomy
intraneural pressure
intraneurosensory learning
intransit disease
intraocular
   Miostat I.
   i. pressure
intraoperative
   i. hearing loss
   i. skin expansion
   i. spatial confirmation
   i. tumor staging
intraoral
   i. anchorage
   i. antrostomy
   i. approach
   i. cone
   i. cyst
   i. film
   i. flap
   i. fracture appliance
   i. impression
   i. incision
   i. Kaposi sarcoma
   i. light-curing unit
   i. lining deficiency
   i. meloplasty
   i. mucosal defect

   i. occlusal film
   i. orthodontic appliance
   i. pressure
   i. radiograph
   i. radiography
   i. source radiography
   i. survey
   i. telemetry
   i. tracing
   i. wire
intraosseous
   i. ameloblastoma
   i. carcinoma
   i. cyst
   i. drill
   i. fixation
   i. ganglion cyst
   i. implant
   i. injection
   i. lesion
intraparotideal metastasis
intraparotid mesenchymal tumor
intrapartum
intraperiapical
   i. injection
   i. pressure
intraperiosteal implant
intrapleural
   i. pressure
intrapulmonic
intrapulpal
   i. anesthesia
   i. injection
   i. pressure
intraregional steroid
intraseptal alveoloplasty
intrasulcular
intrathoracic
   i. pressure
intratracheal
   i. intubation
   i. tube
intratreatment
intratubular
   i. calcification
   i. nerve
intratympanic
   i. gentamicin
intravelar veloplasty
intravenous (IV)
   i. antibiotic
   i. antibiotic

NOTES

intravenous *(continued)*
    i. drug use (IVDU)
    immune globulin, i.
intravenous-human
    cytomegalovirus immune
      globulin i.-h.
intraverbal
    i. acceleration
    i. operant
intraversion
intravesical
    i. instillation
    i. therapy
intrinsic
    i. brainstem lesion
    i. color
    i. coloring
    i. feedback
    i. mechanism
    i. muscles of larynx
    i. muscle of tongue
    i. staining
introducer
    stent i.
introitus
    neovaginal i.
Intron A
    I. A. therapy
introversion
introvert
intruded tooth
intrusion
    incisor i.
    ineffective i.
    linguistic i.
    maxillary i.
intubate
intubation
    blind nasotracheal i.
    endotracheal i.
    intratracheal i.
    nasotracheal i.
    orotracheal i.
    retromolar i.
    retrotuberosity i.
    submental i.
intubator
Inula helenium
invaded
    i. furca
    i. furcation
invaginate
invagination
    epithelial i.
    Oehlers type 3 dens i.
    skin envelope i.
invaginatus
    dens i.

invasion
    furca i.
    laryngotracheal i.
    perineural i. (PNI)
    perivascular i.
invasive
    i. *Aspergillus* infection
    i. fungal infection
    i. fungal infection of temporal
      bone
    i. keratitis
    i. lobular carcinoma
inventory
    Basic Concept I.
    Bowen-Chalfant Receptive
      Language I.
    Carrow Elicited Language I.
      (CELI)
    Clark Picture Phonetic I.
    communicative development i.
      (CDI)
    consonant i.
    Dizziness Handicap I. (DHI)
    Environmental Language I. (ELI)
    limited phonetic i.
    MacArthur Communicative
      Development I.'s
    Oral Language Sentence Imitation
      Diagnostic I. (OLSIDI)
    phonetic i.
    Temple University Short Syntax I.
      (TUSSI)
inverse
    i. bevel incision
    i. feedback
    i. square law
inversion
    nipple i.
    penile skin i.
    i. recovery pulse sequence
    rubber dam i.
inversus
    situs i.
invertase
inverted
    i. bevel incision
    i. cone bur
    i. ductal papilloma
    i. schneiderian papilloma
    i. teardrop
    i. T scar
    i. T skin excision
inverted-L osteotomy
inverted T
inverted-U incision
inverting papilloma

investing
- i. the pattern
- vacuum i.

investment
- cast i.
- i. cast
- casting i.
- cristobalite i.
- dental i.
- i. expansion
- phosphate-bonded i.
- quartz i.
- refractory i.

inviscation

invisible
- i. brace
- i. calculus

involuntary
- i. whispering

involution

involvement
- bifurcation i.
- furca i.
- pulp i.
- trifurcation i.

Iodex
- I.-p

iodide
- echothiophate i.
- thymol i.

iodinated glycerol
iodination
iodine
- i.-123, -125, -131
- i.-125 seeding
- i. bush
- i. ^{131}I
- Lugol i.
- radioactive i.

iodism
iodophor
- i. disinfectant

iodoquinol and hydrocortisone
Iofed
Iomed Phoresor electrode
ion
- i. collection monitoring device
- I. crown
- i. crown form
- i. phosphate fluoride topical solution
- thiocyanate i.

ion-collecting chamber
ionization
- i. chamber
- i. chamber pocket
- root canal i.

ionized air
ionizing
- i. irradiation
- i. radiation

ionomer
- glass i.

iontophoresis
Iopidine
iotacism
iothalamate
- meglumine i.

Iowa Pressure Articulation Test
IP
- interphalangeal
- IP joint

IPA
- International Phonetic Alphabet

I-Paracaine
I-Pentolate
I-Phrine Ophthalmic Solution
iproplatin
ipsilateral
- i. frontal routing of signals (IFROS)
- i. molar
- i. routing of signals (IROS)
- i. total lobectomy and contralateral subtotal lobectomy

Ipsoclip attachment
IQ
- intelligence quotient

IR
- incisal ridge
- HydroStat IR

Iradicav acidulated phosphate fluoride solution
IRC
- implant related complications
- Instrument Recirculation Center

iridium
iridodental dysplasia
iris
- blue flag i.
- i. forceps

Iris versicolor
IRM
- intermediate restorative material

NOTES

IRMA
immunoradiometric analysis
iron
i. deficiency
i. hematoxylin
i. hydroxide
i. oxide
i. oxide abrasive
iron-binding protein
IROS
ipsilateral routing of signals
irradiated homologous costal cartilage
irradiation
elective neck i. (ENI)
ionizing i.
telecobalt i.
irregular
i. dentin
i. dentinal sclerosis
i. rod
irreplaceable tooth
irreversible
i. hydrocolloid
i. hydrocolloid impression
i. hydrocolloid impression material
i. pocket
i. pulpitis
Irri-Cath suction system
irrigant
intracanal i.
irrigation
antral i.
bacitracin i.
caloric i.
canal i.
endodontic i.
frontal i.
heparin i.
oral i.
pulsatile saline i.
pulsating nasal i.
root canal i.
sinus i.
i. syringe
i. system
irrigator
Hydrofloss electronic oral i.
LySonix 250 i.
LySonix Delta Tip i.
oral i.
Stopko i.
irrigator/aspirator
LySonix series 250 i.
irritability
electric i.
myotatic i.

irritant
primary i.
secondary i.
irritation
counter i.
i. dentin
i. fibroma
i. index
pulpal i.
thermal i.
irritative receptor
Irrivac syringe
IRV
inspiratory reserve volume
^{123}I scan
ischemia
hand i.
ischemic
i. necrosis
i. neuropathy
i. ulatrophy
ischial pressure sore
ISG Viewing wand
island
i. adipofascial flap in Achilles tendon resurfacing
attached i.
cartilage i.
epimyoepithelial i.
i. fasciocutaneous flap
i. frontalis muscle transfer
myoepithelial cell i.
septocutaneous i.
septofasciocutaneous i.
skin i.
teres major skin i.
Ismotic
ISO
International Standard Organization
ISO sizing
isobutyl
isochronal
Isoclor Expectorant
Isocom
isodense
isodose curve
isoflurophate
isogeneic graft
isogloss
isognathous
isograft
isolated
i. abutment
i. laryngeal candidiasis
i. naso-ocular cleft
i. orbital hypertelorism
i. Pierre Robin sequence
i. sphenoid sinusitis

isolation
    i. aphasia
    carotid i.
    i. technique
isologous graft
isolyte S multielectrolyte solution
Isomet
    I. low speed saw
    I. Plus precision saw
Isopap
isoperistaltic
isoplastic graft
isopropyl alcohol
isoproterenol
Isopto
    I. Atropine
    I. Carbachol Ophthalmic
    I. Carpine Ophthalmic
    I. Cetamide Ophthalmic
    I. Cetapred Ophthalmic
    I. Homatropine Ophthalmic
    I. Hyoscine Ophthalmic
    I. Plain Solution
    I. Tears Solution
Iso-Shields obstructor
Isosit N
isosulfan blue dye
isotransplantation
isotretinoin
isotype
ISP
    input signal processor
Ispaghula
israelii
    Actinomyces i.
Isse endo brow instrument
Isshiki
    I. thyroplasty
    I. thyroplasty type I
isthmus, pl. isthmi
    i. of fauces
    i. faucium
    i. tympani anticus
    i. tympani posticus
    velopharyngeal i.
Italian
    I. cypress
    I. flap

    I. method
    I. operation
    I. rhinoplasty
itch
    Absorbine Jock I.
    Aftate for Jock I.
    Tinactin for Jock I.
ITE
    in-the-ear
    ITE hearing aid
    ITE listening device
item
    lexical i.
iter
    i. chordae posterioris
    i. dentis
    i. dentium
ITI
    I.-Bonefit endosseous implant
    I. dental implant
    I. dental implant system
    I. type-F endosseous implant
Ito
    I. nevus
ITPA
    Illinois Test of Psycholinguistic Abilities
itraconazole
I-Tropine
IV
    intravenous
I.V.
    Gammar-P I.V.
    Merrem I.V.
Ivalon sponge
IVDU
    intravenous drug use
ivory
    i. clamp
    i. membrane
    i. rubber dam clamp
    i. rubber dam clamp forceps
IVRF
    incomplete vertical root fracture
Ivy
    I. loop
    I. loop wiring
    I. wire

NOTES

J

joule
- J wire

jacket
- j. appliance
- j. crown
- porcelain j.
- j. regainer-maintainer
- yellow j.

jackscrew
- j. appliance
- j. regainer-maintainer

Jackson
- J. anterior commissure laryngoscope
- J. appliance
- J. approximation forceps
- J. broad staple forceps
- J. button forceps
- J. conventional foreign body forceps
- J. crib
- J. cross-action forceps
- J. cylindrical object forceps
- J. double-prong forceps
- J. dull rotation forceps
- J. esophagoscope
- J. flexible upper lobe bronchus forceps
- J. globular object forceps
- J. laryngoscope
- J. papilloma forceps
- J. ring jaw globular object forceps
- J. sharp-pointed rotation forceps
- J. steel-stem woven filiform bougie
- J. syndrome
- J. triangular brass dilator

jacksonian seizure
Jackson-Pratt drain
Jacobsen template
Jacobson
- J. nerve
- J. organ
- J. plexus

Jadassohn-Lewandowski syndrome
Jaeger
- J. bone plate
- J. lid plate

Jako laryngoscope
James Language Dominance Test
Jameson face lift scissors
Janar
- J. acidulated phosphate fluoride rinse
- J. sodium fluoride rinse

Jandel Scientific Sigma Image software

Jannetta retractor
Jansen-Middleton punch forceps
Jansen operation
Japanese cedar
Japan Facial Score
Jaquette scaler
Jarabak
- J. analysis
- J.-type archwire

jargon
- j. aphasia

Jarisch-Herxheimer reaction
jaundice
jaw
- bird-beak j.
- j. bone
- j. brace
- cleft j.
- Cox regression analysis of partially edentulous j.
- crackling j.
- j. grading
- Hapsburg j.
- lumpy j.
- j. movement
- multiple exostoses of j.
- parrot j.
- progonoma of j.
- j. protrusion
- j. radiograph
- ramus of j.
- j. reflex
- j. relation
- j. relation record
- j. repositioning
- j. separation
- j. stabilization
- upper j.
- wide j.

jawline
jaw-to-jaw
- j.-t.-j. position
- j.-t.-j. relation

jaw-winking
- j.-w. phenomenon

J/cm²
- joules per centimeter squared

Jebsen test
JedMed TRI-GEM microscope
jejunal
- j. free flap
- j. interposition

jejunoplasty
Jelenko
- J. arch bar

Jelenko *(continued)*
    J. Durocast gold alloy
    J. Modulay gold alloy
    J. special inlay
    J. super wire
    J. surveyor
Jel-Span alloy
Jena method
Jenamicin Injection
Jenkins porcelain
Jesberg esophagoscope
Jessner
    J. solution
    J. solution peel
jet
    j. insufflation anesthesia
    j. ventilation
jeweler's forceps
Jewett wave
Jiffy tube
jig
    acrylic j.
    transosteal implant j.
jigsaw blade
jitter
    frequency j.
jitter-related measure
JND
    just noticeable difference
Jo Dandy disk
Jod-Basedow disease
Joe Hall-Morris external fixator
Johnson
    J. cheek retractor
    J. endo-bam instrument
    J. grass
    J. root canal filling method
    J. twin wire appliance
Johnston method
joint
    Ackerman bar j.
    j. arthrodesis
    axial rotation j.
    ball and socket j.
    bar j.
    butt j.
    capsule of temporomandibular j.
    CMC j.
    j. contracture
    cranial suture j.
    cricoarytenoid j.
    cricothyroid j.
    diarthrodial synovial j.
    DIP j.
    frozen knee j.
    incudostapedial j.
    intercalated j.
    IP j.

    Lisfranc j.
    MCP j.
    metacarpophalangeal j.
    metatarsal j.
    metatarsophalangeal j.
    MTP j.
    proximal interphalangeal j.
    rotation j.
    j. sepsis
    single sleeve bar j.
    socket j.
    j. space
    Steiger j.
    temporomandibular j. (TMJ)
Joliet 3-Minute Speech and Language Screen
Jolly-Thomas palsy
Jonah word
Joseph
    J. clamp
    J. knife
    J. periosteal elevator
    J. rhinoplasty
    J. saw
joule (J)
    j. counter
joules per centimeter squared (J/cm^2)
jowl
    j. fat
    neck j.
Jr
    Children's Dynafed Jr
    Congess Jr
J-receptor
J-scar
JS Quick-fill system
Juberg-Marsidi syndrome
judgment
    metalinguistic j.
juga (*pl. of* jugum)
jugal bone
jug-handle view
jugomasseteric mutilation
jugomaxillary point
jugular
    j. bulb
    j. bulb decompression
    j. chain lymph node
    j. foramen
    j. foramen syndrome
    j. foramen tumor
    j. fossa
    j. lymph node
    j. vein
    j. venography
jugulare
    glomus j.

jugulodigastric
    j. node
    j. region
jugulo-omohyoid node
jugum, pl. **juga**
    juga alveolaria mandibulae
    juga alveolaria maxillae
jumbling
jump flap
jumping
    j. the bite
    j. genioplasty
jumping-the-bite
    j.-t.-b. appliance
    j.-t.-b. plate
junction
    adhering j.
    alar-facial j.
    amelodental j.
    amelodentinal j.
    cementodentinal j.
    cemento-enamel j. (CEJ)
    chondroethmoidal j.
    communicating j.
    dentinoblastic-predentin j.
    dentinoblastic-subdentinoblastic j.
    dentinocemental j.
    dentinoenamel j. (DEJ)
    dentoepithelial j.
    dentogingival j.
    gap j.
    hard-soft palate j.
    impermeable j.
    intermediate j.
    mucocutaneous j.
    mucogingival j. (MGJ)
    neuromuscular j.
    nexus-type j.
    pontomedullary j.
    pulpoperiodontal j.
junctional
    j. complex
    j. epithelium
    j. nevus
junctural feature
juncture
    closed j.

    internal j.
    open j.
    phonetics of j.
    plus j.
    terminal j.
June
    J. grass
    J. grass antigen
Junior
    J. Strength Motrin
    J. Strength Panadol
juniper
    j. berries
    j. mix
    Western j.
Juniperus communis
Juri
    J. flap
    J. II, III degree of male pattern
    baldness
jurisprudence
    dental j.
just
    j. noticeable difference (JND)
    J. Tears Solution
    J. Treatment reliner
Justi resin cement
jute
juvenile
    j. angiofibroma
    j. hemangiofibroma
    j. nasopharyngeal angiofibroma
    j. nevus
    j. ossifying fibroma
    j. papillomatosis
    j. periodontitis
    j. periodontitis syndrome
    j. thyrotoxicosis
    j. xanthogranuloma
juxta-articular ankylosis
juxtabrow skin
juxtacapillary receptor
juxtacortical
    j. chondroma
    j. osteogenic sarcoma
juxtaposition

J

NOTES

K3-7991 Thornton 360 degree arcuate marker

KA
keratoacanthoma

Kaderavek-Sulzby Bookreading Observational Protocol (KSBOP)

Kadian Capsule

Kadon primer

Kahler forceps

kale

Kalginate calcium alginate wound dressing

kallikrein

Kallmann syndrome

kanamycin

Kangaroo gastrostomy feeding tube

Kanner syndrome

kansasii
Mycobacterium k.

Kantrex

kaolin

Kaplan-Feinstein comorbidity grade

kapok

Kaposi
K. sarcoma
K. sarcoma of mastoid
K. varicelliform eruption

kappacism

Kappa test

Kapp surgical instrument

Karapandzic
K. flap
K. method
K. technique

karat (*var. of* carat)

Karaya gum

Karidium
K. fluoride
K. liquid
K. phosphate fluoride topical gel

Karigel
K.-N
K. Professional

Kari rinse

Karisma carbamide peroxide bleaching agent

Karl
K. Storz light source connector
K. Storz pediatric bronchoscopy system

Karman cannula

Karnofsky performance status scale

Karolyi effect

Kartagener
K. syndrome
K. triad

Kasabach-Merritt phenomenon

Kathon-CG

Kaufman Assessment Battery for Children

kava-kava

KaVo oral surgery system

Kawamoto technique

Kawasaki disease

Kaye
K. face lift scissors
K. minimal-incision anterior approach

Kay rhinolaryngeal stroboscope

Kazangia
K. and Converse facial fracture classification
K. and Converse mandibular fracture classification

Kazanjian
K. forceps
K. operation
K. splint
K. T bar
K. vestibuloplasty
K. vestibuloplasty technique
K. vestibulotomy

kc
kilocycle

K cell

K-Cide 10

K-complex

KD chin prosthesis

keel
Montgomery laryngeal k.

Keeler
K. fiberoptic headlamp
K. Lightsource stand
K. panoramic loupe

Keeler-Galilean surgical loupe

Keel tip

Keflex

Keftab

Kefurox Injection

Kefzol

Keinböck disease

Keith needle

Kelly
K. forceps
K. hemostat

Kelocote

keloid
earlobe k.

keloid *(continued)*
>k. formation
>k. scar
>k. tumor

keloplasty

Kenacort

Kenaject-40

Kenalog
>K.-10
>K.-40
>K. in Orabase

Kennedy
>K. bar
>K. classification

Kenonel

Kentucky bluegrass

Kent-Vitek mandibular prosthesis

Kent zinc cement

keratin
>k. filament
>k. pearl

keratinization
>intracellular k.

keratinized
>k. epithelium
>k. tissue

keratinizing
>k. epithelial odontogenic cyst
>k. epithelial odontogenic tumor
>k. squamous cell carcinoma

keratinocyte
>cultured autologous k.

keratitis
>exposure k.
>invasive k.
>xerotic k.

keratoacanthoma (KA)
>nodulo-vegetating k.
>subungual k. (SUKA)

keratoconjunctivitis
>bacterial k.
>k. sicca

keratocyst
>odontogenic k.

keratocyte

keratohyalin
>k. granule

keratolytic agent

keratoma

keratonocyte

keratopachyderma

keratopathy

keratosis, pl. **keratoses**
>actinic k.
>focal k.
>focal (oral) k.
>k. follicularis
>k. labialis

>k. obliterans
>k. obturans
>papillary k.
>seborrheic k.
>senile k.

keratotic papilloma

Kerckring
>valves of K.

Kerlone Oral

Kernecht red stain

kernel
>k. sentence

kernicterus

Kernig sign

Kerr
>K. antiseptic root canal sealer
>K. Endopost
>K. equalizing paste
>K. hard wax
>K. K-Flex file
>K. Luralite paste
>K. M4 safety handpiece
>K. Permplastic material
>K. Pulp Canal sealer
>K. reamer
>K. regular wax
>K. Snow White plaster No. 1
>K. Spher-A-Caps amalgam
>K. Spheraloy amalgam
>K. Topical Flura-Gel gel
>K. Traycon material

Kerrison
>K. forceps
>K. rongeur

Kesling
>K. appliance
>K. spring

Kesselring
>K. aspirative lipoplasty
>K. curette technique

Kessler suture technique

Ketac
>K. Fil cement
>K. Silver cement

Ketac-Endo
>K.-E. glass-ionomer-based sealer
>K.-E. glass-ionomer root canal
>sealer
>K.-E. root canal sealer

Ketac-Silver glass-ionomer cement

ketamine

ketoacidosis

ketoconazole

ketone
>methyl ethyl k.

ketoprofen

ketorolac tromethamine

key
k. attachment
dental k.
Fitzgerald K.
k. ridge
k. stitch
torquing k.
k. word method
key-and-keyway attachment
keyhole
keyhole limpet hemocyanin (KLH)
keyhole shape
keyhole-shaped rod
Key-Pred-SP Injection
keyway
k. attachment
K-file
Mity K.-f.
Nitinol K.-f.
K-Fix Fixator system
K-Flex
K-Flexofile
K.-F. Batt tip
Khan-Jaeger clamp
KHN
Knoop hardness number
kidney bean
Kiel graft
kieselguhr
Kiesselbach
K. area
K. plexus
K. triangle
killer cell
lymphokine-activated k. c. (LAK)
natural k. c. (NK)
Killian
K. frontoethmoidectomy procedure
K. incision
K. nasal speculum
K. operation
Killian-Lynch suspension laryngoscope
kilocycle (kc)
kilovolt (kV)
Kimura cartilage graft
Kinder Design pedo forceps
Kindergarten
K. Auditory Screening Test
K. Language Screening Test
(KLST)
Phonetically Balanced K. (PBK)

kinematic
k. face-bow
kinesia
kinesics
kinesiographic analysis
kinesiology
kinesthesia, kinesthesis
kinesthetic
k. analysis
k. cue
k. feedback
k. method
k. motor aphasia
k. perception
k. technique
kinetic
k. analysis
k. energy
k. motor aphasia
King operation
Kingsley
K. appliance
K. plate
K. splint
kinin
k. system
kininogen
kink
kinked tooth
kinking
pedicle k.
Kinn-Air bed
kinocilium, pl. kinocilia
Kinzie method
Kirkland
K. cement
K. cement dressing
K. instrument
K. knife
K. periodontal pack
Kirkland-Kaiser pack
Kirschner wire
Kisch reflex
kissing
k. disease
k. tonsils
kit
Ace bone screw tacking k.
acrylic color correction k.
Apdyne phenol applicator k.
Cyfra 21-1 IRMA k.
ERx Avulsed Tooth k.

K

NOTES

kit *(continued)*
Fer-Will Object K.
Gel-Kam FluoroCare dual rinse k.
Genius 4/Digoxigenin RNA
labeling k.
Lang jet adjustor k.
McGhan fill k.
micro-bicinchoninic acid protein
assay k.
polycarbonate crown k.
Roche Z gel k.
Roydent silver point extractor k.
Save-A-Tooth k.
Set-Op myringotomy k.
Sigma TMB assay k.
Skintech Postoperative Skin
Care K.
Taub minute stain k.
temporization k.

Kitano and Okada method
Klammt activator
Klebanoff factor
Klebsiella
K. rhinoscleromatis
kleeblattschädel
k. anomaly
k. craniosynostosis
k. syndrome
Kleenite denture cleanser
Kleen-Needle system
Klein
K. cannula
K. cannula tip
K. Delrin Luer lock handle
K. 1-hole infiltrator tip
K. infiltration needle
K. infiltrator
K. multihole infiltrator tip
K. pump
Kleinert-Kutz bone-cutting forceps
Kleinsasser anterior commissure
laryngoscope
Klerist-D Tablet
Klestadt cyst
KLH
keyhole limpet hemocyanin
Kligman
K. formula
K. solution
Klinefelter syndrome
Kling gauze
Klippel-Trénaunay syndrome
Kloehn
K. cervical extraoral orthodontic
appliance
K. face-bow
K. headgear

KLS-Martin modular osteosynthesis
system
KLST
Kindergarten Language Screening Test
Klumpke
K. palsy
K. score
Knapp
K. gold alloy
K. No. 2 gold
knee salvage
knife, *pl.* **knives**
Austin k.
Blair k.
Buck k.
cautery k.
Cottle k.
diathermy k.
electronic k.
endotherm k.
finishing k.
free-hand k.
gamma k.
gold k.
Goldman-Fox k.
Goulian k.
Humby k.
interdental k.
Joseph k.
Kirkland k.
Merrifield k.
Monahan-Lewis k.
myringotomy k.
Orban k.
periodontal k.
plaster k.
sickle k.
straight tympanoplasty k.
tympanoplasty k.
knife-edged finishing line
Knight nasal scissors
knives *(pl. of* knife*)*
knob
olfactory k.
Knoop
K. hardness
K. hardness indenter point
K. hardness number (KHN)
K. hardness scale
K. hardness test
knot
Ahern k.
enamel k.
knowledge
k. of performance (KP)
k. of result (KR)
knurled handle
Kobayashi tie

Kocher incision
kochia
Kodak X-Omatic C-1 cassette
Koerner flap
kojic
    k. acid
    k. acid cream
Kole procedure
Kolmogorov-Sirnov Two Sample Test
Konakion Injection
Kondon Nasal
Konȳne 80
Koplik spot
Korff
    K. fiber
Körner septum
koronion (*var. of* coronion)
Korsakoff disease
Ko-type reamer
KP
    knowledge of performance
KR
    knowledge of result
Kramer-Rhodes periodontal collection
  system
Krause
    K. corpuscle
    K. graft
    K. method
Krause-Wolfe graft
Krebs-Ringer solution
Krex impression corrective paste
Kronfeld mountain pass concept
Krönlein orbitotomy
Krueger
    K. instrument stop
    K. stop
Krukenberg procedure

Kruskal-Wallis test
Kryptex dental cement
KSBOP
    Kaderavek-Sulzby Bookreading
    Observational Protocol
KT
    Orudis KT
KTD Dentvision
KTP
    potassium titanyl phosphate
    KTP laser
KTP/532 laser
KTP/Nd:YAG XP surgical laser system
KTP/YAG laser
K-type
    K.-t. file
    K.-t. reamer
    K.-t. tile
Kuhnt-Szymanowski
    K.-S. ectropion repair procedure
    K.-S. technique
Kulzer
    K. inlay
    K. inlay system
Kurer
    K. anchor
    K. anchor system
Küttner tumor
kV
    kilovolt
kymogram
kymograph
kyphectomy
kyphos
    bony k.
kyphosis
    basilar k.

K

NOTES

lab

computerized speech l. (CSL)

earmold l.

Laband syndrome

Labbé

L. vein

label

Alert L.

biohazard l.

labeling

labia

labial

l. angle

l. arch

l. artery

l. assimilation

l. bar

l. cavity

l. cleft

l. commissure

l. curve

l. edema

l. embrasure

l. filter

l. flange

l. flaring

l. frenum

l. gingiva

l. gland

l. hypertrophy

l. lamina

l. line

l. and lingual arches

l. minor salivary gland

l. movement

l. notch

l. occlusion

l. pad

l. pit

l. region

l. splint

l. stent

l. surface

l. teeth

l. torque

l. tubercle

l. vestibule

l. wire

labial-buccal sulcus

labialis

facies l.

herpes l.

keratosis l.

labialism

labialization

labicolumellar crease incision

labioalveolar

labioaxiogingival

labiocervical

labiochorea

labioclination

labiodental

l. area

l. sulcus

labiogeniomandibular mutilation

labiogingival (LAG)

labioglossolaryngeal

l. paralysis

labioglossopharyngeal

labiograph

labioincisal (LAI)

l. edge (LIE)

l. line angle

labiolingual

l. diameter of crown

l. fixed orthodontic appliance

l. plane

l. splint

l. technique

labiolingually

labiomandibular

l. glossotomy

l. ligament

labiomarginal sulcus

labiomaxilloseptocolumellar amputation

labiomental

l. amputation

l. fold

l. groove

labionasal

labiopalatal amputation

labiopalatine

labioplacement

labioplasty

labioproximal

labiotenaculum

labioversion

labium

l. inferius oris

l. mandibulare

l. maxillare

l. oris

l. superius oris

laboratory

l. core

mobile anaerobic l.

l. plaster

labrale

l. inferius

L

labrale (*continued*)
 l. superioris
 l. superius
labrum, pl. **labra**
labyrinth
 bony l.
 ethmoidal l.
 membranous l.
 osseous l.
 otic l.
 vestibular l.
labyrinthectomy
 chemical l.
 mechanical l.
labyrinthine
 l. angiospasm
 l. aplasia
 l. artery
 l. cryptococcosis
 l. fenestration
 l. fistula
 l. gusher
 l. hydrops
 l. membrane
 l. nystagmus
 l. ossification
 l. righting reflex
 l. segment
 l. torticollis
 l. vertigo
labyrinthitis
 circumscribed l.
 congenital luetic l.
 diffuse serous l.
 diffuse suppurative l.
 obliterative l.
 suppurative l.
 viral l.
labyrinthotomy
lacerated wound
laceration
lacerum
 foramen l.
Lac-Hydrin
Laclede Fluoride Foam
Lacril Ophthalmic Solution
Lacri-Lube
 L.-L. opthalmic ointment
lacrimal
 l. bone
 l. duct
 l. fossa
 l. gland
 l. groove of maxilla
 l. lake
 l. probe
 l. process

 l. sac
 l. sulcus of maxilla
lacrimation
 gustatory l.
 l. test
lacrimoauriculodentodigital (LADD)
 l. syndrome
β-lactamase
lactation
lacteus
 dens l.
lactic
 l. acid
 l. acid and sodium-PCA
 l. acid with ammonium hydroxide
 l. dehydrogenase
LactiCare
Lactobacillus
 L. acidophilus
 L. casei
lactoferrin
lactoperoxidase
LactoSorb
 L. copolymer
 L. resorbable craniomaxillofacial
 fixation
 L. resorbable fixation system
lactulose
lacuna, pl. **lacunae**
 absorption l.
 l. of cementocyte
 Howship l.
 osteocytic l.
 repaired l.
 resorbed l.
 resorption l.
lacunar tonsillitis
LAD
 language acquisition device
Ladamore plugger
LADD
 lacrimoauriculodentodigital
ladder
 abstraction l.
laddergram
Ladmore plastic filling instrument
Laënnec cirrhosis
LAER
 late auditory evoked response
 LAER audiometry
laesa
 functio l.
laeso
 vertigo ab aure l.
LAG
 labiogingival
lag
 forehead l.

initial l.
maturational l.
l. screw
l. screw fixation
terminal l.
lagophthalmos, lagophthalmia
peretic l.
LaGrange scissors
Lahey clamp
LAI
labioincisal
lait
café au l.
LAK
lymphokine-activated killer cell
lake
lacrimal l.
venous l.
laliatry
lallation
lalling
lalognosis
Lalonde
L. extra fine skin hook forceps
L. skin hook forceps
lalopathy
laloplegia
lamb
lambdacism
lambdoidal
l. suture
l. synostotic plagiocephaly
lambdoid synostosis deformity
Lambert-Eaton myasthenic syndrome
Lambone
L. demineralized laminar bone
L. freeze dried bone
lamb's quarter
lamella, pl. lamellae
basal l.
cemental l.
circumferential l.
enamel l.
ground l.
interstitial l.
lateral l.
lamellar
l. bone
l. cementum
l. granule

lamellated
l. bone
lamina, pl. laminae
basal l.
buccal l.
buccogingival l.
dental l.
l. dentalis
l. dentalis dentogingival
dentogingival l.
l. dura
l. dura-like appearance
hamartoma of dental l.
labial l.
l. limitans
l. lucida
l. medialis
nuclear l.
palatine l.
l. papyracea
l. profunda
l. propria
reticular l.
l. of Rexed
spiral l.
successional l.
vestibular l.
lamina-bud stage
laminagraph
laminagraphy
cephalometric l.
laminar
l. bone
l. fat
laminate
Paste L.
l. veneer
laminated
l. esthetic veneer
l. gold foil
l. layer
l. radiopacity
lamination
laminin
laminography
LaminOss
L. implant
L. Implant System
Lamisil Cream
lamp
annealing l.

L

NOTES

lamp (*continued*)
    halogen l.
    mouth l.
Lamprene
Lanacort
Lanaphilic Topical
lancet
    l. blade
    gingival l.
    gum l.
    Lipectron ultrasonic l.
    ultrasonic l.
lancinating
lancing
landmark
    cephalometric l.
    cranial base l.
    facial l.
Landry-Guillain-Barré syndrome
Lane plate
Lang
    L. bridge
    L. crown
    L. jet adjustor kit
Langenbeck repair
Langer
    L. cleavage line
Langerhans
    L. cell eosinophilic granuloma
    L. cell granulomatosis
    L. cell histiocytosis
    L. cells
Langhans cells
Langhans-type giant cells
language
    l. acquisition device (LAD)
    American Indian Sign L.
    (AMERIND)
    American Sign L. (Ameslan, ASL)
    L. Assessment, Remediation, and
    Screening Procedure
    automatic l.
    body l.
    l. boundary
    l. center
    Clark-Madison Test of Oral L.
    l. clinician
    Coarticulation Assessment in
    Meaningful L. (CAML)
    l. code
    computer l.
    confused l.
    l. content
    delayed l.
    l. development
    deviant l.
    l. difference
    l. disorder

    dominant l.
    egocentric l.
    emergent l.
    l. expansion technique
    expressive l.
    figurative l.
    l. form
    l. function
    gesture l.
    Grammatical Analysis of
    Elicited L. (GAEL)
    home l.
    hypercorrect l.
    l. impairment (LI)
    implicit l.
    inner l.
    integrative l.
    mathetic function of l.
    L. Modalities Test for Aphasia
    native l.
    nonspecific l.
    nonstandard l.
    oral l.
    l. pathologist
    l. pathology
    prelinguistic l.
    Procedures for the Phonological
    Analysis of Children's L.
    l. processing
    L. Processing Test
    L. Proficiency Test (LPT)
    rationalist theory of l.
    receptive l.
    Receptive-Expressive Emergent L.
    (REEL)
    l. register
    l. sample
    L. Sampling, Analysis, and
    Training
    school l.
    Screening Test of Adolescent L.
    Screening Test for Auditory
    Comprehension of L.
    sign l.
    standard l.
    l. structure
    subcultural l.
    substandard l.
    Test of Adolescent L.
    Tests for Auditory Comprehension
    of L.-R (TACL-R)
    l. theory
    l. therapist
    true l.
    twin l.
    written l.
language-learning impaired

lanolin, cetyl alcohol, glycerin, and
    petrolatum
lanthanum hydroxide
lap
    l. pad
    l. ridge
laparoscope
laparotomy pad
L-approach
Lap Vacu-Irrigator
large
    l. canal
    l. interarch distance
    l. radiolucency
    l. restoration
large-caliber nonabsorbable suture
large-cell lymphoma
large-pore polyethylene implant
Larmor
    L. equation
    L. frequency
LaRoe undermining forceps
Larrea tridentata
Larsen syndrome
laryngeal
    l. abscess
    l. anesthesia
    l. angioleiomyoma
    l. anomaly
    l. artery
    l. atresia
    l. blastomycosis
    l. burn
    l. cancer
    l. carcinoid
    l. carcinoma
    l. cartilage
    l. cartilage fracture
    l. chondroma
    l. chondroradionecrosis
    l. chorea
    l. cleft
    l. cramp
    l. crisis
    l. diversion
    l. edema
    l. epilepsy
    external branch of the superior l.
        (EBSL)
    l. fold
    l. framework surgery
    l. granuloma

l. hemangioma
l. hemorrhage
l. hyperesthesia
l. image biofeedback
internal branch of the superior l.
    (IBSL)
l. lipoma
l. mask
l. mask airway (LMA)
l. melanosis (LM)
l. motor paralysis
l. neoplasm
l. nerve
l. neuroendocrine carcinoma
l. obstruction
l. oscillation
l. papillomatosis
l. paraganglioma
l. paresthesia
l. perichondritis
l. polyp
l. prominence
l. reflex
l. release
l. respiration
l. saccular cyst
l. saccule of Hilton
l. sensory paralysis
l. spasm
l. stenosis
l. stent
l. stridor
l. stuttering
l. syncope
l. syringe
l. tension
l. tuberculosis
l. vein
l. ventricle
l. vertigo
l. vestibule
l. web
laryngectomy
    anterior partial l.
    frontolateral l.
    horizontovertical l.
    narrow-field l.
    near-total l.
    salvage l.
    subtotal l.
    subtotal supraglottic l. (SSL)
    supracricoid l.

L

NOTES

laryngectomy *(continued)*
  supraglottic l.
  total l.
  wide-field total l.
larynges (*pl. of* larynx)
laryngis
  ictus l.
  myasthenia l.
  pachyderma l.
  ventriculus l.
laryngismus
  l. stridulus
laryngitic
laryngitis
  acute l.
  acute supraglottic l.
  chronic l.
  chronic hyperplastic l.
  chronic subglottic l.
  croupous l.
  hemorrhagic l.
  hyperplastic l.
  hypertrophic l.
  membranous l.
  l. sicca
  spasmodic l.
  l. stridulosa
  traumatic l.
laryngocele
  symptomatic l.
laryngofissure
  l. with tracheotomy
Laryngoflex reinforced endotracheal tube
laryngograph
laryngography
laryngology
laryngomalacia
laryngoparalysis
laryngopathy
laryngopharyngeal sensation
laryngopharyngectomy
  partial l. (PLP)
  total l. (TLP)
laryngopharyngitis
laryngopharyngoesophagectomy procedure
laryngopharynx
laryngophthisis
laryngoplasty
  sternothyroid muscle flap l.
laryngoplegia
laryngoptosis
laryngopyocele
laryngoscope
  Benjamin binocular slimline l.
  Benjamin-Lindholm
    microsuspension l.
  Benjamin pediatric operating l.
  Dedo l.
  Holinger anterior commissure l.
  Jackson l.
  Jackson anterior commissure l.
  Jako l.
  Killian-Lynch suspension l.
  Kleinsasser anterior commissure l.
  Lindholm operating l.
  Lynch suspension l.
  Weerda distending operating l.
laryngoscopic
  l. view
laryngoscopist
laryngoscopy
  direct l.
  flexible fiberoptic l.
  indirect l.
  laser l.
  microdirect l.
  suspension l.
laryngospasm
laryngospastic reflex
laryngostenosis
laryngostomy
laryngostroboscope
laryngotomy
  inferior l.
  median l.
  superior l.
  transepiglottic l.
laryngotracheal
  l. diversion
  l. invasion
  l. reconstruction (LTR)
  l. stenosis
  l. trauma
laryngotracheitis
laryngotracheobronchitis
laryngotracheoesophageal cleft
larynx, pl. **larynges**
  artificial l.
  chondromalacia of l.
  Cooper-Rand intraoral artificial l.
  electrical artificial l.
  electronic artificial l.
  extrinsic muscles of l.
  glottic l.
  intrinsic muscles of l.
  neuroendocrine tumor of l.
  neurofibroma of l.
  Nu-Vois artificial l.
  pneumatic artificial l.
  supraglottic l.
Laschal scissors
LaseAway
  L. ruby laser system

L. ruby and Q-switched Nd:YAG laser
L. Smooth Touch laser

laser

alexandrite l.
ALEXlazr l.
argon green l.
argon tuneable dye l.
Candela l.
carbon dioxide l.
CB Erbium/2.94 l.
char-free carbon dioxide l.
CLR 2940 erbium l.
CO_2 l.
l. coagulation
Coherent UltraPulse l.
cold beam l.
continuous wave l.
copper vapor l.
Cynosure l.
Derma 20 l.
Derma K combination l.
diode pumped Nd:YAG l.
l. dissection technique
l. Doppler flowmeter
l. Doppler flowmetry
l. Doppler perfusion monitor
l. endoforeheadplasty
EpiLaser hair removal l.
Erbium CrystaLase l.
esthetic CO_2 l.
excimer ultraviolet l.
l. festoon reduction
flashlamp pulse-dye l. (FLPD)
flashlamp pumped pulsed dye l. (FPPDL)
25 Gold portable CO_2 l.
l. hair transplant
l. hair transplantation
helium-neon l.
HGM Spectrum K1 krypton yellow & green l.
holmium:YAG l.
l. holography
I.L.MED l.
l. incisional blepharoplasty
2.5 joule Erbium resurfacing l.
KTP l.
KTP/532 l.
KTP/YAG l.
l. laryngoscopy

LaseAway ruby and Q-switched Nd:YAG l.
LaseAway Smooth Touch l.
l. lower lid transconjunctival blepharoplasty
Luxar NovaPulse CO_2 l.
MedLite Q-Switched neodymium-doped yttrium-aluminum-garnet l.
MedLite Q-Switched YAG l.
l. meloplasty
MultiLase D copper vapor l.
NaturaLase Erbium l.
NaturaLase Er:YAG l.
Nd:YAG l.
neodymium:yttrium-aluminum-garnet l.
510-nm pigmented lesion dye l.
NovaPulse l.
NovaPulse CO_2 l.
Paragon l.
PBI Medical copper vapor l.
PBI MultiLase D copper vapor l.
PhotoDerm PL l.
PhotoDerm VL l.
PhotoGenica LPIR with TKS l.
PhotoGenica T^{10} l.
PhotoGenica V l.
PhotoGenica VLS pulsed dye l.
Polytec LaseAway Q-switched ruby l.
potassium titanyl phosphate l.
pulsed-dye l.
pulsed tunable dye l.
pulsed yellow dye l.
QS alexandrite l.
QS Nd:YAG l.
QS ruby l.
Q-switched alexandrite l.
Q-switched neodymium YAG l.
Q-switched neodymium:yttrium aluminum-garnet l.
Q-switched ruby YAG l.
resurfacing l.
l. resurfacing
ruby l.
Sharplan l.
SharpLase Nd:YAG l.
Silhouette endoscopic l.
Silktouch l.
Skinlight erbium yttrium-aluminum-garnet l.
l. skin resurfacing

NOTES

laser *(continued)*
>l. smoke evacuation
>SoftLight l.
>Spectrum K1 l.
>l. stapedectomy
>l. stapedotomy
>l. stereolithography process
>l. surgery
>Surgica K6 l.
>Surgipulse XJ 150 CO_2 l.
>l. system
>TKS l.
>L. Trach wrapped endotracheal tube
>Tru-Pulse carbon dioxide l.
>Tru-Pulse CO_2 skin resurfacing l.
>tunable dye l.
>two-joule Erbium l.
>ubm Erbium Renaissance l.
>UltraPulse carbon dioxide l.
>UltraPulse CO_2 l.
>ultrapulsed l.
>UltraPulse surgical l.
>Unilase CO_2 l.
>VersaLight l.
>l. welding
>YAG l.

laser-assisted uvulopalatoplasty (LAUP)
laserbrasion
>ultrapulse carbon dioxide l.

Lasercare
>Elysee L.

Laserflo BPM laser Doppler monitor
Laserscope
Laser-Shield XII wrapped endotracheal tube
LaserSite
>L. facial mask
>L. wound dressing

Lasertubus
lasing
Lassus technique
lata
>fascia l.

latae
>tensor fasciae l.

latanoprost
late
>l. auditory evoked response (LAER)
>l. auditory evoked response audiometry
>l. bloomer
>l. infection
>l. obstetric brachial plexus palsy
>l. tooth

latency
>acoustic reflex l.

>facial nerve l.
>interpeak l.

latent
>l. image
>l. image film
>l. image spot
>l. period

lateral
>l. abscess
>l. accessory ligament of Henle
>l. adenoidectomy
>l. alveolar abscess
>l. antebrachial cutaneous nerve
>l. batten
>l. bulbar fossa
>l. canal
>l. canthal raphe
>l. canthopexy
>l. canthoplasty
>l. canthotomy
>l. canthus
>l. capsule
>l. caries
>l. cartilage
>l. checkbite
>l. check-bite interocclusal record
>l. collateral ligament
>l. condensation
>l. condensation root canal filling method
>l. condylar inclination
>l. condylar pole of the TMJ
>l. condyle
>l. cricoarytenoid muscle
>l. crural steal (LCS)
>l. crus
>l. cutaneous thigh flap
>l. cyst
>dark l.
>l. deviation on opening
>l. distally based fasciocutaneous flap
>l. dominance
>l. enamel strand
>l. excursion
>l. excursion test
>l. facial cleft deformity
>l. facial extraoral radiography
>l. femoral cutaneous nerve
>l. fissure
>l. galea aponeurotica
>l. glossoepiglottic fold
>l. head extraoral radiography
>l. hemifacial lesion
>l. incisal guide angle
>l. incisor
>l. incisor tooth
>l. incudal fold

l. intercostal flap
l. interocclusal record
l. jaw extraoral radiography
l. jaw film
l. jaw and occlusal survey
l. jaw panoramic series
l. jaw projection
l. jaw radiograph
l. jaw radiography
l. lamella
l. lemniscus
l. ligament of temporomandibular articulation
light l.
l. lisp
l. mallear fold
l. mallear ligament
l. mandibulectomy
l. mastoid bone
l. maxillary ligament
l. medullary syndrome
l. movement
l. neck crease
l. oblique jaw roentgenogram
l. oblique projection of mandible
l. oblique radiograph
l. oblique transcranial view
l. occlusal position
l. occlusion
l. occlusion relation
l. oral commissure
l. orbitotomy
l. parotidectomy
l. pedicle graft
l. perforation
l. periodontal abscess
l. periodontal cyst
l. pharyngeal space
l. pharyngotomy
l. projection
l. protrusion
l. pterygoid muscle
l. pterygoid plate
l. radiolucency
l. ramus radiograph
l. ramus roentgenogram
l. rectus capitis
l. rectus muscle
l. scar
l. sinus
l. sinus radiograph
l. sinus thrombophlebitis (LST)

l. sinus thrombosis
l. skull radiograph
l. skull roentgenogram
l. smasectomy
l. spinothalamic
l. spinothalamic tract
l. stress
l. sulcus
l. supramalleolar flap
l. surface of zygomatic bone
l. synechia syndrome
l. tarsal artery
l. tarsal strip procedure
l. thigh free flap
l. thyrohyoid ligament
l. TMJ ligament
l. trapezius flap
l. trim of the adenoid
l. upper arm flap
l. upper lip vermilion border
l. venous sinus (LVS)
l. vestibular nucleus
l. wall sphenoid
l. warp

laterale
orbitale l. (ol)

lateralis
musculus vastus l.
proboscis l. (PL)
sinus l.

laterality
crossed l.
mixed l.
l. theory of stuttering

lateralization
cortical l.

lateralizing
Weber l.

lateris
nevus unius l.

laterognathia
laterognathism
lateronasal process
lateroposition
lateroprotrusive
lateroretrusive
laterotrusion
procurrent l.

laterotrusive movement
late-talking
latex
l. agglutination

L

NOTES

latex *(continued)*
    l. glove
    rubber l.
Latham-Georgiade pin-retained presurgical orthopaedic appliance
lathe
    dental laboratory l.
latissimus
    l. dorsi breast reconstruction
    l. dorsi muscle
    l. dorsi muscle flap
    l. dorsi musculocutaneous flap
    l. dorsi myocutaneous flap (LDMCF)
    l. dorsi/scapular bone flap
    l. dorsi segmental musculovascular pedicle
    l. fasciocutaneous turnover flap
    l. muscle flap
    total autogenous l. (TAL)
LATS
    long-acting thyroid stimulator
lattice
    l. fiber
    l. space
laundry
    contaminated l.
LAUP
    laser-assisted uvulopalatoplasty
laurel fever
Laurence-Moon-Biedl syndrome
LAV
    lymphadenopathy-associated virus
lavage
    antral l.
    arthroscopic lysis and l.
    dual-port l.
    high-pressure pulsatile l.
    pulsatile jet l.
Lavandula officinalis
lavender
law
    Beer l.
    Bernoulli l.
    Fourier l.
    Gerhardt-Semon l.
    Hooke l.
    inverse square l.
    Ohm l.
    Semon l.
    Semon-Rosenbach l.
lawn chair position
lax
    l. consonant
    l. phoneme
    l. vowel

laxity
    horizontal lid l.
    orbicularis l.
layer
    adamantine l.
    ameloblastic l.
    basal l.
    cementogenic l.
    cornified l.
    dentinoblastic l.
    Dermanet wound contact l.
    facial fascial l.
    germinal l.
    granular l.
    half-value l. (HVL)
    inner fibrous l.
    intercellular l.
    intermediate l.
    laminated l.
    musculoaponeurotic l.
    odontoblastic l.
    outer fibrous l.
    oxide l.
    palisaded dentinoblastic l.
    parakeratotic l.
    parietal l.
    prickle cell l.
    second half-value l.
    silica-carbon l.
    smear l.
    submucous l.
    subodontoblastic l.
    surface cell l.
    Tomes granular l.
    Weil basal l.
LC
    lingual cusp
LCE
    lower completely edentulous
LCS
    lateral crural steal
LD
    learning disability
    linguodistal
LDD
    low drain class D
LDG
    lingual developmental groove
LDMCF
    latissimus dorsi myocutaneous flap
LDS
    Licentiate in Dental Surgery
Le
    L. Fort III craniofacial dysjunction
    L. Fort I, II, III fracture
    L. Fort I, II, III procedure
    L. Fort I, II osteotomy
    L. Fort I impaction

L. Fort II-type midface osteotomy
L. Fort I-type osteotomy
L. Fort maxillary osteotomy

lead
l. apron
l. collimator
l. disk
l. line
l. shield
l. stomatitis

leaded protective apron
lead-impregnated plastic
lead-lined cone
leaf
l. gauge
silver l.

leak
cerebrospinal fluid l.
chyle l.
halo test for CSF l.
retrosternal esophagocolonic
anastomotic l.
salivary l.

learning
l. disability (LD)
escape l.
integrative l.
interneurosensory l.
intraneurosensory l.
operant l.
paired associate l.
serial list l.
l. theory

leash
subcutaneous l.

leather wheel
LeCron carver
lectin
Ledercillin-VK
Ledermix paste
ledge
crown l.
dental l.
enamel l.

ledging
wall l.

leech
medicinal l.
L. Mobile Home

Lee denture
leek
leeway space

Leff
L. "C" gold
L. hard gold
L. light inlay
L. medium soft gold

left
l. hemisphere brain damage (LHD)
l. lateral excursion

legal dentistry
Leibinger
L. 3-D bone plate
L. E-Z flap
L. Micro Plus plate
L. Micro Plus screw
L. mini Würzburg plate
L. Mini Würzburg screw
L. plating
L. plating system
L. titanium Würzburg mandibular
reconstruction system
L. Würzburg screw

Leigh syndrome
leiomyoma
leiomyosarcoma
mandibular l.

leishmaniasis
American l.
mucocutaneous l.
nasopharyngeal l.
New World l.

Leitz 1600 Saw microtome
Lejour
L. breast reduction
L. mammaplasty
L. mastoplasty
L. technique

Lekholm-Zarb classification system
Leksell rongeur
Lell bite block
LeMesurier repair
lemniscus
lateral l.

Lemoflur fluoride
lemon
l. balm
l. bioflavonoid complex

length
anterior arch l.
arch l.
available arch l.
basialveolar l.
l. of crown

L

NOTES

length *(continued)*
>   dental l.
>   l. of mandible
>   mandibular body l.
>   maxilloalveolar l.
>   mean sentence l. (MSL)
>   muscle moment arm l.
>   Nance analysis of arch l.
>   l. of palate
>   physiognomic l.
>   required arch l.
>   l. of root
>   sill l.
>   upper lip l.

lengthened-off-time (LOT)
lengthener
>   Synthes l.

lengthening
>   distraction l.
>   l. genioplasty
>   levator-Müller complex l.
>   surgical crown l.
>   surgically assisted mandibular
>   arch l.
>   V-Y advancement for columellar l.

lengthening/advancing genioplasty
lenis
>   l. consonant
>   l. phoneme

lens
>   contact l.
>   parfocal defraction l.

lenticular process
lentigo, pl. **lentigines**
>   l. maligna melanoma
>   l. senilis

lentil
lentula, lentulo
>   l. carrier
>   l. paste carrier
>   l. root canal filler
>   l. spiral
>   l. spiral carrier
>   l. spiral drill

lentum
>   *Eubacterium l.*

Leon
>   L. cobra cannula
>   L. cobra tip

leonine facies
leontiasis ossea
leprae
>   l. cell
>   *Mycobacterium l.*

leproma
leprosy
leprous pulpitis
leptodontous

leptophonia
leptophonic
leptothrica
>   mycosis l.

Leptotrichia buccalis
Lermoyez syndrome
Leser-Trelat sign
lesion
>   aggressive l.
>   benign epidermal pigmented l.
>   benign lymphoepithelial l. (BLL)
>   caviar l.
>   cemental l.
>   combined-flow l.
>   cutaneous vascular l.
>   cylindromatous l.
>   cystic l.
>   cystic lymphoepithelial AIDS-
>   related l.
>   epulis-like l.
>   erythroplakic l.
>   fibromyxomatous l.
>   fibro-osseous l.
>   floor-of-mouth l.
>   giant cell l.
>   gross l.
>   ground-glass l.
>   high-flow l.
>   hyperplastic l.
>   hyperplastic epithelial l.
>   inflammatory l.
>   interradicular l.
>   intrabony l.
>   intraosseous l.
>   intrinsic brainstem l.
>   lateral hemifacial l.
>   lymphoepithelial l.
>   melanocytic l.
>   monostotic l.
>   mucoepidermoid l.
>   neurapraxic l.
>   nonneoplastic tumor-like l.
>   oromandibular l.
>   osteoporotic l.
>   periodontal l.
>   pigmented l.
>   precancerous l.
>   primary l.
>   pulpoperiapical l.
>   radiolucent l.
>   radiopaque l.
>   sessile l.
>   skip l.
>   spiculated l.
>   spongiotic l.
>   systemic l.
>   verrucous l.
>   vesiculobullous l.

white-spot l.
wraparound periapical l.

lesser
> l. horn
> l. palatine artery
> l. petrosal nerve
> l. superficial petrosal nerve
> l. wing of sphenoid

lesson
> trial l.

LET
> linear energy transfer

lethal midline granuloma
Letterer-Siwe disease
lettuce
leucovorin
Leudet tinnitus
leukemia
leukemic hyperplastic gingivitis
leukocyte
> neutrophilic l.
> polymorphonuclear l.

leukocytic infiltration
leukodontia
leukoedema
leukokeratosis
> l. nicotina palati

leukopenia
leukoplakia
> l. buccalis
> dyskeratotic l.
> friction/trauma-associated l.
> hairy l. (HL)
> idiopathic/tobacco-associated l.
> l. lingualis
> nondyskeratotic l.
> oral l.
> oral hairy l.
> speckled l.
> verruciform l.
> verrucous l.

leukotriene
levamisole
Levaquin
levarterenol
LeVasseur-Merrill retractor
levator
> l. anguli oris muscle
> l. aponeurosis surgery
> l. complex
> l. costae muscle
> l. dehiscence

l. disinsertion
l. glandulae thyroidea muscle
l. labii superioris alaeque nasi muscle
l. labii superioris muscle
l. muscle
l. muscle of angle of mouth
l. palatini muscle
l. palpebrae superioris
l. resection
l. veli palatini muscle

levator-Müller complex lengthening
Levbid
level
> acoustic reference l.
> L. Anchorage appliance
> L. Anchorage system
> bone conduction l.
> Chopart l.
> Clark l.
> effort l.
> hearing l. (HL)
> hearing threshold l. (HTL)
> loudness l.
> noise interference l. (NIL)
> operant l.
> overall sound l.
> Pirogoff amputation l.
> pressure pain tolerance l. (PPTL)
> reference zero l.
> saturation sound pressure l. (SSPL)
> sensation l. (SL)
> sensorineural acuity l. (SAL)
> signal sound pressure l.
> silicon blood l.
> sound l.
> sound pressure l. (SPL)
> speech interference l. (SIL)
> Syme amputation l.
> threshold hearing l.
> tolerance l.
> uncomfortable l. (UCL)
> uncomfortable listening l. (UCLL)
> uncomfortable loudness l. (UCLL)
> zero hearing l.

leveling
> l. archwire

lever
> dental l.

leverage
> denture l.

levobunolol

L

NOTES

levocabastine
Levo-Dromoran
levofloxacin
Levophed
Levoprome
levorphanol
levo-tryptophan (Lt, L-tryptophan)
levo-tryptophan-containing product
    (LTCP)
Levsin
    L./SL
Levsinex
Levy articulating retractor
Lewis bracket
Lewis-Resnik punch
Lewis-Tanner esophagectomy
Lewy
    L. laryngoscope holder
    L. suspension device
lexical
    l. access
    l. ambiguity
    l. category
    l. cohesion
    l. composition
    l. connotation
    l. denotation
    l. intervention
    l. item
    l. meaning
    l. morpheme
    l. word
lexicography
lexicon
    verb l.
Lezinski Flex-HA PORP ossicular chain
    prosthesis
LF
    lingual fossa
    low frequency
L-form osteotomy, inverted
LG
    lingual groove
LHD
    left hemisphere brain damage
LI
    language impairment
    linguoincisal
LIA
    local infiltrative anesthesia
libitum
    ad l.
Libra
    L. II crown and inlay
    L. III bridge and crown
    L. IV extra hard gold
Librium
Licentiate in Dental Surgery (LDS)

lichen planus
    atrophic l. p.
    bullous l. p.
    erosive l. p.
    oral (erosive) l. p.
    oral (nonerosive) l. p.
    l. p. pemphigoides
    pigmented l. p.
Licon
licorice
    gastrointestinal l.
lid
    l. retraction
    l. retractor
    scalloping of lower l.
Lida-Mantle HC Topical
Lidex
    L.-E
lid-loading technique
lidocaine
    bacitracin, neomycin, polymyxin B,
        and l.
    l. and hydrocortisone
    l. and prilocaine
Lido Multi Joint II isokinetic
    dynamometer
lid-sharing technique
LIE
    labioincisal edge
    linguoincisal edge
life
    quality of l. (QOL)
    reuse l.
    shelf l.
    use l.
lifeboat flap
LifeCell AlloDerm acellular dermal
    graft
Lifecore
    L. cutting advance technology
    L. Restore wide diameter implant
        system
Lifemask infant resuscitator
lift (See also face-lift, face-lift, face lift,
    face lift, face lift)
    biplanar forehead l.
    breast l.
    brow l.
    brow-forehead l.
    coronal brow l.
    deep-plane face l.
    endoforehead l.
    endoforehead-endomidface l.
    endoforehead-periorbital-cheek l.
    endomidface l.
    endoscopic brow l.
    endoscopic face l.
    endoscopic forehead l.

endoscopic subperiosteal forehead l.
endoscopic subperiosteal forehead
  and midface l.
endoscopic subperiosteal midface l.
endotemporal l.
endotemporal-endomidface l.
eyebrow l.
face l., face-lift, facelift
facial subcutaneous l.
FAME midface l.
functional l.
mask l.
midface l.
palatal l.
significative l.
SMAS l.
subcutaneous temporo-facial face l.
subcutaneous temporo-malar face l.
subperiosteal brow l.
subperiosteal face l.
subperiosteal malar cheek l.
subplatysmal face l.
temporomalar endoscopic l.
thigh l.
transblepharoplasty forehead l.

lifting
face l.
Ligaclip
ligament
alveolodental l.
annular l.
anterior mallear l.
anterior suspensory l.
apical dental l.
Berry l.
Broyle l.
cemental l.
circular dental l.
Cleland l.
collateral l.
cricothyroid l.
dentoalveolar l.
gingival l.
gingivodental l.
hammock l.
hypoepiglottic l.
incudal l.
interdental l.
intermetatarsal l.
labiomandibular l.
lateral accessory l. of Henle
lateral collateral l.

lateral mallear l.
lateral maxillary l.
lateral thyrohyoid l.
lateral TMJ l.
Lockwood l.
mallear l.
maxillary l.
medial collateral l.
median thyrohyoid l.
nasolabial l.
nasomandibular l.
peridental l.
periimplant l.
periodontal l. (PDL)
petroclinoid l.
posterior incudal l.
posterior suspensory l.
l. reinsertion
Sappey l.
sphenomandibular l.
spiral l.
stylohyoid l.
stylomandibular l.
superior incudal l.
superior mallear l.
suspensory l.
temporomandibular l.
thyroepiglottic l.
thyrohyoid l.
transseptal l.
transverse carpal l. (TCL)
Treitz l.
vestibular l.
vocal l.
ligamental anesthesia
ligamentous facial fence
ligate
ligation
endoscopic band l. (EBL)
endoscopic variceal l. (EVL)
interdental l.
parotid duct l.
sling l.
surgical l.
teeth l.
tooth l.
transesophageal varix l.
ligature
l. cutter
elastic l.
grass-line l.
occluding l.

L

NOTES

ligature *(continued)*
    orthodontic l.
    plastic l.
    steel l.
    l. tie wire
ligatureless bracket
ligature-locking pliers
ligature-tying pliers
light
    l. around wire technique
    l. body impression material
    cold l.
    cone of l.
    l. contact
    fiberoptic l. (FOL)
    Floxite mirror l.
    l. lateral
    l. microscopy (LM)
    l. photon
    pyramid of l.
    l. reflex
    l. round wire appliance
    ultraviolet l.
    l. voice
    l. vowel
    l. white frosting
    l. wire appliance
    l. wire torque
    l. wire torque force
light-activated
    l.-a. resin
    l.-a. sealant
light amplification by stimulated emission of radiation
light-cured
    l.-c. dimethacrylate
    l.-c. resin
light-curing resin
lighting
    Fastrac l.
lightning strip
light-reflecting wedge
lightsource
    halogen dual l.
Lightspeed
    L. canal preparation technique
    L. file
    L. rotary root canal instrument
Ligmajet syringe
lignite wax
Lignospan Forte
Ligusticum porterii
lilac
Lillie-Crow test
lima bean
limb
    l. bud

complete cutaneous syndactyly of all four l.'s
    l. duplication
    horizontal l.
    l. hypertrophy
    l. salvage
    supernumerary l.
Limberg flap
Limberg-type cutaneous flap
limb-sparing procedure
limbus
    l. alveolaris mandibulae
    l. alveolaris maxillae
limen, pl. limina
    difference l. (DL)
    l. nasi
    temporal difference l. (TDL)
limit
    elastic l. (EL)
    proportional l.
limitans
    lamina l.
limited
    l. phonetic inventory
    l. pocket
    l. range audiometer
    l. retention
limiter
    noise l.
Linc alloy
Linco
Lincomycin
Lindamood Auditory Conceptualization Test
Lindeman
    L. bone cutter
    L. bur
Lindholm operating laryngoscope
Line
line
    accretion l.
    L. alloy
    alveolar point-basion l.
    alveolar point-nasal point l.
    alveolar point-nasion l.
    alveolobasilar l.
    alveolonasal l.
    l. angle
    anterior axillary l.
    arcuate l.
    bismuth l.
    blue l.
    Burton l.
    calcification l.
    calcification l.'s of Retzius
    calciotraumatic l.
    Camper l.
    cement l.

cemental l.
cementing l.
cerebral reference l.
cervical l. (CL)
Clapton l.
contour l.
craze l.
cross arch fulcrum l.
demarcation l.
developmental l.
developmental l.
external oblique l.
feather-edged proximal finishing l.
fine l.
finish l.
Frankfort horizontal light l.
fulcrum l.
gingival l.
gingival finishing l.
glabellar l.
glabellar frown l.
gum l.
hemiclavicular l.
high lip l.
high smile l.
His l.
Holdaway l.
Hunter-Schreger l.
hyperfunctional facial l.
hyperfunctional glabellar l.
imbrication l.'s of von Ebner
incremental l.
incremental l.'s of von Ebner
infraciliary l.
innominate l.
knife-edged finishing l.
labial l.
Langer cleavage l.
lead l.
lip l.
load l.
low lip l.
marionette l.
median l.
mercurial l.
methylene blue l.
middle cranial fossa l.
milk l.
mucogingival l.
mylohyoid l.
nasion-alveolar point l.
nasolabial l.

neonatal l.
oblique l.
l. of occlusion
Ohngren l.
orbital l.
Owen l.'s
Pickerill imbrication l.
protrusive l.
radiolucent l.
recessional l.
Reid base l.
relaxed skin tension l. (RSTL)
resting l.
retentive fulcrum l.
l.'s of Retzius
reversal l.
Salter incremental l.'s
S-BP l.
Schreger l.'s
sinus l.
S-N l.
stabilizing fulcrum l.
submammary l.
survey l.
Tatagiba l.
temporal l.
Thompson l.
Tycos pressure infusion l.
vertical corrugator l.
vibrating l.
von Ebner l.
l.'s of von Ebner

linea

l. alba
l. alba buccalis
l. aspera
l. temporalis

linear

l. energy transfer (LET)
l. graft
l. hearing aid
l. IgA bullous disease
l. osteotomy
l. scleroderma
l. silicone rubber polymer
l. tan-brown-black pigmentation
l. thermal expansion
l. thermal expansion coefficient

lined flap
linen strip
liner

Accu-Spense cavity l.

L

NOTES

liner *(continued)*
    asbestos l.
    Cavidry base l.
    cavity l.
    Hydroxyline cavity l.
    Hypo-Cal cavity l.
    Plastodent cavity l.
    Pulpdent cavity l.
    resilient l.
    soft l.
    Speed l.
line-to-nipple
    midclavicular l.-t.-n. (MCL-N)
lingua, gen. and pl. **linguae**
    l. alba
    copula linguae
    l. dissecta
    l. fissurata
    l. frenata
    frenulum linguae
    l. geographica
    l. nigra
    nigrities linguae
    pityriasis linguae
    l. plicata
    tylosis linguae
    l. villosa alba
    l. villosa nigra
linguadental *(var. of* linguodental)
linguagram
lingual
    l. alveolus
    l. angle
    l. approach
    l. apron
    l. arch
    l. arch-forming pliers
    l. artery
    l. attachment
    l. bar
    l. bar major connector
    l. bone
    l. button
    l. canine-to-canine retainer
    l. cavity
    l. clasp
    l. cortical plate
    l. crib
    l. crossbite
    l. cusp (LC)
    l. cyst
    l. developmental groove (LDG)
    l. dovetail
    l. duct
    l. embrasure
    l. flange
    l. follicle
    l. foramen

    l. fossa (LF)
    l. frenulum
    l. frenum
    l. gingiva
    l. gland
    l. groove (LG)
    l. hemiatrophy
    l. hypoplasia
    l. inclination
    l. lisp
    l. lobe
    l. lymph follicle
    l. lymph node
    l. mandibular periosteum
    l. movement
    l. mucoperiosteal flap
    l. mucosa
    l. nerve
    l. occlusion
    l. papilla
    l. paralysis
    l. peak
    l. periosteum
    l. placement
    l. plate
    l. plexus
    l. premolar-to-premolar retainer
    l. quinsy
    l. ramping
    l. raphe
    l. resin
    l. rest
    l. ridge (LR)
    l. root (LR)
    l. saliva
    l. salivary gland depression
    l. septum
    l. shield
    l. splint
    l. split-bone technique
    l. strap
    l. sulcus
    l. surface
    l. surface of tooth
    l. thyroid
    l. thyroid carcinoma
    l. tongue flap
    l. tonsil
    l. trophoneurosis
    l. wire
lingualis, pl. **linguales**
    papilla l.
lingually
linguapalatal contact
linguine sign
linguist
linguistic
    l. ambiguity

l. aspect
l. competence
l. component
l. determinism
l. intrusion
l. performance
l. phonetics
l. relativity
l. retention
l. universals
l. variation
linguistics
anthropological l.
applied l.
comparative l.
contrastive l.
descriptive l.
diachronic l.
general l.
historical l.
structural l.
synchronic l.
theoretical l.
lingula, pl. lingulae
l. of mandible
l. mandibulae
lingulectomy
linguoalveolar
l. area
linguoangular
linguoaxial
linguoaxiogingival
linguocervical
l. ridge
linguoclination
linguoclusion
linguodental, linguadental
l. area
linguodistal (LD)
linguogingival
l. fissure
l. ridge
l. shoulder
linguoincisal (LI)
l. edge (LIE)
l. line angle
linguomesial (LM)
linguo-occlusal (LO)
l.-o. line angle
linguopapillitis
linguoplacement
linguoplasty

linguoplate
l. major connector
palatal l.
linguoproximal
linguopulpal (LP)
linguotrite
linguoversion
lining
cavity l.
mucoperiosteal l.
l. mucosa
oral mucosal l.
linking verb
Linkow blade implant
Link-Plus retention pin
linters
cotton l.
lion jaw bone holder
lip
l. augmentation
l. biting
l. border advancement
l. bumper
cleft l., cleft-lip
l. competency
complete cleft l.
l. curtain
double l.
l. elevator
l. enhancement
frenulum of superior l.
l. furrow band
l. habit appliance
Hapsburg l.
l. hypertonia
incisive muscle of lower l.
incisive muscle of upper l.
l. incompetence
incompetent upper l.
inferior l.
l. line
lower l.
median cleft l.
mucous membrane of l.
l. paresthesia
l. pit
l. plumper
l. pucker
quadrate muscle of lower l.
quadrate muscle of upper l.
red zone of l.
l. retractor

L

NOTES

lip *(continued)*
    l. rounding
    square muscle of lower l.
    square muscle of upper l.
    superior l.
    l. switch flap
    tubercle of upper l.
    unilateral cleft l.
    upper l.
    vermilion border of l.
lipase
lipectomy
    blunt suction l.
    orbital l.
    suction l.
    suction-assisted l. (SAL)
    transjunctival l.
    ultrasound-assisted l. (UAL)
Lipectron
    L. ultrasonic lancet
    L. ultrasonic scalpel
lipexeresis
lipid
    l. droplet
lip-lip flap
lipoaspirated material
lipoaspiration
lipoatrophy
lipoblast
lipoblastoma
    benign l.
lipoblastomatosis
    benign l.
lipocontour
lipocrit
lipocyte
lipodystrophy
    facial l.
    posttraumatic l.
lipofilling
Lipoflavonoid
lipogen
lipogenic tumor
lipogranuloma
lipogranulomastosis
    sclerosing l.
lipohypertrophic mass
lipohypertrophy
    insulin-induced l.
lipoidica
    necrobiosis l.
lipoidosis cutis et mucosae
lipoid proteinosis
lipoinfiltration
    periorbital l.
lipoinjection technique
lipo layering technique
lipolysis

lipoma
    l. arborescens
    l. aspiration
    hypopharyngeal l.
    laryngeal l.
    posttraumatic l.
    salivary l.
    subcutaneous l.
lipomatosis
Lipo-Medi girdle
lipomyxoma
liponecrosis
liponecrotic pseudocyst
Lipopanty girdle
lipophagic granuloma
lipophilic virus
lipoplasty
    blunt suction-assisted l.
    Fischer aspirative l.
    Illouz aspirative l.
    Kesselring aspirative l.
    Schrudde aspirative l.
    Teimourian aspirative l.
    traditional l.
lipopolysaccharide (LPS)
liporestructure
liposarcoma
    adult-type well-differentiated l.
    myxoid l.
    pleomorphic l.
    round-cell l.
liposculpture
    superficial l.
    syringe l.
liposculpturing
    ultrasonic l.
lipostructure
liposuction
    l. cannula
    l. divot
    extended l.
    l. fat fillant implant
    massive all layer l. (MALL)
    submental l.
    syringe-assisted l.
    l. technique
    tumescent l.
    ultrasonic l.
    ultrasound l.
    ultrasound-assisted l.
liposuctioning
lipotropic agent
Lipovacutainer canister
lipoxygenase
lipreading
lip-splitting incision
lipstick sign
lip-sucking habit crib

liquefaction
> bone l.
> l. necrosis

liquefactive necrosis
liquefying
Liqui-Caps
> Vicks 44 Non-Drowsy Cold &
> Cough L.-C.

liquid
> Anaplex L.
> l. chemical sterilization
> Chlorafed L.
> Ed A-Hist L.
> Fluorident l.
> Fluoritab l.
> gliding of l.'s
> Gordofilm L.
> Hayfebrol L.
> Hurricaine l.
> Karidium l.
> Lotrimin AF Spray L.
> Mosco L.
> Naldecon DX Adult L.
> Nebs analgesic l.
> l. nitrogen
> Occlusal-HP L.
> L. Pred
> Prometh VC Plain L.
> Pulpdent l.
> Rescon L.
> Rhinosyn-PD L.
> Rhinosyn-X L.
> Rolatuss Plain L.
> Ru-Tuss L.
> Ryna-C L.
> l. scintillation spectrometer
> Sudafed Plus L.
> Topicale l.

liquidambar
Liquifilm
> Betagan L.
> L. Forte Solution
> HMS L.
> L. Tears Solution

Liqui-Gels
> Alka-Seltzer Plus Flu & Body
> Aches Non-Drowsy L.-G.
> Robitussin Severe Congestion L.-G.

Liquiprin
Lisch nodule
Lisfranc joint

lisp
> dental l.
> frontal l.
> interdental l.
> lateral l.
> lingual l.
> nasal l.
> occluded l.
> protrusion l.
> strident l.
> substitutional l.

lisping
list
> PBK Word L.'s
> Phonetically Balanced Kindergarten
> Word L.'s

listening
> auditory selective l.
> dichotic l.
> diotic l.
> selective l.
> visual l.

Listermint with Fluoride
lite
> Floxite mirror l.

Lite blade
Lite-fil A, P
Lite-Pipe
> Millard L.-P.

literalis
> dysarthria l.
> paralalia l.

literal paraphasia
Literature
> Index to Dental L. (IDL)

lithectomy
lithiasis
> extraglandular l.
> salivary l.

lithium
Lithoclast ballistic energy generator
lithotomy
> l. position
> l. procedure

lithotripsy
> electrohydraulic extracorporeal l.
> intracorporeal l.

lithotriptor
> electromagnetic l.
> piezoelectric l.
> pneumoballistic l.

Littauer suture scissors

L

NOTES

Little
  L. area
  L. Secret CIC
Littler neurovascular island flap
live
  l. oak
  l. voice audiometry
liver
  l. function
  l. spot
living
  activity of daily l. (ADL)
  Communicative Abilities in
    Daily L. (CADL)
Livostin
LJP
  localized juvenile periodontitis
LLETZ/LEEP loop electrode
LM
  laryngeal melanosis
  light microscopy
  linguomesial
LMA
  laryngeal mask airway
LMD
  low-molecular-weight dextran
LO
  linguo-occlusal
load
  gold lid l.
  l. line
  occlusal l.
loadbearing
load-deflection rate
loading
  axial l.
  torsional l.
lobe
  deep parotid l.
  deformity of ear l.
  flocculonodular l.
  frontal l.
  lingual l.
  occipital l.
  parietal l.
  parotid deep l.
  supplemental l.
  temporal l.
lobectomy
  deep l.
  ipsilateral total lobectomy and
    contralateral subtotal l.
  thyroid l.
  total ipsilateral l.
lobster
lobular carcinoma
lobulated tongue
lobulation

lobule
  ear l.
  myxoid l.
  prominent l.
lobuli
  coloboma l.
local
  l. analgesia
  l. anesthesia
  l. anesthetic
  l. argyria
  l. decongestion
  l. excision
  l. infiltrative anesthesia (LIA)
  l. nerve block
  l. rotation flap
  l. vasodilation
localization
  auditory l.
  cerebral l.
  l. technique
localized
  l. amnesia
  l. gingivitis
  l. juvenile periodontitis (LJP)
  l. scleroderma
locally invasive congenital cellular blue
  nevus of scalp
locating canal
locative
locator
  apex l.
  Apit electronic apex l.
  electronic apex l. (EAL)
  Endex apex l.
  Neosono MC apex l.
  Odontometer electronic apex l.
  Root ZX apex l.
  Staodyn Insight point l.
loci
  paracusis l.
lock
  l. pin
  universal Luer l.
locked
  l. bite
  l. occlusion
  l. root
locking
  l. gate
  l. pliers
lockjaw
Lockwood
  L. ligament
Locoid
locomotion
locoregional
  l. control

l. disease
l. treatment oral fistula
loculation
locus minoris resistentiae
locust
black l.
locution
lodgepole pine
Lodine
L. XL
lodoxamide tromethamine
Loeb sliding pad technique
Löe and Silness index
loft register
Logan bow
logaphasia
logarithm
logarithmic graph
logical
l. method
l. operation
logopathy
logopedia
logopedics
logopedist
logoplegia
logorrhea
logospasm
log relative exposure
Lombard voice-reflex test
Lombardy poplar
lomefloxacin
long
l. axis
l. centric
l. cone
l. cone technique
l. face syndrome
l. term memory
l. tongue
l. tooth
Longacre graft augmentation
long-acting
l.-a. somatostatin analog
l.-a. thyroid stimulator (LATS)
long-axis technique
long-bone reconstruction
long-cone radiograph
long-handled
l.-h. foil condenser
l.-h. instrument

longitudinal
l. cerebral fissure
l. melanonychia
l. muscle of tongue
l. raphe
l. raphe of tongue
l. ridge of hard palate
l. suture
l. suture of palate
l. wave
longitudinalis
l. inferior muscle
l. superior muscle
long-scale contrast
long-skin flap blepharoplasty
long-span rigid plate
long-standing radiolucency
longus
l. capitis muscle
l. colli muscle
palmaris l.
Look and Say Articulation Trainer
loop (*See also* loupe)
arterial l.
bitewing l.
cervical l.
flow l.
Hyrtl l.
induction l.
Ivy l.
offending vascular l.
l. pliers
sentinel l.
terminal capillary l.
vascular l.
venous l.
vertical l.
loop-forming pliers
loose premaxilla
lop ear
lophodont
Loprox
loquacity
Lorabid
loracarbef
loratadine
l. and pseudoephedrine
Lorcet
L. 10/650
L.-HD
L. Plus

NOTES

Lorenz

L. gauze packer
L. Micro-Power dense bone drilling and cutting system
L. PC/TC scissors
L. plating system

Lortab

L. ASA
L. Tablet

loss

autoimmune hearing l.
central hearing l.
cochlear hearing l.
conductive hearing l.
l. of contact point
crestal bone l.
discrimination l.
drill-induced hearing l.
extreme hearing l.
familial hearing l.
flat fluctuating hearing l.
fluctuating hearing l.
functional hearing l.
l. of gloss
hearing l.
iatrogenic hearing l.
insertion l.
intraoperative hearing l.
low-frequency sensorineural fluctuating hearing l.
mild hearing l.
moderate hearing l.
moderately severe hearing l.
nerve l.
noise-induced hearing l.
nonsyndromic hearing l. (NSHL)
occupational hearing l.
perceptive hearing l.
postlingual profound sensorineural hearing l.
profound hearing l.
sensorineural hearing l. (SNHL)
severe hearing l.
slight hearing l.
subtotal pulp l.
sudden hearing l. (SHL)
total pulp l.
unilateral hearing l.
vertical bone l.
weight l.
X-linked albinism and sensorineural hearing l.

lost

L. Cord Club
l. wax
l. wax pattern technique
l. wax process

LOT

lengthened-off-time

Lothrop frontoethmoidectomy procedure

lotion

Lotrimin AF L.
M.D. Forté skin rejuvenation l. II
vitamin C facial l.

Lotrimin

L. AF Cream
L. AF Lotion
L. AF Solution
L. AF Spray Liquid
L. AF Spray Powder

loudness

Békésy comfortable l. (BCL)
l. growth perception
l. level
most comfortable l. (MCL)
prosodic feature of l.
l. unit

loudspeaker

loupe (*See also* loop)

binocular l.
Galilean l.
Keeler-Galilean surgical l.
Keeler panoramic l.
l. magnification
panoramic l.

louse

love

l. handles
L. retractor

low

l. biscuit
l. biscuit firing
l. frequency (LF)
l. glaze
l. lip line
l. magnification scanning electron micrograph
l. margin standard abutment
l. oxyhemoglobin saturation (LSAT)
l. profile plate
l. socioeconomic status (low-SES)
l. tone deafness
l. vowel

low-copper alloy

low drain class D (LDD)

Löwenberg forceps

lower

l. anterior dental height
l. anterior forceps
l. arch
l. completely edentulous (LCE)
l. half headache of Sluder
l. impression
l. incisor
l. incisor angulation

l. lateral cartilage
l. lip
l. lip-splitting incision
l. partially edentulous (LPE)
l. ridge slope
l. teeth
l. trapezius flap
l. universal forceps
low-flow anesthetic
low-flying bird incision
low-frequency
l.-f. pulp tester
l.-f. response
l.-f. sensorineural fluctuating
hearing loss
low-fusing
l.-f. alloy
l.-f. porcelain
lowlight area
low-lying tegmen
low-molecular-weight dextran (LMD)
low-pass filter
low-pressure voice prosthesis
low-SES
low socioeconomic status
low-speed
l.-s. Christmas tree diamond bur
l.-s. handpiece
l.-s. tapered carbide bur
low-strength base
**Loyola University classification for
pulpoperiapical pathosis**
lozenge
Flura-Loz l.
Lozi-Tab
Luride L.-T.
Luride-SF L.-T.
LP
linguopulpal
LPE
lower partially edentulous
L-plasty
LPS
lipopolysaccharide
LPT
Language Proficiency Test
LR
lingual ridge
lingual root
LR needle
L&R X-ray film dryer

LSAT
low oxyhemoglobin saturation
L-scar
L-shaped
L.-s. miniplate
L.-s. skin excision
LST
lateral sinus thrombophlebitis
Lt
levo-tryptophan
LTCP
levo-tryptophan-containing product
LTR
laryngotracheal reconstruction
L-tryptophan
levo-tryptophan
lubricant
die l.
ophthalmic l.
silicone l.
lubrication
Lubriderm
LubriTears Solution
Lucas alveolar curette
lucida
camera l.
lamina l.
Luc operation
Ludwig angina
Luer
L. lock fitting
Luer-Lok
L.-L. adapter
L.-L. B-D syringe
L.-L. needle
lug
occlusal l.
retention l.
Lugol iodine
Luhr
L. fixation plate
L. implant
L. maxillofacial fixation system
L. microfixation system
L. pan fixation system
L. Vitallium micromesh plate
L. vitallium screw
Lukens
L. collecting tube
L. needle
L. trap
Luks plugger

L

NOTES

lumbar
- l. drainage
- l. periosteal turnover flap
- l. puncture
- l. roll

lumen, pl. **lumina**
- acinar l.
- intercalated duct l.

Lumex
- L. recliner
- L. Tub Guard Tall

Luminal
luminal ameloblastoma
Luminex post system
lumpectomy
lumpy jaw
lunate
- l. bone
- l. excision

Lund-Browder burn diagram
lung
- l. abscess
- l. capacity
- l. volume
- l. window

lungwort
lupus
- l. erythematosus
- l. pernio
- l. vulgaris

lurching gait
Luride
- L. acidulated phosphate fluoride paste
- L. Drops
- L. Lozi-Tab
- L.-SF Lozi-Tab
- L. topical gel
- L. topical solution

Luschka tonsil
lusoria
- dysphagia l.

lute
luting
- l. agent
- l. cement

Lux
- Brilliant L.

Luxar
- L. NovaPulse CO$_2$ laser
- L. Silhouette noninvasive body appearance equipment

luxated
luxation
- habitual temporomandibular joint l.
- temporomandibular l.
- traumatic l.

Luxator extractor

5 lux color video camera
LVS
- lateral venous sinus

Lyme disease
lymph
- l. capillary
- dental l.
- dentinal l.
- l. node
- l. nodule

lymphadenectomy
lymphadenitis
- mycobacterial l.
- toxoplasma l.

lymphadenoma
- sebaceous l.

lymphadenopathy
- infectious l.
- persistent generalized l. (PGL)

lymphadenopathy-associated virus (LAV)
lymphangiohemangioma
- cavernous l.

lymphangioma
- capillary l.
- cavernous l.
- l. circumscriptum
- cystic l.

lymphangioplasty
lymphangitis
lymphatic
- afferent l.
- l. capillary
- l. drainage
- l. fistula
- l. follicle
- l. follicles of tongue
- l. malformation
- l. massage
- l. metastasis
- l. nodule
- l. vessel
- l. vessels of mouth
- l. vessels of tongue

lymphaticovenous anastomosis
lymphedema
- l. grade II, III

lymphocele
lymphocinesis (*var. of* lymphokinesis)
lymphocutaneous
lymphocyte
- l. activation factor
- B l.
- l. immune globulin
- pulpal l.
- T l.
- T cytotoxic/suppressor l.
- T-helper l.

T helper/inducer l.
T-suppressor l.
lymphocytic choriomeningitis
lymphoepithelial
>   l. cyst
>   l. lesion
>   l. proliferation
lymphoepithelioma
>   malignant l.
lymphoid
>   l. hyperplasia
>   l. wandering cell
lymphokine
lymphokine-activated
>   l.-a. killer cell (LAK)
lymphokinesis, lymphocinesis
lymphoma
>   Burkitt l.
>   Castleman l.
>   cutaneous T-cell l. (CTCL)
>   diffuse large cell l.
>   endemic Burkitt l. (EBL)
>   extranodal malignant l.
>   extranodal non-Hodgkin l.
>   follicular l.
>   giant follicle l.
>   Hodgkin l.
>   large-cell l.
>   malignant l.
>   non-Hodgkin l.
>   sporadic Burkitt l.
lymphomatosa
>   struma l.
lymphomatosum
>   cystadenoma l.
>   papillary cystadenoma l.
lymphonodular pharyngitis
lymphoplasty
lymphoproliferative
>   l. disorder
lymphoreticular tumor
lymphorrhea
lymphosarcoma
lymphoscintigraphy

lymphotoxin
lymphovenous malformation
Lynch
>   L. frontoethmoidectomy procedure
>   L. procedure
>   L. suspension laryngoscope
lyophilization
lyophilized
>   l. botulinum toxin A
>   l. dura
>   l. dura graft
>   l. dural patch
>   l. Transderm Scop transdermal
>   patch
Lyphocin
lysing effect
lysis
LySonix
>   L. 250 aspirator
>   L. 2000 complete ultrasonic
>   surgical system
>   L. Delta Tip irrigator
>   L. Diamond Tip scavenger
>   L. ImageFX patient imaging
>   software
>   L. 250 irrigator
>   L. 2000 Micro ultrasonic surgical
>   system
>   L. 250 operative workstation
>   L. Post-Operative patient system
>   L. series 250 irrigator/aspirator
>   L. Series 250 operative system
>   L. 2000 Standard ultrasonic
>   surgical system
>   L. TTD Cannula Systems
>   L. TTD Design Mercedes
>   L. TTD Design pyramid
>   L. TTD Design Standard
>   L. 2000 ultrasonic surgical system
>   L. 2000 ultrasound device
lysosome
lysozyme
lysyl-bradykinin

L

NOTES

3M
3M CTRS device
3M microvascular anastomotic coupling device

M4
M4 Kerr Safety Hedstrom instrument
M4 safety handpiece

MA
main arteriole
mental age

mA
milliampere

MAA
mandibular advancement appliance

MAC
Minimum Auditory Capabilities Test
Mycobacterium avium complex
Mycobacterium avium-intracellulare complex

MacArthur Communicative Development Inventories

maceration
skin m.

Macewen triangle

MacFee incision

Machida light source connector

machine
casting m.
electric casting m.
MDA ultrasound-assisted lipoplasty m.
Medicamat ultrasound-assisted lipoplasty m.
Mentor ultrasound-assisted lipoplasty m.
Morwel ultrasound-assisted lipoplasty m.
Orthopantomograph-3 panoramic x-ray m.
Orthopantomograph-10 panoramic x-ray m.
OsteoPower drilling and cutting m.
Panelipse panoramic x-ray m.
Panex-E (Panoral) panoramic x-ray m.
panoramic rotating m.
Panorex panoramic x-ray m.
pantomography m.
PC-1000/Laser 1000 panoramic cephalometric x-ray m.
PC-1000 panoramic x-ray m.
Planmeca panoramic x-ray m.
Sebbin ultrasound-assisted lipoplasty m.

SMEI ultrasound-assisted lipoplasty m.
Sono-stat Plus EMG m.
Status-X m.
Surgitron ultrasound-assisted lipoplasty m.

machineable apatite-free glass ceramic

machining
computer assisted design/computer assisted m.

machinist's gauge

MacKenty septal elevator

MacKenzie syndrome

Macleans dentifrice

macrocalcification

macrocephaly

macrocheilia, macrochilia
port-wine m.

macrodactyly

macrodont

macrodontia
relative generalized m.
single-tooth m.
true generalized m.

macrodontic

macrodontism

macrofilled resin

macrofiller

macrogenia

macrogingivae

macroglobulin
alpha$_2$-m.

macroglobulinemia
Waldenström m.

macroglossia
amyloid m.
unilateral m.

macroglossic

macrognathia
mandibular m.
maxillary m.

macrognathic

macroinjection of autologous fat

macromastia

macrophage
blood-borne m.
chemotactic factor for m. (CFM)
pulpal m.
tissue m.
tissue-borne m.

macrophage-activating factor (MAF)

macrophage-inhibiting factor (MIF)

macrophallus

macrophonia

Macroplastique material

M

macrorhinia
macroscopic
    m. concavity
macrosmatic
macrosomia
macrostomia
macrotia
macrotooth
macrotrauma
macula, pl. maculae
    acoustic m.
    m. adherens
    m. cribrosa media
    m. flava
    medial cribrose m.
macular hair cell
macule
    café au lait m.
MAD
    maximum accumulated dose
Madsen OB822 clinical audiometer
Maestro implant
MAF
    macrophage-activating factor
    master apical file
    minimum acceptable field
    minimum audible field
mafenide
Maffucci syndrome
Magan
magenta tongue
Magitot disease
Maglite
Magna-Finder locating device
Magna-Site locating system
magnesium
    m. oxide
    m. salicylate
magnet
    denture m.
    foreign body m.
magnetic
    m. implant
    m. jaw tracking device
    m. resonance angiography (MRA)
    m. resonance imaging (MRI)
    m. source imaging (MSI)
magnetoencephalography (MEG)
Magnevist
magnification
    loupe m.
magnitude
    response m.
magnum
    foramen m.

MAGPI
    meatal advancement and glanduloplasty procedure
    meatoplasty and glanulopasty
MAI
    Mycobacterium avium-intracellulare
Maico Gamma hearing aid
main
    m. arteriole (MA)
    m. venule (MV)
mainstreaming
maintainer
    band and bar space m.
    band and crib space m.
    bonded space m.
    broken-stress space m.
    cantilever space m.
    m. cast space
    crown and bar space m.
    crown and crib space m.
    fixed-removable space m.
    fixed space m.
    Gerber space m.
    Mayne space m.
    removable space m.
    space m.
maintenance
major
    m. anchorage
    aphthae m.
    m. connector
    m. histocompatibility complex (MHC)
    musculus zygomaticus m.
    pectoralis m. (PM)
    thalassemia m.
make-up
    camouflage m.-u.
mal
    grand m.
    petit m.
malacotic
    m. teeth
maladaptive response
Malaga flap
malaise
malaleuca
malaligned tooth
malalignment
    vermilion-white line m.
malar
    m. alloplastic augmentation
    m. arch
    m. bag
    m. bag suctioning
    m. bone
    m. deficiency
    m. elevator

m. eminence
m. facial augmentation
m. flatness
m. fracture
m. gland
m. hypoplasia
m. ligament complex
m. margin
m. mound
m. pad
m. periosteum-SMAS flap fixation suture
m. prominence
m. shell augmentation
m. surface of zygomatic bone
m. tuberosity
malare
malarplasty procedure
malar-zygomatic region
Malassez
M. debris
M. epithelial rests
male
m. abdominoplasty
m. compression girdle
m. flank
m. forehead plasty
m. soprano voice
maleate
ergonovine m.
methysergide m.
male-pattern baldness
maleruption
male-to-female transsexual
malformation
adult Chiari m.
arhinia m.
Arnold-Chiari m.
arteriovenous m. (AVM)
Bing-Siebenmann m.
capillary vascular m.
Chiari type I, II, III, IV m.
congenital m.
Dandy-Walker m.
high-flow arteriovenous m.
lymphatic m.
lymphovenous m.
Michel m.
Mondini m.
Mondini-Alexander m.
osseous craniofacial arteriovenous m.

rugose frontonasal m.
Scheibe m.
split hand/split foot m.
vaginal m.
vascular m.
venous m.
malformed tooth
malfunction
malfunctional occlusion
Malherbe
calcifying epithelioma of M.
epithelioma of M.
malic dehydrogenase
malignancy
malignant
m. blue nevus
m. chondroma
m. dyskeratosis
m. external otitis
m. fibroma
m. fibrous histiocytoma (MFH)
m. granular cell myoblastoma
m. hemangiopericytoma
m. lymphoepithelioma
m. lymphoma
m. melanoma (MM)
m. midline reticulosis
m. necrotizing otitis externa (MNOE)
m. neoplasm
m. odontogenic tumor
m. pemphigus
m. pleomorphic adenoma
m. reticulosis
m. transformation
malignoma
thyroid m.
malinger
malinterdigitation
MALL
massive all layer liposuction
Mallazine Eye Drops
malleability
malleable
mallear
m. fold
m. ligament
mallei
Pseudomonas m.
malleolus
malleostapedial assembly
malleotomy

NOTES

malleovestibulopexy
mallet
>   m. finger
>   hard m.
Mallet scale shoulder external rotation
malleus
>   caput m.
>   fixed m.
>   handle of m.
>   m. head
>   head of m.
>   m. nipper
>   osteoma of m.
malleus-footplate assembly
malleus-stapes assembly
Mallisol
Mallory-Weiss syndrome
mallow
>   marsh m.
malocclusion
>   Ackerman-Proffitt classification
>   of m.
>   Angle classification of m.
>   class I, II, III m.
>   closed-bite m.
>   deflective m.
>   m. index
>   open bite m.
>   Simons classification of m.
>   teeth m.
malodor
malomaxillary suture
Maloney bougie
malpighian cell
malposed tooth
malposition
>   bilateral m.
>   functional m.
>   implant m.
>   inferior m.
>   superior m.
>   teeth m.
malpositioned
>   m. tooth
malrelation
malrotation
malt
Malta fever
maltase
malturned
malunion
mamelon
mammaplasty, mammoplasty
>   Arie-Pitanguy m.
>   augmentation m.
>   bilateral McKissock reduction m.
>   devil's incision m.

endoscopic transaxillary submuscular
  augmentation m.
Lejour m.
periareolar m.
m. procedure
reconstructive m.
reduction m.
m. reduction technique
Toronto two-stage m.
vertical m.
mammary
>   m. artery
>   m. gangrene
>   m. implant
>   m. prosthesis explantation
mammillaplasty
mammography
Mammopatch
>   M. gel self adhesive
>   M. gel self adhesive dressing
>   M. gel self-adhesive scar treatment
mammoplasty (*var. of* mammaplasty)
management
>   airflow m.
>   airway m.
>   contingency m.
>   endovascular m.
mandible
>   alveolar limbus of m.
>   alveolar margin of m.
>   alveolar process of m.
>   alveolar surface of m.
>   articular fossa of m.
>   ascending ramus of the m.
>   breadth of m.
>   cant of occlusal plane of m.
>   condyle of m.
>   coronoid process of m.
>   disappearing m.
>   hypoplastic m.
>   incisive fossa of m.
>   lateral oblique projection of m.
>   length of m.
>   lingula of m.
>   mental tubercle of m.
>   mylohyoid sulcus of m.
>   neck of m.
>   m. panogram
>   peripheral osteoma of the m.
>   (POM)
>   protruding m.
>   pterygoid tuberosity of m.
>   m. radiography
>   ramus of m.
>   retrognathic m.
>   retruded m.
>   m. rim
>   sagittal splitting of m.

short m.
space of body of m.
symphysial height of m.
temporal process of m.
vertical osteotomy of ramus of m.
mandibula, gen. and pl. **mandibulae**
arcus alveolaris mandibulae
capitulum mandibulae
mandibular
m. advancement
m. advancement appliance (MAA)
m. alveolar mucosa
m. alveolus
m. angle
m. angle fracture intraoral open reduction microplate
m. angle fracture intraoral open reduction screw
m. anteroposterior ridge slope
m. arch
m. artery
m. articulation
m. axis
m. base
m. bicuspid
m. bicuspid radiograph
m. block
m. body fracture
m. body length
m. body retractor
m. border
m. bridging plate
m. canal
m. cartilage
m. centric relation
m. condylar hypoplasia
m. condyle
m. condyle fracture
m. contour
m. crest
m. cuspid
m. cuspid-first bicuspid radiograph
m. cuspid radiograph
m. cyst
m. defect
m. deficiency
m. dentition
m. depth
m. deviation
m. dislocation
m. distraction osteogenesis
m. equilibration

m. excess
m. fissure
m. foramen
m. forceps
m. fossa
m. functional reconstruction
m. gland
m. glide
m. gliding movement
m. guide-plane prosthesis
m. guide prosthesis
m. head
m. hinge position
m. hypoplasia
m. impression
m. incisor
m. incisor crowding
m. incisor radiograph
m. leiomyosarcoma
m. lingual flange
m. lymph node
m. macrognathia
m. median cyst
m. micrognathia
m. miniplate
m. molar
m. molar radiograph
m. nerve
m. neurovascular canal
m. notch
m. occlusal view
m. osteotomy-genioglossus advancement
m. overdenture
m. plane
m. plane angle
m. plane to hyoid (MPH)
m. premolar
m. process
m. prognathism
m. prognathism/protrusion
m. protraction
m. protrusion
m. ramus
m. ramus fracture
m. ramus osteotomy
m. range of motion
m. reflex
m. rest position
m. restriction
m. retraction
m. retrognathia

M

NOTES

mandibular *(continued)*
  m. retrognathism
  m. retrognathism/retrusion
  m. retroposition
  m. retrusion
  m. ridge
  m. sagittal deficiency
  m. sagittal split osteotomy
  m. sieving
  m. sling
  m. space
  m. spine
  m. splint
  m. split
  m. staple bone plate (MSBP)
  m. sulcus
  m. surgery
  m. swing approach
  m. swing operation
  m. symphysis
  m. symphysis comminution
  m. symphysis fracture
  m. teeth
  m. torus
  m. trusion
  m. vestibule
  m. visceral arch
  m. wiring
mandibulectomy
  anterior m.
  lateral m.
  marginal m.
  right segmental m.
  segmental m.
mandibulofacial
  m. dysostosis
mandibulomasseteric
mandibulomaxillary fixation
mandibulo-oculofacial dyscephaly
mandibulotomy
Mandol
mand operant
mandrel, mandril
  disk m.
  endosseous implant needle m.
  Moore m.
  Morgan m.
  snap-on m.
maneuver
  Cairns m.
  Cottle m.
  deglutition m.
  Dix-Hallpike m.
  Frenzel m.
  Hallpike m.
  Heimlich m.
  Hueter m.
  Mendelsohn m.

Moore head-tilt m.
Schartzmann m.
Valsalva m.
maneuverability
Mangat curvilinear chin prosthesis
manic reaction
manipulation
  digital m.
  interceptive orthodontic m.
  skin-subcutaneous dissection with SMAS m.
manipulator
  Microbeam m.
  Ramirez m.
mannitol
manometer
manometric flame
manometry
  esophageal m.
Mantel-Haenszel analysis
mantle
  blue m.
  m. dentin
manual
  m. alphabet
  m. English
  m. method
  m. t. former
  m. volume control
manubrium, pl. **manubria**
manudynamometer
manufacture
  computer assisted design/computer assisted m. (CAD/CAM)
MAP
  minimum audible pressure
  Muma Assessment Program
Mapap
maple
  box elder m.
  red m.
  sugar m.
mapping
  auditory brain m.
  brain m.
  cognitive m.
  electrophysiologic m.
  nerve m.
  sentinel lymphatic m.
mappy tongue
Maranox
marble bone disease
Marcaine
marcescens
  Serratia m.
Marcillin
Marena by LySonix compression garment

Marezine
Marfan syndrome
Margesic H
margin
alveolar m.
bone m.
carious restoration m.
cavity m.
cavosurface m.
ceramo-metal m.
cervical m.
enamel m.
free gingival m.
free gum m.
frontal m.
gingival m. (GM)
incisal m.
infraorbital m.
malar m.
metal crown m.
temporal m.
m. of tongue
m. trimmer
zygomatic m.
marginal
m. adaptation
m. bevel
m. crest
m. excess
m. gingiva
m. gingivitis
m. incision
m. integrity of amalgam
M. Line Calculus Index (MLC)
m. mandibular branch
m. mandibular nerve
m. mandibular resection
m. mandibulectomy
m. nevus
m. periodontitis
m. process of malar bone
m. ridge
m. ridge fracture
m. spinning
m. tubercle
m. tubercle of zygomatic bone
m. zone
marginalis
arcus m.
crista m.
margination
margines (*pl. of* margo)

marginis (*gen. of* margo)
marginoplasty
marginotomy
inferior m.
superior m.
supplementary m.
margo, gen. **marginis**, pl. **margines**
m. alveolaris
m. incisalis
m. temporalis
Margraf beam aligning film holder
marinum
Mycobacterium m.
marionette line
Marjolin ulcer
marked falling curve
markedness theory
marker
Accu-line Products skin m.
Allskin m.
cytokeratin m.
epithelial m.
fiducial m.
I m.
intentional m.
K3-7991 Thornton 360 degree
arcuate m.
MIB-1 and PC10 as
prognostic m.'s for esophageal
squamous cell carcinoma
neuroendocrine m.
neuropeptide m.
periodontal pocket m.
phenotypic m.
Richey condyle m.
sign m.
Squeeze-Mark surgical m.
T4/Leu2a m.
T4/Leu3a m.
tumor m.
Vismark skin m.
X-act cutaneous x-ray m.
marking pocket
Mark May sinus disease criteria
Marlex
M. mesh
M. mesh closure
Maroteaux-Lamy
mucopolysaccharidosis type VI M.-
L. (MPS-VI)
Marquette monitor
Marquis probe

M

NOTES

Marritt dilator
marrow
> bone m.
> cancellous cellular m.
> fatty m.
> particulate cancellous bone and m. (PCBM)
> m. space

Mars Black artist's acrylic paint
marsh
> m. elder
> m. mallow

Marshall syndrome
marsupialization
> m. method

Marthritic
Martin
> M. incision
> M. plane

Marx protocol for ORN treatment
Maryland bridge
Marzola hair restoration surgery
Masera septal organ
mask
> laryngeal m.
> LaserSite facial m.
> m. lift
> Petit facial m.
> Swiss Therapy eye m.

masker
> tinnitus m.
> tunable tinnitus m.

masking
> backward m.
> central m.
> effective m.
> m. efficiency
> forward m.
> initial m.
> m. level difference
> maximum m.
> peripheral m.
> m. technique
> upward m.

masklike facies
masoprocol
masque
> Nouvisage acne m.
> Nouvisage anti-aging m.
> Nouvisage M. for damaged or sunburned skin
> Nouvisage M. for normal to dry skin
> Nouvisage M. for normal to oily skin

mass
> exophytic m.
> hyperintense m.

> incudomalleolar m.
> infra-auricular m.
> lipohypertrophic m.
> multilocular m.
> radiopaque m.
> retroareolar m.
> retromammilar m.
> sclerotic cemental m.
> soft-tissue m.
> Stent m.

massage
> gingival m.
> glandular m.
> gum m.
> lymphatic m.

Massé Breast Cream
Masseran trepan bur
masseter
> m. abscess
> m. muscle
> m. muscle flap
> m. muscle hypertrophy
> m. muscle transfer
> m. tendon

masseteric
> m. artery
> m. hypertrophy
> m. nerve
> m. space

masseter-mandibulopterygoid space
massive
> m. all layer liposuction (MALL)
> m. hemoptysis
> m. resorption

Masson
> M. trichrome stain

mast cell
mastectomy
> Halstead radical m.
> modified radical m.
> radical m.
> simultaneous latram and m. (SLAM)
> m. skin flap
> skin-sparing m.
> subcutaneous m.
> transareolar m.

master
> m. apical file (MAF)
> m. cast
> m. cone

Master of Dental Surgery (MDS)
masticate
masticating
> m. apparatus
> m. cycle
> m. surface

mastication
    component of m.
    force of m.
    m. muscle
    prosthesis-mediated m.
masticator
    m. nerve
    m. space
masticatoria
    facies m.
    monoplegia m.
masticatory
    m. adaptation
    m. apparatus
    m. bone
    m. efficiency
    m. fat pad
    m. force
    m. mandibular movement
    m. mucosa
    m. muscle
    m. muscle disorder
    m. process
    m. reflex
    m. silent period
    m. space
    m. surface
    m. system
mastic varnish
Mastisol
mastitis
    silicone m.
mastocele
    transareolar m.
mastoid
    m. abscess
    m. antrum
    artificial m.
    m. bowl
    m. cavity
    m. cortex
    m. emissary vein
    m. empyema
    m. foramen
    Kaposi sarcoma of m.
    m. node
    m. notch
    m. obliteration operation
    m. pneumatization
    m. pressure
    m. process

    m. tip
    m. tip cell
mastoid-conchal suture
mastoidectomy
    canal wall-down m.
    canal wall-up m.
    cortical m.
    modified radical m.
    radical m.
    tympanoplasty m.
    tympanoplasty with m. (TPWM)
    tympanoplasty without m.
      (TPWOM)
mastoideum
    tegmen m.
mastoiditis
    Bezold m.
    coalescent m.
    Pneumocystis carinii m.
    sclerosing m.
    sclerotic m.
mastopathy
mastopexy
    dual-pedicle dermoparenchymal m.
      (DPM)
    IMF wedge excision m.
    internal m.
    modified Kiel m.
    purse string m.
    pursestring m.
    Wise pattern m.
mastopexy-breast augmentation
mastoplasty
    integrative m.
    Lejour m.
mat
    m. foil
    gingival m.
    m. gold
    Secur-Its silicon cushion m.
match
    perceptual-motor m.
matching
    impedance m.
    sentence-picture m.
mater
    dura m.
materia, pl. **materiae**
    m. alba
    m. dentica
material
    Absorb-its m.

NOTES

material *(continued)*

agar-alginate impression m.
agar hydrocolloid impression m.
agar impression m.
6AI/4V ELI alloy implant m.
alginate impression m.
alloplastic graft m.
American Society for Testing and M.'s
Aquaplast alloplastic m.
Aquaplast rapid setting splint m.
autophagocytosed cellular m.
base m.
baseplate m.
biocompatible spacing m.
Bioglass bone substitute m.
BioMend periodontal m.
Bioplastique augmentation m.
Biovert implant m.
block-out m.
brittle m.
Canals-N root canal filling m.
Canals root canal filling m.
cast m.
CeraMed bone grafting m.
chrome-cobalt-molybdenum m.
coating m.
Collastat OBP microfibrillar collagen hemostat m.
colloid impression m.
composite m.
Cyano-Dent m.
dental m.
devascularized m.
ductile m.
Durafill dental restorative m.
Dur-A-Sil ear impression m.
elastic impression m.
elastomeric impression m.
eosinophilic proteinaceous m.
Epoxy Die m.
Fermit-N occlusal hole blockage m.
filling m.
Finapec APC root canal filling m.
Flexicon m.
Frosted Flex earmold m.
Geristore repair m.
glass ionomer restorative m.
glycolide trimethylene carbonate m.
Gore subcutaneous augmentation m.
Gore-Tex alloplastic m.
Gore-Tex augmentation m. (GTAM)
Gore-Tex periodontal m.
Gore-Tex regenerative m.
Hapex bioactive m.
heavy-bodied m.
heavy body impression m.
heterologous m.

Hydrocal cast m.
hydrocolloid impression m.
impression m.
inelastic impression m.
Insta-Mold silicone ear impression m.
intermediate restorative m. (IRM)
irreversible hydrocolloid impression m.
Kerr Permplastic m.
Kerr Traycon m.
light body impression m.
lipoaspirated m.
Macroplastique m.
MediFlex earmold m.
Medpor allograft m.
Medpor alloplastic m.
Medpor block facial structure building m.
Opotow Jelset m.
osteoconductive bone grafting m.
OsteoGen bone grafting m.
OsteoGen HA Resorb implant m.
Osteograf bone grafting m.
Osteograf/D dense bone grafting m.
Osteograf/LD low density bone grafting m.
Osteograf/N natural bone grafting m.
Pacific Coast demineralized bone grafting m.
PerioGlas m.
PermaSoft reline m.
plaster impression m.
plastic restoration m.
plastic wax m.
polyether impression m.
polyether rubber impression m.
polysulfide impression m.
polysulfide rubber impression m.
polyurethane elastomer m.
Polyviolene polyester suture m.
Proplast-Teflon m.
provisionally acceptable m.
radar absorbent m. (RAM)
regular body impression m.
reline m.
restorative m.
restorative dental m.'s
reversible hydrocolloid impression m.
root-end filling m.
rubber impression m.
semisolid m.
silicate restorative m.
silicone impression m.
silicone rubber impression m.
Sta-Tic impression m.

subcutaneous augmentation m.
  (SAM)
Surgamid polyamide suture m.
Teflon m.
temporary m.
temporary endodontic restorative m.
  (TERM)
thermoplastic impression m.
tissue-equivalent m.
tridodecylmethylammonium chloride
  graft coating m. (TDMAC)
two-paste polysulfide rubber
  impression m.
unacceptable m.
Uroplastique m.
vinyl polysiloxane impression m.
Vitremer glass-ionomer
  restorative m.
wash impression m.
Xantopren impression m.
zinc oxide-eugenol impression m.
Materialise computer aided design
  software
mathetic
  m. function of language
  m. text
Matricaria recutita
matrix, pl. **matrices**
  amalgam m.
  m. band
  bone m.
  celluloid m.
  Class V cervical m.
  Coloured Progressive Matrices
  custom m.
  demineralized bone m.
  dentin m.
  dentinal m.
  direct porcelain m.
  enamel m.
  extracellular m. (ECM)
  m. metalloproteinase (MMP)
  Mylar m.
  myxochondroid m.
  nuclear m. (NM)
  organic m.
  perilacunar mineral m. (PMM)
  PermaMesh hydroxyapatite woven
    sheet m.
  plastic m.
  platinum foil m.
  m. pliers

predentin m. (PDM)
resin m.
resin shell m.
m. retainer
m. sentence
T-band m.
Matsura preparation
matter
  particulate m.
Matthew forceps
mattress
  Akros m.
  D.A.D. m.
  m. stitch
  m. suture
  m. suture otoplasty
mattressed onlay graft
maturation
  enamel m.
  rate of m.
maturational lag
maturative stage
mature
  m. bite
  m. dentin
  m. teratoma
maturing temperature
max
  PB m.
Maxaquin
Maxicide
Maxidex
Maxiflor
Maxigold alloy
maxilla, gen. and pl. **maxillae**
  alveolar limbus of m.
  alveolar process of m.
  alveolar surface of m.
  anterior surface of m.
  arcus alveolaris maxillae
  conchal crest of m.
  crista conchalis maxillae
  crista ethmoidalis maxillae
  facial surface of m.
  greater palatine sulcus of m.
  incisive fossa of m.
  infraorbital ridge of m.
  infraorbital sulcus of m.
  infratemporal surface of m.
  juga alveolaria maxillae
  lacrimal groove of m.
  lacrimal sulcus of m.

M

NOTES

maxilla *(continued)*
    limbus alveolaris maxillae
    medial surface of m.
    palatine groove of m.
    palatine lamina of m.
    palatine process of m.
    palatine sulcus of m.
    posterior surface of m.
    m. radiograph
    retrodisplaced maxillae
    septum interalveolaria maxillae
    spine of m.
    superolateral surface of m.
    zygomatic process of m.

maxillary
    m. alveolar protrusion
    m. alveolus
    m. angle
    m. anterior tooth
    m. antrum
    m. antrum closure
    m. arch
    m. artery
    m. bicuspid
    m. bicuspid radiograph
    m. bite plate
    m. bone
    m. buttress
    m. canal
    m. canine
    m. cuspid
    m. cuspid radiograph
    m. cyst
    m. deficiency
    m. dentition
    m. depth
    m. division
    m. downgrafting
    m. excess
    m. expansion
    m. first molar alveolus
    m. fissure
    m. foramen
    m. forceps
    m. fossa
    m. fracture
    m. impression
    m. incisor
    m. incisor radiograph
    m. incisor retraction
    m. intrusion
    m. ligament
    m. lymph node
    m. macrognathia
    m. malignant mesenchymoma
    m. median anterior cyst
    m. micrognathia
    m. molar

    m. molar radiograph
    m. neoplasm
    m. nerve
    m. occlusal view
    m. osteotomy
    m. ostium
    m. posterior tooth
    m. process
    m. process of zygomatic bone
    m. prognathism/protrusion
    m. prominence
    m. prosthesis
    m. protraction
    m. protrusion
    m. rampart
    m. removable implant-retained
      denture
    m. removal and reinsertion
    m. restoration
    m. retardation
    m. retrognathia
    m. retroposition
    m. retrusion
    m. sinus
    m. sinus carcinoma
    m. sinuscopy
    m. sinus cyst
    m. sinus Foley catheter balloon
      placement technique
    m. sinusitis
    m. sinus mucocele
    m. sinus radiograph
    m. sinus roentgenogram
    m. stent
    m. surface
    m. surface of great wing
    m. surface of perpendicular plate
      of palatine bone
    m. surgery
    m. teeth
    m. trusion
    m. tuberosity
    m. vein

maxillary-zygomatic hypoplasia
maxillectomy
    composite bilateral infrastructure m.
    endoscopic medial m.
maxillitis
maxilloalveolar
    m. breadth
    m. index
    m. length
maxillodental
maxillofacial
    m. abnormality
    m. anomaly
    m. and facioproximal surface
      toothbrushing

m. fracture
m. injury
m. prosthesis
m. prosthetics
m. prosthodontics
m. reconstruction
m. skeletal advancement
m. surgery
maxillofrontale
maxillojugal
maxillolabial
maxillomandibular
m. anchorage
m. disharmony
m. dysplasia
m. elastic
m. fixation (MMF)
m. record
m. registration
m. relation
m. traction
maxillonasal dysostosis
maxillopalatal and palatoproximal surface toothbrushing
maxillopalatine
maxillotomy
maxillozygomatic complex
maximal
m. contrast
M. Static Response Assay (MSRA)
m. static response assay of facial motion
m. stress
maximum
m. accumulated dose (MAD)
m. acoustic output
m. amplitude
m. bite force
m. duration of phonation
m. duration of sustained blowing
m. frequency range
m. intercuspation
m. interincisal distance (MID)
m. masking
m. movement
m. permissible dose (MPD)
m. power output (MPO)
m. stimulation test (MST)
M. Strength Anbesol
M. Strength Desenex Antifungal Cream

maximus
gluteus m.
Maxipime
Max-I-Probe endodontic irrigation syringe
Maxitrol
Maxivate
Maxon suture
Mayer
M.-Rokitansky-Küster-Hauser syndrome (MRKHS)
M. view
Mayer-Rokitansky syndrome
mayfly
Mayne
M. muscle control appliance
M. space maintainer
Mayo
M. scissors
M. stand
mazopexy
MB
mesiobuccal
MBC
mesiobuccal cusp
MBCR
mesiobuccal cusp ridge
MBD
minimal brain dysfunction
minimal brain dysfunction syndrome
MBDG
mesiobuccal developmental groove
MBO
mesiobucco-occlusal
MBP
mesiobuccopulpal
MBR
mesiobuccal root
MC
mesenchymal chondrosarcoma
MCA
mesial contact area
McBernie point
McCall
M. curette
M. festoon
M. instrument
M. scaler
McCarthy Scales of Children's Abilities
McCollum attachment
McComb procedure
McCraw technique

M

NOTES

McCune-Albright syndrome
McGhan
468 M. Biocel anatomical breast implant
M. fill kit
McGill Pain Questionnaire
McGivney forceps
McGoon technique
McIndoe
M. inlay graft
M. method
M. and Reese alar cartilage suture fixation
M. skin graft
M. technique
MCL
most comfortable loudness
MCL-N
midclavicular line-to-nipple
MCLR
most comfortable loudness range
MCP
metacarpophalangeal
MCP joint
MCR
mesial cusp ridge
m-cresyl acetate
McShirley
M. electromallet
M. electromallet condenser
McSpadden
M. compactor
M. endodontic technique
M. method
MCT
motor coordination test
mucociliary transport
McXIM file
M.D.
M.D. Forte
M.D. Forté glycolic acid-based skin care system
M.D. Forté glycolic-based skin care product
M.D. Forté rejuvenating eye cream
M.D. Forté skin rejuvenation lotion II
MDA ultrasound-assisted lipoplasty machine
MDD
mesial developmental depression
MDS
Master of Dental Surgery
MDVP 4305
Multi-Dimensional Voice Program 4305
Mead forceps

meadow
m. fescue
m. foxtail
meal
rye m.
soybean m.
mean
m. foundation plane
m. hearing
m. length of response (MLR)
m. length of utterance (MLU)
m. rejection grading (MRG)
m. relational utterance (MRU)
m. residual gap (MRG)
m. sentence length (MSL)
meaning
grammatical m.
idiosyncratic m.
lexical m.
transferred m.
meaningful speech
measles
German m.
three-day m.
m. virus
measure
Bilingual Syntax M. (BSM)
jitter-related m.
online m.
perturbation m.
shimmer-related m.
measurement
acoustic immittance m.
anthropometric m.
bite force m.
m. control handle
facial excursion m.
m. film
MPH distance m.
nasion-pogonion m.
PAS m.
PNSP m.
Real Ear m.
tooth m.
measuring
precise lesion m. (PLM)
m. wire
meatal
m. advancement and glanduloplasty procedure (MAGPI)
m. atresia
m. stenosis
meatoplasty
m. and glanulopasty (MAGPI)
meatorrhaphy
meatoscope
meatoscopy
meatotome

meatotomy
meatus, pl. **meatus**
    acoustic m.
    anterior middle m.
    external auditory m.
    inferior m.
    internal acoustic m.
    internal auditory m. (IAM)
    middle m.
    superior m.
mebendazole
MEC
    mucoepidermoid carcinoma
mechanical
    m. amalgamator
    m. avulsion
    m. condenser
    m. creep of skin
    m. impedance
    m. labyrinthectomy
    m. perforation
    m. pulp exposure
    m. retention
    m. separator
    m. strain
    m. tooth separation
    m. triturator
mechanically balanced occlusion
mechanism
    balance m.
    cough m.
    extrinsic m.
    hydrodynamic m.
    inhibitory-excitatory m.
    intrinsic m.
    respiratory control m.
    speech m.
mechanoactivation
mechanoreceptor
mechanotherapy
    multibanded m.
Meckel
    M. cartilage
    M. cave
    M. ganglion
meclizine
meclofenamate
Mectra irrigation/aspiration system
Med
    Perio M.
MedDev gold eyelid implant

media
    acute otitis m. (AOM)
    adhesive otitis m.
    aerotitis m.
    barotitis m.
    catarrhal otitis m.
    chronic cholesteatomatous otitis m.
    chronic granulation otitis m.
    chronic otitis m. (COM)
    chronic suppurative otitis m.
     (CSOM)
    macula cribrosa m.
    mucoid otitis m.
    necrotizing otitis m.
    noncholesteatomatous chronic
     suppurative otitis m.
    nonsuppurative otitis m.
    otitis m.
    Pneumocystis carinii otitis m.
    purulent otitis m.
    reflux otitis m.
    scala m.
    secretory otitis m.
    serous otitis m. (SOM)
    suppurative otitis m.
    tuberculous otitis m.
    tunica m.
medial
    m. antebrachial cutaneous nerve
    m. brachial cutaneous nerve
    m. canthal fissure
    m. canthoplasty
    m. canthus
    m. collateral ligament
    m. cribrose macula
    m. crus
    m. cutaneous thigh flap
    m. distally based fasciocutaneous
     flap
    m. elevation
    m. geniculate
    m. incisor
    m. incudal fold
    m. nasal concha
    m. oblique and low lateral
     osteotomy
    m. plantar sensory flap
    m. pterygoid muscle
    m. pterygoid plate
    m. rectus muscle
    m. slip
    m. surface

M

NOTES

medial *(continued)*
  m. surface of maxilla
  m. turbinated bone
  m. upper arm flap
  m. vestibular nucleus
  m. wall of agger nasi cell
medialis
  lamina m.
  vastus m.
medialization
  fracture m.
  greenstick m.
  incomplete m.
  vocal cord m.
medialized
medial-to-lateral tumor removal
median
  m. alveolar cyst
  m. anterior maxillary cyst
  m. cleft face syndrome
  m. cleft lip
  m. facial cleft
  m. forehead flap
  m. glossoepiglottic fold
  m. jaw relation
  m. labiomandibular glossotomy
  m. laryngotomy
  m. line
  m. lingual sulcus
  m. longitudinal raphe
  m. mandibular cyst
  m. mandibular point
  m. maxillary anterior alveolar cleft
  m. nerve (MN)
  m. nerve compression test
  m. occlusal position
  m. palatal cyst
  m. palatine suture
  m. raphe plane
  m. retruded relation
  m. rhinoscopy
  m. rhomboid glossitis
  m. sagittal plane
  m. thyrohyoid fold
  m. thyrohyoid ligament
mediastinal dissection
mediastinitis
  descending necrotizing m. (DNM)
  fulminant m.
mediastinoscope
  Carlens m.
  Tucker m.
mediastinoscopy
mediastinum
mediation
  verbal m.
mediator
  pain-related m.

Medicago sativa
medical
  M. Research Council muscle
    strength scale system
  m. waste
Medicamat
  M. ultrasound-assisted lipoplasty
    machine
  M. ultrasound device
medicamentosa
  dermatitis m.
  rhinitis m.
  stomatitis m.
medicated
  Zilactin-B M.
medication
  ototoxic m.
  Red Cross Canker Sore m.
medication-induced hyperplasia
medicinal
  m. leech
  m. preparation
medicinalis
  Hirudo m.
medicine
  Doctor of Dental M. (DMD)
  evidence-based m. (E-BM)
medicodental
Medicon
  M. ultrasonic liposuction device
  M. US liposuction device
MediFlex earmold material
mediodens
medionasal process
mediotrusion
Medipain 5
Medipatch Gel Z adhesive dressing
Mediplast Plaster
Medipore H surgical tape
Medi-Quick Topical Ointment
Mediterranean fever
medium
  m. biscuit
  m. biscuit firing
  m. bisque firing
  m. disk
  Dulbecco modified Eagle m.
    (DMEM)
  Hypaque contrast m.'s
  resorbable blast m.'s (RBM)
  separating m.
  m. temperature maturing porcelain
medium-fusing porcelain
MedLite
  M. Q-Switched neodymium-doped
    yttrium-aluminum-garnet laser
  M. Q-Switched YAG laser

MedMorph
    M. III patient video imaging
    M. III software
Medpor
    M. allograft material
    M. alloplastic material
    M. Biomaterial wedge
    M. block facial structure building
        material
    M. facial implant
    M. malar implant
    M. reconstructive implant
    M. surgical implant
Medrol
    M. Dosepak
medroxyprogesterone acetate
medrysone
Medtronics Sequestra 1000
    autotransfusion system
medulla
    m. oblongata
medullary
    m. artery
    m. fixation
medullated nerve fiber
medullogram
    sternal puncture m.
Med-Wick nasal pack
MEE
    middle ear effusion
mefenamic acid
Mefoxin
MEG
    magnetoencephalography
megadont
megadontia
megadontism
megadontismus
MegaDyne
    M. arthroscopic hook electrode
    M. electrocautery pencil
megaesophagus
megaglossia
megagnathia
megahertz (MHz)
megalodont
megalodontia
megaloglossia
megalourethra
megavoltage
meglumine iothalamate
meibomian gland

Meige
    M. disease
    M. syndrome
meiopragic bone
Meissner tactile corpuscle
Meisterschnitt incision
mel
Melanex
melanin
melaninogenica
    Prevotella m.
melaninogenicus
    Bacteroides m.
melanization
melanoameloblastoma
melanocyte
    cultured autologous m.
melanocyte-stimulating hormone
melanocytic
    m. atypia
    m. lesion
melanogenesis
melanoglossia
melanoma
    acral lentiginous m.
    cutaneous m.
    desmoplastic m.
    lentigo maligna m.
    malignant m. (MM)
    neurotropic m.
    nodular m.
    sinonasal m.
    m. in situ (MIS)
    subungual m.
    superficial spreading m.
melanonychia
    longitudinal m.
    m. striata (MS)
melanoplakia
melanosarcoma
melanosis
    dermal m.
    laryngeal m. (LM)
    mucocutaneous m.
melanosome
melanotic
    m. neuroectodermal tumor
    m. neuroectodermal tumor of
        infancy
    m. whitlow
melanotrichosis
    m. linguae

M

NOTES

melasma
melatonin
Melissa officinalis
melitis
Melkersson-Rosenthal syndrome
Melkersson syndrome
mellitus
    diabetes m.
melocervicoplasty
melody of speech
melolabial flap
meloplasty, melonoplasty
    intraoral m.
    laser m.
    m. procedure
melphalan
MEM
    minimal essential solution
    Eagle MEM
membrana, gen. and pl. membranae
    m. adamantina
    m. eboris
    m. eboris of Kölliker
    m. preformata
    m. preformativa
membranaceous ampulla
membrane
    adamantine m.
    alveolodental m.
    barrier m.
    basement m.
    basilar m.
    biobarrier m.
    Bio-Gide resorbable barrier m.
    BioMend m.
    bioresorbable guided tissue m.
    cloacal m.
    cricothyroid m.
    cricovocal m.
    dentinoenamel m.
    drum m.
    enamel m.
    ePTFE m.
    ePTFE augmentation m.
    fibroelastic m.
    Golgi m.'s
    Gore Resolut regenerative tissue m.
    Gore-Tex m.
    Gore-Tex augmentation m. (GTAM)
    hyoglossal m.
    Imtec BioBarrier m.
    internal elastic m.
    ivory m.
    labyrinthine m.
    mucous m.
    Nasmyth m.
    oropharyngeal m.
    otolithic m.

    peridental m.
    periodontal m. (PM)
    plasma m.
    pseudoserous m.
    pulpodentinal m.
    quadrangular m.
    Reissner m.
    resorbable bilayer collagen m.
    Rivinus m.
    salpingopalatine m.
    salpingopharyngeal m.
    schneiderian m.
    Shrapnell m.
    stylomandibular m.
    subepithelial m.
    subimplant m.
    submucous m.
    synovial m.
    tectorial m.
    TefGen-FD guided tissue
      regeneration m.
    TefGen-FD plastic m.
    thyrohyoid m.
    tympanic m.
    unit m.
    vestibular m.
membranous
    m. gingivostomatitis
    m. labyrinth
    m. laryngitis
    m. pharyngitis
    m. stomatitis
Meme implant
memocouple
memory
    auditory m.
    m. cell
    immunologic m.
    long term m.
    odor recognition m.
    rote m.
    sequential m.
    short-term m.
    m. span
    visual m.
    working m.
men
    Rogaine for M.
Menadol
mendelian theory
Mendelsohn maneuver
Menetrier disease
Meni-D
Ménière, Meniere
    M. disease
    M. quadrad
    M. syndrome
meningeal artery

meningioma
> cutaneous m.
> m. en plaque
> extracranial m.
> posterior cranial fossa m.

meningismus
meningitidis
> *Neisseria m.*

meningitis
> AIDS-related cryptococcal m.
> bacterial m.
> cryptococcal m.
> otitic m.

meningocele
meningoencephalocele
> frontoethmoidal m.

meningoencephalomyelitis
> mumps m.

meningothelial cell
meningovascular syphilis
meniscus, pl. menisci
menogingivitis
> periodic transitory m.

menopausal gingivostomatitis
menstruation gingivitis
mental
> m. age (MA)
> m. artery
> m. block injection
> m. extraoral radiography
> m. foramen
> m. height
> m. muscle
> m. nerve
> m. point
> m. process
> m. projection
> m. protuberance
> m. region
> m. retardation
> m. ridge
> m. spine
> m. tubercle
> m. tubercle of mandible
> m. V-Y island advancement island flap

mentalis
> m. band
> m. muscle

mentally
> m. impaired (MI)
> m. retarded (MR)

Mentha piperita
mentolabial
> m. sulcus

menton
mentoplasty
Mentor
> M. breast implant
> M. Contour Genesis ultrasonic assisted lipoplasty system
> M. H/S Siltex implant
> M. 1600 implant
> M. ultrasound-assisted lipoplasty machine
> M. ultrasound device

mentum
mepenzolate
Mepergan
meperidine
> m. hydrochloride
> m. and promethazine

mephentermine
Mephyton Oral
Mepitel
> M. dressing
> M. nonadherent silicone dressing

mepivacaine
> m. HCl injection
> m. with levonordefrin

meprobamate
merbromin
mercaptan
> m. impression

mercaptopurine
6-mercaptopurine (6-mp)
Mercedes
> M. cannula
> M. incision
> LySonix TTD Design M.
> M. tip

mercurial
> m. line
> m. stomatitis

mercuric oxide
mercurochrome
mercuroscopic expansion
mercury
> m.-alloy ratio
> dental m.

Merendino technique
Merit-B periodontal probe
Merkel
> M. cell

M

NOTES

Merkel *(continued)*
    M. cell carcinoma
    M. corpuscles
Merocel epistaxis packing
meropenem
Merrem I.V.
Merrifield knife
Merrill Language Screening Test
Mershon arch
Mersilene mesh
Mersol
Merthiolate
Mesalt sodium chloride impregnated dressing
mesencephalon
mesenchyma
mesenchymal
    m. cell
    m. chondrosarcoma (MC)
    m. cleft
    m. neoplasm
    m. sarcoma
    m. tumor
mesenchyme
    m. papilla
    perifollicular m.
mesenchymoma
    maxillary malignant m.
mesenteric arcade
mesh
    Dexon surgically knitted m.
    Dumbach mini m.
    Dumbach regular m.
    Dumbach titanium m.
    Gore-Tex m.
    m. graft
    m. graft urethroplasty
    Marlex m.
    Mersilene m.
    micro m.
    mixed m.
    polyamide m.
    polypropylene m.
    polytetrafluoroethylene m.
    Supramid polyamide m.
    synthetic m.
    TiMesh cranial m.
    TiMesh orbital m.
    TiMesh titanium m.
    Vicryl m.
meshed split-thickness skin graft
mesial
    m. angle
    m. caries
    m. contact area (MCA)
    m. curvature
    m. cusp ridge (MCR)

    m. developmental depression (MDD)
    m. displacement
    m. drift
    m. marginal developmental groove (MMDG)
    m. marginal ridge (MMR)
    m. movement
    m. and occlusal
    m., occlusal, and distal (MOD)
    m. occlusion
    m. pit (MP)
    m. radiolucency
    m. root
    m. surface
    m. triangular fossa (MTF)
mesioangular
    m. impaction
    m. position
mesioaxial
mesioaxiogingival
mesioaxioincisal
mesiobuccal (MB)
    m. alveolus
    m. canal
    m. cusp (MBC)
    m. cusp ridge (MBCR)
    m. developmental groove (MBDG)
    m. line angle
    m. root (MBR)
mesiobucco-occlusal (MBO)
    m.-o. point angle
mesiobuccopulpal (MBP)
mesiocervical
mesioclination
mesioclusion
    bilateral m.
    class III m.
    unilateral m.
mesiodens, pl. **mesiodentes**
mesiodistal
    m. clasp
    m. diameter of crown
    m. fracture
    m. plane
    m. width
mesiodistocclusal (MOD)
mesiogingival (MG)
mesiognathic
mesioincisal
mesioincisodistal (MID)
mesiolabial (MLA)
    m. bilobed transposition flap
    m. line angle
mesiolabioincisal (MLAI)
    m. point angle
mesiolingual (ML)
    m. cusp (MLC)

m. cusp ridge (MLCR)
m. developmental groove (MLDG)
m. fossa (MLF)
m. groove (MLG)
m. line angle
mesiolinguoincisal (MLI)
m. point angle
mesiolinguo-occlusal (MLO)
m.-o. point line angle
mesiolinguopulpal (MLP)
mesio-occlusal (MO)
mesio-occlusal line angle
mesio-occlusion
mesio-occlusodistal (MOD)
mesiopalatal
mesioplacement
mesiopulpal (MP)
mesiopulpolabial (MPLA)
mesiopulpolingual (MPL)
mesioversion
mesoderm
mesodermal
m. core
m. somite
m. tumor
mesodont
mesodontia
mesodontic
mesodontism
mesognathic
mesognathous
mesons
pi m.
mesostomia
mesostructure
m. bar
m. conjunction bar
implant m.
m. implant
integral intraoral bilateral
posterior m.
mesotaurodontism
mesotympanum
mesquite
messages
competing m.
dichotic m.
diotic m.
Messerklinger technique
Messing
M. gun
M. root canal gun

META
methacryloxyethyl trimellitic anhydride
citric acid-ferric chloride/4 META
metabolic sialadenosis
metacarpal
rudimentary m.
metacarpophalangeal (MCP)
m. joint
metachronous
m. metastasis
m. tumor
metacognition
metacommunication
metacone
metaconid
metaconule
metacresol
metacresyl acetate
Metadent
metaidoioplasty, metoidioplasty
metal
alloy-forming m.
Babbitt m.
m. base
m. base denture
m. bracket
m. bucket-handle prosthesis
m. crown
m. crown margin
d'Arcet m.
m. frame reinforced plastic bracket
m. handle mixing spatula
implant m.
m. insert tooth
m. interface
m. opaquer
m. reconstruction plate
m. and rubber block
m. scleral shield
wrought m.
metal-ceramic
m.-c. crown
m.-c. restoration
metalinguistic
m. assessment
m. judgment
metallic
m. frontal needle
m. implant
m. oxide paste
m. restoration
m. stain

NOTES

metallic-dense shadow
metalloproteinase
    matrix m. (MMP)
metal-plated die
metamerism
metamorphosis
    calcific m.
Metamucil
metaphor
metaphysis
metaplasia
    cystic oncocytic m.
    m. of pulp
    sebaceous m.
metapragmatic
metaproterenol
metarteriole
metastasis, pl. metastases
    cervical m.
    cutaneous m.
    hematogenous m.
    intraparotideal m.
    lymphatic m.
    metachronous m.
    precocious m.
    septic m.
    skip m.
    synchronous m.
    tumor-to-tumor m.
metastasize
metastatic
    m. basal cell carcinoma
    m. carcinoma
    m. neoplasm
metatarsal
    m. bone
    m. free vascularized graft
    m. joint
metatarsophalangeal (MTP)
    m. joint
metathesis
metaxalone
meter
    Endodontic M. SII
    noise exposure m.
    Pocketpeak peak flow m.
    sound level m.
    vibration m.
    volume unit m. (VU meter)
    VU m.
       volume unit meter
    Youlten nasal inspiratory peak
      flow m.
methacholine
methacrylate
    bisphenol A-glycidyl m. (bis-GMA)
    butyl m.
    dimethyl m.

    ethyl m.
    hydroxyethyl m.
    2-hydroxyethyl m. (HEMA)
    methyl m.
    poly-(2-hydroxyethyl m.) (poly-
      HEMA)
    polymethyl m. (PMMA)
    vinyl ethyl m.
methacryloxyethyl trimellitic anhydride
(META)
methadone
methantheline bromide
methanthelinium
methazolamide
methemoglobinemia
methicillin
methicillin-resistant *Staphylococcus*
  aureus **(MRSA)**
methimazole
methocarbamol
    m. and aspirin
method
    acoupedic m.
    acoustic m.
    analytic m.
    ANOVA m.
    apneic m.
    artificial m.
    auditory m.
    Bass m.
    bimodal m.
    biotechnologic m.
    bisensory m.
    Blue Peel chemical m.
    Bobath m.
    breathing m.
    Brown-Brenn staining m.
    Bruhn m.
    Callahan m.
    Callahan root canal filling m.
    carbon dioxide snow m.
    Carpue m.
    Charters m.
    Chayes m.
    chewing m.
    chloropercha m.
    combined m.
    consonant-injection m.
    conventional m.
    cross-consonant injection m.
    crown-contouring m.
    Dieffenbach m.
    diffusion root canal filling m.
    Eicken m.
    ethnographic m.
    finite element m. (FEM)
    foam and dome m.
    Fones m.

formal m.
French m.
French-line m.
fusion temperature wire m.
German m.
grammatic m.
Gruber m.
hanging chain m.
Hirschfeld m.
Howe silver precipitation m.
Indian m.
indirect restorative m.
informal m.
inhalation m.
injection m.
injection-molded m.
Italian m.
Jena m.
Johnson root canal filling m.
Johnston m.
Karapandzic m.
key word m.
kinesthetic m.
Kinzie m.
Kitano and Okada m.
Krause m.
lateral condensation root canal
  filling m.
logical m.
manual m.
marsupialization m.
McIndoe m.
McSpadden m.
modified Frost m.
modified Wardill m.
mother m.
Mueller-Walle m.
multiple cone root canal filling m.
natural m.
Needles split cast m.
ninhydrin-Schiff m.
Nitchie m.
numerical cipher m.
odd-even m.
Ollier m.
online assessment m.
oral-aural m.
Partsch I m.
plateau m.
plosive-injection m.
Politzer m.
prolabial unwinding flap m.

retrofilling m.
retrograde root canal filling m.
Reverdin m.
Rochester m.
Roux m.
Sargenti m.
sectional root canal filling m.
segmentation root canal filling m.
shadowing m.
silver cone m.
silver point root canal filling m.
simultaneous m.
single cone root canal filling m.
sniff m.
Song and Song m.
split cast m.
Stillman m.
swallow m.
synthetic m.
systematic m.
Thiersch m.
threshold shift m.
Tweed m.
verbotonal m.
vertical condensation root canal
  filling m.
vertical-cut m.
visual m.
von Koss m.
Warthin-Starry staining m.
water sorption/desorption m.
Weber-Ferguson m.
Wolfe m.
zigzag m.

methodology
  Cutler-Ederer life-table m.
methohexital anesthesia
methotrexate (MTX)
methotrimeprazine
methoxycinnamate and oxybenzone
methscopolamine
  chlorpheniramine, phenylephrine,
    and m.
methyl
  m. cellulose paste
  m. ethyl ketone
  m. methacrylate
  m. methacrylate ear stent
  m. methacrylate polymer
methylcellulose
  gelatin, pectin, and m.
  hydroxypropyl m.

M

NOTES

369

methyldopa
methylene
    m. blue
    m. blue line
methylprednisolone
methylsulfate
    diphemanil m.
methysergide
    m. maleate
Meticorten
Metimyd Ophthalmic
metipranolol
metoclopramide
metodontiasis
metoidioplasty (*var. of* metaidoioplasty)
Metol
metonymy
metopic
    m. synostosis
    m. synostosis reoperation
metopoplasty
metrizamide
MetroGel Topical
Metro I.V. Injection
metronidazole
metroplasty
Mettelman pre jowl chin implant
Metz
    M. recruitment test
    M. test for loudness recruitment
Meurmann external ear anomaly grade
Meyenburg-Altherr-Uehlinger syndrome
Meyenburg disease
Meyer organ
Mezlin
mezlocillin
MF
    mitogenic factor
M/F
    moment-force ratio
MFC
    Micro-Flow compactor
MFH
    malignant fibrous histiocytoma
MF-Y gold
MG
    mesiogingival
MGJ
    mucogingival junction
MHC
    major histocompatibility complex
MHN
    Mohs hardness number
MHz
    megahertz
MI
    mentally impaired

Miacalcin
    M. Injection
    M. Nasal Spray
MIB-1 and PC10 as prognostic markers for esophageal squamous cell carcinoma
Micatin Topical
Michel malformation
Michigan probe
miconazole
micracoustic, microcoustic
micro
    M. Link endoscope fiber
    m. mesh
    M. oral surgery handpiece
    M. OSH
    M. Plus plating system
microabrasion
microabscess
micro-adaption plate
microanastomosis
microbar
Microbeam manipulator
microbial
    m. pathogen
    m. plaque
micro-bicinchoninic acid protein assay kit
microbiology
microbiota
    dental m.
microblade
    Sharptome m.
Microbond NP
microbrachycephaly
microcephaly
microcheilia, microchilia
microcinematography of the dental pulp
microcirculation
    peripheral m.
    pulp m.
microclamp
    disposable m.
micrococcus, pl. micrococci
microcoil
    platinum m.
microcoustic (*var. of* micracoustic)
microcrack
microcrystalline wax
microcystic
    m. adnexal carcinoma
microdebrider
    Hummer m.
microdensitometric
microdentium
    Treponema m.
MicroDigitrapper
microdirect laryngoscopy

microdissection
microdont
microdontia
    relative generalized m.
    single-tooth m.
    true generalized m.
microdontism
microdrill
microdrilling guide
microdroplet
    silicone m.
microembolization
microetcher
microetching technique
microfibrillar
    m. collagen
    m. collagen hemostat
Microfil
    M. injection
    M. silicone-rubber injection
      compound
    M. solution
microfilled
    m. adhesive
    m. composite
    m. composite resin
Microfine
    Prisma M.
microfixation
Micro-Flow compactor (MFC)
microfoam
microfracture
microgenia
microglossia
microglossic
micrognathia
    adult acquired m.
    mandibular m.
    maxillary m.
    m. with peromelia
micrognathic
    m. appearance
micrograft
    m. dilator
    m. punctiform technique
micrograph
    electron m.
    low magnification scanning
      electron m.
    scanning electron m. (SEM)
    transmission electron m.
microgravity

Micro-Halogen otoscope
microhandpiece
microischemia
microknife
microlaryngeal surgery
microlaryngoscopy
    suspension m.
microleakage
Micro-Lok implant
MicroLux video camera system
micromandible
micromanipulator
    microscope mounted m.
    microspot m.
    UniMax 2000 laser m.
micromat
micromaxilla
MicroMax speed drill
micromechanical retention
micrometastasis, pl. micrometastases
micrometastatic disease
MicroMirror gold sensor
micro-mosquito
    m.-m. curved scissors
    m.-m. straight scissors
microneurolysis
microneurorrhaphy
microneurosurgery
Micronor
microorganism
    gram-negative m.
    gram-positive m.
    pathogenic m.
microparticle
MicroPeel
micropenis
microphallus
microphone
    directional m.
    nondirectional m.
    omnidirectional m.
    pressure zone m. (PZM)
    probe tube m.
    Sennheiser electric condenser m.
      ME 40-3
microphonia
microphonic
    cochlear m.
microphonics
microphonoscope
microphthalmos
micropigmentation handpiece

M

NOTES

micropipette
microplate
    AO-Titanium m.
    m. fixation
    mandibular angle fracture intraoral
    open reduction m.
Micropolyspora
Micropore
    M. dressing
    M. tape
microporosity
microprocessor
microradiograph
microradiography
microreconstruction
micros
    Peptostreptococcus m.
microscope
    confocal m.
    EIE 150F operating m.
    electron m.
    JedMed TRI-GEM m.
    m. mounted micromanipulator
    operating m.
    Protégé Plus m.
    scanning electron m.
    Seiler MC-M900 surgical m.
    stereoscopic m.
    tonsillectomy with operating m.
    (TE$_{mic}$)
    transmission electron m. (TEM)
    Welch Allyn LumiView portable
    binocular m.
    Wild operating m.
    Zeiss m.
    Zeiss/Jena surgical m.
    Zeiss operating m.
microscopy
    binocular m.
    light m. (LM)
    scanning electron m. (SEM)
    transmission electron m. (TEM)
microscrew
microsmatic
microsomia
    craniofacial m.
    hemifacial m. (HFM, HM)
microsomy
microspectroscopy
Microsponge delivery system
Microsporum
microspot micromanipulator
Microstat handpiece
microstomia
Microstone
microsurgery

microsurgical
    m. free pulp flap
    m. procedure
microsyringe
Microtek Heine otoscope
microtia
microtome
    Leitz 1600 Saw m.
microtrauma
microtubule
microvascular
    m. anastomosis
    m. bone transfer
    m. clip
    m. decompression (MVD)
    m. free flap transfer
    m. free posterior interosseous flap
    m. free tissue transfer
    m. graft
    m. surgery
    m. thrombosis
microvascularize
Micro-Vent
    M.-V. implant
    M.-V.^{2} implant
    M.-V. implant system
microvesicle
    Novasome m.
microvessel density (MVD)
microvillar cell
microvillus, pl. **microvilli**
microwave
micturition
MID
    maximum interincisal distance
    mesioincisodistal
Midas
    M. alloy
    M. Rex instrumentation
midazolam
midbrain
Midchlor
midclavicular line-to-nipple (MCL-N)
midconcha cymba
mid-dentin
middle
    m. constrictor pharyngeal muscle
    m. cranial fossa
    m. cranial fossa line
    m. ear
    m. ear cleft
    m. ear effusion (MEE)
    m. ear infection
    m. ear muscle reflex
    m. ear neoplasm
    m. fossa approach
    m. fossa plate
    m. fossa retractor

m. fossa syndrome
m. fossa vestibular neurectomy
m. latency response (MLR)
m. meatal antrostomy
m. meatus
m. meningeal artery
m. nasal concha
m. pharyngeal constrictor
m. thyroid vein
m. turbinate
m. vault deformity
m. zone
midface
m. alloplastic augmentation
m. avulsion flap
m. fracture
m. hypoplasia
m. lift
m. trauma
midfacelift
subperiosteal m.
midfacial
m. breadth
m. degloving
m. fracture
m. hypoplasia
m. retrusion
midfoot
midge
nimitti m.
Midigold alloy
midlamellar cicatricial retraction
midline
m. cranio-orbital clefting
m. disharmony
m. forehead flap
m. lethal granuloma
m. malignant reticulosis granuloma
Midol
M. IB
M. PM
midpalatal
m. opening
m. suture opening
midpalatine raphe
mid-penile hypospadias
Midrin
midroot
midsagittal
mid-to-deep dermal peel
mid vowel
Miege syndrome

MIF
macrophage-inhibiting factor
migration-inhibiting factor
migraine
basilar artery m.
m. equivalent
m. headache
migrans
erythema m.
glossitis m.
migrated tooth
Migratine
migrating teeth
migration
epithelial m.
physiologic mesial m.
postoperative m.
tooth m.
m. of tooth
migration-inhibiting factor (MIF)
Mikamo double-eyelid operation
Mikulicz
M. aphthae
M. cells
M. disease
M. syndrome
mild
m. hearing impairment
m. hearing loss
silver protein, m.
Miles Magic Mixture
milium, pl. milia
milk
cow m.
goat m.
m. line
m. teeth
m. thistle
Millar asthma
Millard
M. bilateral cleft lip repair
M. clamp
M. creed
M. forked flap technique
M. graft augmentation
M. Lite-Pipe
M. mouth gag
milled-in
m.-i. curves
m.-i. occlusion
m.-i. path

M

NOTES

Miller
- M. Apexo elevator
- M. chemicoparasitic theory
- M. collutory
- M. index
- M. mobility index
- M. organism
- M. scale
- M. theory

Miller-Fisher variant of Guillain-Barré syndrome

Miller-Yoder Comprehension Test

milliamperage

milliampere (mA)

milling-in

milliroentgen

millisecond (msec)

Miltown

mimetic
- m. hyperkinesis
- m. modulation
- m. muscle

mimic
- facial m.
- m. speech

mimicry
- molecular m.

mimmation

mineral
- m. salt
- m. trioxide aggregate (MTA)
- m. wax

mineralization
- calcospherite m.
- capsular m.
- dystrophic m.

mineralized tissue

Mini
- M. Cliplamp
- M. Inventory of Right Brain Injury (MIRBI)
- M. speech processor

mini
- m. trephine
- m. Würzburg Flexplates craniomaxillofacial plating system
- m. Würzburg standard craniomaxillofacial plating system

miniabdominoplasty
- open m.

miniature
- m. carrier
- m. plugger

miniblade
- Beaver m.

Minidyne

Mini-Fibralux pocket otoscope

Minigold alloy

minigraft
- m. dilator

Minilux pocket otoscope

minimal
- m. anchorage
- m. brain dysfunction (MBD)
- m. brain dysfunction syndrome (MBD)
- m. contrast
- m. essential solution (MEM)
- m. instrumentation
- m. pair

minimally
- m. invasive sinus surgery

minimastopexy

Mini-Matic implant

Mini-Mental State Examination (MMSE)

minimum
- m. acceptable field (MAF)
- m. audible field (MAF)
- m. audible pressure (MAP)
- M. Auditory Capabilities Test (MAC)

MiniOX V pulse oximeter

miniplate
- Champy m.
- m. fixation
- 8-hole m.
- L-shaped m.
- mandibular m.
- Storz m.
- titanium m.
- two-holed m.

miniscrew

Minnesota
- M. Preschool Scale
- M. retractor
- M. Test for Differential Diagnosis of Aphasia
- M. thermal disk temperature testing device

Minocin
- M. IV Injection
- M. Oral

minocycline
- m. HCl

minor
- aphthae m.
- m. connector
- m. gland obstruction
- m. salivary gland
- teres m.

minoxidil

minute
- breaths per m. (BPM)

Minute-Gel

Miochol-E

Miostat Intraocular

mirabilis
>*Proteus m.*

Mirage Bond II
Mira-Guard mouth protector
MIRBI
>Mini Inventory of Right Brain Injury

mirror
>curved laryngeal m.
>curved magnifying m.
>DenLite illuminated hand-held m.
>dental m.
>fiberoptic lighted m.
>frontal m.
>head m.
>mouth m.
>Neovision micro m.
>m. speech
>straight laryngeal m.
>straight magnifying m.

mirror-based reflective optics
MirrorOffice software
MIS
>melanoma in situ

misarticulation
misdirection
>facial nerve m.

mismatch
>m. negativity (MMN)
>vessel caliber m.

misphonia
mispronunciation
missile-caused wound
missing tooth
mist
>GraftCyte hydrating m.

misuse
>vocal m.

Mitchella repens
mite
>elevator grain dust m.
>house dust m.
>house dust m. F
>house dust m. P
>soybean grain dust m.
>wheat grain dust m.

Mitek
>M. anchor
>M. GII suture anchor
>M. Mini GII anchor

Mithracin
mitigated echolalia

mitis
>*Streptococcus m.*

mitochondrial oxidative enzyme
mitochondrion, pl. mitochondria
mitogenic factor (MF)
mitomycin-C
mitosis
mitotic figure
mitoxantrone
Mittelman implant
Mitutoyo Digimatic caliper
Mity
>M. engine H-file
>M. engine T-file
>M. Gates Glidden file
>M. Hedström file
>M. K-file
>M. plugger
>M. Roto 360 instrument
>M. Roto rotary instrument
>M. spreader
>M. Turbo File file

Mitz procedure
mix
>juniper m.
>normal m.

mixed
>m. deafness
>m. dentition
>m. dentition analysis
>m. failure
>m. feathers
>m. hemangioma
>m. hypertrophy
>m. laterality
>m. mesh
>m. nasality
>m. odontoma
>m. tumor
>m. tumor of salivary gland
>m. type parapharyngeal schwannoma

mixer
>amalgam m.

mixing slab
mixture
>Carnoy m.
>Miles Magic M.
>m. theory

ML
>mesiolingual

NOTES

MLA
    mesiolabial
Mladick abdominoplasty
MLAI
    mesiolabioincisal
MLB
    Monaural Loudness Balance Test
MLC
    Marginal Line Calculus Index
    mesiolingual cusp
ML-composite
    ML-composite restoration
MLCR
    mesiolingual cusp ridge
MLDG
    mesiolingual developmental groove
MLF
    mesiolingual fossa
MLG
    mesiolingual groove
MLI
    mesiolinguoincisal
MLO
    mesiolinguo-occlusal
MLP
    mesiolinguopulpal
MLR
    mean length of response
    middle latency response
MLR+ camera
MLU
    mean length of utterance
MM
    malignant melanoma
MM 3000
MMC
    myelomeningocele
MMDG
    mesial marginal developmental groove
MMF
    maxillomandibular fixation
MMN
    mismatch negativity
MMP
    matrix metalloproteinase
MMR
    mesial marginal ridge
MMS
    Mohs micrographic surgery
MMSE
    Mini-Mental State Examination
MN
    median nerve
MND
    modified neck dissection
MNOE
    malignant necrotizing otitis externa

MO
    mesio-occlusal
    myositis ossificans
    MO cavity
Moberg pickup test
Mobidin
mobile
    m. anaerobic laboratory
    m. septum
    m. tooth
mobility
    abnormal tooth m.
    normal tooth m.
    pathologic tooth m.
    physiologic tooth m.
    tooth m.
    m. of tooth
mobilization
    bony m.
    stapes m.
Möbius syndrome
moccasin
    water m.
MOD
    mesial, occlusal, and distal
    mesiodistocclusal
    mesio-occlusodistal
    MOD cavity
modal
    m. auxiliary
    m. frequency
    m. phonation
    m. tone
    m. voice
modality
    auditory m.
mode
    MPEAK stimulation m.
    pulsed cutting m.
    SPEAK cochlear stimulation m.
    transverse electromagnetic m.
     (TEM)
    vocal m.
model
    casting m.
    dental m.
    m. denture wax
    immunocompetent squamous cell
     cancer m.
    implant m.
    m. plaster
    m. plaster Grade A
    m. trimmer
    m. wax denture
    Westmore m.
modeling
    bilateral fronto-orbital m.
    m. composition

m. compound
m. plastic
m. plastic impression
moderate
m. hearing impairment
m. hearing loss
moderately
m. differentiated neuroendocrine carcinoma
m. severe hearing impairment
m. severe hearing loss
modification
activator m.
appliance m.
behavior m.
bracket m.
cingulum m.
Goldner m.
interference m.
O'Leary m.
modified
m. abdominoplasty
m. anterior scoring technique
m. Bernard-Burow technique
m. cast
m. Chopart amputation
m. desmosome
m. flap operation
m. Frost method
m. Frost suture
m. junctional complex
m. Kiel mastopexy
m. Krukenberg procedure
m. lateral pharyngotomy
m. Mallet scale
m. metal crown
m. neck dissection (MND)
m. pen grasp
m. polymer
m. radical mastectomy
m. radical mastoidectomy
m. Singapore flap
m. Skoog technique
m. somatic perception questionnaire (MSPQ)
m. submental retractor, flared tip
m. Wardill method
m. Weber-Ferguson incision
m. Weber-Fergusson procedure
m. zinc oxide-eugenol cement
modifier
biologic response m.

color m.
composite resin color m.
nonrestrictive m.
restrictive m.
modiolus labii
modular theory
modulation
amplitude m. (AM)
frequency m. (FM)
immune m.
mimetic m.
module
AIM 7 thermocouple input m.
600 series PDT dye m.
modulus
M. CD anesthesia system
dynamic m.
elastic m.
Moeller glossitis
mogiarthria
mogilalia
mogiphonia
mohair dander
Mohr-Tranebjaerg syndrome
Mohs
M. chemosurgery
M. defect
M. excision
M. hardness
M. hardness number (MHN)
M. hardness scale
M. hardness test
M. index
M. micrographic surgery (MMS)
M. micrographic surgery by fixed-tissue technique
M. resection
M. surgery
M. wound
moiety
carbohydrate m.
moiré topography index
moisture
M. Ophthalmic Drops
moisturizer
Betadine First Aid Antibiotics + M.
molar
anchor m.
m. band
m. bite position
m. bracket

M

NOTES

molar *(continued)*
    m. crowding
    deciduous m.
    deeply placed, unerupted maxillary
      third m.
    first m.
    fourth m.
    m. gland
    m. hook
    impacted m.
    ipsilateral m.
    mandibular m.
    maxillary m.
    Moon m.'s
    mulberry m.
    primary m.
    second m.
    m. sheath
    sixth-year m.
    supernumerary m.
    supraerupted m.
    m. teeth
    third m.
    m. tooth
    m. tube
    m. tubercle
    twelfth-year m.
molariform
molaris, pl. **molares**
    dens m.
    dentes molares
mold, mould
    AquaNot swim m.
    casting m.
    m. guide
    inlay m.
    mother matrix m.
    Swyrls swim m.
    Teflon m.
molding
    border m.
    compression m.
    injection m.
    m. temperature
    tissue m.
mole
    m. melanoma syndrome
    pigmented m.
molecular mimicry
molecule
    cell adhesion m. (CAM)
    collagen m.
    neurotransmitter m.
    polymerized mucopolysaccharide m.
    tropocollagen m.
molilalia

Molina
    M. mandibular distractor
    M. mandibular distractor set
Möller disease
Mollifene Ear Wax Removing Formula
molluscum contagiosum
Mölnlycke
Molt
    M. mouth gag
    M. No. 4 elevator
molybdenum
moment
    activation m.
    pure m.
    residual m.
moment-force ratio (M/F)
momentum
    nuclear angular m.
mometasone
    m. furoate
    m. furoate monohydrate
    m. furoate monohydrate nasal spray
Monahan-Lewis knife
Mona Lisa smile
monangle
    m. hoe
monaural
    m. hearing aid
monauralis
    diplacusis m.
Monaural Loudness Balance Test (MLB)
Mondini
    M. deafness
    M. deformity
    M. dysplasia
    M. malformation
Mondini-Alexander malformation
Mondor disease
mongolism
Monilia
moniliasis
    oral m.
Monistat
    M.-Derm Topical
    M. i.v. Injection
    M. Vaginal
monitor
    Accutorr bedside m.
    Colin STBP-780 stress test blood
      pressure m.
    Criticare m.
    Criticare comprehensive vital
      sign m.
    Criticare 507N noninvasive blood
      pressure m.
    Criticare 507O pulse
      oximeter/NIBP m.

Criticare POET TE end-tidal CO_2 respiration m.
Criticare 507S vital sign m.
Dinamap Plus multiparameter m.
Haemogram blood loss m.
laser Doppler perfusion m.
Laserflo BPM laser Doppler m.
Marquette m.
MRL blood pressure m.
Multinex ID gas m.
m. muscle flap
Neurosign 100 nerve m.
Passport bedside m.
perfusion m.
Porta-Resp m.
Stat-Temp II liquid crystal temperature m.
Transonic laser Doppler perfusion m.
VISA multi-patient m.

monitored live voice audiometry
monitoring
m. audiometry
photoplethysmographic m.
radiation m.
video m.

monkey dander
monoangle chisel
monoangled
monobloc
m. appliance

monochromatic radiation
Monocid
monoclonal antibody
monocortical
m. bone
m. screw

Monocryl suture
monocyte
monocytoid cell
Monodox Oral
monofascicular nerve
monofilament
m. nylon suture
Semmes-Weinstein m. (SWMF)
m. suture
m. test

monofluorophosphate dentifrice
Mono-Gesic
monohydrate
beclomethasone dipropionate, m.
mometasone furoate m.

monologue, monolog
collective m.

monomaxillary
monomer
acrylic m.
hydrophobic m.
residual m.

monomorphic
m. adenoma
m. pattern

Mononine
mononucleosis
infectious m.

mono-parachlorophenol
camphorated m.-p. (CMCP)

monophosphate
cyclic adenosine m.
cyclic adenosine 3′,5′-m. (cAMP)

monophyodont
m. dentition

monoplegia
m. masticatoria

monopodal
m. ankylotic stapes

monostotic
m. fibrous dysplasia
m. lesion

monostructure implant
monosyllabic word
monothermal caloric test
monotone
Monson curve
mons pubis
Montague plane
montan wax
Monterey cypress
Montgomery
M. laryngeal keel
M. speaking valve
M. thyroplasty implant system
M. T tube
M. tubercles

mood
imperative m.
indicative m.
subjunctive m.

Moon
M. molars
M. teeth

Moore
M. head-tilt maneuver
M. mandrel

M

NOTES

moorean ulcer
Moorehead retractor
Moraxella catarrhalis
morbidity
> perinatal m.

morbid obesity
morbillorum
> *Gemella m.*
> *Streptococcus m.*

morcel
morcellation
Morel ear
Morgagni
> sinus of M.
> M. ventricle

Morganella
Morgan mandrel
morning glory configuration
Moro reflex
morphea
morpheaform
> m. basal cell carcinoma

morpheme
> bound m.
> free m.
> grammatical m.
> lexical m.
> m. structure rule
> zero m.

morphine
> m. sulfate

morphodifferentiation
morphogen
morphogenic stage
morphographemic rule
morphological
> m. element

morphology
> Antoni classification of schwannoma m.
> determinants of occlusal m.
> Test for Examining Expressive M. (EEM)
> tooth m.

morphometric
> m. analysis
> m. study
> m. video analysis

morphophonemic component
morphophonemics
morphotactics
morphotype
Morquio
> mucopolysaccharidosis type IV M. (MPS-IV)
> M. syndrome

Morrell crown remover
morsal teeth

morselized cartilage
morsicatio
mortality
> perinatal m.

Morwel
> M. ultrasound-assisted lipoplasty machine
> M. ultrasound device

Mosco Liquid
Mosetig-Moorhof filling
mosquito
> m. forceps
> m. hemostat

Moss balloon triple-lumen gastrostomy tube
most
> m. comfortable loudness (MCL)
> m. comfortable loudness range (MCLR)

moth dander
mother
> m. matrix mold
> m. method

motility
motion
> active range of m. (AROM)
> brownian m.
> cartwheel m.
> ciliary m.
> mandibular range of m.
> maximal static response assay of facial m.
> range of m. (ROM)
> scapholunate m.
> m. sickness
> simple harmonic m. (SHM)

motivating operation
motivation
motokinesthetics
motor
> m. aphasia
> m. area
> m. control test
> m. coordination test (MCT)
> m. disorder
> m. endplate
> fine m.
> gross m.
> m. impairment
> m. nerve
> m. nerve of tongue
> m. neuron
> m. roots of submandibular ganglion
> m. root of trigeminal nerve

Moto-tool
> Dremel M.-t.

Motrin
> Children's M.

M. IB
M. IB Sinus
Junior Strength M.

mottled
m. enamel
m. teeth

mottling

moulage
facial m.

mould (*var. of* mold)

Moult curette

mound
malar m.

mount
Adamount pocket m.'s
film m.
split cast m.
x-ray m.

mountain
m. cedar
m. cedar antigen

mounted
m. diamond points
m. point stone
m. stone

mounting
centric m.
film m.
split cast m.

mouse
m. dander
m. serum protein (MSP)
m. urine protein (MUP)

moustache, mustache
m. dressing

moustache-like flap

mouth
m. breathing
carp m.
denture sore m.
m. denture wax
depressor muscle of angle of m.
dry m.
floor of m. (FOM)
m. flora
m. gag
m. guard
m. hygiene
m. lamp
levator muscle of angle of m.
lymphatic vessels of m.
m. mirror

numerary m.
orbicular muscle of m.
orifice of the m.
phlegmon of floor of m.
m. preparation
m. prop
putrid sore m.
m. rehabilitation
m. rinse
roof of m.
m. stick
trench m.
vestibule of m.
white m.

Mouth-Aid
Orajel M.-A.

mouthguard bleaching

Mouthkote

mouth protector
custom-made m. p.
external m. p.
internal m. p.
Mira-Guard m. p.
polyvinylacetate-polyethylene m. p.
Proform m. p.
Sta-Guard m. p.
stock and mouth-formed m. p.

mouthrinse
Fluorigard m.
Point-Two m.

mouthstick, mouth stick
m. appliance
m. prosthesis

mouthwash
antibacterial m.
astringent m.
buffered m.
concentrated m.
deodorizing m.
therapeutic m.

movability

movable-arm clasp

movement
ballistic m.
Bennett m.
bodily m.
border tissue m.
brownian m.
compensatory m.
cutting m.
dentogenic m.
distal m.

M

NOTES

movement *(continued)*
 empty m.
 eruptive tooth m.
 extraneous m.
 Facial Grading System
  voluntary M. (FGSM)
 free mandibular m.
 functional mandibular m.
 gliding m.
 grinding m.
 hinge m.
 intermediary m.
 jaw m.
 labial m.
 lateral m.
 laterotrusive m.
 lingual m.
 mandibular gliding m.
 masticatory mandibular m.
 maximum m.
 mesial m.
 nonfunction mandibular m.
 opening mandibular m.
 oral commissure m.
 orthodontic tooth m.
 pendulum m.
 posterior border m.
 posteruptive tooth m.
 preeruptive tooth m.
 protrusive m.
 random m.
 retrusive m.
 rotational m.
 sagittal mandibular m.
 smooth-pursuit eye m.
 tipping m.
 tooth m.
 translatory m.
 volition oral m.
moving two-point discrimination
Mowrey
 M. 695 amalgam
 M. B inlay
 M. gold
 M. No. 1 wire
 M. 12% wire
Mozart ear
MP
 mesial pit
 mesiopulpal
6-mp
 6-mercaptopurine
MPAPC
 mucus-producing adenopapillary
  carcinoma
MPD
 maximum permissible dose

myofacial pain-dysfunction
 MPD syndrome
MPEAK
 multipeak
  MPEAK stimulation mode
MPH
 mandibular plane to hyoid
  MPH distance measurement
MPL
 mesiopulpolingual
MPLA
 mesiopulpolabial
M-plasty
MPO
 maximum power output
M-Prednisol Injection
MPS
 mucopolysaccharidoses
 mucopolysaccharidosis
 myofascial pain syndrome
 MPS-IH
  mucopolysaccharidosis type I
   Hurler
 MPS-IHS
  mucopolysaccharidosis type I
   Hurler-Scheie
 MPS-II
  mucopolysaccharidosis type II
   Hunter
 MPS-IIIA
  mucopolysaccharidosis type III
   Sanfilippo A
 MPS-IIIB
  mucopolysaccharidosis type III
   Sanfilippo B
 MPS-IIIC
  mucopolysaccharidosis type III
   Sanfilippo C
 MPS-IS
  mucopolysaccharidosis type I
   Scheie
 MPS-IV
  mucopolysaccharidosis type IV
   Morquio
 MPS-VI
  mucopolysaccharidosis type VI
   Maroteaux-Lamy
 MPS-VII
  mucopolysaccharidosis type VII
   Sly
MQ cement
MR
 mentally retarded
MRA
 magnetic resonance angiography
MRG
 mean rejection grading
 mean residual gap

MRI
    magnetic resonance imaging
    FISP-3D MRI
        fast-imaging steady precession
        sequence three-dimensional
        magnetic resonance imaging
    surface-coil MRI

MRKHS
    Mayer-Rokitansky-Küster-Hauser
    syndrome

MRL
    M. blood pressure monitor
    M. oximeter
    M. Pacette

MRSA
    methicillin-resistant *Staphylococcus aureus*

MRU
    mean relational utterance

MS
    melanonychia striata
    MS Contin Oral

MSBP
    mandibular staple bone plate

MSD

msec
    millisecond

MSI
    magnetic source imaging

MSIR Oral

MSL
    mean sentence length

MS/L

MSP
    mouse serum protein

MSPQ
    modified somatic perception
    questionnaire

MSRA
    Maximal Static Response Assay

MS/S

MST
    maximum stimulation test

MTA
    mineral trioxide aggregate

***m*-tetra(hydroxyphenol) chlorin (*m*-THPC)**

MTF
    mesial triangular fossa

***m*-THPC**
    m-tetra(hydroxyphenol) chlorin

MTP
    metatarsophalangeal
    MTP joint

MTX
    methotrexate

M-type reamer

mucicarmine

mucigen granule

mucin
    allergic m.
    m. granule
    m. plaque

mucinase

mucinosis
    cutaneous focal m.
    oral focal m.

mucinous
    m. cell adenocarcinoma
    m. plaque

mucobuccal
    m. fold
    m. reflection

mucocele
    frontal sinus m.
    maxillary sinus m.
    retention m.
    sinus m.

mucochondrocutaneous flap

mucociliary
    m. drainage pathway
    m. flow
    m. transport (MCT)

mucocutaneous
    m. junction
    m. leishmaniasis
    m. lymph node syndrome
    m. melanosis

mucoepidermoid
    m. carcinoma (MEC)
    m. carcinoma of parotid
    m. carcinoma of the tongue
    m. lesion
    m. tumor

mucogingival
    m. junction (MGJ)
    m. line
    m. surgery

mucoid
    m. otitis media

mucolabial fold

Mucolube

mucolytic

M

NOTES

mucoperichondrial
m. elevation
m. flap
mucoperichondrium
septal m.
mucoperiosteal
m. flap technique
m. lining
m. periodontal flap
m. periodontal graft
m. sliding flap
mucoperiosteum
mucopolysaccharide
acid m.
m. keratin dystrophy
mucopolysaccharidosis,
pl. **mucopolysaccharidoses (MPS)**
m. type I Hurler (MPS-IH)
m. type I Hurler-Scheie (MPS-IHS)
m. type II Hunter (MPS-II)
m. type III Sanfilippo A (MPS-IIIA)
m. type III Sanfilippo B (MPS-IIIB)
m. type III Sanfilippo C (MPS-IIIC)
m. type I Scheie (MPS-IS)
m. type IV Morquio (MPS-IV)
m. type VII Sly (MPS-VII)
m. type VI Maroteaux-Lamy (MPS-VI)
mucopurulent
m. hemorrhagic effusion
mucopus
mucopyelocele
mucopyocele
Mucor
mucormycosis
rhinocerebral m.
rhinoorbital m.
rhinoorbitocerebral m.
mucosa
alveolar m.
alveolar ridge m.
bladder m.
buccal m.
conchal m.
dorsal lingual m.
ethmoidal m.
free graft from urinary bladder m.
gastric m.
gingival m.
hypermobile m.
hyperplastic m.
lingual m.
lining m.
mandibular alveolar m.
masticatory m.

nasal m.
nevus spongiosus albus m.
oral m.
palatine m.
reflecting m.
respiratory m.
retromolar m.
retrotuberosity m.
specialized m.
sublingual m.
vestibular m.
vomer m.
mucosa-borne denture
mucosae
lipoidosis cutis et m.
mucosal
m. blood vessel
m. coat
m. collar
m. cyst
m. excision
m. grafting
m. horn
m. implant
m. insert
m. patch replacement
m. periodontal flap
m. periodontal graft
m. prelaminated flap
m. relaxing incision technique
m. transudate
mucosalize
mucositis
radiation m.
xerostomic m.
mucosobuccal fold
mucostatic
mucosum
Treponema m.
mucous
m. alveolus
m. blanket
m. cell
m. cyst
m. gland
m. membrane
m. membrane of lip
m. membrane of tongue
m. otitis
m. patch
m. plaque
m. plug
m. retention cyst
m. retention phenomenon
m. tubule
mucoviscidosis
mucus
glairy m.

nasal m.
olfactory m.
salivary m.
mucus-producing adenopapillary carcinoma (MPAPC)
mucus-secreting cell
mud
dentin m.
Mueller test
Mueller-Walle method
muffled voice
muffle furnace
mugwort
Muhlmann
M. appliance
M. periodontometer
mulberry
black m.
m. molar
paper m.
red m.
m. tooth
white m.
müllerian
m. dimple
m. duct
m. duct aplasia
mulling
multibanded
m. appliance
m. mechanotherapy
multicanaled tooth
Multicenter Selective Lymphadenectomy trial
multicentric glomus tumor
multichannel cochlear implant
Multicide
multicultural family
multicuspid
m. tooth
multicuspidate
multidentate
Multidimensional Body-Self Relations Questionnaire
Multi-Dimensional Voice Program 4305 (MDVP 4305)
multidirectional distractor
Multi-fil
multifluted carbide
multifocal
m. lymphocytic infiltrate

Multi-Form dual purpose impression paste
multiforme
erythema m.
MULTIGUIDE mandibular distractor
multilaminar
MultiLase D copper vapor laser
multilocular
m. cyst
m. mass
multiloculated
Multinex ID gas monitor
multinodular goiter
multinucleated
m. dentinoblastic cell
m. giant cell
multipara
multipeak (MPEAK)
m. cochlear stimulation code
multiphase
m. appliance
m. attachment
m. bracket
multiplanar
m. endoscopic facial rejuvenation technique
m. upper facial rejuvenation technique
multiple
m. abutment
m. abutment support
m. anchorage
m. clasp
m. cone root canal filling method
m. diastemata
m. endocrine neoplasia
m. exostoses of jaw
m. foramina
m. hamartoma syndrome
m. loop archwire
m. loop wiring
m. myeloma
m. papillomatosis
m. primary
m. retainer
m. sclerosis
multiplex
dysostosis m.
m. dysostosis
steatocystoma m.
multiply handicapped
multipoint contact plate

M

NOTES

multipolar neuron
multiprong rake retractor
multirooted
    m. abutment
    m. tooth
multiscope
    roaming optical access m. (ROAM)
multisensory
multivacuolated
multivesicular body
multiword combination
Muma Assessment Program (MAP)
Mummery
    pink tooth of M.
mummification
    pulp m.
mummified pulp
mumps
    m. encephalitis
    m. meningoencephalomyelitis
    m. virus
MUP
    mouse urine protein
mupirocin
mural ameloblastoma
Murine
    M. Ear Drops
    M. Plus Ophthalmic
    M. Solution
Murocel Ophthalmic Solution
Murocoll-2 Ophthalmic
muromonab-CD3
muscle
    abductor hallucis m.
    abductor pollicis longus m.
    adductor longus m.
    adductor magnus m.
    Aeby m.
    alar m.
    anconeus m.
    ansa hypoglossus m.
    antagonistic m.
    anterior superficialis m.
    aryepiglottic m.
    arytenoid m.
    auricular m.
    m. belly
    bipennate m.
    brachialis m.
    brachioradialis m.
    buccal m.
    buccinator m.
    canine m.
    cheek m.
    chin m.
    chondroglossus m.
    constrictor pharyngeal m.
    m. contraction

    m. contraction headache
    corrugator m.
    corrugator supercilii m.
    cremaster m.
    cricoarytenoid m.
    cricopharyngeus m.
    cricothyroid m.
    dartos m.
    denervated m.
    depressor anguli oris m.
    depressor labii inferioris m.
    depressor labii oris m.
    depressor septi m.
    digastric m.
    dilator naris m.
    epicranius m.
    extensor carpi radialis brevis m.
    extensor carpi radialis longus m.
    extensor carpi ulnaris m.
    extensor digiti minimi m.
    extensor digitorum m.
    extensor digitorum longus m.
    extensor hallucis longus m.
    extensor indicis m.
    extensor pollicis brevis m.
    extensor pollicis longus m.
    extralaryngeal m.
    extraocular m.
    extrinsic m. of tongue
    facial m.
    facial mimetic m.
    fast-twitch fatigable skeletal m.
    flexor carpi ulnaris m.
    flexor digitorum brevis m.
    flexor digitorum longus m.
    flexor digitorum profundus m.
    flexor digitorum superficialis m.
    flexor hallucis longus m.
    flexor pollicis longus m.
    frontalis m.
    genioglossus m.
    geniohyoglossus m.
    geniohyoid m.
    glossopalatine m.
    gracilis m.
    m. hernia
    hyoglossal m.
    hyoglossus m.
    hyperactive m.
    hypertonic m.
    hypotonic m.
    iliocostalis dorsi m.
    iliocostalis lumborum m.
    m. implantation
    incisive m.
    inferior constrictor pharyngeal m.
    inferior oblique m.
    inferior rectus m.

infrahyoid m.
infrahyoid strap m.
infraspinatus m.
interarytenoid m.
intercostalis externus m.
intercostalis internus m.
internal pterygoid m.
intrinsic m. of tongue
lateral cricoarytenoid m.
lateral pterygoid m.
lateral rectus m.
latissimus dorsi m.
levator m.
levator anguli oris m.
levator costae m.
levator glandulae thyroidea m.
levator labii superioris m.
levator labii superioris alaeque
  nasi m.
levator palatini m.
levator veli palatini m.
longitudinalis inferior m.
longitudinalis superior m.
longitudinal m. of tongue
longus capitis m.
longus colli m.
masseter m.
mastication m.
masticatory m.
medial pterygoid m.
medial rectus m.
mental m.
mentalis m.
middle constrictor pharyngeal m.
mimetic m.
m. moment arm length
musculus transversus menti m.
mylohyoid m.
nasal m.
nasalis m.
nasolabial m.
oblique m.
oblique arytenoid m.
obliquus abdominis externus m.
obliquus abdominis internus m.
obliquus inferior m.
obliquus superior m.
occipitofrontalis m.
omohyoid m.
orbicularis m.
orbicularis oculi m.
orbicularis oris m.

orbicular m. of mouth
palatal m.
palatoglossus m.
palatopharyngeal m.
palatopharyngeus m.
palmaris longus m.
paravertebral m.
pectoralis major m.
pectoralis minor m.
perioral m.
periorbital orbicularis oculi m.
peroneus tertius m.
pharyngeal constrictor m.
pharyngopalatinus m.
platysma m.
posterior cricoarytenoid m.
procerus m.
pronator quadratus m.
pronator teres m.
pterygoid m.
quadrate m. of lower lip
quadrate m. of upper lip
quadratus labii superioris m.
quadratus lumborum m.
rectus abdominis m.
rectus capitis m.
rectus femoris m.
rectus labii m.
rectus medialis m.
rectus superioris m.
m. relaxant
m. repositioning
risorius m.
salpingopharyngeal m.
salpingopharyngeus m.
sartorius m.
scalenus anterior m.
scalenus medius m.
scalenus posterior m.
scalp m.
semimembranosus m.
semimembranous m.
serratus anterior m.
serratus posterior inferior m.
serratus posterior superior m.
m. sling
slow-twitch fatigue-resistant
  skeletal m.
soleus m.
spastic m.
m. spindle
splenius capitis m.

M

NOTES

muscle *(continued)*
    square m. of lower lip
    stapedius m.
    sternoclavicularis m.
    sternocleidomastoid m.
    sternocleidomastoideus m.
    sternohyoid m.
    sternohyoideus m.
    sternomastoid m.
    sternothyroid m.
    sternothyroideus m.
    strap m.
    styloglossus m.
    stylohyoid m.
    stylopharyngeus m.
    subclavius m.
    subcostalis m.
    superior constrictor m.
    superior constrictor pharyngeal m.
    supinator m.
    suprahyoid m.
    temporal m.
    temporalis m.
    m. tension headache
    tensor tympani m.
    tensor veli palatini m.
    teres major m.
    teres minor m.
    thyroarytenoid m.
    thyroepiglottic m.
    thyrohyoid m.
    tibialis anterior m.
    tibialis posterior m.
    m. tonus
    trachealis m.
    m. transfer
    transpalpebral corrugator m.
    m. transposition
    transverse arytenoid m.
    transverse rectus abdominis m. (TRAM)
    transverse m. of tongue
    transversus abdominis m.
    transversus linguae m.
    transversus perinei profundus m.
    transversus thoracis m.
    trapezius m.
    triangular m.
    m. trimming
    tympanic m.
    uvular m.
    verticalis linguae m.
    vertical m. of tongue
    vocal m.
    vocalis m.
    zygomatic m.
    zygomaticomandibular m.
    zygomaticus m.
    zygomaticus major m.
    zygomaticus minor m.
muscle-access abdominoplasty
muscle-periosteal flap
muscle-trimming
muscular
    m. bolster
    m. dystrophy
    m. graft
    m. sclerosis
    m. torticollis
musculature
    contralateral m.
musculoaponeurotic
    m. control
    m. layer
    m. plication
    m. system
musculocutaneous
    m. flap
    m. perforator
    rectus abdominis m. (RAM)
    transverse rectus abdominis m. (TRAM)
musculofascial flap
musculomucosal
    facial artery m. (FAMM)
musculoperitoneal
    transverse rectus abdominis m. (TRAMP)
    transversus and rectus abdominis m. (TRAMP)
musculotendinous aponeurosis
musculovascular pedicle
musculus
    m. levator anguli oris
    m. levator labii superioris
    m. risorius
    m. transversus menti muscle
    m. vastus lateralis
    m. zygomaticus major
Musgrave and Dupertuis graft augmentation
mush bite, mushbite
mustache *(var. of* moustache*)*
mustard
    nitrogen m.
    yellow m.
Mustardé, Mustarde
    M. lateral cheek rotation flap
    M. otoplasty
    M. rotation-advancement flap
    M. suture
    M. technique
mutacism
mutagen
mutagenic

mutans
>Streptococcus *m.*

mutation
>p53 gene m.
>m. voice

mute
mutilation
>jugomasseteric m.
>labiogeniomandibular m.
>orbitopalpebral m.

mutism
>elected m.
>elective m.
>voluntary m.

Muti technique
MV
>main venule

MVD
>microvascular decompression
>microvessel density

Myambutol
myasthenia
>m. gravis
>m. laryngis

My-Bond Carbo cement
Mycelex
>M.-7
>M.-G
>M. Troche

mycelium, pl. mycelia
mycetoma
Mycifradin
>M. Sulfate Oral
>M. Sulfate Topical

Mycitracin Topical
mycobacteria (*pl. of* mycobacterium)
mycobacterial
>m. infection
>m. lymphadenitis
>m. nodal infection

Mycobacterium
>M. *avium*
>M. *avium* complex (MAC)
>M. *avium-intracellulare* (MAI)
>M. *avium-intracellulare* complex (MAC)
>M. *bovis*
>M. *chelonei*
>M. *fortuitum*
>M. *intracellulare*
>M. *kansasii*
>M. *leprae*

M. *marinum*
M. *scrofulaceum*
M. *terrae*
M. *tuberculosis*

mycobacterium, pl. mycobacteria
>atypical m.
>nontuberculous m. (NTM)

Mycobutin
Mycocide
>M. NS
>M. NS antimicrobial solution

Mycogen II Topical
Mycolog
>M.-II Topical

mycomyringitis
Myconel Topical
mycophenolate
Mycoplasma
>M. *hominis*
>M. *pneumoniae*

mycosis
>antral m.
>m. fungoides
>m. leptothrica
>systemic m.

Mycostatin
>M. Pastilles

mycotic
>m. disease
>m. stomatitis

Myco-Triacet II
Mydfrin Ophthalmic Solution
Mydriacyl
mydriasis
mydriatic
myectomy
myelinated
>m. axon
>m. nerve fiber
>m. sensory nerve fiber

myelination
myelinization
myelin sheath
myeloblastoma
>granular cell m.

myeloma
>multiple m.

myelomeningocele (MMC)
myiasis
>aural m.
>nasal m.
>oral m.

M

NOTES

389

Mylar
 M. matrix
 M. strip
mylohyoid
 m. line
 m. muscle
 m. nerve
 m. region
 m. ridge
 m. sulcus
 m. sulcus of mandible
Myminic Expectorant
Mynol cement
myoblastoma
 granular cell m.
 malignant granular cell m.
myocardial infarction
myocutaneous
 m. flap
 transverse rectus abdominis m.
 (TRAM)
myodermal flap
myoelastic-aerodynamic theory of
 phonation
myoelastic theory
myoepithelial
 m. cell
 m. cell island
 m. cell process
 m. sialadenitis
myoepithelioma
myofacial
 m. pain-dysfunction (MPD)
 m. pain-dysfunction disorder
 m. pain-dysfunction syndrome
myofascial
 m. flap
 m. pain syndrome (MPS)
myofasciitis
 necrotizing m.
myofiber atrophy
myofibrositis
myofunctional
 m. therapy
myogaleal
myogenic
myognathus
myograph
 palate m.
myography
myoma
Myo-Monitor centric
myomucosal flap
myonecrosis
myoneural blocking agent
myoneurotization
myopathic
 m. paralysis

myopathy
 thyrotoxic m..
myoplastic
myoplasty
myosarcoma
 angiomatoid m.
myositis
 m. ossificans (MO)
 m. ossificans progessiva
myospherulosis
myotactic
myotatic
 m. irritability
 m. reflex
myotomy
 cricopharyngeal m.
 hyoid m.
 procerus muscle m.
myotonia
 acquired m.
 congenital m.
 dystrophic m.
Myphetane DC
Myrica cerifera
Myrica pensylvanicum
myringeal web
myringectomy
myringitis
 m. bulbosa
 bullous m.
myringodermatitis
myringomycosis
myringoplasty
myringostapediopexy
myringotome
myringotomy
 m. and grommet insertion
 m. knife
myrinx
myrtle
 wax m.
mytacism
Mytrex F Topical
Mytussin DAC
myxedema
 m. voice
myxochondroid
 m. matrix
 m. stroma
myxofibroma
 odontogenic m.
myxoid
 m. crystal
 m. liposarcoma
 m. lobule
 m. neurofibroma
 m. stroma
myxolipoma

myxoma
    fibro-osteogenic m.
    nerve-sheath m. (NSM)
    odontogenic m.
    osteogenic m.

myxomatous degeneration
myxosarcoma

NOTES

N
newton
N2
second nerve
N2-Sargenti technique
Nabers probe
nabumetone
NAC
nerve-approximating clamp
nipple-areola complex
NaCl solution
nadolol
Naegleria fowleri
naeslundii
Actinomyces n.
Nafazair Ophthalmic
Nafcil Injection
nafcillin
NaFpak powder
NaFrinse
N. acidulated solution
N. rinse
naftifine
Naftin
Nager
N. acrofacial dysostosis
N. syndrome
nail
n. bed
n. fold
gamma locking n.
Grosse & Kempf locking n.
Seidel humeral locking n.
nalbuphine
Naldecon
N. DX Adult Liquid
N.-EX Children's Syrup
Naldelate
Nalfon
Nalgest
nalidixic acid
Nallpen Injection
naloxone
Nalspan
naming
online cross-modal n.
Nance
N. analysis of arch length
N. leeway space
nanoid enamel
8NAP
eighth nerve action potential
nape of neck flap
naphazoline
n. and pheniramine

Naphcon
N.-A Ophthalmic
N. Forte Ophthalmic
naphthylamide
benzol-arginine n.
napier, neper
Naprelan
Naprosyn
naproxen
napsylate
propoxyphene n.
Narcan
narcosis
narcotic
n. antagonist
naris, pl. nares
anterior n.
nares constriction
nares interna
posterior n.
narrative
n. speech
narrow
n. fissure bur
n. range audiometer
n. tooth
n. transcription
n. vowel
narrow-band noise
narrow-field laryngectomy
Nasabid
Nasacort
N. AQ
N. nasal inhaler
Nasahist B
nasal
n. accessory artery
n. airstream
n. airway
n. airway obstruction
n. airway resistance
n. ala
n. antrostomy
n. artery
n. assimilation
n. bone
n. calculus
n. capsule
n. catarrh
n. cavity
n. chondroma
n. concha
n. congestion
n. consonant
n. coupling

N

nasal *(continued)*
    n. CPAP
    n. cross-sectional area
    n. dome
    n. dorsum
    n. duplication
    n. dysplasia
    n. emission
    n. endoscopy
    n. escape
    n. floor
    n. fossa
    n. fracture
    n. Fraser suction technique
    n. glioma
    n. height
    n. hemorrhage
    n. hump
    n. index
    Kondon N.
    n. lisp
    n. mucosa
    n. mucosal congestion
    n. mucus
    n. muscle
    n. myiasis
    n. nerve
    n. obstruction
    Otrivin N.
    n. packing
    n. patency
    n. polyp
    n. polyposis
    n. port
    Privine N.
    n. process
    n. pyramid
    n. recess
    n. reflex
    n. regurgitation
    n. resonance
    n. respiration
    n. root
    n. rustle
    n. sebaceous gland
    n. septal abscess
    n. septal perforation
    n. septa reconstruction
    n. septum
    n. sill
    n. snort
    n. sound
    n. speculum
    n. speech
    n. spinal point
    n. spine
    n. spur
    n. stenosis

    n. swell body
    n. synechia
    n. tamponade
    n. tip
    n. tip deformity
    n. tip-plasty
    n. tract
    n. trumpet
    n. tube switch
    n. turbulence
    n. twang
    Twice-A-Day N.
    Tyzine N.
    n. uncoupling
    n. valve
    n. valve collapse
    n. valve suspension
    n. vault
    n. vestibule
    n. vestibulitis
    n. vibrissa
    n. volume
    n. vowel
    n. wing
nasalance
Nasalcrom
    N. Nasal Solution
Nasalide
    N. Nasal Aerosol
nasalis muscle
nasality
    assimilated n.
    excessive n.
    mixed n.
nasalization
    n. of vowel
nasalized speech
nasal-labial furrow
nasal-septal fracture
Nasarel
    N. Nasal Spray
nasendoscope
nasendoscopy
nasi
    agger n.
    ala n.
    apex n.
    cancrum n.
    limen n.
    radix n.
nasion
    orbitale n.
    n. perpendicular
    n. point
    n. soft tissue
nasion-alveolar point line
nasion-pogonion measurement

Nasmyth
- N. cuticle
- N. membrane

nasoalveolar cyst
nasoantral window
nasociliary nerve
nasoethmoidal fracture
naso-ethmoid-orbital fracture
nasofacial
- n. analysis
- n. groove

nasofrontal
- n. angle
- n. duct
- n. orifice
- n. suture

nasogastric
- n. tube
- n. tube retrocricoid ulceration

nasogram
- n. curve

nasojugal fold
nasolabial
- n. angle
- n. cyst
- n. fold (NLF)
- n. ligament
- n. line
- n. muscle
- n. rotation flap
- n. stigma
- n. sulcus

nasolacrimal duct
nasomalarmaxillary
nasomandibular
- n. fixation
- n. ligament

nasomaxillary
- n. balloon
- n. buttress
- n. dysplasia

nasomental reflex
nasometer
Nasonex
naso-ocular
- n.-o. cleft

naso-oral
naso-orbito-ethmoid (NOE)
- n.-o.-e. fracture

nasopalatine
- n. cyst
- n. duct
- n. duct cyst
- n. foramen
- n. injection
- n. nerve

nasopharyngeal
- n. abscess
- n. angiofibroma
- n. bursa
- n. carcinoma (NPC)
- n. cyst
- n. fibroma
- n. leishmaniasis
- n. secretion
- n. stenosis (NPS)

nasopharyngectomy
nasopharyngolaryngoscope
nasopharyngoscope
- Smith and Nephew ENT n.

nasopharyngoscopy
- n. biofeedback therapy

nasopharynx
- carcinoma of n.
- carcinoma of n. type a, b, c

nasoplasty
nasosinusitis
nasotracheal
- n. catheter
- n. intubation
- n. tube (NTT)

Natacyn
Nataf lateral flap
natal
- n. cleft
- n. teeth

natamycin
National Temporal Bone, Hearing and Balance Pathology Registry
native
- n. condyle
- n. language

nativist theory
natural
- n. bristle
- n. dentition
- n. frequency
- n. human interferon-γ (nHuIFN-γ)
- n. human interferon-β (nHuIFN-β)
- n. killer cell (NK)
- n. method
- n. phonological process
- n. pitch
- n. process analysis

N

NOTES

NaturaLase
    N. Erbium laser
    N. Er:YAG laser
    N. holistic skin care program
natural-feel breast prosthesis
Natural Profile abutment system
nature's
    n. root canal filling
    N. Tears Solution
Naugle exophthalmometer
navel
    enamel n.
navigator
navy bean
NCS
    numb chin syndrome
NDGA
    nordihydroguaiaretic acid
ND-Stat
NDT
    neurodevelopmental treatment
    noise detection threshold
Nd:YAG
    neodymium:yttrium-aluminum-garnet
    Nd:YAG laser
    Nd:YAG laser system
Nealon technique
near pulp
near-total laryngectomy
Nebcin Injection
Nebs analgesic liquid
nebulizer
    Acorn II n.
    AeroSonic personal ultrasonic n.
neck
    adenoid cystic carcinoma of head
      and n. (ACCHN)
    bur n.
    condylar n.
    n. of condyle
    congenital cartilaginous rest of
      the n. (CCRN)
    n. dissection
    n. flap
    functional assessment of cancer
      therapy–head and n. (FACT-HN)
    implant n.
    n. implant substructure
    implant superstructure n.
    n. jowl
    n. of mandible
    n. of middle turbinate
    osteotomy of condylar n.
    n. plucking
    ridge of mandibular n.
    squamous cell carcinoma of head
      and n. (SCCHN)
    sulcus of mandibular n.

    n. support
    n. of tooth
    n. torsion
necrobiosis lipoidica
necrophorum
    Fusobacterium n.
necropsy
necrosis
    acute tubular n.
    aseptic n.
    avascular n. (AVN)
    avascular scaphoid n.
    caseous n.
    coagulation n.
    colliquative n.
    coronal n.
    cortical n.
    coumadin n.
    epidermal n.
    fat n.
    flap n.
    gangrenous pulp n.
    gingival n.
    gummatous n.
    ischemic n.
    liquefaction n.
    liquefactive n.
    periodontal membrane n.
    pulp n.
    pulpal n.
    radiation n.
    rim n.
    skin edge n.
    spot n.
    tumor-like n.
    warfarin-induced n.
    wound n.
necrotic
    n. angina
    n. caries
    n. cementum
    n. hyalinized tissue
    n. predentin
    n. pulp
    n. ulcerative peri-implantoclasia
    n. zone
necrotizing
    n. external otitis
    n. fasciitis (NF)
    n. gingivitis
    n. granuloma
    n. myofascial fungal infection
    n. myofasciitis
    n. otitis media
    n. sialometaplasia
    n. soft tissue infection (NSTI)
    n. tracheobronchitis (NTB)
    n. ulcerative gingivitis (NUG)

n. ulcerative gingivostomatitis
n. ulcerative stomatitis
NED
no evidence of disease
needle
ACCUJECT sterile disposable
dental n.
anesthetic n.
n. aspiration
n. aspiration cytology
atraumatic n.
Colorado MicroDissection n.
cut taper n.
diathermal n.
disposable n.
Double D n.
n. endosseous implant
n. endosteal implant
Entree disposable CO_2
insufflation n.
Ethicon ST-4 straight taper-point n.
Gillmore n.
Grice suture n.
n. holder
Hunstad infusion n.
hypodermic n.
Keith n.
Klein infiltration n.
n. localization breast biopsy
LR n.
Luer-Lok n.
Lukens n.
metallic frontal n.
NoKor n.
Permark micropigmentation n.
PermaSharp suture and n.
polypropylene n.
precision lancet cutting n.
Protect.Point n.
Reverdin n.
Rosen n.
n. shape crystal
Stabident ultrashort n.
surgical n.
swaged n.
Vicat n.
needle-point
n.-p. electrocautery
n.-p. tracer
n.-p. tracing
Needles split cast method

needlestick
contaminated n.
negation
negative
n. correlation
n. culture
n. emotion
n. feedback
n. politzerization
n. practice
n. reinforcer
n. response
n. spike
n. spike-wave
negativity
mismatch n. (MMN)
NegGram
Neisseria
N. catarrhalis
N. gonorrhoeae
N. meningitidis
Nellcor
N. N-20PA, N-20 pulse oximeter
N. Symphony N-3000 pulse
oximeter
Nembutal
N. Sodium
neoadjuvant chemotherapy
neoclitoris, pl. **neoclitorides**
vascularized sensate n.
neoclitoroplasty
sensate pedicled n.
Neo-Cobefrin
neocolpopoiesis
rectosigmoid n. (RSC)
Neo-Cortef
NeoDecadron
N. Ophthalmic
N. Topical
Neo-Dexameth Ophthalmic
neodymium:yttrium-aluminum-garnet
(Nd:YAG)
neoformans
Cryptococcus n.
neoformation
Neo-fradin Oral
neoglottic reconstruction
neoglottis
neologism
neomeatus urethrae
Neomixin Topical

N

NOTES

neomycin
>n. and dexamethasone
>n. and hydrocortisone
>n. and polymyxin B
>n., polymyxin B, and dexamethasone
>n., polymyxin B, and gramicidin
>n., polymyxin B, and hydrocortisone
>n., polymyxin B, and prednisolone
>n. sulfate

neonatal
>n. audiometry response cradle
>n. auditory response cradle
>n. dentition
>n. line
>n. ring
>n. teeth

Neonatal Y TrachCare
neonate
neonatorum
>nevus flammeus n.
>tetany n.

neo-osteogenesis
Neopap
neophallus
neoplasia
>endocrine n.
>multiple endocrine n.

neoplasm
>benign epithelial n.
>benign mesenchymal n.
>central neurogenic n.
>connective tissue n.
>cranial base n.
>epithelial n.
>expansible osseous n.
>glandular n.
>infratentorial n.
>laryngeal n.
>malignant n.
>maxillary n.
>mesenchymal n.
>metastatic n.
>middle ear n.
>neural sheath n.
>neuroendocrine n.
>odontogenic n.
>salivary n.
>salivary gland n.
>vascular n.

neoplastic
neoprene glove
neopulp
Neoral Oral
neo-round window
Neosar Injection

Neosonic
>N. piezo ultrasonic unit
>N. (P-5) SPM super powered mini retroprep/endo system

Neosono
>N. MC apex locator
>N. Ultima apex locator/pulp tester

neosphincter
>electrically stimulated anal n.

Neosporin
>N. Cream
>N. Ophthalmic Ointment
>N. Ophthalmic Solution
>N. Topical Ointment

NeoStrata
>N.-15
>N. skin rejuvenation system

neosulcus
>submammary n.

Neo-Synephrine
>N.-S. 12 Hour Nasal Solution
>N.-S. Ophthalmic Solution

Neo-Tabs Oral
Neotricin HC Ophthalmic Ointment
Neotrode II neonatal electrode
neoumbilicoplasty
NeoV0$_2$R volume control resuscitator
neovagina
neovaginal
>n. cavity
>n. introitus

neovaginoplasty
neovascularization
neovasculature
Neovision micro mirror
neper (*var. of* napier) **(Np)**
nephritic gingivitis
nephritis
Neptazane
nerve
>abducent n.
>acoustic n.
>acousticofacial n.
>n. action potential
>afferent n.
>alveolar n.
>ampullary n.
>n. anastomosis
>anterior ethmoidal n.
>n. approximator
>Arnold n.
>auditory n.
>auricular n.
>auriculotemporal n.
>n. block
>n. branch
>branchial n.
>buccal n.

buccinator n.
n. bundle
n. cell
cervical sympathetic n.
chorda tympani n.
cochlear n.
cochleovestibular n.
n. compression
n. compression syndrome
n. of Cotunnius
cranial n.
n. crush injury
dead n.
n. deafness
deep peroneal n.
deep petrosal n.
dental n.
dentinal intratubular n.
dorsal antebrachial cutaneous n.
EBSL n.
efferent n.
eighth cranial n.
eleventh cranial n.
n. ending
ethmoidal n.
n. evulsion
n. excitability test (NET)
external branch of the superior
  laryngeal n.
external nasal n.
facial n. (FN)
n. factor
n. fascicle
femoral cutaneous n.
n. fiber
n. fiber bundle
fibroma of n.
fifth cranial n.
first cranial n.
n. force
fourth cranial n.
frontal n.
furcal n.
Galen n.
n. gap
genitofemoral n.
gingival n.
glossopharyngeal n.
n. graft
great auricular n.
greater petrosal n.
greater superficial petrosal n.

n. growth factor (NGF)
gypoglossal n.
hypoglossal n.
IBSL n.
iliohypogastric n.
ilioinguinal n.
n. impulse
incisive n.
inferior alveolar n. (IAN)
inferior laryngeal n.
inferior nasal n.
infraorbital n.
infratrochlear n.
intercostal n.
intermediary n.
intermediate n.
internal branch of the superior
  laryngeal n.
intertubular n.
intratubular n.
Jacobson n.
laryngeal n.
lateral antebrachial cutaneous n.
lateral femoral cutaneous n.
lesser petrosal n.
lesser superficial petrosal n.
lingual n.
n. loss
mandibular n.
n. mapping
marginal mandibular n.
masseteric n.
masticator n.
maxillary n.
medial antebrachial cutaneous n.
medial brachial cutaneous n.
median n. (MN)
mental n.
monofascicular n.
motor n.
motor root of trigeminal n.
mylohyoid n.
nasal n.
nasociliary n.
nasopalatine n.
ninth cranial n.
nonmyelinated n.
nonrecurrent laryngeal n.
obturator n.
ocular n.
oculomotor n.
olfactory n.

NOTES

N

nerve *(continued)*
    ophthalmic n.
    optic n.
    palatine n.
    palmar cutaneous n.
    peroneal n.
    petrosal n.
    phrenic n.
    polyfascicular n.
    posterior ampullary n. (PAN)
    posterior ethmoidal n.
    posterior inferior nasal n.
    posterior superior nasal n.
    posterosuperior alveolar n.
    postganglionic n.
    predentinal n.
    pterygoid n.
    radial n.
    recurrent laryngeal n. (RLN)
    saccular n.
    saphenous n.
    second n. (N2)
    second cranial n.
    sensory n.
    sensory root of trigeminal n.
    seventh cranial n.
    n. sharing
    n. sheath
    n. sheath tumor
    sixth cranial n.
    somatic motor n.
    special somatic sensory n.
    spinal accessory n.
    spinal tract of trigeminal n.
    splayed facial n.
    n. stump
    sublingual n.
    submaxillary n.
    superficial petrosal n.
    superficial radial n.
    superior laryngeal n. (SLN)
    superior maxillary n.
    superior nasal n.
    supraorbital n.
    supratrochlear n.
    sural n.
    sympathetic n.
    temporal n.
    temporofacial n.
    temporomalar n.
    tensor tympani n.
    tenth cranial n.
    terminal n.
    third cranial n.
    thoracic n.
    thoracodorsal n.
    n. transfer
    trigeminal n.

    trochlear n.
    n. trunk
    twelfth cranial n.
    n. twig
    tympanic n.
    upper cervical n.
    vagus n.
    variant n.
    vestibular n.
    vestibulocochlear n.
    vidian n.
    zygomatic frontal n.
    zygomaticofacial n.
    zygomaticotemporal n.
nerve-approximating clamp (NAC)
nerve-sheath myxoma (NSM)
nervosa
    dysphagia n.
    rhinitis n.
nervous
    n. cough
    n. system
nervus intermedius
Nesacaine
nest
    cell n.
NET
    nerve excitability test
netilmicin
Netromycin Injection
netting
    Dacron n.
nettle
network
    dermal n.
    n. hypothesis
    terminal capillary n. (TCN)
Neumann
    N. cell
    N. sheath
neural
    n. architecture
    n. crest cell
    n. element
    n. filament
    n. impulse
    n. plate
    n. sheath neoplasm
    n. sheath tumor
    n. tube
neuralgia
    atypical facial n.
    auriculotemporal n.
    buccal n.
    causalgia n.
    facial n.
    n. facialis vera
    geniculate n.

geniculate ganglion n.
genitofemoral n.
glossopharyngeal n.
Hunt n.
iliohypogastric n.
ilioinguinal n.
occipital n.
paratrigeminal n.
paroxysmal n.
postherpetic n.
postsurgical n.
posttraumatic n.
Sluder n.
sphenopalatine n.
temporomandibular n.
trifacial n.
trigeminal n.
vidian n.

neuralgia-inducing cavitational osteonecrosis (NICO)
neuralgic
    n. disorder
neurapraxia
neurapraxic lesion
neurectomy
    cochleovestibular n. (CVN)
    middle fossa vestibular n.
    pharyngeal plexus n.
    retrolabyrinthine n.
    retrolabyrinthine/retrosigmoidal vestibular n. (RRVN)
    retrolabyrinthine vestibular n. (RVN)
    retrosigmoid vestibular n.
    transcochlear cochleovestibular n.
    transcochlear vestibular n.
    transtympanic n.
    tympanic n.
    vestibular n. (VN)
neurilemma
neurilemmatosis
    familial n.
neurilemoma
    acoustic n.
neurinoma
    acoustic n.
    facial n.
neuritis
    peripheral n.
    retrobulbar n.
    vestibular n.

neuroadventitia
    perivascular n.
neuroaudiology
neuroblastoma
    olfactory n.
neurochronaxic
    n. theory
    n. theory of phonation
neurocutaneous flap
neurodevelopmental treatment (NDT)
neuroendocrine
    n. carcinoma
    n. marker
    n. neoplasm
    n. tumor
    n. tumor of larynx
neuroepithelioma
    olfactory n.
neuroepithelium
    olfactory n.
neurofibroma
    n. of larynx
    myxoid n.
    paranasopharyngeal n.
    plexiform n.
    solitary n.
neurofibromatosis (NF)
    bilateral acoustic n.
    cranio-orbital n.
    n. type 1 (NF 1)
    n. type 2 (NF 2)
    von Recklinghausen n.
neurofibrosarcoma
neurogenic
    n. dysarthria
    n. dysphagia
    n. factor
    n. language disorder
    n. sarcoma
    n. tumor
Neurohr spring-lock attachment
Neurohr-Williams rest shoe
neurolinguistics
neurologic
    n. embarrassment
neurological
    n. dysfunction
    n. pinwheel
neurolysis
neuroma
    acoustic n. (AN)
    amputation n.

N

NOTES

neuroma *(continued)*
    n. excision
    palisaded encapsulated n.
    subcutaneous n.
    traumatic n.
Neuromeet soft tissue approximator
neuromotor
neuromuscular
    n. choristoma
    n. hamartoma
    n. junction
    n. pacification (NMP)
    n. pedicle graft
    n. retraining
neuromyography
neuron
    afferent n.
    bipolar n.
    motor n.
    multipolar n.
    postganglionic n.
    preganglionic n.
    pseudounipolar n.
    sensory n.
    unipolar n.
neuronal
    n. circuit
    n. survival
neuronitis
    vestibular n.
neuron-specific enolase
neuro-otologic *(var. of* neurotologic)
neuro-otology *(var. of* neurotology)
neuropathic incontinence
neuropathy
    diabetic n.
    ischemic n.
    optic n.
    postherniorrhaphy n.
neuropeptide
    n. marker
    n. Y (NPY)
neurophonia
neurophrenia
neuroplasty
neuropolyendocrine syndrome
Neuropulse unit
neurorrhaphy
neurosarcoidosis (NS)
neurosensorial free medial plantar flap
neurosensory flap
Neurosign 100 nerve monitor
neurosis, pl. neuroses
    occlusal habit n.
neurosome
Neurospora

neurosurgical
    n. cottonoid
    n. pledget
neurosyphilis
neurotensin
neurothekeoma
neurotic
    n. profit
    n. theory of stuttering
neurotization
neurotmesis
neurotmetic injury
neurotologic, neuro-otologic
    n. complication
    n. examination
neurotologist
neurotology, neuro-otology
neurotomy
    bilateral temporal n.
    vestibular n.
neurotoxic effect
neurotoxin
neurotransmitter
    n. molecule
neurotrophic
neurotropic
    n. environment
    n. melanoma
neurovascular
    n. bundle
    n. cross compression (NVCC)
    n. free flap
    n. infrahyoid island flap for tongue reconstruction
    n. pulpal plexus
neurulation period
neutral
    n. axis of straight beam
    n. occlusion
    n. stimulus
    n. vowel
    n. zone
neutralization
    vowel n.
neutroclusion
neutron
    n. beam therapy
neutropenia
    cyclic n.
neutrophil
neutrophilic leukocyte
nevocellular
    n. nevus
nevus, pl. nevi
    agminated blue n.
    Becker n.
    benign n.
    benign cellular blue n.

blue n.
blue rubber bleb n.
common blue n.
compound n.
congenital n.
cutaneous blue n.
developmental n.
dysplastic n.
epidermal n.
eruptive blue n.
extensive blue n.
n. flammeus
n. flammeus neonatorum
giant n.
hairy n.
halo blue n.
inflammatory linear verrucous
  epidermal n. (ILVEN)
intradermal n.
Ito n.
junctional n.
juvenile n.
malignant blue n.
marginal n.
nevocellular n.
oral epithelial n.
organoid n.
Ota n.
pigmented cellular n.
plaque-type blue n.
n. sebaceous
spider n.
Spitz n.
n. spongiosus albus mucosa
strawberry n.
n. unius lateris
white sponge n.

New
N. Beginnings GelShapes silicone
  gel sheeting
N. Decongestant
N. Vision magnification system
N. World leishmaniasis

new
n. dermis
n. skin

newborn
congenital epulis of n.
epulis of n.

newsprint
newton (N)
nexin

nexus-type junction
Ney
N. articulator
N. gold color elastic gold wire
  alloy
N. surveyor

Ney-Oro
N.-O. elastic No. 4 gold wire
  alloy
N.-O. gold alloy

NF
necrotizing fasciitis
neurofibromatosis

NF 1
neurofibromatosis type 1

NF 2
neurofibromatosis type 2

NGF
nerve growth factor

NG strip nasal tube fastener
N.G.T. Topical
NGVB
night guard vital bleaching

NHR
noise-to-harmonic ratio

nHuIFN-γ
natural human interferon-γ

nHuIFN-β
natural human interferon-β

Niamtu
N. video imaging
N. Video Imaging System

nib
instrument n.

N'ice Vitamin C Drops
niche
enamel n.
round window n.

nickel
n. alloy
n. titanium alloy

nickel-chromium alloy
nickel-titanium
n.-t. file

NICO
neuralgia-inducing cavitational
  osteonecrosis

nicotina
stomatitis n.

nicotine stomatitis
nicotinic
n. acid

NOTES

N

Nicotrol NS
nidus
        vascular n.
niger
        Aspergillus n.
        Peptococcus n.
night-grinding
nightguard
night guard vital bleaching (NGVB)
nigra
        dermatosis papulosa n.
        lingua n.
nigrescens
        Prevotella n.
nigricans
        onychomycosis n.
nigrities
        nigrities linguae
Nigrospora
nihilism
Nikolsky sign
NIL
        noise interference level
Nilstat
nimitti midge
ninhydrin-Schiff method
ninth cranial nerve
Niplette
nipper
        bone n.
        malleus n.
        wire n.
nipple
        boxing of n.
        donor n.
        n. inversion
        shared n.
        n. sharing
        supernumerary n.
nipple-areola complex (NAC)
nipple-areolar
        n.-a. amputation
        n.-a. reconstruction
Nissenbaum surgical exposure
Nissen fundoplication
Nitchie method
Nite
        N. White carbamide peroxide
          bleaching agent
        N. White NSF
NiTi nickel-titanium endodontic files
Nitinol
        N. arch
        N. K-file
        N. subglottic stenosis stent
nitrate
        5% potassium n.
        silver n.

nitrated cellulose
nitrile latex utility glove
nitrofurantoin
nitrofurazone
nitrogen
        liquid n.
        n. mustard
nitroglycerin
nitroimidazole
nitrous oxide
Nizoral
NK
        natural killer cell
NLF
        nasolabial fold
NM
        nuclear matrix
NMP
        neuromuscular pacification
NMR
        nuclear magnetic resonance
        NMR scan
N-nitroso compound
Nobelpharma
        N. gold prosthetic retaining screw
        N. implant
        N. implant system
Noble gold alloy
Nocardia
        N. asteroides
        N. brasiliensis
nocardiosis
        primary soft-tissue n.
        soft-tissue n.
nociceptive
        n. circuit
        n. pain stimulus
node
        accessory n.
        buccal lymph n.
        calcified lymph n.
        deep facial lymph n.
        deep lateral n.
        deep parotid n.
        delphian n.
        draining lymph n.
        facial n.
        hot n.
        inferior deep cervical n.
        jugular chain lymph n.
        jugular lymph n.
        jugulodigastric n.
        jugulo-omohyoid n.
        lingual lymph n.
        lymph n.
        mandibular lymph n.
        mastoid n.
        maxillary lymph n.

nuchal n.
occipital lymph n.
parotid lymph n.
periparotid lymph n.
postauricular n.
posterior auricular n.
postglandular n.
preauricular lymph n.
preglandular n.
prelaryngeal n.
pretracheal n.
Ranvier n.
regional lymph n.
retroauricular lymph n.
retroparotid lymph n.
retropharyngeal lymph n.
sentinel lymph n. (SLN)
singer's n.'s
speaker's n.'s
spinal accessory chin lymph n.
subdigastric lymph n.
submandibular n.
submandibular lymph n.
submaxillary lymph n.
submental lymph n.
subparotid lymph n.
superficial parotid n.
superior deep cervical n.
supraclavicular lymph n.
suprahyoid n.
supramandibular n.
teachers' n.'s
tonsillar-subdigastric n.
transverse cervical n.

nodosa
chorditis n.
polyarteritis n.

nodosum
erythema n.

nodular
n. fasciitis
n. melanoma

nodularity

nodule
Bohn n.'s
calcified n.
enamel n.
Lisch n.
lymph n.
lymphatic n.
polypoid vocal n.
pulp n.

satellite n.
screamer's n.
sessile vocal n.
singer's n.
thyroid n.
vocal n.
vocal cord n.

nodulo-vegetating keratoacanthoma

nodulus elasticus

NOE
naso-orbito-ethmoid
NOE fracture

no-echo chamber

no evidence of disease (NED)

Nogenol sealer

noise
ambient n.
n. analyzer
automobile airbag impulse n.
background n.
complex n.
n. detection threshold (NDT)
environmental n.
n. exposure
n. exposure meter
extraneous n.
gaussian n.
n. generator
n. interference level (NIL)
n. limiter
narrow-band n.
pink n.
n. pollution
random n.
saw-tooth n.
speech n.
Speech Discrimination in N.
thermal n.
tone in n. (TIN)
white n.
wide-band n.

noise-induced
n.-i. damage
n.-i. deafness
n.-i. error
n.-i. hearing loss

noise-related variation

noise-to-harmonic ratio (NHR)

NoKor needle

Nolahist

Nolamine

Nolex LA

NOTES

N

noma
nomenclature
> American Dental Association
> Uniform Code on Dental
> Procedures and N.

nominal
> n. aphasia
> n. compound
> n. strain

no-mix adhesive
non-A
> n.-A. hepatitis
> n.-A. hepatitis virus

nonabsorbable
> n. mattress suture

non-A-G hepatitis virus
nonanatomic teeth
non-arcon articulator
nonautologous implant
non-B
> n.-B. hepatitis
> n.-B. hepatitis virus

nonbiofeedback therapy
noncariogenic
noncarious
nonchanger
noncholesteatomatous chronic
suppurative otitis media
nonchromaffin paraganglioma
noncohesive
> n. gold
> n. gold foil

noncompressible
nonconsanguineous parent
noncontrastive distribution
noncornified epithelium
nondirectional microphone
nondistinctive feature
Non-Drowsy
> Comtrex Maximum Strength N.-D.
> Drixoral N.-D.

nondyskeratotic leukoplakia
nonendoscopic sinus surgery
nonepithelial bone cyst
noneugenol paste
nonexcisional anterior approach
nonextraction
nonfaller
nonfebrile-associated vesicular eruption
nonferromagnetic
nonfluctuant
nonfluency
nonfluent aphasia
nonfunctional
> n. grinding
> n. parathyroid cyst

nonfunction mandibular movement
nonhealing wound

nonhemolytic streptococcus
non-Hodgkin
> n.-H. lymphoma
> n.-H. lymphoma of middle ear
> cleft

nonhornified epithelium
nonimmune
nonimmunized
noninflamed
noninflammatory hyperplasia
noninterfering separator
noninvasive *Aspergillus* infection
nonirritating
nonkeratinization
nonkeratinize
nonkeratinized epithelium
nonkeratinizing
> n. carcinoma

nonkernel sentence
nonlinear distortion
nonmedullated nerve fiber
nonmetallic spatula
nonmicrosurgical reattachment
nonmyelinated
> n. axon
> n. nerve

nonnasal sound
nonneoplastic
> n. tumor-like lesion

nonobtrusive text
nonoccluding earmold
nonocclusion
nonoculoplastic surgeon
nonodontogenic cyst
nonopportunistic infection
nonoral communication
nonorganic deafness
nonosteogenic fibroma
nonpainful pulpitis
nonparallel post
nonpenicillin antibiotic
nonpercutaneous dental transmission
nonperiodic wave
nonprecious alloy
nonpropositional speech
nonpulsatile
nonpulsed-current stimulus
nonpurulent
nonrecurrent laryngeal nerve
nonreduplicated babbling
nonreinforcement
nonresorbable
> n. hydroxyapatite
> n. suture

nonrestorable tooth
nonrestrictive modifier
nonrigid connector
nonsecreting mucosal cyst

nonsense
- n. syllable
- n. word

nonseptate cavity
nonsonorant
- n. sound

nonspecific
- n. gingivitis
- n. granulomatous disease
- n. language
- n. stomatitis

nonspeech
- n. respiratory task
- n. sound

non-S-phase specific drug
nonstandard language
nonsteroidal anti-inflammatory drug (NSAID)
nonstimulated gracilis transposition
nonstrategic tooth
nonsuppurative
- n. osteomyelitis
- n. otitis media

nonsurgical
nonsyllabic speech sound
nonsyndromic
- n. craniosynostosis
- n. hearing loss (NSHL)
- n. hereditary hearing impairment

nonsynostotic plagiocephaly
nontender
nontoxic
nontrauma
nontraumatized full-thickness specimen
nontuberculous mycobacterium (NTM)
nonunion
- fibrous n.

nonvascularized
- n. bone graft (NVBG)
- n. fibular strut graft

nonverbal
- n. communication skill
- n. test

nonviable
nonvital
- n. bleaching
- n. pulp
- n. tooth

nonvocal
- n. communication

nonvolitional facial expression
non-weight-bearing tissue

Noonan syndrome
Norcet
Norco
Nord
- N. appliance
- N. expansion plate

nordihydroguaiaretic acid (NDGA)
norepinephrine
norethindrone
Norflex
Norgesic
- N. Forte

norm
- cultural n.

normal
- n. bite
- n. distribution
- n. hearing
- n. mix
- n. occlusion
- n. phonology
- n. probability curve
- n. pulp
- n. swallowing habit
- n. tooth mobility
- n. transition

normally posed tooth
normative phonetics
Normlgel protective wound dressing
normodivergent facial pattern
normosmic
norm-referenced test
NOR-Q.D.
Norrie disease
Northampton charts
Northwestern
- N. Syntax Screening Test (NSST)
- N. University Children's Perception of Speech Test

Norwegian system
nose
- bifid n.
- bilateral cleft-lip-associated n.
- bottom-shaped n.
- brandy n.
- n. cleft
- cleft lip n.
- columellar jut of n.
- copper n.
- Cyrano n.
- dog n.
- external n.

N

NOTES

nose *(continued)*
    hammer n.
    Pinocchio n.
    platyrrhine n.
    potato n.
    rum n.
    saddle n.
    toper's n.
nosebleed
nosocomial infection
nostril
    N. Nasal Solution
    n. rim
    n. sill
    n. stenosis
    supernumerary n.
Nostrilla
notation
    Palmer n.
notch
    acoustic n.
    antegonial n.
    buccal n.
    Carhart n.
    n. correction
    craniofacial n.
    ethmoidal n.
    n. filter
    hamular n.
    Hutchinson crescentic n.
    interarytenoid n.
    intertragic n.
    labial n.
    mandibular n.
    mastoid n.
    palatine n.
    pterygomaxillary n.
    rivinian n.
    Rivinus n.
    sigmoid n.
    supraorbital n.
    supratragal n.
    thyroid n.
    tragal n.
    trigeminal n.
notchcord plate
notched
    n. teeth
    n. wave
notcher
    point n.
notching
    antegonial n.
    vermilion n.
notch-shaped erosion
notch-to-nipple
    sternal n.-t.-n. (SN-N)

No-Touch delivery and mounting system
Nouvisage
    N. acne masque
    N. anti-aging masque
    N. Deep Hydration body patch
    N. Deep Hydration glove
    N. Deep Hydration neck patch
    N. Masque for damaged or sunburned skin
    N. Masque for normal to dry skin
    N. Masque for normal to oily skin
    N. transdermal beauty product
Novack special extraction/injection set
NOVA DPM 9003 skin testing instrument
Novagold mammary implant
NovaPulse
    N. CO_2 laser
    N. laser
    N. laser system
Novascan scanning headpiece
Novasome microvesicle
novel stimulus
Novocain
nov-ovalis
    fenestra n.-o.
noxious stimulus
noy
NP-27
Np
    neper
NPB-295 pulse oximeter
NPC
    nasopharyngeal carcinoma
NPS
    nasopharyngeal stenosis
N-180, -200 pulse oximeter
NPY
    neuropeptide Y
NS
    neurosarcoidosis
    Mycocide NS
    Nicotrol NS
    Stadol NS
NSAID
    nonsteroidal anti-inflammatory drug
NSF
    Nite White NSF
NSHL
    nonsyndromic hearing loss
NSM
    nerve-sheath myxoma
NSST
    Northwestern Syntax Screening Test
NSTI
    necrotizing soft tissue infection

NTB
necrotizing tracheobronchitis
N-terface software
NTM
nontuberculous mycobacterium
NTT
nasotracheal tube
NTZ Long Acting Nasal Solution
NU
NU Auditory Test Lists 4 and 6
Nubain
nuchal node
nuclear
n. angular momentum
n. chromation
n. complex
n. envelope
n. lamina
n. magnetic resonance (NMR)
n. matrix (NM)
n. matrix protein
n. paralysis
nucleatum
Fusobacterium n.
nucleus, pl. **nuclei**
n. ambiguus
angular vestibular n.
Bechterew n.
cochlear n.
N. 22 cochlear implant
Deiters n.
dentinoblastic n.
descending vestibular n.
droplet n.
Edinger-Westphal n.
eosinophilic n.
facial motor n.
n. fasciculus solitarius
inferior vestibular n.
intralaminar thalamic n.
lateral vestibular n.
medial vestibular n.
N. multichannel cochlear implant
periolivary n.
n. prepositus hypoglossi
principal vestibular n.
pyknotic n.
n. salivatorius superior
Schwalbe n.
serous cell n.
spinal vestibular n.
superior vestibular n.

triangular vestibular n.
ventroposteroinferior n.
vestibular n.
Nucofed
N. Pediatric Expectorant
Nucotuss
Nufluor gel
NUG
necrotizing ulcerative gingivitis
Nuhn gland
null
nulliparous
numb chin syndrome (NCS)
number
attenutation n.
Brinell hardness n. (BHN)
Knoop hardness n. (KHN)
Mohs hardness n. (MHN)
Rockwell hardness n. (RHN)
Vickers hardness n.
numbness
numerary mouth
numerical cipher method
Numorphan
Numzitdent
Numzit Teething
nunnation
Nuprin
Nupro Fine paste
Nürnberg gold alloy
Nurolon suture
nursery
stepdown n.
nursing bottle caries
NuSmile
nut
Brazil n.
Nu-Tears II Solution
Nutracort
Nu-Trake Weiss emergency airway system
Nutraplus Topical
nutrient canal
nutrition
parenteral n.
nutritive
Nuva-Lite ultraviolet activator
Nuvaseal resin
Nuva-System tooth conditioner
Nuva-Tach resin
Nu Voice Club
Nu-Vois artificial larynx

NOTES

N

NVBG
    nonvascularized bone graft
NVCC
    neurovascular cross compression
NX
    Talwin NX
Nygaard-Otsby frame
nylon
    n. bristle
nystagmus
    caloric n.
    gaze n.
    horizontal n.
    horizontal-gaze n.

    labyrinthine n.
    optokinetic n.
    palatal n.
    paroxysmal n.
    pharyngolaryngeal n.
    positional n.
    rotationally-induced n.
    spontaneous n.
    n. test
    vestibular n.
Nystar Plus ENG
nystatin
    n. and triamcinolone
Nystex

OAE
  otoacoustic emission
OAF
  osteoclast-activating factor
oak
  o. antigen
  Gambel o.
  live o.
  poison o.
OAS
  orbital apex syndrome
oat
  o. cell carcinoma
  o. grass
Obagi
  O. Blue peel
  O. Blue Peel skin peel treatment
  O. controlled variable-depth peel
  O. Nu-Derm skin care program
  O. Nu-Derm system
  O. sign
Oberto mouth prop
obesity
  morbid o.
object
  o. concept
  o. consistency
  indirect o.
  o. permanence
objective
  behavioral o.
  o. complement
  elements of performance o.
  instructional o.
  operational o.
  performance o.
  predicate o.
  o. quantity
  Ricketts visualized treatment o.
  surgical treatment o. (STO)
  o. test
  visualized treatment o. (VTO)
obligatory occurrence
oblique
  o. arytenoid muscle
  o. facial cleft
  o. fiber
  o. flap in mucogingival surgery
  o. lateral jaw roentgenogram
  o. line
  o. muscle
  o. occlusal intraoral radiography
  o. ridge (OR)
  o. septum
  o. subcondylar ramus ostectomy

obliquus
  o. abdominis externus muscle
  o. abdominis internus muscle
  o. inferior muscle
  o. superior muscle
obliterans
  keratosis o.
  thromboangiitis o.
obliteration
  posterior sulcus o.
  total ear o.
obliterative labyrinthitis
oblongata
  medulla o.
O'Brien
  O. fixation forceps
  O. tissue forceps
obscuration
obscure vowel
observation
  Receptive-Expressive O. (REO)
obsessive compulsive reaction
obstetric
  o. brachial plexus injury
  o. brachial plexus palsy
obstruction
  airway o.
  ductal o.
  gastric outlet o.
  laryngeal o.
  minor gland o.
  nasal o.
  nasal airway o.
  ostial o.
  papillary o.
  parotid o.
  respiratory o.
  salivary duct o.
  sublingual o.
  submandibular o.
  upper airway o. (UAO)
  upper respiratory o. (URO)
obstructive
  o. airway disease
  o. apnea
  o. sialadenitis
  o. sleep apnea (OSA)
  o. sleep apnea syndrome (OSAS)
obstructor
  Dri-Angles o.
  Iso-Shields o.
obstruent
  o. omission
  o. sound
obtainer space

O

obtrusive text
obtunded
Obtura
    O. II
    O. injectable technique
obturans
    keratosis o.
obturation
    canal o.
    retrograde o.
    root canal filling technique o.
obturator
    o. appliance
    o. nerve
    palatal o.
    Thermafil Plus o.
obturatoria stapedis fold
Obwegeser
    O. orthognathic surgery instrument
    O. sagittal split osteotomy
OC
    occlusocervical
OCC
    oral cavity cancer
occipital
    o. anchorage
    o. artery
    o. bone
    o. condyle
    o. condyle syndrome
    o. lobe
    o. lymph node
    o. neuralgia
occipitofrontalis
    o. muscle
    venter frontalis musculi o.
occipitomeatal view
occipitosphenoidal synchondrosis
occipitotemporal
occlude
occluded lisp
occludens
    zonula o.
occluder
occluding
    o. centric relation record
    o. frame
    o. ligature
    o. paper
    o. relation
occlusal
    o. adjustment
    o. adjustment armamentarium
    o. adjustment instrument
    o. amalgam
    o. analysis
    o. appliance therapy
    o. balance

o. bite force
o. cant
o. canting
o. caries
o. cavity
o. cephalometric analysis
o. clearance
o. climate
o. contouring
o. correction
o. cross section radiograph
o. curvature
deflective o.
o. disharmony
o. disturbance
o. dovetail
o. embrasure
o. equilibration
o. facet
o. film
o. film radiography
o. form
o. function
o. glide
o. guard
o. habit neurosis
o. harmony
o. imbalance
interceptive o.
o. interference
o. load
o. lug
mesial and o.
o. pad
o. path
o. pattern
o. perception
o. pivot
o. plane
o. plane angle
o. plane plate
o. position
o. prematurity
o. pressure
o. projection
o. quadrant view
o. recontouring
o. registration
o. registration dye
o. rehabilitation
o. relation
o. relationship
o. rest
o. rest angle
o. rest bar
o. rim
o. scheme
o. scheme system

o. spillway
o. splint
o. stability
o. stent
o. stop
o. stress
o. sulcus
o. surface
o. surface of denture
o. surface toothbrushing
o. table
o. template
o. therapy
o. trauma
o. vertical dimension (OVD)
o. wear
Occlusal-HP Liquid
occlusion
abnormal o.
acentric o.
adjusted o.
adjustment o.
afunctional o.
o. analysis
anatomic o.
Andrews six keys to normal o.
anterior o.
anterior determinants of cusp o.
attritional o.
o. balance
balanced o.
balloon o.
bilateral balanced o.
bimaxillary protrusive o.
buccal o.
central o.
centric o.
centrically balanced o.
centric relation o.
centric relation-centric o. (CR/CO)
class I, II, III o.
class I molar and canine o.
convenience o.
crossbite o.
curve of o.
cuspid protected o.
dental o.
distal o.
eccentric o.
edge-to-edge o.
o. effect
end-to-end o.

faulty centric o.
functional o.
gliding o.
habitual o.
height of o.
hyperfunctional o.
ideal o.
labial o.
lateral o.
line of o.
lingual o.
locked o.
malfunctional o.
mechanically balanced o.
mesial o.
milled-in o.
neutral o.
normal o.
o. of occlusion
pathogenic o.
physiologic o.
physiologically balanced o.
posterior o.
postnormal o.
prenormal o.
protrusive o.
o. rest
retrusive o.
rim o.
o. rim
skeletal o.
spherical form of o.
table o.
terminal o.
torsive o.
transfemoral balloon o.
trauma from o.
traumatic o.
traumatogenic o.
two-plane o.
working o.
occlusive
o. artery disease
o. dressing
o. semipermeable dressing
occlusocervical (OC)
occlusogingival
occlusometer
occlusorehabilitation
occuloglandular syndrome
occult
o. cholelithiasis

O

NOTES

occult *(continued)*
  o. cleft palate
  o. malformation of the skull base
  o. primary
  o. trauma
occupational
  o. abrasion
  o. deafness
  o. disease
  o. exposure
  o. hearing loss
Occupational Safety and Health
  Administration (OSHA)
occurrence
  obligatory o.
OCD
  osteochondritis dissecans
Ochsenbein gingivectomy
Ochsenbein-Luebke flap
Ochterlony gel diffusion technique
OCN
  osteocalcin
Ocoee scalp cleansing unit
Octa-Hex implant
octave
  o. band analyzer
  o.-band filter
  o. frequency
  o. twist
Octicair Otic
OCTR
  open carpal tunnel release
octreoscan
octreotide
  indium 111-diethyltriaminepentaacetic
    acid-D-Phe-1 o.
  ^{111}In-DTPA-D-Phe 1 o.
  ^{111}In-labeled o.
OcuClear Ophthalmic
OcuCoat PF Ophthalmic Solution
Ocufen Ophthalmic
ocular
  o. adnexa
  o. dysmetria
  o. dysmetria test
  o. headache
  o. nerve
  o. prosthesis
  o. torticollis
ocular-mucous membrane syndrome
oculi
  orbicularis o.
oculo-auriculo-vertebral syndrome
oculocardiac reflex
oculodento-osseous dysplasia
oculomandibulodyscephaly
oculomotor
  o. nerve

oculopharyngeal syndrome
oculoplastic surgeon
oculovestibulo-auditory syndrome
Ocupress Ophthalmic
Ocusert
  O. Pilo-20 Ophthalmic
  O. Pilo-40 Ophthalmic
Ocusulf-10 Ophthalmic
Ocutricin Topical Ointment
odd-even method
odontagra
odontalgia
  o. dentalis
  phantom o.
odontalgic
odontatrophia
odontectomy
odontexesis
odontiasis
odontic
odontinoid
odontitis
odontoameloblastoma
odontoblast
  adjacent o.'s
  process of o.
  o. process
odontoblastic
  o. layer
  o. process
odontoblastoma
odontobothrion
odontobothritis
odontobothrium
odontocele
odontoceramic
odontocia
odontoclamis
odontoclasia
odontoclasis
odontoclast
odontoclastoma
odontocyte
odontodynia
odontodysplasia
  regional o.
odontogen
odontogenesis
  o. imperfecta
odontogenic
  o. adenomatoid tumor
  o. cervical necrotizing fasciitis
  o. cyst
  o. dysplasia
  o. fiber
  o. fibroma
  o. fibrosarcoma
  o. gingival epithelial hamartoma

o. keratocyst
o. myxofibroma
o. myxoma
o. neoplasm
o. tumor
odontogenous
odontogeny
odontoglyph
odontogram
odontograph
odontography
odontohyperesthesia
odontohypophosphatasia
odontoid
o. peg
o. process
o. process of epistropheus
odontolith
odontolithiasis
odontologist
odontology
forensic o.
odontoloxia, odontoloxy
odontolysis
odontoma
o. adamantinum
ameloblastic o.
complex o.
composite o.
compound o.
compound composite o.
coronal o.
coronary o.
cystic o.
dens invaginatus gestant o.
dilated o.
embryoplastic o.
fibrous o.
gestant o.
mixed o.
radicular o.
soft mixed o.
Odontometer electronic apex locator
odontonecrosis
odontoneuralgia
odontonomy
odontonosology
odontoparallaxis
odontopathy
odontoperiosteum
odontophobia

odontoplast
odontoplasty
odontoplerosis
odontoprisis
odontoprogenitor cell
odontoptosis
odontoradiograph
odontorrhagia
odontoschism
odontoscope
odontoscopy
odontoseisis
odontosis
odontosteophyte
odontotheca
odontotherapy
odontotomy
prophylactic o.
odontotripsis
odor
o. blindness
foul o.
o. recognition memory
odorant
odorata
Chromolaena o.
odoriferous
odorimeter
odorimetry
odorivection
odorography
odorous
O'Dwyer tube
odynacusis
odynophagia
odynophonia
Oehlers type 3 dens invagination
off effect
offending vascular loop
Off-Ezy Wart Remover
off-glide
office diagnostic rechargeable otoscope
offline
o. cloze task
ofloxacin
o. otic solution
Ogston-Luc operation
OHI
Oral Hygiene Index
Ohio Tests of Articulation and
Perception of Sounds (OTAPS)

O

NOTES

OHI-S
Oral Hygiene Index, Simplified
Simplified Oral Hygiene Index
Ohl elevator
ohm
O. law
Ohmeda
O. continuous vacuum regulator
O. intermittent suction unit
O. thoracic suction regulator
Ohngren line
OI
osteogenesis imperfecta
oi
orbitale inferius
oil
clove o.
o. of cloves
o. cyst
o. of eucalyptol
glycerin, lanolin, and peanut o.
o. granuloma
hyaluronic acid based o.
o. pseudocyst
squalene o.
trypsin, balsam peru, and castor o.
oil-free pumice
ointment
A and D o.
AK-Spore H.C. Ophthalmic O.
Aureomycin o.
bacitracin o.
Catrix 10 o.
chlortetracycline o.
Cortisporin Ophthalmic O.
Cortisporin Topical O.
Eupolin o.
o. granuloma
Lacri-Lube ophthalmic o.
Medi-Quick Topical O.
Neosporin Ophthalmic O.
Neosporin Topical O.
Neotricin HC Ophthalmic O.
Ocutricin Topical O.
Prevacare extra protective o.
Septa Topical O.
Terak Ophthalmic O.
Terramycin w/Polymyxin B
Ophthalmic O.
OKT3
Orthoclone O.
ol
orbitale laterale
old man's beard
O'Leary modification
oleate-condensate
triethanolamine polypeptide o.-c.

oleogranuloma
olfactie, olfacty
olfaction
o. and sensory asymmetry
olfactology
olfactometer
olfactometry
olfactoria
fila o.
olfactory
o. acuity
o. bulb
o. cell
o. cilium
o. cleft
o. disorder
o. epithelium
o. fatigue
o. glomeruli
o. hypesthesia
o. knob
o. mucus
o. nerve
o. neuroblastoma
o. neuroepithelioma
o. neuroepithelium
o. placode
o. reflex
o. tract
o. vesicle
olfacty (*var. of* olfactie)
oligodontia
oligomer
oligoptyalism
oligosialia
olivary complex
olive
Russian o.
olivocochlear bundle
Ollier
O. disease
O. graft
O. method
Ollier-Thiersch graft
olopatadine
olophonia
Olsen stiffness tester
OLSIDI
Oral Language Sentence Imitation
Diagnostic Inventory
Olympus
O. endocamera
O. light source connector
OME
otitis media with effusion
Omega compression hip screw

OMENS
    orbit, mandible, ear, cranial nerves, and
      soft tissue
      OMENS score
omental
      o. filler
      o. skin graft
      o. transposition
      o. transposition flap
omentoplasty
omentum
      transposed o.
omission
      obstruent o.
      postvocalic obstruent singleton o.
Omnicide
Omniderm dressing
omnidirectional microphone
Omni II
Omni laser tip
Omniloc
OmniMedia XRS scanner
Omnipen
Omnipen-N
Omniprep
Omnivac
omocervical flap
omohyoid
      o. muscle
OMS
    oral and maxillofacial surgery
      OMS Oral
OMU
    ostiomeatal unit
ON
    onlay
oncocyte
oncocytic
      o. epithelial cell
      o. schneiderian papilloma (OSP)
oncocytoid
      o. carcinoid
      o. change
oncocytoma
      o. adenoma
oncocytosis
oncogene
oncologic
      o. mandibular resection
oncologist
      surgical o.

oncotaxis
      inflammatory o.
Ondine curse
one-buttress defect
on effect
one-phase subperiosteal implant
    technique
one-piece lip retractor
one-pour technique
one-sitting endodontics
one-stage esthetic correction
one-way drainage
on-glide
onion
onion-peel appearance
onlay (ON)
      o. bone graft
      o. bone grafting
      cast gold o.
      ceramic o.
      composite o.
      o. denture
      o. splint
      o. technique
      o. tip graft
online
      o. assessment method
      o. cross-modal naming
      o. measure
      o. task
Onodi cell
onomatopoeia
onset
      gentle o.
ontogenesis
ontogeny
onychomycosis nigricans
onychoplasty
Ony-Clear Spray
Onyx-R NiTi file
oomycosis
oophoroplasty
OP-3
    Orthopantomograph-3
OP-10
    Orthopantomograph-10
opacification
opacified frontal sinus
opacifier
opacity

O

NOTES

417

opalescence
    O. carbamide peroxide bleaching agent
opalescent dentin
opaque
    o. enamel
    o. porcelain
    o. waterproof wrapper
opaquer
    composite resin color o.
    metal o.
Opcon Ophthalmic
opeidoscope
open
    o. apex
    o. bite
    o. bite malocclusion
    o. capsulotomy
    o. carpal tunnel release (OCTR)
    o. cavity
    o. cell foam
    o. class
    o. coronal browlift
    o. earmold
    o. flap
    o. flap technique
    o. foreheadplasty
    o. fracture
    o. juncture
    o. miniabdominoplasty
    o. osteotomy
    o. pulpitis
    o. quotient
    o. reduction
    o. reduction internal fixation (ORIF)
    o. rhinoplasty
    o. sky procedure
    o. sky rhinoplasty
    o. spring
    o. structure rhinoplasty
    o. syllable
    o. vowel
    o. word
open-end cone
opener
    dynamic bite o.
open-face crown
opening
    access o.
    o. axis
    bony caval o.
    choanal o.
    o. flap
    interincisal o.
    lateral deviation on o.
    o. mandibular movement
    midpalatal o.

    midpalatal suture o.
    posterior movement on o.
    o. stroke
    vertical o.
    vertical displacement on o.
    voluntary interincisal o.
open-set speech-recognition performance
Operand
operant
    autoclitic o.
    o. behavior
    o. behavior theory
    o. conditioning
    echoic o.
    intraverbal o.
    o. learning
    o. level
    mand o.
    o. procedure
    tact o.
    textual o.
    o. therapy
    verbal o.
operated cleft
operating
    o. field
    o. microscope
operation
    Abbe o.
    Abbe-Estlander o.
    accessory feminizing o.
    Arie-Pitanguy o.
    Auclair o.
    Blaskovics o.
    Brophy o.
    Burow o.
    Caldwell-Luc o.
    Carmody-Batson o.
    combined o.
    commando o.
    Dupuy-Dutemps o.
    Edlan-Mejchar o.
    effector o.
    Esser o.
    Estlander o.
    fenestration o.
    flap o.
    Foley o.
    Gillies o.
    Hinsberg o.
    Indian o.
    Italian o.
    Jansen o.
    Kazanjian o.
    Killian o.
    King o.
    logical o.
    Luc o.

mandibular swing o.
mastoid obliteration o.
Mikamo double-eyelid o.
modified flap o.
motivating o.
Ogston-Luc o.
orthognathic o.
palatoplasty push back o.
Partsch o.
pedicle flap o.
plastic o.
pull-through o.
Ridell o.
Schönbein o.
sensor o.
Sistrunk o.
Sorrin o.
stapes mobilization o.
tagliacotian o.
Thiersch graft o.
Toti o.
Veau-Wardill-Kilner pushback o.
operational objective
operative
    o. dentistry
    o. perforation
operator's x-ray exposure guideline
operatory
opercula (*pl. of* operculum)
operculectomy
operculitis
operculum, gen. **operculi**, pl. **opercula**
    dental o.
    Rolando o.
Ophthalgan Ophthalmic
ophthalmic
    Achromycin O.
    Acular O.
    Adsorbocarpine O.
    Akarpine O.
    AK-Chlor O.
    AK-Cide O.
    AK-Dex O.
    AK-Homatropine O.
    AK-Neo-Dex O.
    AK-Poly-Bac O.
    AK-Pred O.
    AKPro O.
    AK-Sulf O.
    AKTob O.
    AK-Tracin O.
    Albalon-A O.

Albalon Liquifilm O.
Alomide O.
Antazoline-V O.
o. artery
Betimol O.
Betoptic S O.
Bleph-10 O.
Blephamide O.
Carbastat O.
Carboptic O.
Cetamide O.
Cetapred O.
Chloroptic-P O.
Ciloxan O.
Collyrium Fresh O.
Comfort O.
Cyclomydril O.
Degest 2 O.
Econopred Plus O.
E-Pilo-x O.
Estivin II O.
Eyesine O.
Floropryl O.
Garamycin O.
Gelfilm O.
Geneye O.
Genoptic S.O.P. O.
Gentacidin O.
Gentak O.
Herplex O.
Humorsol O.
Ilotycin O.
I-Naphline O.
Inflamase Forte O.
Inflamase Mild O.
Isopto Carbachol O.
Isopto Carpine O.
Isopto Cetamide O.
Isopto Cetapred O.
Isopto Homatropine O.
Isopto Hyoscine O.
o. lubricant
Metimyd O.
Murine Plus O.
Murocoll-2 O.
Nafazair O.
Naphcon-A O.
Naphcon Forte O.
NeoDecadron O.
Neo-Dexameth O.
o. nerve
OcuClear O.

O

NOTES

ophthalmic *(continued)*
Ocufen O.
Ocupress O.
Ocusert Pilo-20 O.
Ocusert Pilo-40 O.
Ocusulf-10 O.
Opcon O.
Ophthalgan O.
Optigene O.
OptiPranolol O.
Osmoglyn O.
Paremyd O.
Phospholine Iodide O.
Pilagan O.
Pilocar O.
Pilopine HS O.
Piloptic O.
Pilostat O.
Polysporin O.
Polytrim O.
Pred Forte O.
Pred-G O.
Pred Mild O.
Profenal O.
Propine O.
PxEx O.
Sodium Sulamyd O.
Sulf-10 O.
Tetrasine O.
Tetrasine Extra O.
Timoptic O.
Timoptic-XE O.
TobraDex O.
Tobrex O.
Vasocidin O.
VasoClear O.
Vasocon-A O.
Vasocon Regular O.
Vasosulf O.
Vira-A O.
Viroptic O.
Visine Extra O.
Visine L.R. O.
Voltaren O.
ophthalmicus
herpes zoster o.
ophthalmometer
Hertel o.
ophthalmopathy
Graves o.
ophthalmoplegia
Ophthetic
opiate
opisthocheilia
opisthogenia
opisthognathism
opium
o. alkaloids

belladonna and o.
o. smoker's tongue
o. tincture
Opmilas laser system
OPN
osteopontin
Opotow Jelset material
opponensplasty
opportunistic infection
opposite phase
opposition
o. breathing
o. respiration
OPS
output signal processor
opsonin
opsonization
Optaloy
O. amalgam alloy
O. II copper alloy
optic
o. canal
o. chiasm
o. foramen
2-lens, 2-mirror o.'s
mirror-based reflective o.'s
o. nerve
o. neuropathy
optical
o. biopsy forceps
o. Doppler velocimeter
Opticyl
Optigene Ophthalmic
optimal
o. force
o. pitch
Optimine
optimum orthodontic force
OptiPranolol Ophthalmic
optokinetic
o. nystagmus
o. test
OR
oblique ridge
orienting reflex
ora (*pl. of* os)
Orabase
O.-B
O. HCA
Kenalog in O.
O.-O
O. Plain
O. With Benzocaine
Orajel
O. Brace-Aid Oral Anesthetic
O. Maximum Strength
O. Mouth-Aid
O. Perioseptic

oral

AllerMax O.
Amen O.
o. anomaly
Ansaid O.
o. antibiotic
o. antimicrobial prophylaxis
o. apraxia
o. arch
o. atresia
Banophen O.
Belix O.
Benadryl O.
o. biology
Bio-Tab O.
o. bleeding
Blocadren O.
Calm-X O.
o. cancer
o. candidiasis
Cartrol O.
Cataflam O.
o. cavity
o. cavity cancer (OCC)
Ceftin O.
Chloraseptic O.
Cipro O.
o. cloze procedure
o. commissure
o. commissure movement
o. commisuroplasty
o. communication
Curretab O.
Cycrin O.
Cytoxan O.
o. debris
Delta-Cortef O.
Dimetabs O.
Dormarex 2 O.
Dormin O.
Doryx O.
Doxy O.
Doxychel O.
Dramamine O.
Dynacin O.
E.E.S. O.
E-Mycin O.
o. environment
o. epithelial nevus
o. epithelium
o. (erosive) lichen planus
Eryc O.

EryPed O.
Ery-Tab O.
Erythrocin O.
o. evacuator
o. feeding
o. fissure
o. flora
o. florid papillomatosis
o. fluid
o. focal mucinosis
o. form recognition
o. fossa
o. frowning
Gastrocrom O.
Genahist O.
Gly-Oxide O.
o. hairy leukoplakia
o. hygiene
O. Hygiene Index (OHI)
O. Hygiene Index, Simplified
   (OHI-S)
o. hygiene instruction
o. hygiene score
o. hyperkeratosis
Ilosone O.
o. implant
o. implantology
o. inaccuracy
o. inactivity
o. infection
o. irrigation
o. irrigator
Kerlone O.
o. language
O. Language Sentence Imitation
   Diagnostic Inventory (OLSIDI)
O. Language Sentence Imitation
   Screening Test (ORSIST)
o. leukoplakia
o. and maxillofacial surgery (OMS)
Mephyton O.
Minocin O.
o. moniliasis
Monodox O.
MS Contin O.
MSIR O.
o. mucosa
o. mucosal lining
o. mucosal transudate
o. mucosal transudate test
Mycifradin Sulfate O.
o. myiasis

O

NOTES

oral *(continued)*
Neo-fradin O.
Neoral O.
Neo-Tabs O.
o. (nonerosive) lichen planus
OMS O.
Oramorph SR O.
o. orthopaedics
o. papilloma
o. pathology
o. pathosis
PCE O.
Pedia Care O.
Pediapred O.
o. peripheral examination
o. pharynx
Phendry O.
o. physiotherapy
o. plate
Prelone O.
o. prophylaxis
Protostat O.
Provera O.
Proxigel O.
o. radiograph
o. rehabilitation
o. respiration
Rifadin O.
Rimactane O.
o. rinse
Roxanol SR O.
Salagen O.
Sandimmune O.
O. Scan computer imaging system
O. Scan video imaging system
o. SCC
o. screen
o. sensory discrimination
o. sepsis
o. shield
Siladryl O.
o. sphincter
o. squamous carcinoma
o. squamous cell carcinoma (oral SCC)
o. stereognosis
o. submucous fibrosis
Sumycin O.
o. surface
o. surgeon
o. surgery
o. surgery handpiece (OSH)
o. teeth
Terramycin O.
O. Therapy Control Program
o. tissue
Toradol O.
o. trauma

Unipen O.
o. vestibular depth
Vibramycin O.
O. Video Scope
Voltaren O.
Voltaren-XR O.
oral-aural method
Oral-B
O.-B. Minute Foam
O.-B. Minute Gel
O.-B. soft foam interdental brush
O.-B. toothbrush
orale
Oralet
Fentanyl O.
oral-facial-digital syndrome
oralis
Bacteroides o.
pachyderma o.
Prevotella o.
oralism
oral-like language form
oral-nasal/oral-antral fistula repair
OralVision intraoral camera
Oramorph SR Oral
orange
o. blossom
o. stain
o. wood
Orascoptic acuity system
Orasept
Orasol
Orasone
Ora Tone
Orban
O. file
O. knife
orbicular
o. muscle of mouth
o. retractor
orbicularis
o. laxity
o. muscle
o. oculi
o. oculi muscle
o. oris
o. oris muscle
orbit
exenterated o.
harlequin o.
hollow sunken o.
o., mandible, ear, cranial nerves, and soft tissue (OMENS)
o., mandible, ear, cranial nerves, and soft tissue score
orbital
o. abscess
o. apex

o. apex syndrome (OAS)
o. blow-in fracture
o. blow-out fracture
o. cellulitis
o. compartment syndrome
o. decompression
o. dysmorphology
o. dystopia
o. emphysema
o. enucleation
o. fat
o. fissure
o. height
o. hematoma
o. hypertelorism
o. infection
o. line
o. lipectomy
o. neurovascular bundle
o. plane
o. process
o. rim
o. rim reconstruction
o. roof
o. support
orbitale
o. inferius (oi)
o. laterale (ol)
o. nasion
planum o.
o. sellion
septum o.
o. superius (OS)
orbital-palpebral furrow
orbiting condyle
orbitoethmoid osteoma
orbitomaxillary defect
orbitomaxillectomy
orbitonasal tissue
orbitopalpebral mutilation
orbito-temple distance
orbitotomy
Krönlein o.
lateral o.
orbitozygomaticomalar bone ridge
orchard grass
orchiectomy procedure
orchioplasty
orchitis
order
rank o.
Ordrine AT Extended Release Capsule

Oregon ash
organ
o. of Corti
effector o.
enamel o.
end o.
Jacobson o.
Masera septal o.
Meyer o.
otolith o.
spiral o.
vocal o.
vomeronasal o. (VNO)
organelle
organic
o. articulation disorder
o. deafness
o. dental cement
o. dyslalia
o. matrix
organism
Miller o.
pleuropneumonia-like o.
Vincent o.
organization
International Standard O. (ISO)
organizing stage
organoid nevus
organophosphate toxicity syndrome
Oriental sore
orientation
orienting reflex (OR)
ORIF
open reduction internal fixation
repeat ORIF
orifice
dentinal tubules o.
eustachian tube o.
exocranial o.
o. of the mouth
nasofrontal o.
root canal o.
o. widener
origin
ectomesenchymal o.
intralingual cyst of foregut o.
Original
Doan's O.
Origin PDB 1000 balloon
O-ring attachments
oris
bucca cavum o.

NOTES

oris *(continued)*
    cancrum o.
    fetor o.
    musculus levator anguli o.
    orbicularis o.
    pachyderma o.
ORL
    otorhinolaryngology
Ormazine
Ormco appliance
ORN
    osteoradionecrosis
Ornade Spansule
Ornex No Drowsiness
oroantral
    o. communication
    o. fistula
orocutaneous fistula
orodigitofacial dysostosis
orofacial
    o. dysfunction syndrome
    o. fistula
    o. muscle imbalance
    o. reconstruction
orolingual
oromandibular
    o. defect
    o. dystonia
    o. lesion
    o. rehabilitation
oromaxillary
oronasal
    o. communication
    o. fistula
oro-ocular
oropharyngeal
    o. defect
    o. membrane
    o. pack
    o. ulcer
oropharynx
orostoma
orotracheal
    o. intubation
    o. tube
orphan
    enterocytopathogenic human o.
    (ECHO)
orphenadrine
    o., aspirin and caffeine
orris root
ORSIST
    Oral Language Sentence Imitation
    Screening Test
Orthicide
Ortho
    O. ID
    O. Trans Linear tomography

Orthoceph
    O. x-ray unit
orthoclase
    ceramic o.
    o. ceramic feldspar
Orthoclone OKT3
Ortho-Cycle
orthodentin
orthodontia
    surgical o.
orthodontic
    o. appliance
    o. attachment
    o. band
    o. bracket
    o. camouflage
    o. force
    o. impression tray
    o. instrument
    o. ligature
    o. maintainer space
    o. pliers
    o. procedure
    o. resin
    o. screw
    o. theory
    o. therapy
    o. tooth movement
    o. wire
orthodontics
    corrective o.
    cosmetic o.
    interceptive o.
    preventive o.
    prophylactic o.
    surgical o.
orthodontist
orthodontology
Orthofix lengthening device
orthognathia
orthognathic
    o. occlusal relator
    o. operation
    o. surgery
orthognathism
orthognathous
orthognathus
orthogonal
    o. analysis
    o. axis
    o. projection
orthographic
orthography
orthokeratinization
orthokeratinized
    o. cyst
    o. variant
orthokeratotic stratum corneum

Orthomatrix binder
Orthomite resin
orthopaedic, orthopedic
    o. force
orthopaedics, orthopedics
    Crozat dental o.
    dental o.
    dentofacial o.
    functional jaw o.
    gnathologic o.
    oral o.
    presurgical infant o.
orthopantogram
orthopantograph
orthopantographic view
orthopantomogram
orthopantomograph
    O.-10 (OP-10)
    O.-3 (OP-3)
Orthopantomograph-10 panoramic x-ray machine
Orthopantomograph-3 panoramic x-ray machine
orthopedic (var. of orthopaedic)
orthopedics (var. of orthopaedics)
orthophonic
orthophosphoric
    o. acid
    o. acid etch gel
orthoprosthesis
orthopsychiatry
orthostatic position
orthosurgical
orthotopic graft
orthotropic bone graft
orthovoltage radiation
Orticochea
    O. pharyngoplasty
    O. procedure
    O. scalping technique
Orton enamel cleaver
Orudis
    O. KT
Oruvail
Orzeck Aphasia Evaluation
OS
    orbitale superius
os, pl. ora
os, gen. ossis, pl. ossa
OSA
    obstructive sleep apnea

PSG-proven OSA
    polysomnography-proven obstructive sleep apnea
OSAS
    obstructive sleep apnea syndrome
O-scar
oscheoplasty
Oschler disease
oscillation
    laryngeal o.
oscillator
    bone-conduction o.
oscillopsia
oscitate
oscitation
OSH
    oral surgery handpiece
    Micro OSH
OSHA
    Occupational Safety and Health Administration
osmatic
osmesis
osmics
osmidrosis
Osmitrol Injection
OsmoCyte
    O. island wound care dressing
    O. pillow wound dressing
Osmogen vitamin C and E patch
Osmoglyn Ophthalmic
osmology
OSP
    oncocytic schneiderian papilloma
    output signal processor
osphresiologic
osphresiology
osphresis
osphretic
ossa (pl. of os)
Ossalin fluoride
ossea
    leontiasis o.
osseocartilaginous craniofacial skeleton
osseointegrated
    o. cylinder implant
    o. fixture
    o. implant rehabilitation
    o. oral implant
osseointegration
osseoprosthesis

NOTES

Osseotite
O. dental implant
O. two-stage procedure implant
osseous
o. ampulla
o. coagulum trap
O. Coagulum Trap collecting system
o. craniofacial arteriovenous malformation
o. dysplasia
o. fixation
o. grafting
o. labyrinth
o. surgery
ossicle
auditory o.
o. chain
ossicular
o. chain
o. chain reconstruction
o. prosthesis
o. replacement
ossiculectomy
ossiculoplasty
tympanoplasty o.
ossiculotomy
ossificans
myositis o. (MO)
pseudomalignant myositis o.
ossification
labyrinthine o.
reactive o.
ossifying fibroma
Ossin fluoride
ossis (*gen. of* os)
ossium
fragilitas o.
os symphysis
ostectomy
buccal o.
oblique subcondylar ramus o.
periodontal o.
posterior maxillary segmental o.
osteitis
alveolar o.
condensing o.
focal condensing o.
residual focal o.
sclerosing o.
synovitis, acne, pustulosis, hyperostosis, o. (SAPHO)
osteoadaptic phase
osteoarthritis
generalized o. (GOA)
temporomandibular joint o. (TMJ-OA)

osteoblast
o. stimulation
osteoblastic
o. rimming
o. sinusitis
osteoblastoma
osteocalcin (OCN)
Osteocalcin Injection
osteocartilagenous framework
osteocartilaginous
o. excision
o. exostosis
osteocementum
osteochondritis dissecans (OCD)
osteochondroma
tracheal o.
osteochondromatosis
osteoclasia
interseptal o.
traumatic o.
osteoclast
osteoclast-activating factor (OAF)
osteoclastic
o. cell
o. resorption
osteoclast-like giant cell
osteoclastoma
osteocompetent cell
osteoconduction
osteoconductive
o. bone grafting material
o. phase
osteocutaneous
o. filet flap
o. scapular flap
osteocyte
osteocytic
o. lacuna
o. osteolysis
osteodentin
osteodentinoma
osteodistraction
osteodistractor
Ace/Normed o.
osteodystrophy
Albright hereditary o. (AHO)
osteofibroma
osteofibrosis
periapical o.
OsteoGen
O. bone graft
O. bone grafting material
O. HA Resorb implant material
osteogenesis
distraction o. (DO)
o. imperfecta (OI)
mandibular distraction o.

osteogenic
- o. fibroma
- o. myxoma
- o. sarcoma

Osteogen vitamin and mineral supplement

Osteograf
- O. binder
- O. bone grafting material
- O./D
- O./D dense bone grafting material
- O./LD low density bone grafting material
- O./N
- O./N HA
- O./N natural bone grafting material
- O./N natural hydroxyapatite

osteoid

Osteo implant

osteoinduction
- o. process

osteointegrated dental implant

osteointegration

osteolysis
- osteocytic o.

osteoma, pl. osteomas, osteomata
- dental o.
- o. dentale
- o. of malleus
- orbitoethmoid o.

osteomalacia
- tumor-induced o.

osteomicrotome
- Tessier o.

Osteomin
- O. freeze dried bone
- O. Thermo-Ashed bone powder
- O. Thermo-Ashed bone powder Pulvograft

osteomusculocutaneous flap

osteomyelitis
- chronic diffuse sclerosing o.
- chronic focal sclerosing o.
- chronic recurrent multifocal o. (CRMO)
- diffuse sclerosing o. (DSO)
- Garré o.
- nonsuppurative o.
- o. of the skull base
- suppurative o.
- zygomatic o.

osteomyocutaneous flap

osteon

Osteon drill

osteonecrosis
- neuralgia-inducing cavitational o. (NICO)

osteonectin

osteoperiosteal graft

osteoperiostitis
- alveolodental o.

osteopetrosis

osteopetrotic scar

osteophilic surface

osteophony

osteophyllic phase

osteophyte

osteoplastic
- o. craniotomy
- o. frontal sinus procedure

osteoplastica
- tracheobronchopathia o.
- tracheopathia o.

osteoplasty

Osteoplate implant

osteopontin (OPN)

osteoporosis

osteoporotic
- o. lesion
- o. marrow defect

OsteoPower drilling and cutting machine

osteoprogenitor cell

osteoradionecrosis (ORN)

osteosarcoma
- chondroblastic o.

osteosclerosis
- pulpoperiapical o.

osteosynthesis
- distraction o.
- indirect axial anchor screw o.
- wire o.

osteotome
- Parkes o.
- Rubin o.
- sinus lift o.
- Zeiss o.

osteotomized

osteotomy
- bijaw o.
- bijaw segmental dentoalveolar setback o.
- bilateral mandibular sagittal split o.
- bilateral sagittal split o. (BSSO)

O

NOTES

osteotomy *(continued)*
  bilateral sagittal split
    advancement o. (BSSO)
  blind o.
  block o.
  C-form o.
  closed o.
  o. of condylar neck
  C sliding o.
  cuneiform o.
  cup-and-ball o.
  hinge o.
  horizontal o.
  horseshoe Le Fort I o.
  inverted-L o.
  Le Fort I, II o.
  Le Fort II-type midface o.
  Le Fort I-type o.
  Le Fort maxillary o.
  L-form o., inverted
  linear o.
  mandibular ramus o.
  mandibular sagittal split o.
  maxillary o.
  medial oblique and low lateral o.
  Obwegeser sagittal split o.
  open o.
  perforation o.
  proximal o.
  reverse facial o.
  rotational-advancement o.
  sagittal ramus o.
  sagittal split o. (SSO)
  sagittal split mandibular o.
  sagittal split ramus o. (SSRO)
  segmental alveolar o.
  sliding oblique o.
  subapical o.
  subcondylar oblique o.
  total midface o.
  vertical o.
  visor o.
  zygomaticomaxillary o.
osteotropic hormone
osteotympanic bone conduction
ostial obstruction
ostiomeatal
  o.-m. complex
  o.-m. stent
  o.-m. unit (OMU)
ostium
  accessory o.
  accessory maxillary o.
  accessory maxillary sinus o.
  anterior ethmoidal o.
  ethmoidal o.
  frontal o.
  o. internum

  maxillary o.
  posterior ethmoid o.
  o. seeker
  sphenoidal o.
ostomate
ostomy
Ota
  O. nevus
otalgia
  o. dentalis
  geniculate o.
  postherpetic o.
  referred o.
  reflex o.
otalgic
OTAPS
  Ohio Tests of Articulation and Perception
    of Sounds
otic
  o. abscess
  Acetasol HC O.
  AK-Spore H.C. O.
  Americaine o.
  AntibiOtic O.
  o. barotrauma
  o. capsule
  Cerumenex O.
  Cipro HC o.
  Cortatrigen O.
  Cortisporin O.
  Debrox O.
  O. Domeboro
  Floxin O.
  o. ganglion
  o. labyrinth
  Octicair O.
  Otic-Care O.
  Otobiotic O.
  Otocort O.
  Otosporin O.
  Pediotic O.
  UAD O.
  o. vesicle
  VōSol HC O.
  VŠol O.
oticus
  herpes zoster o.
otitic
  o. hydrocephalus
  o. meningitis
otitis
  acute diffuse external o.
  acute localized external o.
  adhesive o.
  atelectatic o.
  aviation o.
  chronic diffuse external o.
  chronic stenosing external o.

o. desquamativa
eczematoid external o.
o. externa
external o.
o. interna
malignant external o.
o. media
o. media with effusion (OME)
mucous o.
necrotizing external o.
seborrheic external o.
serous o.
otoacoustic emission (OAE)
otobasion
Otobiotic Otic
Otocalm Ear
Otocap myringotomy blade
otoconia
otoconium
Otocort Otic
otocup
otocyst
otodental
o. dysplasia
o. syndrome
Otodynamics model ILO-92 distortion-product otoacoustic emission
otodynia
otogenic
o. pain
otolaryngic
otolaryngologist
otolaryngology
otolith
o. organ
otolithic membrane
otologic
o. pain
otological screening
otologist
otology
otomandibular dysostosis
otomastoiditis
Aspergillus o.
otomicrosurgical transtemporal approach
otomucormycosis
otomycosis
otoneuralgia
otoneurosurgical
otopalatodigital syndrome
otopathy
otophyma

otoplasty
anterior-posterior o.
incisionless o.
mattress suture o.
Mustardé o.
Peled knifeless o.
Stenstrom o.
Tan o.
otorhinolaryngology (ORL)
otorrhea
cerebrospinal fluid o.
otosclerosis
otoscope
Advanced beta 200 o.
Alpha fiberoptic pocket o.
Micro-Halogen o.
Microtek Heine o.
Mini-Fibralux pocket o.
Minilux pocket o.
office diagnostic rechargeable o.
pneumatic o.
Siegle o.
otoscopy
pneumatic o.
otospongiosis
Otosporin Otic
ototoxic
o. drug
o. medication
ototoxicity
ototrophic viral disease
Otrivin Nasal
Otsby
O. dam frame
O. frame
O-type reamer
out
o. of phase
pull o.
shelled o.
time o. (TO)
outer
o. ear
o. enamel epithelium
o. fibrous layer
outfracture
outline
basal seat o.
o. form
outpatient suction cautery tonsillectomy
output
HAIC o.

O

NOTES

output (*continued*)
    o. limiting potentiometer
    maximum acoustic o.
    maximum power o. (MPO)
    peak o.
    radiation o.
    saturation o.
    o. signal processor (OPS, OSP)
outstanding ear
oval
    o. arch
    o. bur
    o. curette
    o. forceps
    o. window
    o. window fistula
    o. window seal
    o. window seal technique
    o. window tensile strength
ovale
    foramen o.
ovalis
    fenestra o.
ovate pontic
OVD
    occlusal vertical dimension
oven
    Coltene o.
    Thermoprep heating o.
    toaster o.
overall sound level
overangulation
overbite
    deep o.
    excessive o.
    horizontal o.
    vertical o.
overbite/overjet relationship
overclosure
    reduced interarch distance o.
overcorrection
overdenture
    mandibular o.
    o.-retained prosthesis
overeruption
overexpose
overexposure
overextend
overextension
overfilled
    o. canal
overfilling
overflow
overgrafting
overhang
    excess o.
    restoration o.
overhanging restoration

overinstrumentation
overinstrumented
    o. tooth
overjet, overjut
    incisor o.
overlap
    acrylic o.
    deep vertical o.
    horizontal o.
    vertical o.
overlapping
    o. pincer
overlay
    acrylic o.
    o. cantilever bone graft
    o. crown
    o. denture
    o. prosthesis
    o. restoration
overlearning
overload
overmasking
overmix
overprojecting nasal tip
overrecruitment
overrestriction
overrotation
overshoot
    calibration o.
overstatement
overt
    o. response
overtone
overzealous flaring
ovoid
    o. arch
    o. pupil
O-V statin
Owen
    contour lines of O.
    interglobular space of O.
    O. lines
    O. view
Owren disease
oxacillin
oxalate
    potassium o.
    o. system
oxaprozin
oxeye daisy
oxiconazole
oxidant
oxidase
    cytochrome o.
    xanthine o.
oxidation
oxidative stress

oxide
      aluminum o. (Al_2O_3)
      ethylene o.
      iron o.
      o. layer
      magnesium o.
      mercuric o.
      nitrous o.
      tin o. (SnO_2)
      zinc o.
oxide-eugenol
      zinc o.-e. (ZOE, ZnOE)
oxidize
oxidized
      o. cellulose
      o. glutathione
oxidizing agent polishing agent
oximeter
      Accusat pulse o.
      Criticare 503 pulse o.
      Datascope pulse o.
      MiniOX V pulse o.
      MRL o.
      Nellcor N-20PA, N-20 pulse o.
      Nellcor Symphony N-3000 pulse o.
      NPB-295 pulse o.
      N-180, -200 pulse o.
oximetry
      cutaneous pulse o.
      pulse o.
Oxisensor II adult adhesive sensor
Oxismart advanced signal processing and alarm management technology
Oxistat Topical
oxyacoia
oxybenzone
      methoxycinnamate and o.

Oxycel
oxycephaly
oxychlorosene
oxycodone
      o. and acetaminophen
      o. and aspirin
OxyContin
oxygen
      hyperbaric o. (HBO)
      o. recovery skin treatment
      o. therapy
Oxyguard
OxyIR
oxylate dentin bonding system
oxymetazoline
      o. HCl
      o. hydrochloride
oxymorphone
oxyphenbutazone
oxyphilic
      o. adenoma
      o. cytoplasm
oxyphonia
oxyphosphate cement
oxytalan
      o. fiber
oxytetracycline
      o. and hydrocortisone
      o. and polymyxin B
oyster splint
ozena
      o. caseosa
ozenous
ozokerite
      purified o.
ozostomia

NOTES

O

P-50

p53

    p53 gene mutation
    p53 tumor suppressor gene

P-700 Color Velocity Imaging system

PA

    pulpoaxial

Pac

    Trichlor Fresh P.

pacemaker

    P. Fluorinse
    P. Nafeen solution
    P. topical fluoride gel
    P. topical fluoride solution

Pacette

    MRL P.

pachycheilia

pachyderma

    p. laryngis
    p. oralis
    p. oris

pachyglossia

pachygnathous

pachymucosa alba

pachyonychia congenita

pachyotia

pachysalpingitis

Pacific

    P. Coast demineralized bone
      grafting material
    P. Coast demineralized cortical
      bone powder
    P. Coast flexible laminar bone
      strip

pacification

    neuromuscular p. (NMP)

Pacini corpuscle

pack

    Cool Comfort cold p.
    eugenol p.
    gauze p.
    gingival tissue p.
    Kirkland-Kaiser p.
    Kirkland periodontal p.
    Med-Wick nasal p.
    oropharyngeal p.
    periodontal noneugenol p.
    pressure p.
    wax p.

packer

    Balshi p.
    dental amalgam p.
    Lorenz gauze p.
    retraction cord p.

packing

    p. chamber
    denture p.
    Merocel epistaxis p.
    nasal p.
    p. process
    p. strip
    Weimert epistaxis p.

paclitaxel

pad

    ABD p.
    adenoidal p.
    AirLITE support p.
    Bichat fat p.
    buccal fat p.
    cheek p.
    gauze p.
    gum p.
    hydropolymer p.
    labial p.
    lap p.
    laparotomy p.
    malar p.
    masticatory fat p.
    P.'s Médipatch Gel Z self-adhesive
      scar treatment
    occlusal p.
    Passavant p.
    Poloris P.'s
    ptotic malar fat p.
    retrodiscal p.
    retromolar p.
    rubber dam p.
    sucking p.
    suctorial p.
    Telfa sterile adhesive p.
    TopiFoam gel-backed self-adhering
      foam p.

padding

paddle

    boomerang-shaped skin p.
    crescentic-shaped skin p.
    cutaneous p.
    fleur-de-lis-shaped skin p.
    horizontal-shaped skin p.
    skin p.
    p. spring
    Y-shaped skin p.

Padgett

    P. dermatome
    P. endoscope

Paecilomyces variotii

PAF

    platelet-activating factor

P

Paget
> P. disease
> P. disease of bone
> P. disease-like mosaic appearance

PAH
> pulmonary artery hypertension

pain
> p. fiber
> ghost p.
> p. impulse
> incisional p.
> otogenic p.
> otologic p.
> phantom p.
> preauricular p.
> pulpal p.
> p. receptor
> referred p.
> referred pulp p.
> sialogenic p.
> p. syndrome
> p. threshold
> unilateral neck p.

Paine carpal tunnel retinaculotome
painful pulpitis
pain-related mediator
paint
> acrylic p.
> Artista II Tempera p.
> p. brushing
> Mars Black artist's acrylic p.

pair
> minimal p.

paired
> p. associate learning
> p. syllables

Pak
> Zone Periodontal P.

palatal
> p. access
> p. aponeurosis
> p. arch
> p. area
> p. bar
> p. connector
> p. dimple
> p. edema
> p. expansion
> p. expansion appliance
> p. fronting
> p. gland
> p. height index
> p. incompetence
> p. index
> p. insufficiency
> p. lengthening procedure
> p. lift
> p. linguoplate

> p. mucoperiosteal flap
> p. mucosa
> p. muscle
> p. nystagmus
> p. obturator
> p. papillomatosis
> p. paralysis
> p. plate
> p. prosthesis
> p. pushback
> p. ramping
> p. reflex
> p. root
> p. seal
> p. shelf
> p. strap

palate
> bilateral cleft p.
> bilateral cleft lip and p.
> p. bone
> bony p.
> breadth of p.
> Byzantine arch p.
> classification of cleft p.
> cleft p.
> cleft lip and p. (CLP)
> complete cleft p.
> falling p.
> Gothic p.
> hard p.
> hard cleft p.
> height of p.
> p. hook
> incomplete cleft p.
> length of p.
> longitudinal ridge of hard p.
> longitudinal suture of p.
> p. myograph
> occult cleft p.
> partial cleft p.
> pendulous p.
> pillar of soft p.
> p. plate
> posterior nasal spine to soft p.
> (PNSP)
> premaxillary p.
> primary p.
> p. reconstruction
> p. retractor
> secondary p.
> soft p.
> soft cleft p.
> submucous cleft p.
> subtotal cleft p.
> total cleft p.
> unilateral cleft lip and p.

palate-splitting appliance
palati (*pl. of* palatum)

palatine
- p. arch
- p. artery
- p. bone
- p. canal
- p. fold
- p. foramen
- p. gland
- p. groove
- p. groove of maxilla
- p. index
- p. lamina
- p. lamina of maxilla
- p. mucosa
- p. nerve
- p. notch
- p. papilla
- p. papilla cyst
- p. process of maxilla
- p. raphe
- p. recess
- p. reflex
- p. ridge
- p. root
- p. ruga
- p. shelf
- p. spine
- p. sulcus
- p. sulcus of maxilla
- p. surface
- p. suture
- p. tonsil
- p. torus
- p. uvula
- vertical plate of p.
- p. vessel

palatini
palatitis
palatization
palatoalveolar fistula
palatoglossal
- p. arch
- p. band

palatoglossus muscle
palatognathous
palatogram
palatograph
palatographic visual biofeedback
palatography
palatomaxillary
- p. arch
- p. canal

- p. cleft
- p. groove
- p. groove of palatine bone
- p. index
- p. suture

palatomyograph
palatomyography
palatopagus
palatopharyngeal
- p. closure
- p. fold
- p. muscle
- p. ring

palatopharyngeus
- p. muscle

palatopharyngoplasty
palatopharyngorrhaphy
palatoplasty
- Furlow double opposing Z-plasty p.
- p. push back operation

palatoplegia
palatoproximal
palatorrhaphy
- p. procedure

palatoschisis
palatovaginal canal
palatum, pl. palati
- p. fissum
- leukokeratosis nicotina palati
- velum palati

palilalia
paliphrasia
palisaded
- p. dentinoblastic layer
- p. encapsulated neuroma

palladium
palladium-copper alloy
palladium-silver alloy
palliation
palliative care
pallidum
- *Treponema p.*

palm
- queen p.

palm-and-thumb grasp
palmar
- p. crease
- p. cutaneous nerve
- p. dysesthesia
- p. flap
- p. incision
- p. skin bridge

NOTES

P

palmaris
    p. longus
    p. longus composite flap
    p. longus muscle
    p. longus tendon
Palmaz stent
Palmer notation
palmetto
    saw p.
palpate
palpation
    tenderness to digital p. (TDP)
palpebral
    p. artery
    p. fissure
palpitation
palsy
    Bell p.
    cerebral p.
    combined p.
    early obstetric brachial plexus p.
    Erb p.
    Erb-Duchenne p.
    Erb-Duchenne-Klumpke p.
    facial p.
    House grade facial p.
    Jolly-Thomas p.
    Klumpke p.
    late obstetric brachial plexus p.
    obstetric brachial plexus p.
    posticus p.
pamidronate
PAN
    posterior ampullary nerve
Panadol
    Junior Strength P.
Panasal 5/500
Panasonic hearing aid battery
Panavia
    P. bonding
    P. OP
Panax ginseng
Panax quinquefolius
Pancoast suture
pancraniomaxillofacial fracture
pancreatic carcinoma
pancreozymin
Pandel
Panelipse
    P. panoramic radiograph
    P. panoramic x-ray machine
panendoscope
panendoscopy
Paneth cell
Panex
    P.-E (Panoral) panoramic x-ray
    machine
    P. panoramic radiograph

panfacial fracture
Panje prosthesis
panniculectomy
panniculitis
panniculus adiposus
pannus
    abdominal p.
panogram
    mandible p.
panographic tracing
panoral radiography
panoramic
    p. extraoral radiography
    p. loupe
    p. radiograph
    p. roentgenogram
    p. rotating machine
    p. series
    p. survey
    p. view
    p. x-ray film
Panoramix
Panorex
    P. panoramic x-ray machine
    P. radiograph
    P. view
panotitis
Panscol
pansinusitis
    hemorrhagic p.
pantaloon sign
pantograph
pantographic radiograph
Pantomatic
pantomogram
pantomograph
pantomographic
pantomography
    p. machine
Pantopon
pantothenic acid
pants-over-vest muscle repair
PAOD
    peripheral arterial occlusive disease
papaverine
paper
    articulating p.
    p. mulberry
    occluding p.
    p. point
    p. wasp
papilla, pl. papillae
    atrophied p.
    calciform papillae
    capitate papillae
    circumvallate papillae
    dental p.
    p. dentis

filiform p.
foliate p.
fungiform p.
gingival p.
p. graft
hypertrophied p.
p. incisiva
incisive p.
interdental p.
interproximal p.
lingual p.
papillae linguales
p. lingualis
mesenchyme p.
palatine p.
retained p.
retrocuspid p.
Stensen p.
sublingual p.
papillae of tongue
p. vallatae
vallate p.
p. of Vater
villous papillae of tongue

papillary
p. adenocarcinoma
p. cyst
p. cystadenoma lymphomatosum
p. dermal peel
p. gingiva
p. gingivitis
p. hyperplasia
p. keratosis
p. obstruction
p. pedicle graft
p. penetration
p. reconstruction
p. thyroid carcinoma
papillary-marginal-attached (PMA)
papillectomy
papilliferum
cutaneous syringocystadenoma p.
sialadenoma p.
papillitis
chronic lingual p.
foliate p.
papilloma, pl. papillomas, papillomata
p. forceps
Hopmann p.
inverted ductal p.
inverted schneiderian p.
inverting p.

keratotic p.
oncocytic schneiderian p. (OSP)
oral p.
schneiderian p.
sinonasal p.
squamous p.
squamous cell p.
tracheal p.
transitional p.
papillomatosis
inflammatory p.
juvenile p.
laryngeal p.
multiple p.
oral florid p.
palatal p.
recurrent respiratory p.
papillomavirus
human p. (HPV)
Papillon-Lefèvre syndrome
papule
split p.
papulosis
bowenoid p.
papyracea
lamina p.
parabiotic flap
parabolic
p. curve
p. flow
Para-Cast
paracentesis
parachlorometaxylenol (PCMX)
paracoccidioidomycosis
paracone
paraconid
paracusis, paracousis, paracusia
false p.
p. loci
Willis p.
paradental
p. cyst
p. pyorrhea
paradentitis
paradentium
paradentosis
paradigm
cross-modal naming p.
paradigmatic
p. response
p. shift
p. word

NOTES

P

437

paradontosis
paradoxic
    p. respiratory effort
    p. retrogenia
    p. turbinate
paradoxical rhinorrhea
paraffin
    p. granuloma
    p. wax
paraffinoma
    penile p.
Paraflex
Parafon Forte DSC
parafunction
paragammacism
paraganglioma
    laryngeal p.
    nonchromaffin p.
    vagal p.
paraganglion cell
parageusia
parageusic
paraglottic space
paragnathus
Paragon
    P. implant
    P. laser
    P. single-stage dental implant
      system
    P. single-stage implant system
paragrammatism
parahemophilia
parainfluenza virus
parakappacism
parakeet feather
parakeratinization
parakeratinized
    p. cyst
    p. epithelium
    p. variant
parakeratosis
parakeratotic
    p. layer
paralalia
    p. literalis
paralambdacism
paralanguage
paralingual sulcus
paralinguistics
parallel
    p. attachment
    p. block-out
    p. distribution
    p. post
    p. talk
    p. technique
parallelae
    striae p.

paralleling
    Begg p.
    p. cone position
    p. coping
    p. instrument
    p. technique
parallelism
    root p.
parallelogram condenser
parallelometer
parallel-sided post
paralysis, pl. paralyses
    abductor p.
    adductor p.
    bilateral abductor p.
    bilateral adductor p.
    bilateral laryngeal p.
    bulbar p.
    central facial p.
    cortical supranuclear p.
    cricothyroid p.
    facial p.
    facial nerve p.
    faucial p.
    flaccid p.
    frontalis muscle p.
    hypoglossal p.
    idiopathic facial p.
    incomplete p.
    incomplete facial p.
    labioglossolaryngeal p.
    laryngeal motor p.
    laryngeal sensory p.
    lingual p.
    myopathic p.
    nuclear p.
    palatal p.
    posticus p.
    pseudobulbar p.
    pseudolaryngeal p.
    Ramsay Hunt facial p.
    recurrent laryngeal nerve p.
    sensory p.
    soft palate p.
    spastic p.
    subcortical supranuclear p.
    supranuclear p.
    trigeminal p.
    twelfth nerve p.
    unilateral abductor p.
    unilateral adductor p.
    unilateral vocal cord p. (UVCP)
    V motor p.
    vocal cord p.
    vocal fold p.
    X p.

paralytic
 p. agent
 p. ectropion
paralytica
 aphonia p.
paramedian forehead flap
paramedical
parameter
paramethasone acetate
paramolar
 p. tubercle
paranasal sinus
paranasopharyngeal neurofibroma
paraneoplastica
 acrokeratosis p.
paraneurium
paranoia
paranoid reaction
paraoral
 p. tissue
parapharyngeal
 p. fat
 p. space (PPS)
 p. space abscess
 p. tumor
paraphasia, paraphrasia
 extended jargon p.
 literal p.
 verbal p.
paraphasic
paraphonia
paraphrasia (*var. of* paraphasia)
paraplegia
Parapost
 P. bur
 Whaledent P.
pararhizoclasia
pararhotacism
PARAS
 postauricular and retroauricular scalping
 PARAS flap
parasalpingitis
Parascan scanning device
parascapular flap
parasellar
 p. and orbital apex syndrome
 p. syndrome
parasigmatism
parasinoidal
parasitic
 p. disease
 p. flap

parasympathetic
 p. drug
 p. pathway
 p. root of submandibular ganglion
parasympatholytic
 p. drug
parasympathomimetic
 p. drug
parasymphyseal region
parasymphysis area
paratenon
parathyroid
 p. adenoma
 p. cyst
 p. gland
 p. hormone
parathyroidectomy
paratope
paratransplantal tissue
paratrigeminal
 p. neuralgia
 p. syndrome
paravariceal
paravertebral muscle
parazone
Par-Cast gold alloy
Par Decon
Pardue technique
Paredrine
paregoric
Paremyd Ophthalmic
parenchyma
parenchymal
 p. cell
 p. scar
parenchymatous glossitis
parent
 nonconsanguineous p.
parent-child dyad
parenteral
 p. feeding
 p. nutrition
paresis
 facial nerve p.
 gaze p.
 vestibular p.
paresthesia
 laryngeal p.
 lip p.
parfocal
 p. defraction lens
 p. spot size

NOTES

P

439

parietal
- p. abscess
- p. bone
- p. layer
- p. lobe

parieto-occipital
- p.-o. flap

Parinaud syndrome
park-bench position
Parkes osteotome
Parkes-Weber syndrome
Parkinson disease
parkinsonian dysarthria
parkinsonism
Park-O-Tron drill system
Parodi technique
parodontal
parodontid
parodontitis
parodontium
paronychia
parosmia
parosphresia
parosteal osteogenic sarcoma
parotid
- p. capsule
- p. carcinoma
- p. collector
- p. cyst
- p. deep lobe
- p. duct
- p. duct ligation
- p. duct transposition
- p. fascia
- p. gland
- p. gland abscess
- p. gland exposure guideline
- p. lymph node
- p. lymph node hyperplasia
- mucoepidermoid carcinoma of p.
- p. obstruction
- p. resection
- p. saliva
- p. sialodochoplasty
- p. space

parotid-derived pleomorphic adenoma
parotidectomy
- facial nerve-preserving p.
- lateral p.
- p. procedure
- radical p.
- superficial p.
- total p.

parotiditis
- epidemic p.
- postoperative p.
- punctate p.

parotid-masseteric area

parotidomasseteric fascia
parotin
parotitis
- acute suppurative p.
- chronic recurrent p.
- suppurative p.

paroxysmal
- p. neuralgia
- p. nystagmus
- p. positional vertigo

parrot
- p.-beak deformity
- p. feather
- p. jaw
- p. tongue

pars
- p. flaccida (PF)
- p. flaccida defect
- p. tensa

parsing
- syntactic p.

parsley
parsnip
Parsons Language Sample
part
- p. implant substructure
- vascularized spare p.
- velopharyngeal p.

partial
- p. alveolectomy
- p. anodontia
- bridge p. IV-D
- p. cleft palate
- p. crown
- p. denture, distal extension
- p. denture impression
- p. denture prosthesis
- p. denture prosthetics
- p. denture retention
- p. denture unit
- p. dural resection
- p. ethmoidectomy
- p. glossectomy
- p. laryngeal reconstruction procedure
- p. laryngopharyngectomy (PLP)
- p. ossicular replacement prosthesis
- p. prosthodontics
- p. pulpectomy
- p. pulpitis
- p. pulpotomy
- p. recruitment
- p. reinforcement
- p. stapedectomy
- p. stress-breaker
- p. subfascial abdominoplasty
- p. tone

upper p.
p. veneer crown
partially
p. dissolved gutta-percha
p. edentulous dental arch
partial-thickness
p.-t. flap
p.-t. periodontal graft
particle
p. velocity
particular grammar
particulate
Bioglass synthetic bone graft p.
p. cancellous bone and marrow
(PCBM)
p. matter
PerioGlas synthetic bone graft p.
partition
cochlear p.
Partsch
P. I method
P. operation
parts of speech
Partuss LA
parulis, pl. **parulides**
parvula
Veillonella p.
PAS
periodic acid-Schiff
posterior airway space
PAS measurement
PASES
Performance Assessment of Syntax
Elicited and Spontaneous
Passavant
P. bar
P. cushion
P. pad
P. ridge
pass-band filter
Passe Muir valve
passer
foil p.
Hoefflin suture p.
Passiflora incarnata
passionflower
passivation procedure
passive
p. bilingualism
p. eruption
p. immunity
p. lingual arch

p. reciprocation
p. voice
passivity
Passport bedside monitor
paste
Abbot p.
base p.
Calasept sterile calcium
hydroxide p.
calcium hydroxide p.
Calxyl calcium hydroxide p.
p. carrier
Caulk impression p.
Coe-Pak p.
Coral Plus fluoride p.
denture adherent p.
desensitizing p.
filler p.
hydrocalcium calcium hydroxide p.
impression p.
Kerr equalizing p.
Kerr Luralite p.
Krex impression corrective p.
P. Laminate
Ledermix p.
Luride acidulated phosphate
fluoride p.
metallic oxide p.
methyl cellulose p.
Multi-Form dual purpose
impression p.
noneugenol p.
Nupro Fine p.
PeroxiCare p.
polishing p.
pressure-indicating p.
Preventodontic AF p.
Pro Care p.
prophylactic p.
pumice p.
RC2B p.
p. removal
Teflon p.
tooth p.
Wach p.
zinc oxide-eugenol impression p.
Zircate p.
Ziroxide prophylactic p.
Pastegraft
Dembone demineralized cortical
powder P.

NOTES

P

Pasteur
    P. pipette
    P. strain
Pastilles
    Mycostatin P.
past-pointing
PAT
    Photo Articulation Test
Patanol
patch
    Gore-Tex soft-tissue p.
    lyophilized dural p.
    lyophilized Transderm Scop
      transdermal p.
    mucous p.
    Nouvisage Deep Hydration body p.
    Nouvisage Deep Hydration neck p.
    Osmogen vitamin C and E p.
    salmon p.
    smoker's p.
    test p.
    Transderm Scop P.
    vascularized fascial p.
patency
    nasal p.
patent suture
Paterson-Kelly syndrome
path
    condyle p.
    generated occlusal p.
    idling p.
    incisal p.
    incisor p.
    p. of insertion
    milled-in p.
    occlusal p.
    p. of placement
    p. of removal
    working p.
pathfinder
    p. broach
Pathocil
pathodontia
pathogen
    blood-borne p.
    microbial p.
pathogenesis
pathogenic
    p. microorganism
    p. occlusion
pathognomonic
pathologic
    p. perforation
    p. recession
    p. sclerosis
    p. tooth mobility
    p. tooth wandering

pathologist
    language p.
    speech p.
    speech and language p.
    voice p.
pathology
    dental p.
    language p.
    oral p.
    speech p.
    speech and language p.
patho-occlusion
pathophysiology
    pulpal p.
pathosis, pl. pathoses
    apical p.
    Ingle classification of
      pulpoperiapical p.
    Loyola University classification for
      pulpoperiapical p.
    oral p.
    periapical p.
    pulpal p.
    pulpoperiapical p.
pathway
    afferent-efferent p.
    apoptotic p.
    auditory p.
    ciliary p.
    extrapyramidal p.
    mucociliary drainage p.
    parasympathetic p.
    spinoreticulothalamic p.
    supranuclear p.
    vestibular p.
patient
    edentulous p.
    p. exposure guideline
    facially aging p.
pattern
    acanthomatous p.
    acoustic reflex p.
    auditory p.
    bipenniform morphological p.
    blood-stained p.
    class III ring avulsion injury p.
    cribriform p.
    follicular p.
    Fu Manchu p.
    gullwing p.
    Hader bar p.
    herringbone p.
    hyperdivergent facial p.
    incremental appositional p.
    investing the p.
    monomorphic p.
    normodivergent facial p.
    occlusal p.

plexiform p.
pressure p.
secretion-clearance p.
stress p.
stuttering p.
p. theory
type I vascular p.
variegated p.
p. wax
wax p.
wear p.
whorled cellular p.
Wise p.
Zellballen p.

Patterned Elicitation Syntax Screening Test (PESST)

patterning

patulous abdomen

pau d'arco

Paul-Bunnell test

Paulus
P. chin plate
P. midfacial plate
P. trocar system

pause
tense p.
vocalized p.

pavlovian conditioning

PB
phonetically balanced
PB max
PB word

PBA
pulpobuccoaxial

PBHA
porous block hydroxyapatite

PBI
P. Medical copper vapor laser
P. MultiLase D copper vapor laser

PBK
Phonetically Balanced Kindergarten
PBK Word Lists

PBMC
peripheral blood mononuclear cell

PBS
phosphate-buffered saline

PBSC
penicillin, bacitracin, streptomycin, caprylate

PBZ-SR

PC
pulp canal

PC-1000
PC-1000/Laser 1000 panoramic cephalometric x-ray machine
PC-1000 panoramic x-ray machine

P.C.A.
P. E-Series hip replacement
P. mid stem

PCBM
particulate cancellous bone and marrow

PCD
primary ciliary dyskinesia

PCE
P. Oral
P. Tablet

PCF
posterior cranial fossa

PCH
pulp chamber

PCMX
parachlorometaxylenol

PCNA
proliferating cell nuclear antigen

PCR
polymerase chain reaction
progressive condylar resorption

PCS
pulp canal sealer

PC/TC
power cut/tungsten carbide

PCV
postcapillary venule

PD
probing depth
pulpodistal
2 PD
two-point discrimination

PDD
pervasive developmental disorder

PDGF
platelet-derived growth factor

PDI
Periodontal Disease Index

PDL
periodontal ligament

PDM
predentin matrix

PDS
polydioxanone suture
PDS II suture

NOTES

P

PDT
> photodynamic therapy

PE
> pharyngoesophageal
> pressure equalization
>> Guiatuss PE
>> Halotussin PE
>> PE tube

pea

Peabody Picture Vocabulary Test

peach

peak
> p. acoustic gain
> buccal p.
> p. clipping
> Cupid's bow p.
> p. expiratory flow rate (PEFR)
> p. inspiratory pressure (PIP)
> lingual p.
> p. output
> spectral p. (SPEAK)
> p. tension
> voltage p. (Vp)

peanut

pear
> p. bur
> p.-shaped area

pearl
> cholesteatoma p.
> P. Drops
> enamel p.
> epithelial p.
> Epstein p.
> gouty p.
> keratin p.
> Serres p.
> p. tumor

Pearson product-moment coefficient of correlation

peau d'orange

pecan tree antigen

Peck purple hard wax

pectoral catheter

pectoralis
> p. major (PM)
> p. major flap
> p. major muscle
> p. major myocutaneous flap
> p. minor muscle
> p. myofascial flap

pectoris
> angina p.

pedagogical grammar

Pedia Care Oral

Pediacof

Pediaflor

PediaPatch
> Trans-Ver-Sal P.

Pediapred Oral

pediatric
> p. audiology
> p. circle system
> Cleocin P.
> Codamine P.
> Cycofed P.
> p. dentistry
> Fedahist Expectorant P.
> Hycomine P.
> p. hyperfunctional dysphonia
> p. rhinosinusitis

pediatrics

Pediatric Speech Intelligibility Test (PSI)

Pediazole

pedicle
> circumflex scapular p.
> p. clamp
> dermal vascularized p.
> fasciovascular p.
> Filatov-Gillies tubed p.
> p. flap
> p. flap in mucogingival surgery
> p. flap operation
> p. graft
> inferior p.
> p. kinking
> latissimus dorsi segmental musculovascular p.
> musculovascular p.
> Ponten-type tubed p.
> popliteal musculovascular p.
> posterior p.
> superior dermal p.
> transferred mesenteric vascular p.
> transverse cervical p.
> vascular p.

pedicled
> p. cartilage graft
> p. colon transfer
> p. compound rib-latissimus dorsi osteomusculocutaneous flap
> p. enteric donor site
> p. galeal frontalis flap
> p. groin flap
> p. jejunal reconstruction
> p. latissimus flap
> p. mucosa flap
> p. myocutaneous flap
> p. pericranial flap
> p. polyp
> p. skin graft
> p. tibial bone flap

Pediotic Otic

Pedituss

pedodontia

pedodontic
    p. endodontics
    p. stent
pedodontics
pedodontist
pedolalia
peduncle
pedunculated polyp
peel
    Blue Peel chemical p.
    chemical p.
    chemosurgical superficial
      dermatologic p.
    full-face p.
    glycolic skin p.
    Jessner solution p.
    mid-to-deep dermal p.
    Obagi Blue P.
    Obagi controlled variable-depth p.
    papillary dermal p.
    phenol p.
    p. product
    TCA p.
    trichloroacetic acid p.
    upper reticular dermal p.
peeling
    chemical face p.
    glycolic acid p.
    phenol p.
peenash
PEEP
    positive end-expiratory pressure
Peeso
    P. drill
    P. pliers
    P. reamer
Peet
    P. forceps
    P. nasal rasp
PEFR
    peak expiratory flow rate
peg
    epithelial p.
    epithelial rete p.
    p. flap
    p. lateral incisor
    p. latissimus dorsi flap breast
      reconstruction
    odontoid p.
    rete p.'s
    p. tooth
Pegasus Airwave pressure relief system

pegged tooth
peg-shaped tooth
Peled knifeless otoplasty
pellagra
pellagrous glossitis
pellet
    Beechwood p.
    cotton p.
    gold foil p.
Pell and Gregory classification
pellicle
    acquired p.
    brown p.
    enamel p.
pellucida
    zona p.
pelvic peritoneal graft
Pemberton sign
pemphigoid
    benign mucous membrane p.
      (BMMP)
    bullous p.
pemphigoides
    lichen planus p.
pemphigus
    benign p.
    malignant p.
    p. vegetans
    p. vulgaris
PEMS
    pulsed electromagnetic stimulator
penalty, frustration, anxiety, guilt, and
  hostility (PFAGH)
penciclovir cream
pencil
    p. drain
    MegaDyne electrocautery p.
pencil-point tattoo
Pendred syndrome
pendulous
    p. abdomen
    p. palate
    p. uvula
pendulum movement
Penecort
penetrating wound
penetration
    p. coefficient
    papillary p.
    p. test
    upper reticular dermal p.
pen grasp

NOTES

P

445

penicillamine
penicillin
  p., bacitracin, streptomycin, caprylate (PBSC)
  p. G
  p. G benzathine
  p. G benzathine and procaine combined
  p. G, parenteral, aqueous
  p. G procaine
  penicillinase-resistant p.
  potassium p.
  p. V
  p. V potassium
penicillinase
penicillinase-resistant penicillin
Penicillium
penile
  p. agenesis
  p. flap
  p. hypospadias
  p. paraffinoma
  p. skin inversion
  p. skin inversion vaginoplasty
  p. torsion
peninsula flap
penis
  buried p.
peno-preputial vascularized flap
penoscrotal
  p. edema
  p. transposition
Penrose drain
pentamidine
Pentax light source connector
pentazocine
  p. compound
  p. HCl
pentobarbital
  p. sodium
Pentra-fil II
penumbra
Pen-Vee-K
People
  Self-Help for Hard of Hearing P. (SHHH)
Pepcid
peplomycin
pepper
  black p.
  cayenne p.
  green p.
peppermint
peppertree
  California p.
peptic
  p. esophagitis
  p. ulcer

peptidase
peptide
  vasoactive intestinal p.
Peptococcus niger
Peptostreptococcus
  P. anaerobius
  P. micros
perakeratosis
perborate
  alkaline p.
  sodium p. (SP)
perceived noise decibel (PNdB)
percentage
percentile
  p. rank
perception
  auditory p.
  central auditory p.
  cross-modality p.
  haptic p.
  kinesthetic p.
  loudness growth p.
  occlusal p.
  proprioceptive p.
  rapidly alternating speech p. (RASP)
  Screening Test for Auditory P.
  speech p.
  supramodal p.
  tactile kinesthetic p.
  visual p.
perceptive
  p. deafness
  p. hearing loss
perceptual
  p. analysis
  p. consistency
  p. disorder
  p. distortion
  p. disturbance
  p. immaturity
  p. retardation
perceptually
  p. adequate sound
  p. handicapped
perceptual-motor
  p.-m. match
perch
percha
Percocet
Percodan
  P.-Demi
Percogesic
percolation
percussion
  hard p.
  p. test

percussor
   G5 Neocussor p.
percutaneous
   p. dilational tracheostomy
   p. pencil Doppler probe
   p. stick
   p. tracheotomy
   p. transmission
perennial
   p. antigen
   p. rye grass
peretic lagophthalmos
Perfection
perforans
   folliculitis nares p.
perforata
   habenula p.
perforating
   p. alveolar artery
   p. canal of Zuckerkandl
   p. fiber
perforation
   apical root p.
   Bezold p.
   cortical p.
   furcation p.
   iatrogenic p.
   lateral p.
   mechanical p.
   nasal septal p.
   operative p.
   p. osteotomy
   pathologic p.
   root p.
   sealing p.
   septal p.
   strip p.
   sublabial p.
   tooth p.
perforator
   musculocutaneous p.
   periumbilical p.
   septal p.
   septocutaneous p.
   septomuscular p.
   p. vessel
perforator-based flap
performance
   P. Assessment of Syntax Elicited
      and Spontaneous (PASES)
   knowledge of p. (KP)
   linguistic p.

   p. objective
   open-set speech-recognition p.
   receptive language p.
   p. test
   Test of Articulation P.-Diagnostic
      (TAP-D)
   Test of Articulation P.-Screen
      (TAP-S)
performance-intensity
   p.-i. function
   p.-i. function test
performative
   p. pragmatic structure
perfringens
   Clostridium p.
perfume
perfusion
   flap p.
   p. monitor
pergingival
   p. implant
perhydrol-urea
Periactin
periadenitis
   p. aphthae
   p. mucosa necrotica recurrens
perialar crescentic advancement flap
perialveolar wiring
periapex
periapical
   p. abscess
   p. access
   p. cemental dysplasia
   p. cementum
   p. curettage
   p. cyst
   p. fibroma
   p. film
   p. granuloma
   p. hyperemia
   p. infection
   p. intraoral radiography
   p. osteofibrosis
   p. pathosis
   p. pressure
   p. radiograph
   p. radiographic survey
   p. radiolucency
   p. roentgenogram
   p. sensitivity
   p. surgery

NOTES

P

periapical *(continued)*
    p. tissue
    p. tissues alteration
    p. tooth repair
periaqueductal air cell
periareolar
    p. de-epithelialization
    p. mammaplasty
    p. retractor
    p. technique
peribuccal
pericanal dentin
pericapsular
pericardial patch tracheoplasty
pericemental
    p. abscess
    p. attachment
    p. zone
pericementitis
    apical p.
    chronic suppurative p.
    rarefying p. fibrosa
pericementoclasia
pericementum
perichondrial-periosteal tissue
perichondrial spring
perichondritis
    arytenoid p.
    laryngeal p.
    relapsing p.
perichondrium
perichondrocutaneous graft
periciliary fluid
pericoronal
    p. abscess
    p. flap
pericoronitis
pericranial flap
pericranium
pericyte
peridens
peridental
    p. ligament
    p. membrane
peridentinoblastic space
peridentitis
peridentium
Peridex
    P. Oral Rinse
Peridin-C
peridontoclasia
peridural block
perifascicular proliferation
perifollicular mesenchyme
periglossitis
periglottic
periglottis

periimplant
    p. infection
    p. ligament
    p. space
    p. tissue
periimplantitis
peri-implantoclasia
    exfoliative p.-i.
    necrotic ulcerative p.-i.
    resorption p.-i.
    traumatic p.-i.
    ulcerative p.-i.
perikymata, sing. perikyma
perilabyrinthitis
perilacunar mineral matrix (PMM)
perilymph
    p. fistula (PLF)
    p. gusher
    p. protein
perilymphatic
    p. duct
    p. gusher
perimeter
    arch p.
    dental p.
    p. earmold
perimolysis
perimysium
perinatal
    p. morbidity
    p. mortality
    p. trauma
perineal
    p. artery axial flap
    p. reconstruction
perineoplasty
    single-stage castration, vaginal
      construction, p.
perineorrhaphy
perineoscrotal flap
perineosynthesis
perineural
    p. fibroblastoma
    p. invasion (PNI)
    p. space
perineurial suture
perineurium
perinuclear cytoplasm
Perio-Aid
perioareolar scar
periocular
    p. bulge
    p. festooning
    p. pigmentation
    p. rhytid
period
    concrete operations p.
    decay p.

developmental p.
exposure p.
heat-up p.
latent p.
masticatory silent p.
neurulation p.
preoperational thought p.
refractory p.
sensorimotor intelligence p.
periodic
p. acid-Schiff (PAS)
p. acid-Schiff hematoxylin
p. transitory menogingivitis
p. wave
periodicity
periodontal
p. abscess
p. anesthesia
p. armamentarium
p. atrophy
p. bony defect
p. cement
p. chart
p. chisel
p. cyst
p. defect
p. disease
P. Disease Index (PDI)
p. disease rate
p. disease score
p. dressing
p. file
p. flap
p. hydrodynamic system
P. Index (PI)
p. inflammation
p. infrabony abscess
p. instrument
p. intrabony defect
p. knife
p. lesion
p. ligament (PDL)
p. ligament anesthesia
p. ligament fiber
p. ligament injection
p. membrane (PM)
p. membrane necrosis
p. noneugenol pack
p. ostectomy
p. pitch system
p. pocket
p. pocket marker

p. portrait
p. probe
p. prosthesis
p. resilient system
p. stent
p. support
p. theory
p. therapy
p. traumatism
p. varnish
p. vascular system
periodontalgia
periodontia (*pl. of* periodontium)
periodontics
preventive p.
periodontist
periodontitis
acute p.
apical p.
chronic periapical p.
p. complex
HIV-associated p.
human immunodeficiency virus-
associated p. (HIV-P)
juvenile p.
localized juvenile p. (LJP)
marginal p.
periradicular p.
prepubertal p.
primary p.
secondary p.
simple p.
p. simplex
suppurative p.
suppurative apical p.
periodontium, pl. **periodontia**
p. alteration
periodontoclasia
periodontology
periodontolysis
periodontometer
Muhlmann p.
periodontosis
PerioGard
PerioGlas
P. material
P. synthetic bone graft
P. synthetic bone graft particulate
periolivary nucleus
Perio Med
perioral
p. dermatitis

NOTES

P

perioral *(continued)*
    p. flaw
    p. muscle
    p. wrinkling
periorbita
periorbital
    p. cellulitis
    p. fat
    p. infection
    p. lipoinfiltration
    p. orbicularis oculi muscle
    p. wrinkle
Perioseptic
    Orajel P.
periositis
    florid reactive p.
periostea *(pl. of* periosteum)
periosteal
    p. chondroma
    p. cyst
    p. elevation
    p. elevator
    p. flap
    p. graft
    p. reaction
    p. release
    p. vessel
periosteitis
    gangrenous p.
periosteitis *(var. of* periostitis)
periosteotome
periosteotomy
periosteum, pl. **periostea**
    alveolar p.
    p. alveolare
    dental p.
    lingual p.
    lingual mandibular p.
periostitis, periosteitis
    alveolodental p.
    ethmoidal p.
    Garré p.
    suppurative p.
periotemp system
Periotest
    P. implant
    P. Implant Innovations gold screw
    P. system
    P. value
periotic duct
PerioWise probe
periparotid lymph node
peripharyngeal space
peripheral
    p. ameloblastic fibroma
    p. ameloblastoma
    p. apnea

    p. arterial occlusive disease (PAOD)
    p. blood mononuclear cell (PBMC)
    p. cavity wall
    p. cemental dysplasia
    p. dentin
    p. dysarthria
    p. frame implant substructure
    p. giant cell reparative granuloma
    p. giant cell tumor
    p. glioma
    p. lymphoid tissue
    p. masking
    p. microcirculation
    p. nerve stimulator
    p. nervous system (PNS)
    p. neuritis
    p. neuroectodermal tumor
    p. odontogenic fibroma
    p. odontogenic tumor
    p. ossifying fibroma
    p. osteoma of the mandible (POM)
    p. plexus
    p. pressure
    p. reparative granuloma
    p. seal
    p. temporomandibular joint remodeling
periphery
    denture p.
    p. denture
periprosthetic
    p. breast abscess
    p. fibrous capsule
    p. fluid
    p. space
periradicular
    p. periodontitis
perirhizoclasia
perisinus abscess
perisinusitis
peristalsis
    residual dyskinetic p.
peristaltic pump
peritendinous soft tissue
peritenon
peritoneoplasty
peritonsillar
    p. abscess (PTA)
    p. cellulitis
    p. space
peritonsillitis
peritubular
    p. dentin
    p. zone
periumbilical perforator
periungual tissue

perivascular
    p. invasion
    p. neuroadventitia
Perko technique
perlèche
perlocution
Perma-Bond
PermaMesh hydroxyapatite woven sheet matrix
permanence
    object p.
permanens
    dens p.
permanent
    p. baseplate
    p. deformation
    p. dentition
    p. filling
    p. lip augmentation
    p. pedicle flap
    p. restoration
    p. retention
    p. smile facies
    p. splint
    p. teeth
    p. threshold shift (PTS)
Permapen
PermaRidge alveolar ridge augmentation
Permark
    P. micropigmentation needle
    P. micropigmentation system
PermaSharp
    P. PGA suture
    P. suture and needle
PermaSoft reline material
permeability
    dentin p.
    dentinal p.
permeation
permucosal
    p. endosteal implant
    p. implant system
    p. needle aspiration
permutation
pernicious anemia
pernio
    lupus p.
peromelia
    micrognathia with p.
peroneal
    p. nerve
    p. vessel

peroneus tertius muscle
peroral
    p. endoscopy
PeroxiCare paste
peroxidase
    salivary p.
peroxidative enzyme
peroxide
    alkaline p.
    benzoyl p.
    carbamide p. (CP)
    hydrogen p. (HP)
    urea p.
perpendicular
    p. anterior wall
    nasion p.
    p. plane
    p. plate
perpetually growing tooth
perpetuating factor
perseveration
    infantile p.
    p. theory
persistent
    p. generalized lymphadenopathy (PGL)
    p. lop ear
persistently growing tooth
personification
Personna
    P. Plus disposable Teflon scalpel
    P. prep blades
person with AIDS (PWA)
Perspective dental imaging system
perstimulatory fatigue
perturbation
    dose p.
    p. measure
    pitch period p. (PPR)
    radiation p.
    relative average p. (RAP)
pertussis
    Bordetella p.
Peru
    balsam of P.
pervasive developmental disorder (PDD)
P.E.S.
    Plastic Endosurgical System
pes anserinus
PESS
    powered endoscopic sinus surgery

NOTES

P

PESST
    Patterned Elicitation Syntax Screening
        Test
pestle
petechia, pl. **petechiae**
petechial hemorrhage
PET-FDG
    positron emission tomography with 2-[F-
        18]-fluoro-2-deoxy-D-glucose
        PET-FDG procedure
petiole
petit
    P. facial mask
    p. mal
Petrac hybrid
Petri dish
petroclinoid ligament
petroclival
    p. area
    p. suture
petrolatum
    p. gauze
    lanolin, cetyl alcohol, glycerin,
        and p.
petromastoid
petrosal
    p. artery
    p. nerve
    p. ridge
    p. sulcus
petrosectomy
petrositis
petrosphenoidal syndrome
petrosquamosal
petrotympanic
    p. fissure
    p. suture
petrous
    p. apex tumor
    p. apicectomy
    p. apicitis
    p. bone
    p. pyramid
    p. pyramid fracture
    p. ridge
    p. tip
Peutz-Jeghers syndrome
pexis
    ruptured p.
pexy
    endoscopy brow p.
PF
    pars flaccida
PFA
    profunda femoris artery
PFAGH
    penalty, frustration, anxiety, guilt, and
        hostility

Pfannenstiel incision
Pfaundler-Hurler disease
PFC
    purified fibrillar collagen
Pfeiffer syndrome
Pfizerpen
PFS
    Adriamycin PFS
    Folex PFS
P/G
    Fulvicin P/G
PGA
    polyglycolic acid
PGA-PLLA plating system
PGE
    prostaglandin E
PGF
    prostaglandin F
PGL
    persistent generalized lymphadenopathy
PGSR
    psychogalvanic skin response
PGSRA
    psychogalvanic skin response audiometry
PH
    pulp horn
pH
    critical p.
    salivary p.
PHA
    polyhydroxy acid
phagedenic gingivitis
phagocyte
    granulocytic p.
phagocytic cell
phagocytized dense bodies
phagocytosis
phagodynamometer
phagolysosome
phagosome
phalangization
phalanx, pl. **phalanges**
    distal p.
Phalen sign
phalloplasty
    p. procedure
phallourethroplasty
phallus
phantom
    p. odontalgia
    p. pain
    p. speech
    p. tissue
**pharmacoradiologic disimpaction of
    esophageal foreign bodies**
Pharmaflur
pharyngeal
    p. arch

p. artery
p. bursa
p. calculus
p. cleft
p. constrictor muscle
p. fascia
p. fistula
p. flap
p. flap surgery
p. pituitary
p. plexus neurectomy
p. pouch syndrome
p. raphe
p. recess
p. reflex
p. resonance
p. speech
p. tonsil
p. type parapharyngeal schwannoma
p. vein
p. wall
p. wall augmentation
pharyngectomy
pharynges (*pl. of* pharynx)
pharyngismus
pharyngitic
pharyngitis
atrophic p.
gangrenous p.
lymphonodular p.
membranous p.
p. sicca
ulcerative p.
ulceromembranous p.
pharyngobasilar fascia
pharyngocele
pharyngoconjunctival fever
pharyngocutaneous fistula
pharyngoepiglottic fold
pharyngoesophageal (PE)
p. defect
p. diverticulum
p. reconstruction
pharyngoesophagoplasty
pharyngoesophagus
pharyngoglossus
pharyngoinfraglottic duct
pharyngolaryngeal nystagmus
pharyngolaryngectomy
pharyngolaryngitis
pharyngolith

pharyngomaxillary
p. fissure
p. space
pharyngomycosis
pharyngo-oral
pharyngopalatine
p. arch
pharyngopalatinus muscle
pharyngoplasty
Hynes p.
Orticochea p.
sphincter p.
Wardill p.
pharyngoplegia
pharyngorhinoscopy
pharyngoscope
pharyngoscopy
pharyngospasm
pharyngostenosis
pharyngostoma
pharyngotomy
lateral p.
modified lateral p.
transhyoid p.
pharyngotonsillitis
pharynx, pl. pharynges
oral p.
phase
eruptive p.
functional p.
in p.
opposite p.
osteoadaptic p.
osteoconductive p.
osteophyllic p.
out of p.
posteruptive p.
preeruptive p.
prefunctional p.
proliferative p.
stuttering p.
p.'s of stuttering
phasic
p. bite
p. stretch reflex
phatnorrhagia
pHaze
p. 16 C-Cream
p. 15 Serum-C
PHDPE
porous, high-density polyethylene
Phemister graft

NOTES

phenacetin
Phenahist-TR
Phenaphen With Codeine
Phenazine
Phenchlor S.H.A.
Phendry Oral
Phenerbel-S
Phenergan
    P. VC Syrup
    P. VC With Codeine
Phenhist Expectorant
phenidone
phenindamine
pheniramine
    naphazoline and p.
    p., phenylpropanolamine, and
      pyrilamine
    phenyltoloxamine,
      phenylpropanolamine, pyrilamine,
      and p.
phenobarbital
    p. with belladonna
phenol
    Barker-Gordon p.
    camphorated p.
    camphor, menthol, and p.
    p. cauterization
    complex p.
    p. peel
    p. peeling
phenolic
    p. disinfectant
phenolsulphonic acid
phenomenon, pl. phenomena
    all-or-none p.
    Bell p.
    blind alley p.
    cellulite p.
    dental p.
    Doppler p.
    extravasation p.
    hesitation p.
    jaw-winking p.
    Kasabach-Merritt p.
    mucous retention p.
    Raynaud p.
    reflex p.
    rouleau p.
    Schellong-Strisower p.
    Splendore-Hoeppli p.
    tip-of-the-tongue p.
    Tullio p.
    Wever-Bray p.
    zipper p.
phenothiazine
phenotypic marker
Phenoxine
phenylbutazone

Phenyldrine
phenylephrine
    brompheniramine and p.
    chlorpheniramine and p.
    chlorpheniramine, phenyltoloxamine,
      phenylpropanolamine, and p.
    chlorpheniramine, pyrilamine,
      and p.
    cyclopentolate and p.
    guaifenesin and p.
    guaifenesin, phenylpropanolamine,
      and p.
    p. hydrochloride
    promethazine and p.
    p. and scopolamine
    sulfacetamide sodium and p.
    p. test
Phenylfenesin L.A.
phenylglycine
phenyloxidase
Phenyl-P
phenylphenol
phenylpropanolamine
    brompheniramine and p.
    caramiphen and p.
    chlorpheniramine and p.
    chlorpheniramine, phenindamine,
      and p.
    chlorpheniramine, phenylephrine,
      and p.
    chlorpheniramine, pyrilamine,
      phenylephrine, and p.
    clemastine and p.
    guaifenesin and p.
    hydrocodone and p.
phenyltoloxamine
    acetaminophen and p.
    chlorpheniramine, phenylephrine,
      and p.
    p., phenylpropanolamine, and
      acetaminophen
    p., phenylpropanolamine, pyrilamine,
      and pheniramine
phenyltoloxamine,
phenytoin
pheochromocytoma
Pherazine VC w/ Codeine
pheromone
Philips Gyroscan
philosophy
    Ayurveda p.
    Crozat p.
philtral
    p. column elevation
    p. dimple
    p. height
philtrum, pl. philtra

pHisoHex
> p. facial wash

phlebography
phlebolith
phlebolithiasis
phleboplasty
phlegmon
> Escat p.
> p. of floor of mouth
> Holz p.

phobia
phoenix abscess
Phoma
phonagnosia
phonal
phonasthenia
phonation (Fo)
> p. break
> dysrhythmic p.
> hypervalvular p.
> maximum duration of p.
> modal p.
> myoelastic-aerodynamic theory of p.
> neurochronaxic theory of p.
> posttraumatic ventricular p.
> reverse p.
> speaking p. (SFo)
> p. time
> p. type harshness
> ventricular p.
> voice disorders of p.

phonatory
phoneme
> acute p.
> back p.
> compact p.
> diffuse p.
> front p.
> grave p.
> lax p.
> lenis p.
> segmental p.
> suprasegmental p.
> tense p.

phonemic
> p. analysis
> p. articulation error
> p. regression
> p. synthesis
> p. transcription

phonemics

phonetic
> p. alphabet
> p. analysis
> p. articulation error
> p. context
> p. feature
> p. inventory
> p. placement
> p. power
> p. transcription
> p. variation

phonetically
> p. balanced (PB)
> P. Balanced Kindergarten (PBK)
> P. Balanced Kindergarten Word Lists
> p. balanced word

phonetician
phonetics
> acoustic p.
> applied p.
> articulatory p.
> auditory p.
> descriptive p.
> evolutionary p.
> experimental p.
> general p.
> historical p.
> impressionistic p.
> p. of juncture
> linguistic p.
> normative p.
> physiologic p.

phoniatrics
phoniatrist
phonic
> p. spasm

phonics
> vocal p.

phonogram
phonological
> p. analysis
> p. behavior
> p. conditioning
> p. disorder
> p. error
> p. process
> p. process analysis
> p. rule

phonology
> disordered p.
> normal p.

NOTES

P

phonology *(continued)*
    Slosson Articulation Language Test with P. (SALT-P)
phonometer
phonopathy
phonophobia
phonophotography
phonosurgery
phonotactics
Phos-Flur
    P.-F. daily oral rinse
    P.-F. oral rinse supplement
phosphatase
    acid p.
    alkaline p.
    tartrate-resistant acid p. (TRAP)
phosphate
    p.-300
    p.-40
    aluminum p.
    ammonium p.
    p.-bonded investment
    p.-buffered saline (PBS)
    Cleocin P.
    Decadron P.
    Hexadrol P.
    hexose p.
    Hydrocortone P.
    potassium titanyl p. (KTP)
    resorbable tricalcium p.
    technetium-99m p.
    β-tricalcium p.-300
    β-tricalcium p.-40
phosphaturic mesenchymal tumor
Phospholine Iodide Ophthalmic
phosphonated
    p. dimethacrylate
    p. dimethacrylate/phosphated bis-GMA system
phosphonecrosis
phosphophorin
phosphoprotein
phosphoric
    p. acid
    p. acid gel
    p. acid gel etch
    glacial p. acid
phosphotungstic acid-hematoxylin (PTAH)
phosponated bis-GMA
Photo
    P. Articulation Test (PAT)
    P. Clearfill
photoaging
photocoagulation
    intralesional laser p. (ILP)
photocure

photocured
    p. composite resin
PhotoDerm
    P. PL laser
    P. PL pulsed light device
    P. VL laser
    P. VL/PL hair removal system
photodynamic therapy (PDT)
PhotoGenica
    P. LPIR with TKS laser
    P. T^{10} laser
    P. T laser system
    P. T^{10} tattoo removal system
    P. V laser
    P. VLS pulsed dye laser
photoglottography
photomicrograph
    scanning electron p.
photon
    light p.
    p. radiotherapy
photo-oxidation
    UV p.-o.
photophore
photoplethysmographic monitoring
photoplethysmography (PPG)
photoradiation therapy
photosensitizer
photothermolysis
    selective p.
phrase
    carrier p.
    dual-meaning idiomatic p.
    p. structure grammar
phrenic nerve
phthalate
Phycomycetes
phycomycosis
phylogenesis
phylogenetic, phylogenic
    p. change
    p. theory
phylogeny
physaliphorous cell
physical
    Facial Disability Index P. (FDIP)
    p. therapy
    p. voice handicap score
Physician's Choice skin care product
physicochemical
physiogenic
physiognomic
    p. length
    p. width
physiognomy
physiologic
    p. drift
    p. mesial migration

p. method of toothbrushing
p. occlusion
p. phonetics
p. rest position
p. saline
p. sclerosis
p. tooth mobility
p. wear
physiological
p. crown
p. reconstruction
p. root
physiologically balanced occlusion
physiology
gingival p.
physiomechanical
physiotherapy
oral p.
physis
physostigmine
phytonadione
PI
Periodontal Index
Piaget cognitive development stage
PICA
Porch Index of Communicative Abilities
posterior inferior cerebellar artery
PICAC
Porch Index of Communicative Abilities
in Children
pick
apical p.
crane p.
Rhein p.
root p.
tooth p.
Pickerill
P. imbrication line
picket fence fever
pickle
pickling
p. solution
pickup impression
Picornaviridae
PIC symbol
PICSYMS
picture symbols
pictographs
Pictorial Test of Intelligence
picture
P. Articulation and Language
Screening Test

P. Sound Discrimination
P. Speech Discrimination Test
p. symbols (PICSYMS)
PID
position indicating device
pidgin
p. Sign English (PSE)
piecemeal
pier
PiercingCare solution
Pierre
P. Robin sequence
P. Robin syndrome
Pierse tip forceps
piezoelectric
p. lithotriptor
p. ultrasonic unit
piezoelectricity
pigeon
p. droppings
p. feather
p. serum protein (PSP)
pigment
p. gel
inorganic p.
pigmentation
amalgam p.
bismuth p.
gingival p.
linear tan-brown-black p.
periocular p.
pigmented
p. ameloblastoma
p. cellular nevus
p. epulis
p. lesion
p. lesion of nail bed
p. lichen planus
p. mole
p. villonodular synovitis
p. villonodular tenovagosynovitis
(PVNS)
pigmenti
incontinentia p.
pigmentosum
xeroderma p.
pigtail appearance
pigweed
redroot p.
spiney p.

NOTES

P

Pik
  Grossan nasal irrigator tip with Water P.
Pilagan Ophthalmic
pilar cyst
pillar
  p. of soft palate
  tonsillar p.
Pillo Pro dressing
Pilocar Ophthalmic
pilocarpine
  p. and epinephrine
  p. hydrochloride
pilomatrixoma
pilonidal disease
Pilopine HS Ophthalmic
Piloptic Ophthalmic
pilosebaceous units
Pilostat Ophthalmic
pilot hole
pi mesons
Pimpinella anisum
pin
  p. amalgam
  apex p.
  biphasic p.
  cemented p.
  chrome-cobalt alloy p.
  distraction p.
  endodontic p.
  p. endosseous implant
  friction-retained p.
  p. implant
  incisal guide p.
  intramedullary p.
  p. and ligature cutter
  Link-Plus retention p.
  lock p.
  p. punch
  p. retention
  retention p.
  Roger-Anderson p.
  screw p.
  self-threading p.
  sprue p.
  Steinmann p.
  thread mate system p.
  p. and tube fixed orthodontic appliance
  ZAAG guide and p.
pincer
  overlapping p.
pinch
  fine p.
  p. graft
  p. strength
  p. technique
  p. test

pinching
  supraalar p.
Pin-Dalbo attachment
Pindborg tumor
pine
  Australian p.
  lodgepole p.
  Ponderosa p.
  slash p.
  white p.
pineapple
ping-pong ball crackling
pinhole
  p. retention
pinion head holder
pink
  p. noise
  p. spot
  p. tooth of Mummery
pinlay
pinledge
  p. attachment
  p. crown
pinless teeth
pinna, pl. pinnae
  rudimentary p.
pinned amalgam
pinning
  fixation p.
Pinocchio
  P. nose
  P. tip deformity
pin-retained amalgam
pin-supported
  p.-s. amalgam
  p.-s. restoration
Pinto
  P. dissector tip
  P. superficial dissection cannula
pinwheel
  Clean-Wheel disposable neurological p.
  neurological p.
PIP
  peak inspiratory pressure
piperacillin
  p. and tazobactam sodium
Piper methysticum
pipette, pipet
  Pasteur p.
Pipracil
piriform
  p. angle
  p. aperture stenosis
  p. fossa
  p. rim
  p. sinus
Pirogoff amputation level

piroxicam
pistachio
pistol
  Cameco syringe p.
  harvesting p.
piston
  p. stapes prosthesis
  Teflon p.
pistoning
pit
  basilar p.
  buccal p.
  p. caries
  central p. (CP)
  commissural p.
  distal p. (DP)
  p. and fissure caries
  p. and fissure cavity
  p. and fissure sealant
  labial p.
  lip p.
  mesial p. (MP)
Pitanguy abdominoplasty
pitch
  basal p.
  p. break
  p. elevation
  habitual p.
  natural p.
  optimal p.
  p. period perturbation (PPR)
  prosodic feature of p.
  p. raiser
  p. range
  p. shift
  p. system
Pitressin Injection
pitting
pituita
pituitary
  p. adenoma
  p. dwarf
  p. gland
  pharyngeal p.
  p. tumor
pituitous
pitviper
  p. bite
pityriasis
  p. linguae
pivot
  adjustable occlusal p.

  p. grammar
  occlusal p.
  p. word
PL
  proboscis lateralis
  pulpolingual
PLA
  pulpolabial
  pulpolinguoaxial
place
  p. of articulation
  p. theory
placebo effect
placement
  dowel-core p.
  eyelid sulcus p.
  lingual p.
  path of p.
  phonetic p.
  prefilm p.
  p. scaler
placode
  olfactory p.
plagiocephaly
  compensational frontal p.
  deformational frontal p.
  frontal p.
  lambdoidal synostotic p.
  nonsynostotic p.
  synostotic frontal p. (SFP)
  type I, II, III frontal p.
  unilateral p.
  p. without synostosis
PLAI
  Preschool Language Assessment
    Instrument
plain
plain-line articulator
Plak-Vac oral suction brush
plan
  Exposure Control P.
  Individualized Family Service P.
    (IFSP)
plana (*pl. of* planum)
plane
  alveolar point meatus p.
  auriculoinfraorbital p.
  axial p.
  axiobuccolingual p.
  axiolabiolingual p.
  axiomesiodistal p.
  base p.

NOTES

P

plane *(continued)*
  bipupital p.
  bite p.
  Broca p.
  buccolingual p.
  Camper p.
  cleavage p.
  coronal p.
  cusp p.
  p. of dissection
  extended supraplatysmal p. (ESP)
  eye-ear p.
  facial p.
  fascial p.
  Frankfort horizontal p.
  Frankfort mandibular p.
  French p.
  frontal p.
  guide p.
  guiding p.
  Hamy p.
  His p.
  horizontal p.
  Huxley p.
  labiolingual p.
  mandibular p.
  Martin p.
  mean foundation p.
  median raphe p.
  median sagittal p.
  mesiodistal p.
  Montague p.
  occlusal p., p. of occlusion
  orbital p.
  perpendicular p.
  preglenoid p.
  prepectoral p.
  p.'s of reference
  sagittal p.
  Schwalbe p.
  slant of occlusal p.
  subgaleal p.
  subperiosteal vomerine-ethmoidal p.
  subplatysmal p.
  temporal p.
  terminal p.
  tooth p.
  transumbilical p.
  transverse p.
  vertical p.
  Von Ihring p.
planer
  Rubin bone p.
planes of reference
planification
  inadequate p.
planigraphy

planing
  root p.
Planmeca panoramic x-ray machine
planned ventral hernia
planning
  reverse p.
planometer
plantain
  English p.
plantaris tendon
PlantarPatch
  Trans-Ver-Sal P.
plant wax
planum, pl. plana
  p. orbitale
  p. semilunatum
  p. sphenoidale
  p. temporale
  verruca plana
planus
  lichen p.
  oral (erosive) lichen p.
plaque
  attachment p.
  bacterial p.
  p. control
  P. Control Program
  dental p.
  facial p.
  P. Index
  p. inhibitor
  meningioma en p.
  microbial p.
  mucin p.
  mucinous p.
  mucous p.
  p.-type blue nevus
plasma
  p. cell
  p. cell gingivitis
  p. cell gingivostomatitis
  p. imbibition
  p. membrane
plasmacytoid
plasmacytoma
  extramedullary p.
plasmacytosis
plasma-derived hepatitis B vaccine
plasma-sprayed
plasmin
plasmocytosis
  gingival p.
plaster
  dental p.
  Hapset bone graft p.
  p. headcap
  headcap p.
  impression p.

p. impression
p. impression material
Kerr Snow White p. No. 1
p. knife
laboratory p.
Mediplast P.
model p.
model p. Grade A
p. of Paris splint
Sal-Acid P.
p. spatula
p. trimmer
Plastibell clamp-on device
plastic
    acrylic p.
    p. base
    p. block
    p. bracket
    cold-curing p.
    composite p.
    p. corneal protector
    P. Endosurgical System (P.E.S.)
    Erkoflex p.
    heat-curing p.
    p. instrument
    lead-impregnated p.
    p. ligature
    p. matrix
    p. matrix technique
    modeling p.
    p. operation
    p. restoration material
    p. spatula
    p. splint
    p. strip
    p. surgery
    p. teeth
    unfilled acrylic p.
    vinyl p.
    p. wax material
    p. wedge
plasticity
plasticize
plasticizer
plastisol
    vinyl p.
Plastodent
    P. cavity liner
    P. elastic impression powder
Plastopaste
plasty
    double-eyelid p.

male forehead p.
tendon p.
V-Y p.
plate
    alloplastic p.
    Alta femoral p.
    AO reconstruction p.
    atresia p.
    bandelette p.
    base p.
    basic p.
    Bimler elastic p.
    bite p.
    bone p.
    bony atretic p.
    buccal alveolar p.
    buccal cortical p.
    Coffin split p.
    compression p.
    condylar lag screw p.
    cortical bone p.
    cortical oral p.
    cribriform p.
    3D p.
    dental p.
    2D flat p.
    3D-flat Lactosorb p.
    die p.
    2D railed p.
    3D railed p.
    Dynamic Bridging p.
    dynamic compression p. (DCP)
    ethmoid p.
    ethmoidomaxillary p.
    expansion p.
    fibrocartilage p.
    p. fixation
    genial advancement p.
    Hawley bite p.
    horizontal p.
    horizontal p. of palatine bone
    infraorbital p.
    Jaeger bone p.
    Jaeger lid p.
    jumping-the-bite p.
    Kingsley p.
    Lane p.
    lateral pterygoid p.
    Leibinger 3-D bone p.
    Leibinger Micro Plus p.
    Leibinger mini Würzburg p.
    Leibinger Würzburg p.

NOTES

P

plate *(continued)*
    lingual p.
    lingual cortical p.
    long-span rigid p.
    low profile p.
    Luhr fixation p.
    Luhr Vitallium micromesh p.
    mandibular bridging p.
    mandibular staple bone p. (MSBP)
    maxillary bite p.
    medial pterygoid p.
    metal reconstruction p.
    micro-adaption p.
    middle fossa p.
    multipoint contact p.
    neural p.
    Nord expansion p.
    notchcord p.
    occlusal plane p.
    oral p.
    palatal p.
    palate p.
    Paulus chin p.
    Paulus midfacial p.
    perpendicular p.
    PolyMedics p.
    Profil-O-Plastic preshaped chin p.
    Profil-O-Plastic preshaped
      midfacial p.
    pterygoid p.
    p. punch
    reconstruction p.
    safety p.
    Schwartz p.
    Sherman p.
    six-hole mandibular p.
    split p.
    spring p.
    stainless steel AO p.
    staple bone p.
    Steinhauser p.
    Storz p.
    suction p.
    superior border p.
    supraorbital p.
    Synthes AO reconstruction p.
    Synthes maxillofacial titanium p.
    Synthes stainless steel
      minifragment p.
    Synthes titanium minifragment p.
    tegmen p.
    THORP-type mandibular
      reconstruction p.
    TiMesh orthognathic strap p.
    titanium AO p.
    titanium hollow osseointegrating
      reconstruction p. (THORP)
    vestibular oral p.
    wing p.
    Yaeger p.

plateau
    p. method

plated die

plate-holding clamp

platelet-activating factor (PAF)

platelet-derived growth factor (PDGF)

platelet gel

platform
    force p.
    p. posture test
    PSI-TEC aspiration/irrigation p.

plating
    compression p.
    eccentric dynamic compression p.
      (EDCP)
    Leibinger p.

Platinol
    P.-AQ

platinum
    p. embolization coil
    p. eyelid implant
    p. foil
    p. foil matrix
    p. microcoil

platinum-bonded alumina crown

platinum-iron compound

platinum-silver system

platyglossal

platyrrhine nose

platyrrhinia
    caudal p.

platysma
    p. muscle
    p. myocutaneous flap
    p. rhytidectomy

platysmal
    p. band
    p. imbrication
    p. plication

platysmaplasty
    corset p.

platysmarrhaphy

plausible context

Plaut
    P. angina
    P. ulcer

plauti-vincenti
    Fusobacterium p.-v.

Plaut-Vincent stomatitis

Plax
    P. anti-plaque pre-brushing rinse
    P. Mint Sensation
    P. SoftMINT

play
    p. audiometry
    combinatorial/thematic p.

pretend p.
symbolic p.
p. therapy
verbal p.
vocal p.
Pleasants disease
Pleasure curve
plectrum
pledget
cotton p.
neurosurgical p.
pleomorphic
p. adenocarcinoma
p. adenoma
p. liposarcoma
p. tumor
pleomorphism
cellular p.
plethysmography
respiratory inductive p. (RIP)
pleuripotential
pleurisy root
pleuropneumonia-like organism
plexiform
p. neurofibroma
p. pattern
Plexiglas
P. base
P. tissue equivalency block
plexitis
brachial p.
plexus, pl. plexus
arterial p.
brachial p.
capillary p.
cervical p.
cutaneous nerve of the cervical p.
dermal vascular p.
Haller p.
intermediate p.
Jacobson p.
Kiesselbach p.
lingual p.
p. maxillaris externus
neurovascular pulpal p.
peripheral p.
ranine vein p.
Raschkow p.
subdentinoblastic capillary p.
subepithelial nerve p.
suboccipital p.
subodontoblastic p.

thyroid p.
p. thyroideus impar
tympanic p.
PLF
perilymph fistula
PLGA
polymorphous low-grade adenocarcinoma
plica
p. semilunaris
p. stapedis
p. sublingualis
p. triangularis
plicamycin
plicata
lingua p.
plicate
plicated tongue
plication
buccinator p.
endoscopic muscle p.
fascial p.
fusiform p.
galea-aponeurotic p.
musculoaponeurotic p.
platysmal p.
Psillaki and Appiani crossed
external oblique flap and
horizontal p.
tongue p.
Toronto wide rectus p.
plicature
plicotomy
pliers
Allen root p.
band p.
band-removing p.
band-soldering p.
Becker-Parkin p.
clasp-adjusting p.
clasp-bending p.
contouring p.
cotton p.
crown-crimping p.
cusp-forming p.
debonding p. (DP)
eagle's beak p.
foil-carrying p.
hollow-jawed p.
ligature-locking p.
ligature-tying p.
lingual arch-forming p.
locking p.

NOTES

P

pliers *(continued)*
    loop p.
    loop-forming p.
    matrix p.
    orthodontic p.
    Peeso p.
    serrated p.
    silver point p.
    smooth p.
    Steiglitz p.
    stretching p.
    wire-bending p.
plissé, plisse
PLLA
    poly-l-lactic acid
PLM
    precise lesion measuring
    PLM device
Plomp test
plosive
    p. sound
plosive-injection method
PLP
    partial laryngopharyngectomy
plucking
    neck p.
plug
    Aqua Brites ear p.
    Catamaran swim p.
    Dent-O-Lux Smooth-Flow gutta-
      percha p.
    Insta-Putty silicone ear p.
    mucous p.
    Super punctum p.
    Umbrella punctum p.
plug-finishing bur
plugger
    amalgam p.
    automatic p.
    back-action p.
    Bredall amalgam p.
    endodontic p.
    foil p.
    foot p.
    gold p.
    heated p.
    Ladamore p.
    Luks p.
    miniature p.
    Mity p.
    reverse p.
    root canal p.
    Schilder p.
    serrated amalgam p.
    Zipperer finger p.
plugging instrument
pluglet
plum

PlumeSafe Whisper 602 smoke evacuation system
Plummer
    P. bougie
    P. disease
Plummer-Vinson syndrome
plumper
    lip p.
plunger cusp
plunging ranula
pluridirectional tomography
pluripotential
    p. cell
    p. primordial germ cell
plus
    Atrohist P.
    DHC p.
    Duramist P.
    Extra Strength Bayer P.
    p. juncture
    Lorcet P.
    PreviDent 5000 P.
    Quinsana P.
    Silux P.
PM
    pectoralis major
    periodontal membrane
    pulpomesial
    Midol PM
PMA
    interdental papilla, marginal gingiva and
      attached gingiva
    papillary-marginal-attached
    PMA index
PMM
    perilacunar mineral matrix
PMMA
    polymethyl methacrylate
PMN
    polymorphonuclear
PNdB
    perceived noise decibel
pneumatic
    p. artificial larynx
    p. condenser
    p. otoscope
    p. otoscopy
    p. tourniquet
pneumatization
    mastoid p.
pneumatize
pneumatocele
    extracranial p.
pneumatype
pneumoballistic
    p. energy
    p. lithotriptor

pneumocele
    extracranial p.
pneumocephalus
    tension p.
pneumocisternogram
pneumocisternography
pneumococcal infection
pneumococci
pneumoconiosis
Pneumocystis
    P. carinii
    P. carinii mastoiditis
    P. carinii in middle ear
    P. carinii otitis media
    P. carinii in temporal bone
pneumogram
pneumograph
pneumomassage
pneumomediastinum
pneumonia
pneumoniae
    Mycoplasma p.
    Streptococcus p.
pneumonitis
pneumosialosis
pneumosinus dilatans
pneumotachogram
pneumotachograph
pneumothorax
PNI
    perineural invasion
PNS
    peripheral nervous system
    posterior nasal spine
PNSP
    posterior nasal spine to soft palate
    PNSP measurement
pocket
    absolute p.
    bleeding p.
    bottom p.
    calculus p.
    complex p.
    compound p.
    conchal p.
    Crane-Kaplan marker p.
    deepening p.
    p. depth
    elimination p.
    p. epithelium
    expander p.
    gingival p.

    infrabony p.
    infracrestal p.
    intra-alveolar p.
    intrabony p.
    ionization chamber p.
    irreversible p.
    limited p.
    marking p.
    periodontal p.
    p. probe
    Rathke p.
    relative p.
    retraction p.
    simple p.
    skin p.
    subcrestal p.
    submuscular p.
    suprabony p.
    supracrestal p.
    p. wall
Pockethaler
    Vancenase P.
Pocketpeak peak flow meter
podophyllin and salicylic acid
Pog
    point P.
pogonion
    bony p.
poikilodentosis
poikiloderma
point
    A p.
    p. A
    abrasive p.
    p. of abscess
    absorbent p.
    absorbent paper p.
    alveolar p.
    p. angle
    p. of articulation
    Aufrecht p.
    auricular p.
    B p.
    p. B
    Bolton p.
    Brinell hardness indenter p.
    Broadbent registration p.
    central-bearing p.
    p. centric
    chin p.
    condenser p.
    p. condenser

NOTES

P

465

point *(continued)*
    contact p.
    contact area p.
    convenience p.
    ethmoid registration p.
    faulty contact p.
    p. forceps
    fusing p.
    gingival p.
    gutta-percha p.
    hinge axis p.
    Hirschfeld silver p.
    p. IdI
    p. IdS
    impaction p.
    incisal p.
    p. incisor
    incisor p.
    jugomaxillary p.
    Knoop hardness indenter p.
    loss of contact p.
    McBernie p.
    median mandibular p.
    mental p.
    mounted diamond p.
    nasal spinal p.
    nasion p.
    p. notcher
    paper p.
    p. Pog
    power p.
    preauricular p.
    p. of proximal contact
    purchase p.
    p. removal
    retention p.
    retromandibular p.
    Rockwell hardness indenter p.
    root canal p.
    rotary mounted p.
    sella nasion B p.
    separation p.
    silver p.
    sulfur and silver p.
    trial p.
    trigger p.
    Vickers hardness indenter p.
    white p.
    wood p.
pointed cone bur
pointer
    tragal p.
pointing
Point-Two
    P.-T. mouthrinse
poison
    p. oak
    p. sumac

Poladex
Poland
    P. chest-wall deformity
    P. syndrome
Polaramine
pole
    tonsil p.
    upper p.
Polhemus 3Space digitizer
poliglecaprone 25 suture
poliomyelitis
    p. virus
poliovirus
    p. type 2 virus
    p. virus
polish
    Bendick p.
polished
    p. surface
    p. surface denture
polisher
    rubber p.
polishing
    p. abrasive
    p. brush
    coronal p.
    p. disk
    electro-p.
    p. paste
    p. strip
Politzer
    P. bag
    P. luminous cone
    P. method
politzerization
    negative p.
pollicization
    p. technique
Pollock-Dingman elevator
pollutant
    air p.
pollution
    air p.
    noise p.
polly beak
    p. b. nasal deformity
Polocaine
    P. with levonordefrin
Poloris Pads
poly-(2-hydroxyethyl methacrylate) (poly-HEMA)
polyacrylamide gel electrophoresis
polyacrylic acid
polyamide mesh
polyarteritis nodosa
polycarbonate
    p. crown

p. crown kit
p. resin
polycarboxylate
p. cement
polychondritis
chronic atrophic p.
relapsing p.
polychromaticity
Polycillin
P.-N
polycystic disease
polydactyly
index finger p.
postaxial p. type A, B
preaxial p.
preaxial p. type I, II, III, IV
thumb p.
Polydek suture
polydentate
polydentia
Polydine
polydioxanone
p. sheet
p. suture (PDS)
polyelectrolyte
polyester fiber
polyether
p. impression material
p. rubber
p. rubber base
p. rubber impression
p. rubber impression material
polyethylene
high density p.
porous p.
porous, high-density p. (PHDPE)
ultra-high molecular weight p.
(UHMWPE)
polyfascicular nerve
Polygam
P. S/D
polyglactic acid
polyglactin 910 suture
polyglot
polyglycolic
p. acid (PGA)
p. acid conduit
p. acid suture
Polyglyd suture coating
polygon
Bjork p.

polygonal
p. cell
p. fat cell
polygraph
poly-HEMA
poly-(2-hydroxyethyl methacrylate)
polyhexanide methacrylate resin
Poly-Histine
P.-H. CS
P.-H.-D Capsule
polyhydroxy acid (PHA)
polyisoprene
polylactic acid
poly-l-lactic acid (PLLA)
polymastia
PolyMedics plate
PolyMem dressing
polymer
acrylic p.
Bioplastique p.
cross-linked p.
dimethacrylate p.
p. gel
high-molecular weight network p.
linear silicone rubber p.
methyl methacrylate p.
modified p.
polysulfide p.
polyvinylacetate-polyethylene p.
thermoplastic p.
p. tooth replica implant
unfilled acrylic p.
polymerase
p. chain reaction (PCR)
Sp6 RNA p.
T3 RNA p.
polymeric biomaterial
polymerization
p. shrinkage
polymerize
polymerized mucopolysaccharide
molecule
polymer-reinforced zinc oxide-eugenol
cement
polymethyl
p. methacrylate (PMMA)
p. methacrylate cement
p. methacrylate ear splint
polymicrobial infection
polymorphemic utterance
polymorphic
p. reticulosis

NOTES

P

polymorphism
short tandem repeat p. (STRP)
polymorphonuclear (PMN)
p. leukocyte
polymorphous low-grade adenocarcinoma (PLGA)
Polymox
polymyalgia rheumatica
polymyositis
polymyxin
p. B
bacitracin and p. B
bacitracin, neomycin, and p. B
p. B and hydrocortisone
neomycin and p. B
oxytetracycline and p. B
trimethoprim and p. B
polyneuritis
cranial p.
polyneuropathy
polynitrile glove
polyodontia
polyostotic
p. fibrous dysplasia
polyotia
polyp
adenomatous p.
antral p.
antrochoanal p.
choanal p.
dental p.
granulation p.
gum p.
Hopmann p.
laryngeal p.
nasal p.
pedicled p.
pedunculated p.
pulp p.
tooth p.
vocal p.
polypectomy
intranasal p.
polypeptide
p. chain
polyphyodont
p. dentition
polypoid
p. degeneration of the true fold
p. hyperplasia
p. vocal nodule
polyposis
diffuse vocal p.
nasal p.
vocal p.
Poly-Pred Ophthalmic Suspension

polypropylene
p. mesh
p. needle
polysaccharide
p. molecular chain
polysiloxane
p. impression
polysomnogram
polysomnographic technique
polysomnography (PSG)
polysomnography-proven obstructive sleep apnea (PSG-proven OSA)
Polysporin
P. Ophthalmic
P. Topical
polysulfide
p. impression material
p. polymer
p. rubber
p. rubber base
p. rubber base impression
p. rubber impression material
polysyllabic word
polysyndactyly
complex p.
Polytec LaseAway Q-switched ruby laser
polytef
polytetrafluoroethylene
polytetrafluoroethylene (polytef, PTFE)
expanded p. (ePTFE)
p. implant
p. membrane graft
p. mesh
p. prosthesis
polythelia
familial p.
polytomography
Polytrim Ophthalmic
polyurethane
p. elastomer material
p. foam (PUF)
p. primer
polyurethane-coated silicone breast implant
Poly-Vi-Flor multivitamin mineral and fluoride supplement
polyvinyl
p. chloride (PVC)
p. chloride endotracheal tube
polyvinylacetate-polyethylene
p.-p. mouth protector
p.-p. polymer
polyvinylpyrrolidone (PVP)
polyvinylsiloxane putty
Polyviolene polyester suture material
POM
peripheral osteoma of the mandible

pomette
POMR
    problem-oriented medical record
Ponderosa pine
pons, pl. **pontes**
    inferior lip of p.
Ponstel
Ponten-type
    P.-t. fasciocutaneous flap
    P.-t. tubed pedicle
pontes (*pl. of* pons)
pontic
    bonded p.
    ovate p.
    ridge lap p.
    sanitary p.
    Stein p.
Pont index
Pontocaine
pontomedullary junction
pooling site
poorly differentiated synovial sarcoma
poor take
Pope wick
poplar
    Lombardy p.
    white p.
popliteal
    p. musculovascular pedicle
    pterygium p.
porcelain
    aluminous p.
    Ames plastic p.
    baked p.
    p. carver
    p. cement
    Ceramco p.
    p. cervical contact and single bake
      technique
    p. cervical ditching technique
    p. condensation
    p. crown
    dental p.
    p. denture
    p. enamel
    feldspathic p.
    p. finished bridge
    fired p.
    p. fracture
    p. furnace
    high-fusing p.
    p. inlay

    p. jacket
    p. jacket restoration
    Jenkins p.
    p. laminate veneer
    low-fusing p.
    medium-fusing p.
    medium temperature maturing p.
    opaque p.
    S.S. White new filling p.
    p. stain
    synthetic p.
    p. veneer gold crown
porcelain-bonded restoration
porcelain-faced
    p.-f. dowel crown
porcelain-fused-to-gold alloy
porcelain-fused-to-metal
    p.-f.-t.-m. crown
    p.-f.-t.-m. restoration
    p.-f.-t.-m. splint
porcelain-metal
    p.-m. bonding
    p.-m. failure
Porcelana
    P. Sunscreen
Porch
    P. Index of Communicative
      Abilities (PICA)
    P. Index of Communicative
      Abilities in Children (PICAC)
porcine
    p. skin graft
    p. xenograft
pore
    gustatory p.
    taste p.
Porex implant
Porges Neoflex dilator
porion, pl. **poria**
pork
poroma
    eccrine p.
porosity
porous
    p. block hydroxyapatite (PBHA)
    p. casting
    p., high-density polyethylene
      (PHDPE)
    p. polyethylene
    p. polyethylene implant
porphyria

NOTES

P

Porphyromonas
  P. endodontalis
  P. gingivalis
port
  endoscopic access p. (EAP)
  Hassan-type p.
  nasal p.
  p. protector
  velopharyngeal p.
  p. wine stain (PWS)
  p. wine stain birthmark
portacaval shunt
portal
  p. hypertension
  velopharyngeal p.
Porta-Resp monitor
portepolisher
  contra-angle p.
Portex
  P. Blue Line tracheostomy tube
  P. F29 Blue Line tracheal tube
portio, pl. portiones
  p. major nervi trigemini
  p. minor nervi trigemini
portion
  cisternal p.
portmanteau word
portrait
  periodontal p.
port-wine macrocheilia
porus
  p. acusticus
  p. acusticus internus
position
  4-7 p.
  anomalous tongue p.
  backward p.
  bisecting angle cone p.
  Boyce p.
  centric p.
  condylar hinge p.
  consonant p.
  cuspid-molar p.
  distoangular p.
  diver's p.
  eccentric jaw p.
  final cone p.
  final consonant p.
  first cone p.
  forehead-nose p.
  Fuchs p.
  gingival p.
  half-seated recumbent dorsal p.
  Hallpike p.
  hinge p.
  incisor bite p.
  p. indicating device (PID)
  initial consonant p.

  intercuspal p.
  jaw-to-jaw p.
  lateral occlusal p.
  lawn chair p.
  lithotomy p.
  mandibular hinge p.
  mandibular rest p.
  median occlusal p.
  mesioangular p.
  molar bite p.
  occlusal p.
  orthostatic p.
  paralleling cone p.
  park-bench p.
  physiologic rest p.
  posterior border p.
  postural resting p.
  prone jackknife p.
  protrusive occlusal p.
  pterygoid p.
  RC p.
  recumbent p.
  rest p.
  retruded p.
  Rose p.
  semi-Fowler p.
  semirecumbent p.
  p. sensor
  terminal hinge p.
  p. test
  tonsil p.
  tooth p.
  tooth-to-tooth p.
  Trendelenburg p.
  vertical p.
positional
  p. distortion
  p. nystagmus
  p. test
positioner
  forehead p.
  tooth p.
positioning
  surgical p.
  tooth p.
positive
  p. correlation
  p. culture
  p. emotion
  p. end-expiratory pressure (PEEP)
  p. reinforcer
  p. response
positron emission tomography with 2-[F-18]-fluoro-2-deoxy-D-glucose (PET-FDG)
Pospischill-Feyrter syndrome
possessor-possession

post

abutment p.
p. and core crown
p. dam
p. dam area
fabricating p.
implant p.
p. implant
p. implant substructure
P. Laser Balm
nonparallel p.
parallel p.
parallel-sided p.
Pullen-Warner split p.
p. removal
screw p.
self-threading p.
serrated p.
smooth-sided p.
p. space preparation (PSP)
split-shank screw p.
tapered p.
threaded p.
vented p.

post-ablation defect
postablative

p. template

postage stamp graft
postalveolar cleft
postameloblast
postauricular

p. area
p. artery
p. incision
p. node
p. and retroauricular scalping
(PARAS)

postaxial

p. polydactyly type A, B

postbuccal
postburn

p. scar contracture treatment

postcapillary venule (PCV)
postcarotid air cell
postcementation

p. sensitivity

postcentral

p. gyrus
p. sulcus

post-cervix-crown complex
Post Com II
postconcussion syndrome

postcondensation
postconsonantal vowel
postcore restoration
postcricoid

p. carcinoma
p. squamous cell carcinoma

postcrown
postcuring
postdam
postdeterminer
post-endodontic discoloration
posterior

p. airway space (PAS)
p. ampullary nerve (PAN)
p. arch width
p. auricular artery
p. auricular node
p. band
p. belly
p. border jaw relation
p. border movement
p. border position
p. bridge abutment
p. chisel
p. clinoid process
p. commissure
p. cranial fossa (PCF)
p. cranial fossa meningioma
p. cricoarytenoid muscle
p. crossbite
p. crus
p. divergence
p. ethmoid
p. ethmoidal artery
p. ethmoidal cell
p. ethmoidal foramen
p. ethmoidal nerve
p. ethmoid ostium
p. facial vein
p. fontanel
p. fossa
p. fossa artery aneurysm
p. fossa craniotomy
p. fracture
hiatus semilunaris p.
p. incudal ligament
p. inferior cerebellar artery (PICA)
p. inferior nasal nerve
p. inlay
p. maxillary segmental ostectomy
p. movement on opening
p. naris

NOTES

P

posterior *(continued)*
    p. nasal spine (PNS)
    p. nasal spine to soft palate (PNSP)
    p. occlusal discrepancy
    p. occlusion
    p. open bite
    p. palatal major connector
    p. palatal seal
    p. palatal seal area
    p. palatine artery
    p. pedicle
    p. plagiocephaly deformity
    p. rhinoscopy
    p. semicircular canal (PSC)
    p. septal artery
    p. sinus
    sulcus auriculae p.
    p. sulcus obliteration
    p. superior alveolar artery
    p. superior nasal nerve
    p. surface of maxilla
    p. suspensory ligament
    p. teeth
    p. thigh fasciocutaneous flap
    p. tooth form
    p. tympanic artery
    p. vertical canal
    p. wall of agger nasi cell
posterioris
    iter chordae p.
posteroanterior
    p. extraoral radiography
    p. mandible radiograph
    p. sinus radiograph
    p. skull radiograph
posteroclusion
posterolateral
    p. nasal artery
posterosuperior alveolar nerve
posteruption cuticle
posteruptive
    p. phase
    p. tooth movement
postexcision skin expansion
postexposure
Post-Exposure Evaluation
postextraction
    p. hemorrhage
postganglionectomy
    p. wrist destabilization
postganglionic
    p. nerve
    p. neuron
postgastroplasty diet
postglandular node

postglenoid
    p. process
    p. tubercle
postherniorrhaphy neuropathy
postherpetic
    p. neuralgia
    p. otalgia
posthioplasty
posthole
posticus
    isthmus tympani p.
    p. palsy
    p. paralysis
postirradiation
    p. dental caries
    p. sialadenitis
postlingual
    p. deafness
    p. profound sensorineural hearing loss
postmaxillectomy
    p. collapsed cheek
    p. deformity
postmitotic cell
postnasal
    p. balloon tamponade
    p. drip
postnatal
    p. dentin
    p. enamel
postnormal occlusion
postoperated cleft
postoperative
    p. mammary support
    p. migration
    p. parotiditis
post-op soothing skin treatment
postoral
postpalatal
    p. seal
    p. seal area
postpalatine
postparalytic hemifacial spasm
postperception
postpermanent
    p. dentition
    p. teeth
postpharyngeal flap
postpoliomyelitis syndrome
postponement
postradiation xerostomia
postreconstructive
postresection
    p. defect
    p. filling
    p. filling technique
postretention adjustment
postsclerotherapy hyperpigmentation

postsensation
postsialolithectomy
poststapedectomy related sequela
poststimulus time histogram
postsurgical neuralgia
posttesting
posttraumatic
    p. amnesia (PTA)
    p. ectropion
    p. enophthalmos
    p. exorbitism
    p. lipodystrophy
    p. lipoma
    p. neuralgia
    p. reconstruction
    p. ventricular phonation
posttreatment
postulate
    conversational p.'s
    Sheen p.
postural
    p. resting position
    p. vertical dimension (PVD)
    p. vertigo
posturing
    anterior mandibular p.
    vertical mandibular p.
posturographic
posturography
    computerized dynamic p. (CDP)
    computerized dynamic platform p. (CDPP)
    dynamic p.
    dynamic platform p.
    fixed forceplate p.
    foam p.
    static p.
postvocalic
    p. obstruent singleton omission
postzygomatic space
potassium
    amoxicillin and clavulanate p.
    p. bromide
    p. indoxyl sulfate
    5% p. nitrate
    p. oxalate
    p. penicillin
    p. penicillin G
    penicillin V p.
    ticarcillin and clavulanate p.
    p. titanyl phosphate (KTP)
    p. titanyl phosphate laser

potato
    p. nose
    sweet p.
    white p.
potential
    action p.
    auditory evoked p.
    brainstem auditory evoked p. (BAEP)
    cochlear nerve action p. (CNAP)
    corneoretinal p.
    eighth nerve action p. (8NAP)
    electrical p.
    endocochlear p.
    p. energy
    evoked p.
    nerve action p.
    receptor p.
    resting p.
    p. trauma
    vertex p.
potentiometer
    gain p.
    output limiting p.
    threshold kneepoint p.
    variable compression p.
    variable high cut p.
    variable low cut p.
Pott puffy tumor
Potts elevator
Potts-Smith tissue forceps
pouce flottant
pouch
    cheek p.
    dermal p.
    heat-seal p.
    Rathke p.
    self-seal p.
    visceral p.
poudrage
    talc p.
poultice
pour hole
poverty weed
povidone-iodine
    p.-i. solution
powder
    Absorbine Antifungal Foot P.
    budesonide p.
    Cel Touch white indicator p.
    Co-Re-Ga denture adhesive p.
    Dembone demineralized cortical p.

NOTES

P

powder *(continued)*
demineralized cortical bone p.
denture adherent p.
Goody Headache P.'s
Lotrimin AF Spray P.
NaFpak p.
Osteomin Thermo-Ashed bone p.
Pacific Coast demineralized cortical bone p.
Plastodent elastic impression p.
Prophy Choice polishing p.
Pycopay tooth p.
sulfonamide p.
Ultimatics demineralized cortical bone p.
Youngblood natural mineral p.
Zeasorb-AF P.

powdered
p. gold
p. gold-calcium alloy

power
p. adapter
p. centric
p. contralateral routing of signals
p. CROS
p. cut/tungsten carbide (PC/TC)
high definition p. (HDP)
instantaneous p.
p. peak filter
phonetic p.
p. point
p. stroke

power-assisted adenoidectomy
power-driven mechanical spatulator
powered
p. endoscopic sinus surgery (PESS)
p. toothbrush

PowerProxi Sonic interdental toothbrush system
PowerStar bipolar scissors
PPG
photoplethysmography
PPR
pitch period perturbation
PPS
parapharyngeal space
PPT
pressure pain threshold
PPTL
pressure pain tolerance level
practice
family-centered p.
p. increment
negative p.

Prader-Willi syndrome
praecox
dentia p.

pragmatic
p. anomaly
p. aphasia
P. Screening Test
p. structure
p. text

pragmatics
preabsorptive
prealveolar cleft
preamalgamated alloy
preamplifier
preanesthetic
pre-article
preauricular
p. crease
p. cyst
p. fistula
p. incision
p. lymph node
p. pain
p. point

preaxial
p. polydactyly
p. polydactyly type I, II, III, IV

prebase
precancer
precancerous
p. erythroplakia
p. lesion

precapillary
precarotid air cell
precementum
precentral
p. gyrus
p. sulcus

precession
prechamber
ethmoidal p.

precipitated silver
precipitating factor
precipitation
precise
P. anastomotic coupler
p. lesion measuring (PLM)
p. lesion measuring device

precision
p. anchorage
p. attachment
p. fluence shaping
p. lancet cutting needle
P. Osteolock stem
p. rest
p. retained denture
p. retainer
p. therapy

Pre-Cision miniature and microminiature scalpel
precleaning

precochlear cell
precocious
    p. advanced alveolar atrophy
    p. dentition
    p. metastasis
precollagenous fiber
preconsonantal vowel
precurved file
precurving file
Pred
    P. Forte Ophthalmic
    Liquid P.
    P. Mild Ophthalmic
Predalone Injection
Predcor-TBA Injection
predeciduous
    p. dentition
    p. teeth
predental
predentin
    p. matrix (PDM)
    necrotic p.
    pulp p.
predentinal
    p. nerve
    p. nerve fiber
    p. zone
Predent topical fluoride treatment gel
predeterminer
Pred-G Ophthalmic
predicate
    p. objective
    p. truncation
predictive
    P. Screening Test of Articulation
    p. validity
predilection
predispose
predisposing factor
prednicarbate
prednisolone
    chloramphenicol and p.
    p. and gentamicin
    neomycin, polymyxin B, and p.
    sulfacetamide sodium and p.
prednisone
pre-epiglottic space
preeruptive
    p. phase
    p. stage
    p. tooth movement
    p. translocation

preexcision skin expansion
preextirpative form
preextraction
    p. cast
    p. record
prefabricate
prefabricated
    p. temporoparietal fascial flap
    p. thin flap
prefabrication
    flap p.
    p. flap procedure
preference
    consonant-vowel p.
prefilm placement
prefinishing appliance
preflaring
preformativa
    membrana p.
preformed
    p. band
    p. crown
Prefrin Ophthalmic Solution
prefrontal bone
prefunctional
    p. phase
    p. phase of tooth eruption
preganglionic neuron
preglandular node
preglenoid plane
pregnancy
    p. gingivitis
    p. tumor
prejowl
    p. depression
    p. sulcus
prelacrimal area
prelaryngeal node
preliminary impression
prelingual deafness
prelinguistic
    p. language
    p. requesting
    p. vocalization
Prelone Oral
Prema enamel microabrasion compound
premandible alloplastic augmentation
premandibular
    p. arches
    p. augmentation
premature
    p. contact

NOTES

premature *(continued)*
    p. dentition
    p. eruption
    p. teeth
prematurity
    occlusal p.
premaxilla
    floating p.
    loose p.
    p. peripyriform deficiency
premaxillary
    p. palate
    p. suture
Pre-Meal
    Dexatrim P.-M.
premedication
    dental p.
premilk teeth
premium
    clear sterile MB p.
premolar
    p. band
    p. crowding
    first p.
    mandibular p.
    second p.
    p. tooth
    two-pointed p.
premolaris
    dens p.
pre-mycosis fungoides stage
prenatal
    p. dentin
    p. enamel
prenodular swelling
prenormal occlusion
preoperational thought period
preoperative
    p. cast
    p. pure tone average
    p. record
preoral
preosteoclasts
Prep
    RC-P.
prepalatal
prepalate
preparation
    access p.
    cavity p.
    chamfer p.
    facial butt joint p.
    figure-eight p.
    full shoulder p.
    funnelform p.
    p. GK-101
    P. H
    incisal p.

    initial p.
    Matsura p.
    medicinal p.
    mouth p.
    post space p. (PSP)
    root-end p.
    shoulder with bevel p.
    slice p.
    slot p.
    slot-type p.
    step p.
    surgical p.
    topical otic p.
    ultrasonic p.
    vertical vs. horizontal p.
preparatory set
prepared
    p. cavity
    p. cavity impression
preparotid fascia
prepectoral plane
prepeel conditioning
pre-periosteal tissue release
prephonatory amplitude
preplatysmal fat
preponderance
    directional p. (DP)
preprosthetic
    p. augmentation
    p. grafting
    p. rebuilding
    p. reconstructive armamentarium
    p. surgery
prepsychosis
prepubertal periodontitis
prepuce
preputial
    p. hood
    p. island flap
preputium
presbyacusis, presbyacousia, presbycusis
presbyesophagus
Preschool
    P. Language Assessment Instrument (PLAI)
    P. Language Scale
    P. Language Screening Test
    P. Speech and Language Screening Test
prescription
    p. arch
    P. Strength Desenex
prescriptive grammar
presellar
presenile atrophy
preseptal cellulitis
presialogram
prespeech

presphenoethmoid suture
press
    glossopharyngeal p.
    tongue p.
press-button chuck
Press Lift chin strap
Pressomatic attachment
pressure
    acoustic p.
    Alladin InfantFlow nasal continuous
      positive air p.
    p. anesthesia
    p. area
    p. atrophy
    aural p.
    biting p.
    p. condensation
    continuous positive airway p.
      (CPAP)
    driving p. (DP)
    p. earring
    end expiratory p. (EEP)
    p. equalization (PE)
    p. equalization tube
    high oxygen p. (HOP)
    intraneural p.
    intraocular p.
    intraoral p.
    intraperiapical p.
    intrapleural p.
    intrapulpal p.
    intrathoracic p.
    mastoid p.
    minimum audible p. (MAP)
    occlusal p.
    p. pack
    p. pain threshold (PPT)
    p. pain tolerance level (PPTL)
    p. pattern
    peak inspiratory p. (PIP)
    periapical p.
    peripheral p.
    positive end-expiratory p. (PEEP)
    pulmonary p.
    pulp p.
    p. receptor
    p. resorption
    p. side
    p. sore
    p. splint
    subglottic p.
    p. syringe

    p. technique
    p. technique filling
    p. threshold
    time p.
    tongue p.
    Tranquility Quest continuous
      positive airway p.
    variable positive airway p. (VPAP)
    vascular p.
    p. welding
    p. zone microphone (PZM)
Pressurefuse automatic constant
    pressure device
pressure-indicating paste
pressure-producing earring
prestandardization
PreSun 29
presupposition
presurgical
    p. impression
    p. infant orthopaedics
presuture
presuturing technique
presynaptic
    p. inhibition
    p. terminal
presyntactic device
pretapped
    p. Synthes lag screw
pretarsal fold
pretemporal space
pretend play
pretesting
pretracheal
    p. fascia
    p. node
    p. space
pretraining ability
pretunneling
Pretz-D
Prevacare
    P. extra protective ointment
    P. moisturizing cream
    P. no-rinse personal cleanser
    P. personal protective cream
    P. preventative skin care product
prevention
    extension for p.
preventive
    p. dentistry
    p. orthodontics

NOTES

P

preventive *(continued)*
  p. periodontics
  p. recall
Preventodontic AF paste
prevertebral
  p. fascia
  p. space
  p. space abscess
PreviDent
  P. Brush-On Gel
  P. Dental Rinse
  P. 5000 Plus
prevocal
prevocalic
  p. singleton
  p. voicing of consonant
prevocational deafness
Prevotella
  P. buccae
  P. intermedia
  P. melaninogenica
  P. nigrescens
  P. oralis
Price rule
prickle
  p. cell
  p. cell layer
Pri-Die
prilocaine
  lidocaine and p.
primary
  p. abutment
  p. aerodontalgia
  p. autism
  p. caries
  p. cementum
  p. cerebellar ectopia
  p. ciliary dyskinesia (PCD)
  p. coping
  p. cuticle
  p. dentin
  p. dentition
  p. enamel cuticle
  p. gain
  p. herpetic stomatitis
  p. hue
  p. impression
  p. intraosseous carcinoma
  p. irritant
  p. lesion
  p. molar
  multiple p.
  p. occlusal traumatism
  occult p.
  p. osteoma cutis
  p. palate
  p. peak frequency
  p. periodontitis

  p. pseudoepitheliomatous hyperplasia
  p. radiation
  p. reinforcement
  p. reinforcer
  second p.
  p. skin graft
  p. soft-tissue nocardiosis
  p. stapedectomy
  p. stress
  p. struts implant substructure
  p. stuttering
  p. teeth
  p. thumb reconstruction
  p. tumor
  p. union
  p. varicella-zoster
Primaxin
primer
  Bonfil p.
  Bowen cavity p.
  cavity p.
  Kadon p.
  polyurethane p.
  Scotchbond 1 p.
  Sevriton Cavity Seal P.
  XR p.
priming
  cross-modal p. (CMP)
primitive hemifacial spasm
primordial cyst
primordium
  tooth p.
principal
  p. fiber
  p. fiber bundle
  p. vestibular nucleus
Principen
principle
  ALARA p.
  Bernoulli p.
  binary p.
  Thielemann p.
priori
  a p.
prism
  adamantine p.
  enamel p.
  p. sheath
Prisma
  P. Fill
  P. Microfine
prisma, pl. prismata
  prismata adamantina
Pritchard elevator
privet
  p. cough
Privine Nasal
ProAlloy

probability curve
Pro-Banthine
probe
  acoustic impedance p.
  ADD side-directed p.
  blunt lacrimal p.
  Brackett p.
  calibrated p.
  cDNA p.
  cross p.
  C-Trak handheld gamma p.
  Doppler ultrasonic p.
  Fox-Williams p.
  Gilmore p.
  Glickman periodontal p.
  Goldman Fox p.
  hand-held p.
  lacrimal p.
  Marquis p.
  Merit-B periodontal p.
  Michigan p.
  Nabers p.
  percutaneous pencil Doppler p.
  periodontal p.
  PerioWise p.
  pocket p.
  Probex p.
  pulpal microdialysis p.
  Reddick/Saye Lav-1 irrigating and
    aspirating p.
  root canal p.
  Softflo fiber optic p.
  SpineStat side-directed
    diskectomy p.
  p. syringe
  p. tube microphone
  Ultra-Precision ultrasonic p.
  visual p.
  WHO p.
  Williams periodontal p.
  p. word
Probex probe
probing depth (PD)
problem
  control p.
  gravitational p.
  word-finding p.
problem-oriented medical record
  (POMR)
ProBond dentin bonding agent
proboscis lateralis (PL)

procaine
  penicillin G p.
Pro Care paste
procedure
  abdominoplasty p.
  ablative p.
  adipofascial sural flap p.
  apron flap p.
  autogenous fascia lata sling p.
  BAT p.
  BC p.
  blepharoplasty p.
  burnout p.
  Burow p.
  Caldwell-Luc window p.
  canal-down p.
  canalith repositioning p.
  canal-wall-down p.
  canthoplasty p.
  Cawthorne-Day p.
  cervicofacial rhytidectomy p.
  Clagett p.
  cocked hat p.
  commando p.
  conjunctivodacryocystorhinostomy p.
  crane p.
  dacryocystorhinostomy p.
  Davis-Kitlowski p.
  dental prosthetic laboratory p.
  dermoplasty p.
  dynamic fascial transfer p.
  dynamic muscle transfer p.
  endoscopic p.
  Eve reconstructive p.
  Ewart p.
  facial bipartition p.
  Fasanella Servat p.
  fenestration p.
  fillet flap p.
  free composite lip-switch p.
  free flap p.
  free jejunal graft p.
  frontalis sling p.
  Furlow p.
  genioplasty p.
  Gillies cocked hat p.
  gold-weight p.
  Gunderson conjunctival flap p.
  Halstead radical mastectomy p.
  Hueston flap p.
  Ilizarov p.
  inner ear tack p.

NOTES

P

procedure *(continued)*
> integral-total p.
> Killian frontoethmoidectomy p.
> Kole p.
> Krukenberg p.
> Kuhnt-Szymanowski ectropion repair p.
> Language Assessment, Remediation, and Screening P.
> laryngopharyngoesophagectomy p.
> lateral tarsal strip p.
> Le Fort I, II, III p.
> limb-sparing p.
> lithotomy p.
> Lothrop frontoethmoidectomy p.
> Lynch p.
> Lynch frontoethmoidectomy p.
> malarplasty p.
> mammaplasty p.
> McComb p.
> meatal advancement and glanduloplasty p. (MAGPI)
> meloplasty p.
> microsurgical p.
> Mitz p.
> modified Krukenberg p.
> modified Weber-Fergusson p.
> open sky p.
> operant p.
> oral cloze p.
> orchiectomy p.
> orthodontic p.
> Orticochea p.
> osteoplastic frontal sinus p.
> palatal lengthening p.
> palatorrhaphy p.
> parotidectomy p.
> partial laryngeal reconstruction p.
> passivation p.
> PET-FDG p.
> phalloplasty p.
> P.'s for the Phonological Analysis of Children's Language
> prefabrication flap p.
> pushback p.
> reanimation p.
> reduction-augmentation p.
> Reiger p.
> restorative p.
> reversed extensor digitorum muscle island flap p.
> reversed first dorsal metatarsal artery flap p.
> reversed medialis pedis island flap p.
> reverse filling p.
> rhinotomy p.
> rhytidectomy p.

> Riedel frontoethmoidectomy p.
> sac and tack p.
> Schuchardt p.
> Shea p.
> Sistrunk p.
> Skoog p.
> SMAS plication p.
> Snow p.
> staged p.
> TAT p.
> tip-lifting p.
> toe fillet flap p.
> touch-up p.
> transblepharoplasty p.
> transendoscopic p.
> uvulopalatoplasty p.
> vaginoplasty p.
> Van Nes p.
> Vilkki p.
> voice-preserving p.
> V-tunnel drill p.
> V-Y p.
> V-Y pushback p.
> W p.
> Wardill-Kilner p.
> Wassmund p.
> Weber-Ferguson p.
> Z p.
> Z-plasty p.

Procera system

procerus
> p. and corrugator ablation
> p. muscle
> p. muscle myotomy

process
> alveolar p.
> anterior clinoid p.
> ascending p.
> Assessment of Phonological P.'s
> assimilation phonological p.
> auditory p.
> benign fibroosseous p.
> central auditory p.
> Children's Language P.'s
> clinoid p.
> cochleariform p.
> condyloid p.
> coronoid p.
> cribriform plate of alveolar p.
> cytoplasmic p.
> dental p.
> dentinoblastic p.
> developmental phonological p.
> feature contrasts p.
> fenestration of alveolar p.
> fibroblast p.
> fibro-osseous p.
> fixing p.

frontal p.
hamular p.
harmony p.
horizontal resorptive p.
inflammatory p.
intercellular matrix p.
intrajugular p. of temporal bone
lacrimal p.
laser stereolithography p.
lateronasal p.
lenticular p.
lost wax p.
mandibular p.
marginal p. of malar bone
masticatory p.
mastoid p.
maxillary p.
medionasal p.
mental p.
myoepithelial cell p.
nasal p.
natural phonological p.
p. of odontoblast
odontoblast p.
odontoblastic p.
odontoid p.
odontoid p. of epistropheus
orbital p.
osteoinduction p.
packing p.
palatine p. of maxilla
phonological p.
posterior clinoid p.
postglenoid p.
pterygoid p.
rinsing p.
sphenoid p.
styloid p.
temporal p. of mandible
temporal p. of zygomatic bone
Tomes p. of ameloblast
uncinate p.
washing p.
zygomatic p.
processed denture base
processing
abbreviated rapid p. (ARP)
automatic p.
automatic signal p. (ASP)
darkroom p.
denture p.
digital sound p. (DSP)

discourse p.
film p.
language p.
quick p.
rapid manual p. (RMP)
reticulation p.
p. stain
p. tank
p. wax
processor
Hope p.
input signal p. (ISP)
Mini speech p.
output signal p. (OPS, OSP)
Procomat small-tank
semiautomatic p.
time domain signal p. (TDSP)
processor-machine performance test
processus, pl. processus
p. alveolaris
p. cochleariformis
procheilia, prochilia
procheilon
prochlorperazine
Procide 14, 30
proclination
p. of incisor
procollagen
Procomat small-tank semiautomatic
processor
Procort
ProcoSol
P. sealer
Procrustes rotation
proctocolpoplasty
proctocystoplasty
proctoelytroplasty
proctoperineoplasty
proctoperineorrhaphy
proctoplasty
procumbency
procurrent laterotrusion
Pro-Dentx
P.-D. Home Fluoride
product
Aesthetica C topical vitamin C
skin care p.
Aqua Glycolic skin care p.
BIONÍQ skin care p.
blood p.
DERMED specialty skin care p.
DERMESS specialty skin care p.

NOTES

P

product *(continued)*
　　GlyMed Plus skin care p.
　　Humatrix Microclysmic skin
　　　care p.
　　levo-tryptophan-containing p.
　　　(LTCP)
　　M.D. Forté glycolic-based skin
　　　care p.
　　Nouvisage transdermal beauty p.
　　peel p.
　　Physician's Choice skin care p.
　　Prevacare preventative skin care p.
　　Schuknecht p.'s
　　Skintech after laser skin p.
　　Skintech skin care p.
production
　　constricted vocal p.
　　electrical measurement of speech p.
　　speech p.
productive fibrosis
product-moment correlation
Proetz displacement technique
Profen
　　P. II DM
　　P. LA
Profenal Ophthalmic
professional
　　Karigel P.
ProFile
　　P. file
　　P. orifice shaper
　　P. Variable Taper Rotary
　　　Instruments
profile
　　p. esthetics
　　extraoral radiographic
　　　examination p.
　　p. extraoral radiography
　　facial p.
　　Functional Communication P.
　　prognathic p.
　　p. record
　　retrognathic p.
Profilnine Heat-Treated
profilometer
Profil-O-Plastic
　　P.-O.-P. preshaped chin plate
　　P.-O.-P. preshaped midfacial plate
profit
　　neurotic p.
Proform mouth protector
profound
　　p. hearing impairment
　　p. hearing loss
profunda femoris artery (PFA)
profundi
profundus
progenia

progenitor cell
progessiva
　　myositis ossificans p.
Progestasert
progesterone
proglossis
prognathia
prognathic
　　p. profile
prognathism
　　basilar p.
　　bimaxillary p.
　　mandibular p.
　　retromaxilla p.
prognathism/protrusion
　　mandibular p.
　　maxillary p.
prognathometer
prognathous
prognosis
　　dental p.
　　denture p.
Prognostic Value of Imitative and
　　Auditory Discrimination Test
progonoma
　　p. of jaw
Prograf
program
　　ENZA laser skin care p.
　　Muma Assessment P. (MAP)
　　NaturaLase holistic skin care p.
　　Obagi Nu-Derm skin care p.
　　Oral Therapy Control P.
　　Plaque Control P.
　　Rocabado 6×6 p.
　　Starkey matrix p.
programmed therapy
programming
　　articulation p.
progressive
　　p. bone cavity
　　p. condylar resorption (PCR)
　　p. extraction
　　p. hemifacial atrophy
　　p. relaxation
　　p. spinal muscular atrophy of
　　　childhood
　　p. systemic sclerosis
　　p. temporomandibular joint
　　　remodeling
　　p. vowel assimilation
project
　　Hear Now research p.
projection
　　p. attachment
　　axial p.
　　bregma-menton p.
　　Chausse III p.

coronal oblique p.
cross-sectional p.
enamel p.
extradental p.
frontal p.
horizontal p.
lateral p.
lateral jaw p.
mental p.
occlusal p.
orthogonal p.
reverse topographic p.
Rungstrom p.
sagittal p.
Schüller p.
Stenvers p.
tangential p.
tip p.
topographic p.
Towne p.
transorbital p.
transverse p.
p. of vermilion
projective technique
projector
prolabial
p. unwinding flap method
prolabium
Prolamine
prolapse
axoplasmic p.
Prolene
P. mesh closure
P. mesh sheet
P. mesh silo
P. stitch
P. suture
proliferating cell nuclear antigen (PCNA)
proliferation
chondrocyte p.
clonal p.
epithelial p.
gingival p.
lymphoepithelial p.
perifascicular p.
tumefactive cartilage p.
p. zone
proliferative
p. gingivitis
p. inflammatory zone
p. phase

proline
prolongation
axillary p.
Proloprim
ProMedyne-D
promenton
Prometh
P. VC Plain Liquid
P. VC with Codeine
promethazine
meperidine and p.
p. and phenylephrine
P. VC Plain Syrup
P. VC Syrup
promethazine, phenylephrine, and codeine
Promethist with Codeine
prominarius
prominence
canine p.
laryngeal p.
malar p.
maxillary p.
root p.
prominent
p. ear
p. lobule
promontory
p. stimulation test (PST)
prompt
prompting
pronasale
pronasion
pronator
p. quadratus muscle
p. teres muscle
prone jackknife position
prong
pronglike excementosis
pronoun
anaphoric p.
exophoric p.
pronounce
Pron-Pillo head positioning device
pronunciation
prop
mouth p.
Oberto mouth p.
Propacet
Propagest
proparacaine

NOTES

P

proper
- pulp p.
- temporal fascia p.
- temporalis fascia p. (TFP)

properant

properdin

prophy
- p. angles

Prophy Choice polishing powder

prophylactic
- p. angles
- antiviral p.
- p. dentistry
- p. drug
- p. odontotomy
- p. orthodontics
- p. paste

prophylactodontics

prophylaxis, pl. prophylaxes
- antibiotic p.
- dental p.
- oral p.
- oral antimicrobial p.
- tetanus p.
- tuberculosis p.

Propine Ophthalmic

propionate
- clobetasol p.
- fluticasone p.

Propionibacterium
- P. acnes
- P. avidum

Proplast
- P. allograft
- P. implant

Proplast-Teflon
- P.-T. disk implant
- P.-T. material

Proplex
- P. SX-T
- P. T

propofol
- p. anesthesia

proportion

proportional
- p. facial analysis
- p. limit

proposition

propositional speech

Pro-Post System

propoxyphene
- p. and acetaminophen
- p. and aspirin
- p. HCl
- p. napsylate

propranolol

propria
- lamina p.
- tunica p.

proprioception

proprioceptive
- p. feedback
- p. perception

proprioceptor

proptosis
- p. bulbi

proptotic globe

propulsor

propylene
- fluorinated ethylene p. (FEP)

propylhexedrine

propylthiouracil

propyphenazone

Prorex

Proscar

prosencephalon

ProSeries laparoscopic laser system

prosodeme

prosodic
- p. feature of loudness
- p. feature of pitch

prosody

Prosonic
- Everbest P.

prosopagnosia

prosopospasm

prostaglandin
- p. E (PGE)
- p. E$_2$
- p. F (PGF)

Prostaphlin

prostatic adenocarcinoma

prosthesis, pl. prostheses
- alloplastic p.
- Armstrong p.
- articulated chin p.
- auricular p.
- bisque-baked p.
- Bivona-Colorado voice p.
- Blom-Singer tracheoesophageal p.
- Blom-Singer voice p.
- cement-retained p.
- cleft palate p.
- cochlear p.
- complete denture p.
- p. contourer
- cranial p.
- custom total alloplastic TMJ reconstruction p.
- definitive p.
- dental p.
- dual-chambered p.
- duckbill voice p.
- Dynaflex p.

extraoral p.
facial p.
feeding p.
fixed bridge p.
fixed expansion p.
glottic p.
hybrid p.
implant-borne p.
KD chin p.
Kent-Vitek mandibular p.
Lezinski Flex-HA PORP ossicular
  chain p.
low-pressure voice p.
mandibular guide p.
mandibular guide-plane p.
Mangat curvilinear chin p.
maxillary p.
maxillofacial p.
metal bucket-handle p.
mouthstick p.
natural-feel breast p.
ocular p.
ossicular p.
overdenture-retained p.
overlay p.
palatal p.
Panje p.
partial denture p.
partial ossicular replacement p.
periodontal p.
piston stapes p.
polytetrafluoroethylene p.
provisional p.
Provox voice p.
PTFE p.
removable expansion p.
Robinson stapes p.
screw-retained p.
screw-type implant p.
self-centering p.
shaft p.
silicone gel p.
Singer-Blom p.
single-chambered saline Becker p.
Steri-Oss dental p.
surgical p.
swing-lock p.
Techmedica p.
telescopic p.
temporary p.
total alloplastic TMJ
  reconstruction p.

total ossicular p. (TOP)
total ossicular replacement p.
tracheoesophageal p. (TEP)
UCLA-type-retained p.
Ultra Low resistance voice p.
voice p.
wire-Gelfoam p.
wire-vein p.

prosthesis-mediated mastication
prosthetic
p. appliance
p. dentistry
p. dentition
p. gingiva
p. implant
p. integration
p. restoration

prosthetics
complete denture p.
dental p.
denture p.
facial p.
full denture p.
maxillofacial p.
partial denture p.

prosthetist
prosthion
prosthodontia
prosthodontic
p. care
p. reconstruction

prosthodontics
complete p.
crown and bridge p.
fixed p.
fixed bridge p.
maxillofacial p.
partial p.
removable p.

prosthodontist
Fellow of the American College
of P.'s

protease
ProTech instrument protection tray
protection
barrier p.
radiation p.

protective
p. eyeglasses
p. eyewear
p. stage

Protec-top

NOTES

P

protector
>autogenous corneal p.
>Breast Implant P. (B.I.P.)
>Elmex P.
>hearing p.
>plastic corneal p.
>port p.

Protect.Point needle
Protégé Plus microscope
protein
>p.-2
>antibacterial p.
>BMP-2 p.
>bone morphogenetic p. (BMP)
>bone morphogenic p. (BMP)
>bone morphogenic p.-2 (BMP-2)
>calcium-binding p.
>cyclin D1 p.
>iron-binding p.
>mouse serum p. (MSP)
>mouse urine p. (MUP)
>nuclear matrix p.
>perilymph p.
>pigeon serum p. (PSP)
>purified bone morphogenetic p.
>rat serum p. (RSP)
>rat urine p. (RUP)
>recombinant human bone
> morphogenetic p. (rhBMP-2)
>salivary p.
>SC p.
>T p.

proteinaceous
>p. fluid

proteinase
proteinosis
>lipoid p.

proteins
>heat shock p.

proteoglycan
proteolysis
proteolysis-chelation theory
proteolytic
>p. enzyme
>p. ferment
>p. theory

Proteus
>*P. mirabilis*
>*P. vulgaris*

protocol
>Brånemark restorative p.
>Children's Hospital Medical Center
> sarcoma chemotherapy p.
>inside-job p.
>Kaderavek-Sulzby Bookreading
> Observational P. (KSBOP)
>VPA p.

protocone

protoconid
protolanguage
proton
>p. radiation

Protostat Oral
protoword
protracted
protraction
>mandibular p.
>maxillary p.

protractor
>cephalometric p.

protruded tooth
protruding
>p. ear
>p. mandible
>p. teeth

protrusion
>alveolodental p.
>bimaxillary p.
>bimaxillary dentoalveolar p.
>double p.
>forward p.
>jaw p.
>lateral p.
>p. lisp
>mandibular p.
>maxillary p.
>maxillary alveolar p.

protrusive
>p. checkbite
>p. condyle
>p. excursion
>p. incisal guide angle
>p. interocclusal record
>p. jaw relation
>p. line
>p. movement
>p. occlusal position
>p. occlusion

protuberance
>Bichat p.
>bony p.
>internal occipital p.
>mental p.

protuberans
>dermatofibroma p.
>dermatofibrosarcoma p.

protympanum
Provera Oral
provider
>dental health care p. (DHCP)

provisional
>p. denture
>p. prosthesis
>p. restoration
>p. splint
>p. splinting

provisionally
p. acceptable device
p. acceptable material
p. accepted dental therapeutic
p. accepted dentifrice
provocation
Brown-Gruss p.
provocative
p. food thyroidectomy
p. test
PROVON
P. antimicrobial lotion soap
Provox
P. tracheoesophageal speaking valve
P. voice prosthesis
proxemics
proxetil
cefpodoxime p.
Proxi-Floss
P.-F. cleaning appliance
P.-F. interproximal cleaner
Proxigel
P. carbamide peroxide bleaching agent
P. Oral
proximal
p. cavity
p. contact
p. contour
p. dental caries
p. hypospadias
p. interphalangeal joint
p. osteotomy
p. space
p. subcontact area (PSCA)
p. surface
p. trimmer
proximally based medial gastrocnemius flap
proximate
p. contact
p. space
p. surface
proximobuccal
proximolabial
proximolingual
proximo-occlusal
prune
Prunus serotina
pruritic
pruritus
Prussak space

Pruzansky classification system
psammoma
psammomatoid ossifying fibroma
psammoosteoid fibroma
Psaume syndrome
PSC
posterior semicircular canal
PSCA
proximal subcontact area
PSE
pidgin Sign English
Entex PSE
Guaifenex PSE
PSEF
psellism
Pseudallescheria boydii
pseudallescheriasis
pseudoagrammatism
pseudoaneurysm
pseudoanodontia
pseudoarthrosis
congenital p.
pseudobinaural hearing aid
pseudobotryomycosis
pseudobulbar paralysis
pseudocapsule
pseudocarcinomatous hyperplasia
Pseudo-Car DM
pseudocholinesterase
pseudochromesthesia
pseudocolumella
pseudocopper cement
pseudocroup
pseudocyst
liponecrotic p.
oil p.
pseudodiverticulosis
pseudoephedrine
acetaminophen and p.
acetaminophen, chlorpheniramine, and p.
acetaminophen, dextromethorphan, and p.
acrivastine and p.
azatadine and p.
brompheniramine and p.
carbinoxamine and p.
chlorpheniramine and p.
dexbrompheniramine and p.
p. and dextromethorphan
diphenhydramine and p.
guaifenesin and p.

NOTES

P

pseudoephedrine *(continued)*
    p. HCl
    p. and ibuprofen
    loratadine and p.
    p. sulfate
    terfenadine and p.
    triprolidine and p.
pseudoepithelioma
    squamous cell p.
pseudoepitheliomatous hyperplasia
Pseudo-Gest Plus Tablet
pseudoglottis
pseudohemophilia
pseudohemoptysis
pseudohernia
pseudoherniated fat
pseudohypacusis, pseudohypoacusis
pseudohyperparathyroidism
pseudohypoparathyroidism
pseudo-Kaposi sarcoma
pseudolaryngeal paralysis
pseudolipocyst
pseudolipoma
    traumatic p.
pseudomacrogenia
pseudomalignant
    p. myositis ossificans
    p. osseous tumor
pseudomelanoma
    pseudometastasizing p.
pseudomembranous
    p. angina
    p. gingivitis
pseudometastasizing pseudomelanoma
Pseudomonas
    P. aeruginosa
    P. mallei
pseudomuscular hypertrophy
pseudomycosis
    bacterial p.
pseudoperitoneum
pseudopocket
pseudopodia
pseudoprognathism
pseudopseudohypoparathyroidism
pseudoptosis
pseudoptotic skin
pseudosarcomatous
    p. carcinoma
    p. fasciitis
    p. fibromatosis
pseudoserous membrane
pseudosmia
pseudostratified
pseudostuttering
pseudotumor
    p. cerebri
    fibro-osseous p. (FOPT)

pseudounipolar neuron
PSG
    polysomnography
PSG-proven OSA
PSI
    Pediatric Speech Intelligibility Test
Psillaki and Appiani crossed external oblique flap and horizontal plication
PSI-TEC aspiration/irrigation platform
psomophagia
Psor-a-set Soap
Psorcon
psoriasis
PSP
    pigeon serum protein
    post space preparation
P&S Shampoo
PST
    promontory stimulation test
psychoacoustics
psychoanalysis
psychoauditory
psychodrama
psychodynamic
psychogalvanic
    p. skin resistance
    p. skin response (PGSR)
    p. skin response audiometry (PGSRA)
psychogenic
    p. aphonia
    p. deafness
    p. disorder
psycholinguistic
    P. Rating Scale
psycholinguistics
psychometry
psychomotor
    p. seizure
psychoneurological
psychopathology
psychophysics
psychosedation
    dental p.
psychosis
    childhood p.
psychosomatic
    p. dentistry
psychotherapy
PTA
    peritonsillar abscess
    posttraumatic amnesia
    pure-tone average
    air PTA
PTAH
    phosphotungstic acid-hematoxylin
ptarmic
ptarmus

pteronyssinus
    Dermatophagoides p.
pteroylglutamic acid
pterygium
    p. axillae
    cervical midline p.
    p. colli
    p. cubitale
    p. digitale
    p. popliteal
pterygoid
    p. hamulus
    p. muscle
    p. nerve
    p. plate
    p. position
    p. process
    p. space
    p. tuberosity
    p. tuberosity of mandible
pterygomandibular
    p. fold
    p. raphe
    p. space
    p. space abscess
pterygomasseteric
    p. sling
    p. sling stripping
pterygomaxillare
pterygomaxillary
    p. buttress
    p. dysjunction
    p. fissure
    p. fossa
    p. notch
    p. separation
    p. space
pterygopalatina
    fossa p.
pterygopalatine
    p. fissure
    p. fossa
    p. ganglion
    p. space
PTFE
    polytetrafluoroethylene
    PTFE-containing implant
    PTFE prosthesis
ptomaine
ptosis
    breast p.
    brow p.

    eyebrow p.
    eyelid p.
    grade I–IV breast p.
ptotic
    p. malar fat pad
PTS
    permanent threshold shift
PTT
    pure-tone threshold
ptyalagogue
ptyalectasis
ptyalin
    α-amylase p.
ptyalism
ptyalocele
ptyalography
ptyalolith
ptyalolithiasis
ptyalolithotomy
P-type reamer
puberphonia
puberty gingivitis
pubic tubercle
pubis
    mons p.
public health dentistry
pucker
    lip p.
PUF
    polyurethane foam
pull
    frenum p.
    p. out
    p. screw
    vector of skin p.
pullback
Pullen-Warner
    P.-W. bolt
    P.-W. split post
pulley
pull-out suture
pull-through
    p.-t. operation
    p.-t. technique
pullularia
pulmonale
    cor p.
Pulmonaria officinalis
pulmonary
    p. artery hypertension (PAH)
    p. disease
    p. embolism

NOTES

P

pulmonary *(continued)*
    p. function test
    p. insufficiency
    p. pressure
pulp
    p. abscess
    aging p.
    p. amputation
    atrophic p.
    p. atrophy
    p. border
    p. calcification
    p. calculus
    p. canal (PC)
    p. canal sealer (PCS)
    P. Canal Sealer EBT sealer
    p. canal therapy
    p. capping
    p. cavity
    p. chamber (PCH)
    p. collagen
    p. core
    coronal p.
    dead p.
    p. death
    dental p.
    p. denticle
    dentinal p.
    p. devitalization
    devitalized p.
    enamel p.
    exposed p.
    p. extirpation
    p. fibrosis
    p. gangrene
    p. horn (PH)
    horn of p.
    hyperactive p.
    p. hyperplasia
    hypersensitive p.
    p. hypersensitivity
    p. injury
    p. involvement
    metaplasia of p.
    microcinematography of the
      dental p.
    p. microcirculation
    p. mummification
    mummified p.
    near p.
    p. necrosis
    necrotic p.
    p. nodule
    nonvital p.
    normal p.
    p. polyp
    p. predentin
    p. pressure

    p. proper
    putrescent p.
    radicular p.
    semivital p.
    p. stone
    p. test
    p. tester
    tooth p.
    transitional p.
    vital p.
    p. vitality
    p. vitality test
pulpa
    p. coronalis
    p. dentis
    p. radicularis
pulpal
    p. abscess
    p. anoxia
    p. circulation
    p. collagen
    p. compatibility
    p. fiber
    p. floor
    p. foramen
    p. granuloma
    p. irritation
    p. lymphocyte
    p. macrophage
    p. microdialysis probe
    p. necrosis
    p. pain
    p. pathophysiology
    p. pathosis
    p. vasculature
    p. wall
pulpalgia
    acute p.
    chronic p.
    hyperreactive p.
    hypersensitive p.
Pulpdent
    P. cavity liner
    P. liquid
    P. syringe
pulpectomize
pulpectomy
    complete p.
    partial p.
pulp horn (PH)
pulpitis
    acute p.
    anachoretic p.
    p. aperta
    caries p.
    chronic p.
    chronic hyperplastic p.
    chronic ulcerative p.

p. clausa
closed p.
generalized p.
hyperplastic p.
hypertrophic p.
incipient p.
irreversible p.
leprous p.
nonpainful p.
open p.
painful p.
partial p.
reversible p.
subacute p.
suppurative p.
total p.
ulcerative p.

pulpless
p. tooth

pulpoaxial (PA)
pulpobuccoaxial (PBA)
pulpodentinal
p. complex
p. membrane

pulpodistal (PD)
pulpodontia
pulpolabial (PLA)
pulpolingual (PL)
pulpolinguoaxial (PLA)
pulpoma
pulpomesial (PM)
pulpoperiapical
p. cyst
p. lesion
p. osteosclerosis
p. pathosis

pulpoperiodontal junction
pulposus
atrophic p.
calcific p.
hyperplastic p.

pulpotomy
complete p.
Cvek-type p.
formocresol p.
partial p.
total p.

pulpstone
pulpy
pulsated voice
pulsatile
p. exophthalmos

p. jet lavage
p. saline irrigation
p. tinnitus

pulsating nasal irrigation
pulsation
Pulsatron unit
pulse
alternating p.
chest p.
glottal p.
p. granuloma
p. oximetry

pulsed
p.-current stimulus
p. cutting mode
p.-dye laser
p. electromagnetic stimulator
(PEMS)
p. tunable dye laser
p. yellow dye laser

PulseDose portable compressed oxygen system
pulsion diverticulum
Pulvertaft weave suture technique
Pulvograft
Dembone demineralized cortical
powder P.
Osteomin Thermo-Ashed bone
powder P.

Pulvules
Co-Pyronil 2 P.
Darvon Compound-65 P.

pumice
oil-free p.
p. paste

pump
ALZET continuous infusion
osmotic p.
Compat enteral feeding p.
dental p.
Gomco p.
InfuO.R. drug delivery p.
Klein p.
peristaltic p.
saliva p.
sodium-potassium p.

pumpkin
punch
Ainsworth p.
backbiting bone p.
backward-biting ostrum p.
biopsy p.

NOTES

P

491

punch *(continued)*
    p. biopsy
    Entrease variable depth p.
    p. graft
    hair transplant p.
    Lewis-Resnik p.
    pin p.
    plate p.
    Rathke p.
    rubber dam p.
    side-biting ostrum p.
    S.S. White p.
    Stough p.
punched-out appearance
punctate parotiditis
puncture
    apical p.
    dental p.
    lumbar p.
    tracheoesophageal p. (TEP)
    transesophageal p. (TEP)
    p. wound
punishment
pupil
    ovoid p.
pupillary response
Puralube Tears Solution
purchase point
pure
    p. agraphia
    p. alexia
    p. aphasia
    p. aphemia
    p. aphrasia
    commercially p. (CP)
    p. end-cutting bur
    p. moment
    p. rotation
    p. tone
    p. tone air-conduction threshold
    p. tone audiogram
    p. tone bone-conduction threshold
    p. translation
    p. vowel
    p. wave
    p. word deafness
pure-tone
    p.-t. audiometer
    p.-t. audiometry
    p.-t. average (PTA)
    p.-t. threshold (PTT)
purified
    p. bone morphogenetic protein
    p. bovine collagen
    p. fibrillar collagen (PFC)
    p. ozokerite
purple cone flower

purpose
    general all p. (GAP)
purpura
    p. fulminans
purse
    shepherd's p.
    p. string mastopexy
pursestring
    p. mastopexy
    p. suture
purse-string suture
pursuit
    saccadic p.
purulence
purulent
    p. apical granuloma
    p. discharge
    p. edema
    p. exudate
    p. exudation
    p. inflammation
    p. otitis media
pus
pushback
    Dorrance palatal p.
    palatal p.
    p. procedure
    p. technique
    V-Y p.
pusher
    band p.
putrefaction
putrescence
putrescent pulp
putrescine
putrid
    p. sore mouth
    p. stomatitis
putty
    DynaGraft p.
    polyvinylsiloxane p.
PVC
    polyvinyl chloride
PVD
    postural vertical dimension
PVNS
    pigmented villonodular tenovagosynovitis
PVP
    polyvinylpyrrolidone
P-V-Tussin
PWA
    person with AIDS
PWS
    port wine stain
PxEx Ophthalmic
pyarthrosis
pycnogenol
Pycopay tooth powder

pyeloplasty
    Anderson-Hynes p.
    capsular flap p.
    Culp p.
    disjoined p.
    Foley Y-plasty p.
    Scardino vertical flap p.
pyknophrasia
pyknosis
pyknotic nucleus
pyocele
pyoderma
    p. gangrenosum
pyogenes
    Staphylococcus p.
    Streptococcus p.
pyogenic
    p. granuloma
pyoptysis
pyorrhea
    p. alveolaris
    paradental p.
    Schmutz p.
pyorrheal
pyramid
    p. cannula
    p. of light

    LySonix TTD Design p.
    nasal p.
    petrous p.
    p. Toomey tip
    truncated tetrahedral p.
pyramidal
    p. eminence
    p. fracture
    p. root
    p. system
    p. tract
    p. tuberosity
    p. tuberosity of palatine bone
pyrethrum
pyriform
    p. aperture
    p. aperture wiring
pyrilamine
    pheniramine, phenylpropanolamine,
      and p.
pyroceram
pyrometer
    furnace p.
pyrophosphatase
Pyroplast
PZM
    pressure zone microphone

NOTES

P

quotient *(continued)*
Romberg q.

speed q.

R

roentgen

root

R forceps

RA

retinoic acid

rabbit

r. bush

r. sniffing exercise

Rabinov cannula

racemic epinephrine

Racer handpiece

rad

roentgen absorbed dose

radar absorbent material (RAM)

radectomy

radial

r. artery

r. forearm flap

R. Jaw biopsy forceps

r. nerve

r. wrinkle

radial-landed design

radiation

background r.

r. caries

r. dewlap

electromagnetic r.

r. film badge

r. fog

homogeneous r.

ionizing r.

r. monitoring

monochromatic r.

r. mucositis

r. necrosis

orthovoltage r.

r. output

r. perturbation

primary r.

r. protection

proton r.

scattered r.

secondary r.

r. shield

solar r.

r. survey

r. therapy

tumoricidal r.

useful r.

whole body r.

x r.

radical

r. complete sphenoethmoidectomy

r. excision

r. exenteration

r. hemimaxillectomy

r. mastectomy

r. mastoidectomy

r. neck dissection (RND)

r. parotidectomy

r. subtotal resection

r. surgery

r. synovectomy

radices (*pl. of* radix)

radiciform

radicis (*gen. of* radix)

radicle

radicula

radicular

r. abscess

r. canal

r. cyst

r. dentin

r. dentinogenesis

r. odontoma

r. pulp

r. retainer

r. retention

radicularis

pulpa r.

radiculogenesis

radiculum

r. appendiciforme

radiectomy

radioactive

r. iodine

r. iodine uptake test

radioallergosorbent test (RAST)

radiodontics

radiodontist

radiogram

radiograph

bisected angle r.

bitewing r.

bregma-menton r.

cephalometric r.

composite r.

contrast r.

density r.

distal oblique molar r.

duplicating r.

extraoral r.

inferior-superior zygomatic arch r.

interproximal r.

intraoral r.

jaw r.

lateral jaw r.

lateral oblique r.

lateral ramus r.

radiograph *(continued)*
    lateral sinus r.
    lateral skull r.
    long-cone r.
    mandibular bicuspid r.
    mandibular cuspid r.
    mandibular cuspid-first bicuspid r.
    mandibular incisor r.
    mandibular molar r.
    maxilla r.
    maxillary bicuspid r.
    maxillary cuspid r.
    maxillary incisor r.
    maxillary molar r.
    maxillary sinus r.
    occlusal cross section r.
    oral r.
    Panelipse panoramic r.
    Panex panoramic r.
    panoramic r.
    Panorex r.
    pantographic r.
    periapical r.
    posteroanterior mandible r.
    posteroanterior sinus r.
    posteroanterior skull r.
    sinus r.
    skull r.
    straight-on r.
    temporomandibular joint r.
    Towne projection r.
    transcranial r.
    transcranial temporomandibular
     joint r.
    transpharyngeal temporomandibular
     joint r.
    verification r.
    Waters view r.
    working r.
    Wrightington wrist r. stage 1, 2,
     3, 4
    zygomatic arch r.
radiographic
    r. apex
    r. cephalometer
    r. duplicator
    r. image processing system
    r. imaging system (RIS)
    r. tooth repair
radiography
    alveolar bone r.
    bitewing intraoral r.
    bregma-menton extraoral r.
    cephalometric r.
    cone cutting r.
    Direct Digital r. (DDR)
    extradental intraoral r.
    extraoral r.

    gingival r.
    intraoral r.
    intraoral source r.
    lateral facial extraoral r.
    lateral head extraoral r.
    lateral jaw r.
    lateral jaw extraoral r.
    mandible r.
    mental extraoral r.
    oblique occlusal intraoral r.
    occlusal film r.
    panoral r.
    panoramic extraoral r.
    periapical intraoral r.
    posteroanterior extraoral r.
    profile extraoral r.
    stereoscopic r.
    stereoscopic extraoral r.
    temporomandibular extraoral r.
    true occlusal topographic
     intraoral r.
    Waters extraoral r.
radioimmunoassay
radioisotope
    r. scan
radiolabeled antibody
radiolabeling
radiolocalization
    gamma probe r. (GPRL)
radiologic
radiologist
radiology
radiolucency
    apical r.
    large r.
    lateral r.
    long-standing r.
    mesial r.
    periapical r.
    r. sclerosis
    vertical extension r.
radiolucent
    r. frame
    r. image
    r. lesion
    r. line
    r. skull
radionecrosis
radionecrotic tissue
radionuclide
    r. imaging
    r. scanning
**radionuclide-labeled red blood cell
  imaging**
radiopacity
    laminated r.
radiopaque
    r. calculus

r. composite resin
r. dye
r. image
r. lesion
r. mass
r. skull

radioresistance
radioresistant
radioresponsive
radiosensitive
radiosensitivity
radiosensitizing drug
radiotherapy
photon r.
radiovisiography (RVG)
R. image
radisectomy
radish
radix, gen. **radicis**, pl. **radices**
R. anchor
r. clinica
r. dentis
r. linguae
r. nasi
Raeder syndrome
RAFF
rectus abdominis free flap
Rafluor
R. topical gel
R. topical solution
ragweed
canyon r.
desert r.
false r.
giant r.
short r.
slender r.
Western r.
rag wheel
ragwort
Rainey Ultra-Flex compression wear
Rainville technique
raiser
pitch r.
raisin
raising bite
rake
r. retractor
r. teeth
RAM
radar absorbent material

rectus abdominis musculocutaneous
RAM flap
RAMCF
rectus abdominis myocutaneous flap
Ramfjord index
rami (*pl. of* ramus)
ramification
apical r.
Ramirez
R. manipulator
R. periosteal elevator
rampant dental caries
rampart
maxillary r.
ramping
lingual r.
palatal r.
Rampton face-bow
Ramsay
R. Hunt facial paralysis
R. Hunt syndrome
ramus, pl. **rami**
angular position of the r.
ascending r.
r. blade
r. blade implant
breadth of mandibular r.
r. endosteal implant
r. frame
height of mandibular r.
r. of jaw
r. of mandible
mandibular r.
r. stripper
random
r. fasciocutaneous flap
r. movement
r. noise
r. pattern flap
r. sample
r. temporoparietal fascial flap
Raney clip
range
audible r.
central speech r.
dynamic r.
r. of frequencies
frequency r.
maximum frequency r.
most comfortable loudness r.
(MCLR)
r. of motion (ROM)

NOTES

R

range *(continued)*
    pitch r.
    sound pressure level r.
    tolerance r.
    vocal r.
ranine
    r. artery
    r. tumor
    r. vein
    r. vein plexus
ranitidine
    r. HCl
    r. hydrochloride
rank
    r. order
    percentile r.
Ranke angle
Rankow and Weisman treatment regimen
ranula
    plunging r.
Ranvier
    R. node
    zone of R.
RAP
    relative average perturbation
raphe
    attenuated media r.
    r. cyst
    horizontal r.
    lateral canthal r.
    lingual r.
    longitudinal r.
    median longitudinal r.
    midpalatine r.
    palatine r.
    pharyngeal r.
    pterygomandibular r.
rapid
    r. body shaper (RBS)
    r. manual processing (RMP)
    r. maxillary expansion (RME)
rapidly
    r. alternating speech perception (RASP)
    r. alternating speech perception test
Rapid Stone
rare
    r. cleft
    r. earth screen
rarefaction
rarefying
    r. pericementitis fibrosa
RAS
    recurrent aphthous stomatitis
Raschkow plexus

rash
    varicelliform r.
    wandering r.
Rasmussen
    fibers of R.
RASP
    rapidly alternating speech perception
    RASP test
rasp
    bone r.
    Fischer nasal r.
    Georgiade r.
    Peet nasal r.
    R-type r.
    snow plow r.
    Stenstrom r.
raspatory
raspberry
    red r.
rasping
    r. action
    bony r.
RAST
    radioallergosorbent test
    screening RAST
rat
    r. dander
    r. serum protein (RSP)
    r. urine protein (RUP)
rate
    alternate motion r. (AMR)
    r. control
    crevicular fluid flow r. (CFFR)
    decay r.
    r. of decay
    DEF r.
    diadochokinetic r.
    DMF r.
    load-deflection r.
    r. of maturation
    peak expiratory flow r. (PEFR)
    periodontal disease r.
    response r.
    salvage r.
    sedimentation r.
    r. of speech
    torque-twist r.
ratemeter
Rathke
    R. pocket
    R. pouch
    R. punch
ratio
    alloy-mercury r.
    clinical crown r.
    clinical root r.
    crown-root r.

R

r. of decayed and filled surfaces (RDFS)
r. of decayed and filled teeth (RDFT)
Holdaway r.
mercury-alloy r.
moment-force r. (M/F)
noise-to-harmonic r. (NHR)
the oronasal acoustic r. (TONAR)
signal-to-noise r. (S/N)
S/N r.
speech-noise r.
support-load r.
s/z r.
T4/T8 r.
water-powder r.
W-P r.

rationalist
r. language theory
r. theory of language

rationalization

rat-tail file

rattle
death r.

rattlesnake

RAU
recurrent aphthous ulcer

Ravocaine

raw score

ray
central r.
r. fungus
gamma r.
roentgen r.
supersonic r.
ultrasonic r.
useful r.

Raynaud phenomenon

RBC
red blood cell

RBM
resorbable blast media
RBM implant

RBS
rapid body shaper

RC
retruded contact
RC position

RC2B paste

RC-Prep

RDA
Registered Dental Assistant

RDF
Adriamycin R.

RDFS
ratio of decayed and filled surfaces

RDFT
ratio of decayed and filled teeth

RDH
Registered Dental Hygienist

RDI
respiratory distress index

reabsorption

Reach
R. ACT fluoride anti-cavity treatment
R. Easy Slide shred-resistant floss
R. Floss Gentle Gum Care dental floss

reactance
inductive r.

reaction
allergic r.
anaphylactoid r.
anticipatory r.
conversion r.
dissociative r.
echo r.
escape r.
Feulgen r.
fibroblastic r.
foreign body giant cell r.
granulomatic r.
Herxheimer r.
homograft r.
idiosyncratic allergic r.
Jarisch-Herxheimer r.
manic r.
obsessive compulsive r.
paranoid r.
periosteal r.
polymerase chain r. (PCR)
r. time (RT)
von Kossa r.
whitegraft r.

reactive
r. hyperostosis
r. hyperplasia
r. lymphoid hyperplasia
r. ossification

reading
choral r.
speech r.

reagumentation

NOTES

Real Ear measurement
realignment rhinoplasty
Rea-Lo
real-time, low-intensity x-ray (RTLX)
real-time spectrograph
reamer
    A-type r.
    B-1, B-2 r.
    D-type r.
    endodontic r.
    engine r.
    engine-driven r.
    Gray flexible intramedullary r.
    G-type r.
    K-r.
    Kerr r.
    Ko-type r.
    K-type r.
    M-type r.
    O-type r.
    Peeso r.
    P-type r.
    quarter-turn r.
    Rispi Micromega r.
    T-type r.
reaming
reanimation
    facial r.
    r. procedure
rear resorption
reattachment
    nonmicrosurgical r.
reauditorization
rebase
rebasing
rebonding
rebound
    r. hyperemia
    r. tenderness
rebuilding
    preprosthetic r.
rebus
recalcification
recalcitrant verruca
recall
    preventive r.
recapitulation
recasting
    sentence r.
receipt vessel
receiver
    air-conduction r.
    bone-conduction r.
receptacle
    C-TUB instrument r.
reception
    speech r. (SR)

receptive
    r. aphasia
    r. deficit
    r. language
    r. language performance
    R. One Word Picture Vocabulary Test (ROWPVT)
    r. vocabulary
Receptive-Expressive
    R.-E. Emergent Language (REEL)
    R.-E. Emergent Language Scale
    R.-E. Observation (REO)
    R.-E. Observation Scale
receptive-expressive
    r.-e. gap
receptor
    acetylcholine r.
    α-adrenergic r.
    β-adrenergic r.
    antigen r.
    epidermal growth factor r.
    irritative r.
    juxtacapillary r.
    pain r.
    r. potential
    pressure r.
    sensory r.
    stretch r.
recess
    elliptical r.
    facial r.
    frontal r.
    nasal r.
    palatine r.
    pharyngeal r.
    sphenoethmoidal r.
    spherical r.
    tubotympanic r.
    zygomatic r.
recessed rest
recession
    bone r.
    gingival r.
    pathologic r.
recessional line
recidivist
recipient
    renal allograft r.
    r. vessel
reciprocal
    r. anchorage
    r. arm
    r. arm clasp
    r. assimilation
    r. force
    r. innervation

reciprocation
    active r.
    passive r.
recirculation
    instrument r.
recliner
    Lumex r.
recognition
    oral form r.
    speech r.
recoil
    elastic r.
recombinant
    r. DNA vaccine
    r. erythropoietin
    r. human (rHu, rH)
    r. human bone morphogenetic
      protein (rhBMP-2)
Recombivax HB
reconditioning
reconstruction
    AL r.
    alar r.
    alloplastic r.
    areolar r.
    bell flap nipple r.
    bony r.
    breast r.
    buttress r.
    chondrocutaneous flap for ear r.
    circumferential esophageal r.
    columellar r.
    composite mandibular r.
    costochondral graft r.
    dermal pouch r.
    epiglottic r.
    esthetic breast r.
    extended lateral arm free flap for
      head/neck r.
    facial paralysis r. with rectus
      abdominis muscle
    free bone r.
    free-flap r.
    free-tissue transfer r.
    Goldman nasal tip r.
    gracilis myocutaneous vaginal r.
    hemimandible r.
    implant/flap r.
    laryngotracheal r. (LTR)
    latissimus dorsi breast r.
    long-bone r.
    mandibular functional r.

    maxillofacial r.
    nasal septa r.
    neoglottic r.
    neurovascular infrahyoid island flap
      for tongue r.
    nipple-areolar r.
    orbital rim r.
    orofacial r.
    ossicular chain r.
    palate r.
    papillary r.
    pedicled jejunal r.
    peg latissimus dorsi flap breast r.
    perineal r.
    pharyngoesophageal r.
    physiological r.
    r. plate
    posttraumatic r.
    primary thumb r.
    prosthodontic r.
    secondary ear r.
    septal r.
    sequential bilateral breast r.
    smile r.
    soft tissue r.
    staged r.
    static r.
    subpectoral r.
    sural island flap for foot and
      ankle r.
    TAL breast r.
    total autogenous latissimus breast r.
    tracheal r.
    transmandibular r.
    tubular r.
    urethral r.
    vaginoperineal r.
    vulvovaginal r.
    Zisser-Madden method upper lip r.
reconstructive
    r. cell/polymer construct
    r. dentistry
    r. hand surgeon
    r. mammaplasty
    r. preprosthetic surgery
recontouring
    gingival r.
    occlusal r.
record
    r. base
    centric interocclusal r.
    centric maxillomandibular r.

R

NOTES

record *(continued)*
    centric occluding relation r.
    chew-in r.
    3D r.
    dental r.
    eccentric interocclusal r.
    eccentric maxillomandibular r.
    face-bow r.
    functional chew-in r.
    interocclusal r.
    jaw relation r.
    lateral check-bite interocclusal r.
    lateral interocclusal r.
    maxillomandibular r.
    occluding centric relation r.
    preextraction r.
    preoperative r.
    problem-oriented medical r.
    (POMR)
    profile r.
    protrusive interocclusal r.
    r. rim
    rim r.
    terminal jaw relation r.
    three-dimensional r.
recorder
    Sony video r.
    Visipitch TM digital tape r.
recovery
    creep r.
    silver r.
    spontaneous r.
recovery-enhanced thermography
recrudescence
recrudescent abscess
recruitment
    complete r.
    incomplete r.
    Metz test for loudness r.
    partial r.
    r. response
    r. test
recrystallized kaolinite abrasive
recta
    Wolinella r.
Rectal
    RMS R.
rectangular
    r. collimation
    r. wire
recti
    diastasis r.
rectification
rectify
rectoperineorrhaphy
rectoplasty
rectosigmoid neocolpopoiesis (RSC)

rectus
    r. abdominis free flap (RAFF)
    r. abdominis muscle
    r. abdominis muscle flap
    r. abdominis musculocutaneous
    (RAM)
    r. abdominis myocutaneous flap
    (RAMCF)
    Campylobacter r.
    r. capitis muscle
    r. fascia
    r. femoris muscle
    r. labii muscle
    r. medialis muscle
    r. muscle of eyeball
    r. superioris muscle
    r. turnover flap
    r. turnover repair
recumbent position
recurrens
    periadenitis mucosa necrotica r.
recurrent
    r. aphtha
    r. aphthous stomatitis (RAS)
    r. aphthous ulcer (RAU)
    r. bacterial adenoiditis
    r. dental caries
    r. empyema
    r. ganglion
    r. gingivitis
    r. herpetic stomatitis
    r. infection
    r. laryngeal nerve (RLN)
    r. laryngeal nerve paralysis
    r. pleomorphic adenoma (RPA)
    r. respiratory papillomatosis
    r. scarring aphtha
    r. squamous cell carcinoma
    r. ulcerative stomatitis
recurvatum
recycling
RED
    rigid external distraction
    RED system rigid external
    distractor
red
    r. alder
    r. ant
    r. birch
    r. blood cell (RBC)
    r. cedar
    r. clover
    r. copper cement
    R. Cross Canker Sore medication
    r. flare
    r. maple
    r. mulberry
    r. raspberry

r. rubber endotracheal tube
r. stone
r. zone of lip
Reddick/Saye Lav-1 irrigating and aspirating probe
redeviation
redistribution
redo
redroot pigweed
redtop A grass
reduced
r. enamel epithelium
r. glans
r. glutathione
r. interarch distance
r. interarch distance overclosure
r. screening audiometry
reduction
alar base r.
anterior displacement no r. (ADNR)
anterior displacement with r. (ADWR)
appropriate r.
bilateral asymmetric turbinate volume r.
breast r.
closed r.
cluster r.
crural foot r.
r. genioplasty
interproximal r.
INTRA angled surgical handpiece, 1:1 speed r.
INTRA angled surgical handpiece, 1:2 speed r.
INTRA straight surgical handpiece, 1:1 speed r.
INTRA surgical handpiece, 4:1 speed r.
INTRA surgical shank 1:1 speed r.
INTRA surgical shank 30:1 speed r.
laser festoon r.
Lejour breast r.
r. mammaplasty
open r.
surgical tongue r.
syllable r.
T-breast r.
r. tuberosity

tuberosity r.
unilateral turbinate volume r.
reduction/advancement genioplasty
reduction-augmentation procedure
redundancy
eyelid r.
redundant
r. abdominal apron
r. tissue
reduplicated babbling
reduplication
Redutemp
redwood
reed
r. canary grass
common r.
r. instrument theory
Reed-Sternberg cell
REEL
Receptive-Expressive Emergent Language
REEL scale
Rees
R. dermatome
R. face lift scissors
reexploration
reference
acoustically specified neutral r.
articulatory specified neutral r.
planes of r.
standard r.
r. zero level
referent
referential
r. function
r. semantics
referred
r. otalgia
r. pain
r. pulp pain
reflected wave
reflecting mucosa
reflection
mucobuccal r.
reflex
acoustic contralateral r.
acoustic ipsilateral r.
acousticopalpebral r.
acoustic stapedial r.
r. arc
audito-oculogyric r.
auditory oculogyric r.

NOTES

reflex *(continued)*
    auricular r.
    auriculopalpebral r.
    auropalpebral r. (APR)
    Babinski r.
    Bell r.
    cochlear r.
    cochleo-orbicular r.
    cochleopalpebral r. (CPR)
    cochleostapedial r.
    conditioned orientation r. (COR)
    consensual r.
    corneal r.
    r. cough
    cough r.
    deglutition r.
    direct light r.
    faucial r.
    flexion r.
    flexion-extension r.
    gag r.
    gustatory r.
    Hering-Breuer r.
    intra-aural muscle r.
    jaw r.
    Kisch r.
    labyrinthine righting r.
    laryngeal r.
    laryngospastic r.
    light r.
    mandibular r.
    masticatory r.
    middle ear muscle r.
    Moro r.
    myotatic r.
    nasal r.
    nasomental r.
    oculocardiac r.
    olfactory r.
    orienting r. (OR)
    r. otalgia
    palatal r.
    palatine r.
    pharyngeal r.
    phasic stretch r.
    r. phenomenon
    round window r.
    sensitivity prediction from the
     acoustic r. (SPAR)
    single lens r. (SLR)
    stapedial acoustic r.
    stapedius r.
    startle r.
    stretch r.
    swallowing r.
    r. sympathetic dystrophy (RSD)
    r. time
    tonic vibration r. (TVR)

    trigeminal-facial nerve r.
    trigeminal-vagal r.
    vestibular r.
    vestibulo-ocular r. (VOR)
    vestibulo-oculomotor r.
    vomiting r.
reflux
    gastroesophageal r.
    r. otitis media
    sialo-acinar r.
reformulation
refracted wave
refraction
refractory
    r. cast
    r. flask
    r. investment
    r. period
refracture
Refresh Plus Ophthalmic Solution
regainer
    coil spring space r.
    r. space
    split acrylic spring space r.
regainer-maintainer
    jacket r.-m.
    jackscrew r.-m.
regeneration
    axon r.
    bony r.
    guided bone r. (GBR)
    guided tissue r. (GTR)
REGENTEX GBR-200
regimen
    Furstenberg r.
    Rankow and Weisman treatment r.
regio, pl. **regiones**
    r. buccalis
    r. submandibulare
    r. submaxillaris
    r. submentalis
    r. temporalis
region
    buccal r.
    cervicomastoid r.
    facial r.'s
    femoral artery-saphenous bulb r.
    frontal r.
    frontoparietal r.
    gingivobuccal r.
    glottal r.
    hypervariable r.
    infraorbital r.
    jugulodigastric r.
    labial r.
    malar-zygomatic r.
    mental r.
    mylohyoid r.

parasymphyseal r.
retromolar trigone r.
sphenopetroclival r.
sternocleidomastoid r.
subantral r.
submandibular r.
submaxillary r.
submental r.
temporal r.
trigone r.
zygomaticofrontal r.
zygomaticomaxillary r.

regional
r. anesthesia
r. blocking anesthesia technique
r. dialect
r. disease
r. flap
r. lymph node
r. muscle transfer
r. odontodysplasia

regiones (*pl. of* regio)

register
language r.
loft r.
Salivary Gland R.
vocal r.
voice r.

registered
R. Dental Assistant (RDA)
R. Dental Hygienist (RDH)

registration
functional occlusal r.
maxillomandibular r.
occlusal r.
tissue r.

registry
National Temporal Bone, Hearing and Balance Pathology r.

Regnault
R. abdominoplasty
R. classification

Regranex gel

regression
calcific r. of pulp
focal calcific r. of pulp
phonemic r.

regressive
r. assimilation
r. temporomandibular joint remodeling

regular
r. body impression material
r. determiner
Esoterica R.
R. Strength Bayer Enteric 500 Aspirin

regulated waste

regulating appliance

regulator
Ohmeda continuous vacuum r.
Ohmeda thoracic suction r.
Vacutron suction r.

regurgitation
nasal r.

rehabilitation
aural r.
mouth r.
occlusal r.
oral r.
oromandibular r.
osseointegrated implant r.
speech r.
vestibular r.
vocal r.
voice r.

rehabilitative audiology

reherniation
r. after repair

Reichert Histo-Stat cryostat

Reid base line

Reiger procedure

reimplant

reimplantation
intentional tooth r.

reinforced anchorage

reinforcement
differential r.
partial r.
primary r.
r. schedule

reinforcer
conditioned r.
delayed r.
generalized r.
negative r.
positive r.
primary r.
secondary r.
unconditioned r.

Reinke
R. edema
R. space

NOTES

R

reinnervate
reinnervation
reinsertion
> ligament r.
> maxillary removal and r.

Reissner membrane
Reiter syndrome
rejuvenation
> complete facial r.
> facial r.
> surgical r.
> upper face r.

ReJuveness
> R. pure silicone sheeting
> R. scar treatment

Rekow system
Relafen
relapsing
> r. perichondritis
> r. polychondritis

relation
> acentric r.
> acquired centric r.
> acquired eccentric r.
> acquired eccentric jaw r.
> alar-columella r.
> buccolingual r.
> case r.
> centric jaw r.
> centric occluding r.
> convenience jaw r.
> cusp-fossa r.
> dynamic r.
> eccentric r.
> eccentric jaw r.
> intermaxillary r.
> jaw r.
> jaw-to-jaw r.
> lateral occlusion r.
> mandibular centric r.
> maxillomandibular r.
> median jaw r.
> median retruded r.
> occluding r.
> occlusal r.
> posterior border jaw r.
> protrusive jaw r.
> rest jaw r.
> retruded jaw r.
> ridge r.
> semantic r.
> static r.
> unstrained jaw r.
> vertical r.
> working bite r.

relational word
relationship
> abnormal occlusal r.

> buccolingual r.
> occlusal r.
> overbite/overjet r.
> tissue-base r.
> upper tooth to upper lip r.

relative
> r. average perturbation (RAP)
> r. generalized macrodontia
> r. generalized microdontia
> r. pocket
> r. quantity

relativity
> linguistic r.

relator
> orthognathic occlusal r.

relaxant
> muscle r.

relaxation
> differential r.
> r. difficulty
> progressive r.
> r. time

relaxed skin tension line (RSTL)
release
> Agee carpal tunnel r.
> carpal tunnel r. (CTR)
> chordee r.
> Concept CTS Relief Kit for carpal tunnel r.
> direct-vision carpal tunnel r.
> endoscopic carpal tunnel r. (ECTR)
> galea-frontalis-occipitalis r.
> Guyon canal r.
> laryngeal r.
> open carpal tunnel r. (OCTR)
> periosteal r.
> pre-periosteal tissue r.
> retro-orbicularis fat pad r.
> single-portal endocarpal tunnel r.
> syndactyly r.

releasing consonant
reliability
> r. coefficient

relief
> r. area
> r. chamber
> gingival r.
> r. incision
> R. Ophthalmic Solution
> r. space
> Tylenol Extended R.
> Vicks DayQuil Sinus Pressure & Congestion R.

reliever
> Arthritis Foundation Pain R.
> Cama Arthritis Pain R.

relieving incision

reline
r. material
reliner
Hydro-Cast denture r.
Just Treatment r.
Re-Stor r.
relining
relocation
Barsky alar cartilage r.
Brown and McDowell alar
cartilage r.
Erich alar cartilage r.
Humby alar cartilage r.
rem
roentgen-equivalent-man
remargination
remeasurement
remifentanil
remineralization
remission
remnant
enamel organ r.
remodeling
adaptive temporomandibular joint r.
bone r.
peripheral temporomandibular
joint r.
progressive temporomandibular
joint r.
regressive temporomandibular
joint r.
remounting
removable
r. bridge
r. bridgework
r. denture
r. expansion prosthesis
r. lingual arch
r. maintainer space
r. orthodontic appliance
r. partial denture
r. prosthodontics
r. space maintainer
removal
foreign body r.
hump r.
intracapsular tumor r.
medial-to-lateral tumor r.
r. mesh silo
paste r.
path of r.
point r.

post r.
tattoo r.
wire r.
remover
anterior band r. (ABR)
band r.
crown r.
Crown-A-Matic crown and
bridge r.
Dr Scholl's Wart R.
foreign body r.
Morrell crown r.
Off-Ezy Wart R.
WaxBuster wax r.
remyelination
Renaissance
R. crown
R. Crown system
R. spirometry system
renal
r. allograft recipient
r. cell carcinoma
r. transplant
Renamel
Renata battery
Rendu-Osler-Weber disease
renewal
Renova
R. cream
REO
Receptive-Expressive Observation
REO scale
reoperation
bilateral coronal synostosis r.
metopic synostosis r.
sagittal synostosis r.
repair
r. of alveolar ridge defect
anatomic r.
Brand tendon r.
calvarial r.
cemental r.
cleft palate r.
columellar r.
commissure r.
dog-ear r.
epineurial r.
functional r.
histologic tooth r.
hypospadias one-stage r.
Langenbeck r.
LeMesurier r.

NOTES

repair *(continued)*
>Millard bilateral cleft lip r.
>oral-nasal/oral-antral fistula r.
>pants-over-vest muscle r.
>periapical tooth r.
>radiographic tooth r.
>rectus turnover r.
>reherniation after r.
>r. resin
>Tennison r.
>tension-free r.
>trunk-to-trunk r.
>vascularized double-sided preputial island flap and W flap glanuloplasty hypospadias r.
>Veau-Wardill-Kilner r.
>von Langenbeck r.
>V-Y r.
>Wardill-Kilner V-Y palatal r.

repaired lacuna
reparative
>r. dentin
>r. giant cell granuloma

repeat
>r. open reduction internal fixation
>r. ORIF

repeater
reperfusion injury
repetition
replace
>R. implant system
>R. system tapered implant

replaced tooth
replacement
>Bioplant HTR-24 synthetic bone r.
>cervical skin r.
>glottal r.
>hard tissue r. (HTR)
>head-neck r. (HNR)
>mucosal patch r.
>ossicular r.
>P.C.A. E-Series hip r.
>single-stage r.

replant
replantation
>intentional r.

replica
replication
>Hayflick limit of fibroblast r.

replicator
>gnathic r.

reposition
repositioning
>auricular r.
>gingival r.
>jaw r.
>muscle r.

representational gesture

representative sample
repress
repressed need theory
requesting
>prelinguistic r.

required arch length
RER
>rough endoplasmic reticulum

rerouting
>facial nerve r.

Resaid
Rescaps-D S.R. Capsule
Rescon Liquid
Rescudose
>Roxanol R.

Rescue Squad topical gel
research
>comparative r.

resectability
resection
>abdominoperineal r.
>bone r.
>composite r.
>corrugator r.
>corrugator muscle r.
>craniofacial r.
>en bloc r.
>epidermoid r.
>gum r.
>interdental r.
>levator r.
>marginal mandibular r.
>Mohs r.
>oncologic mandibular r.
>parotid r.
>partial dural r.
>radical subtotal r.
>root end r.
>septal r.
>skull base tumor r.
>submucous r. (SMR)
>total upper lip r.
>tracheal window r.
>transoral r.

reserve
>r. air
>r. cell
>r. cell zone
>cochlear r.
>r. fat
>r. fat of Illouz
>r. tooth germ

reservoir
>internal fill r.

reshaping
residual
>r. adhesive
>r. air

r. carious dentin
r. chordee
r. cyst
r. dental arch
r. dental caries
r. dyskinetic peristalsis
r. expressive language deficit
r. fat
r. focal osteitis
r. inhibition
r. inhibitor
r. moment
r. monomer
r. ridge
r. senile ectropion
r. skin
r. speech
r. stress
r. volume (RV)
residue
resilience
    dynamic r.
resiliency
resilient liner
resin
acrylic r.
activated r.
r. adhesive
r. analogon
Aurafil r.
auto-cured r.
autopolymer r.
autopolymerizing acrylic r.
bis-GMA r.
Bondeze r.
Bowen r.
Celay Tech light curing r.
r. cement
Charisma r.
chemically cured composite r.
cold cure r.
cold-curing r.
Command Ultrafine r.
composite r.
Concise r.
r. condensation
copolymer r.
crown and bridge r.
cyanoacrylate r.
dental r.
dentin/enamel bonding r.
denture base r.

Dexter clear polyester casting r.
diacrylate r.
dimethacrylate r.
direct filling r.
Directon r.
dual-cure r.
dual-cured luting composite r.
Durafill bonding r.
Duralay inlay r.
Dynabond r.
Endur r.
epoxy r.
Epoxy Die r.
Estilux r.
r. filler
Genie r.
r. hardening time
heat-curing r.
Heliosit r.
hybrid composite r.
hydrophilic acrylic r.
light-activated r.
light-cured r.
light-curing r.
lingual r.
macrofilled r.
r. matrix
microfilled composite r.
Nuvaseal r.
Nuva-Tach r.
orthodontic r.
Orthomite r.
photocured composite r.
polycarbonate r.
polyhexanide methacrylate r.
quick cure r.
radiopaque composite r.
repair r.
resorcinol-formaldehyde r.
r. restoration
restorative r.
Riebler r.
self-curing r.
r. shell matrix
Slux r.
small particle composite r.
Solo-Tach r.
ultraviolet light-polymerized r.
unbonded r.
unfilled r.
urethane dimethacrylate luting
    composite r.

R

NOTES

resin *(continued)*
Visioform light-curing r.
Zapit r.
resin-bonded bridge
resistance
abrasion r.
anchorage r.
r. form
galvanic skin r.
hardness r.
host r.
nasal airway r.
psychogalvanic skin r.
solubility r.
r. welding
resistant tube
resistentiae
locus minoris r.
resistor
resolution
resonance
r. disorder
facilitation of r.
nasal r.
nuclear magnetic r. (NMR)
pharyngeal r.
r. theory of hearing
vocal r.
voice disorders of r.
resonant
r. frequency
r. peak control
resonator
subglottic r.
supraglottic r.
resonatory
resorb
resorbable
r. bilayer collagen membrane
r. blast media (RBM)
r. copolymer PGA/PLLA-Lactosorb
miniplate fixation system
r. plate and screw
r. rigid fixation
r. tricalcium phosphate
resorbed lacuna
resorcinol
resorcinol-formaldehyde resin
resorption
apical root r.
bone r.
r. cell
cemental r.
cementum r.
central r.
compensatory bone r.
crestal r.
external apical root r. (EARR)

external root r.
external tooth r.
extracanalicular r.
frontal r.
frontal bone r.
gingival r.
horizontal r.
idiopathic internal r.
internal root r.
internal tooth r.
intracanalicular r.
r. lacuna
massive r.
osteoclastic r.
r. peri-implantoclasia
pressure r.
progressive condylar r. (PCR)
rear r.
ridge r.
root r.
surface root r.
tooth r.
r. tunnel
undermining r.
unerupted tooth r.
vertical r.
resorptive
r. cell
r. defect
Respaire-120 SR
Respaire-60 SR
Respa-1st
respiration
abdominal-diaphragmatic r.
bronchial r.
clavicular r.
cortical r.
diaphragmatic-abdominal r.
laryngeal r.
nasal r.
opposition r.
oral r.
thoracic r.
respirator
respiratory
r. capacity
r. cilium
r. control mechanism
r. control task
r. disorder
r. distress
r. distress index (RDI)
r. disturbance index
r. epithelium
r. frequency
r. inductive plethysmography (RIP)
r. insufficiency
r. mucosa

R

r. obstruction
r. scleroma
r. stridor
r. syncytial virus
r. system
r. tract
r. tract infection
r. volume

respirometer
respondent conditioning
responder

rotation r.
tilt r.

Respond wire
response

anamnestic r.
audiometric brainstem r. (ABR)
auditory brainstem r. (ABR)
auditory evoked r.
auditory middle latency r.
auditory oculogyric r.
autoimmune r.
brainstem auditory evoked r.
  (BAER)
brainstem evoked r. (BSER)
brainstem evoked auditory r.
  (BEAR)
canal resonance r. (CRR)
catastrophic r.
cell-mediated immune r.
cellular and complex-mediated
  immune r.
conditioned r.
cortical auditory evoked r. (CAER)
covert r.
crestal bone r.
delayed r.
differential r.
evoked r.
false-negative r.
false-positive r.
fixed frequency r. (FFR)
frequency r.
galvanic skin r. (GSR)
generalization r.
r. hierarchy
high-frequency r.
host r.
humoral mediated immune r.
IgE-mediated immune r.
immune r.
inflammatory r.

late auditory evoked r. (LAER)
low-frequency r.
r. magnitude
maladaptive r.
mean length of r. (MLR)
middle latency r. (MLR)
negative r.
overt r.
paradigmatic r.
positive r.
psychogalvanic skin r. (PGSR)
pupillary r.
r. rate
recruitment r.
slow vertex r.
somatosensory r.
r. strength
syntagmatic r.
r. system
target r.
r. time
unconditioned r.
vestibular r.
vibrotactile r.

**Resposable Spacemaker surgical balloon
dissector**
rest

r. angle
r. area
auxiliary implant r.
auxiliary occlusal r.
r. bite
chin r.
cingulum r.
epithelial r.
incisal r.
internal r.
intracoronal r.
r. jaw relation
lingual r.
Malassez epithelial r.'s
occlusal r.
occlusion r.
r. position
precision r.
recessed r.
root r.
r. seat
r. seat area
semiprecision r.
r.'s of Serres
surface r.

NOTES

rest *(continued)*
    r. transient
    r. vertical dimension
restbite
resting
    r. line
    r. potential
Reston
    R. foam dressing
    R. polyurethane foam
    R. sponge
restoration
    acid-etched r.
    adhesive resin bonded cast r.
    after root amputation r.
    alloy r.
    amalgam r.
    bonded cast r.
    buccal r.
    ceramic r.
    ceramo-metal r.
    combination r.
    composite resin r.
    compound r.
    contour r.
    r. contour
    r. crown
    crown r.
    cusp r.
    dental r.
    direct acrylic r.
    direct composite resin r.
    direct gold r.
    direct resin r.
    distal extension r.
    esthetic r.
    facial r.
    facilitating r.
    faulty r.
    full cast r.
    Geristore r.
    implant r.
    IMZ type r.
    inlay r.
    intermediate r.
    Interpore IMZ r.   *Photac-fil*
    large r.
    maxillary r.
    metal-ceramic r.
    metallic r.
    ML-composite r.
    r. overhang
    overhanging r.
    overlay r.
    permanent r.
    pin-supported r.
    porcelain-bonded r.
    porcelain-fused-to-metal r.

    porcelain jacket r.
    postcore r.
    prosthetic r.
    provisional r.
    resin r.
    root canal r.
    silicate r.
    silver amalgam r.
    temporary r.
    r. of vertical dimension
restorative
    r. dental materials
    r. dentistry
    r. fixation
    r. material
    r. procedure
    r. resin
restore
    R. bone implant
    R. close tolerance dental implant system
    R. RBM implant
Re-Stor reliner
restrained
    r. beam
    r. support
restricted syllable structure
restriction
    mandibular r.
restrictive modifier
restructured cell
result
    knowledge of r. (KR)
resurfacing
    endoscopic brow lift with simultaneous carbon dioxide laser r.
    full face laser r.
    island adipofascial flap in Achilles tendon r.
    r. laser
    laser r.
    laser skin r.
    skin r.
resuscitation
    cardiopulmonary r. (CPR)
resuscitator
    Lifemask infant r.
    NeoV0$_2$R volume control r.
resuspend
resuture
resynthesis
    binaural r.
retained
    r. papilla
    r. papilla technique
    r. root

R

retainer
>band and spur r.
>bonded r.
>canine-to-canine bonded r.
>C & L r.
>continuous bar r.
>coping r.
>direct r.
>extracoronal r.
>flexible spiral wire r.
>Hawley r.
>indirect r.
>intracoronal r.
>lingual canine-to-canine r.
>lingual premolar-to-premolar r.
>matrix r.
>multiple r.
>precision r.
>radicular r.
>screw r.
>secondary r.
>space r.
>Tach-E-Z r.
>Tofflemire amalgam matrix r.

retaining
>r. orthodontic appliance
>r. ring

retardation
>idiopathic language r.
>maxillary r.
>mental r.
>perceptual r.

retarded
>r. dentition
>educable mentally r. (EMR)
>mentally r. (MR)

retarDent toothpaste

retarder
>gypsum r.

retarDex oral rinse

rete
>r. pegs

retention
>r. area
>r. area of tooth
>r. arm
>r. bar
>circumferential r.
>r. cyst
>r. denture
>denture r.
>differential r.

>direct r.
>extracoronal r.
>r. form
>frictional wall r.
>r. groove
>r. index
>indirect r.
>intracoronal r.
>intracoronal-extracoronal r.
>limited r.
>linguistic r.
>r. lug
>mechanical r.
>micromechanical r.
>r. mucocele
>partial denture r.
>permanent r.
>r. pin
>pin r.
>pinhole r.
>r. point
>radicular r.
>semipermanent r.
>surgical r.
>terminal r.

retentive
>r. arm
>r. circumferential arm clasp
>r. circumferential clasp arm
>r. clasp
>r. fulcrum line
>r. undercut

Rethi incision

reticular
>r. collagen fiber
>r. lamina
>r. pulp atrophy

reticulation
>r. processing

reticulosis
>malignant r.
>malignant midline r.
>polymorphic r.

reticulum
>agranular r.
>r. cell sarcoma
>endoplasmic r. (ER)
>r. fiber
>granular r.
>rough endoplasmic r. (RER)
>stellate r.

retiform stage

NOTES

Retin-A
    R.-A. cream
retina, pl. **retinae**
    commotio retinae
retinaculotome
    Paine carpal tunnel r.
retinaculum, gen. **retinaculi**, pl. **retinacula**
    retinacula cutis
    endoplasmic r.
    inferior extensor r.
retinae (*pl. of* retina)
retinal
    r. anlage tumor
    r. detachment
    r. tear
retinitis
retinoblastoma
retinoic acid (RA)
retinoid dermatitis
retire
retraction
    r. cord
    r. cord packer
    double cord r.
    gingival r.
    lid r.
    mandibular r.
    maxillary incisor r.
    midlamellar cicatricial r.
    r. pocket
    r. space
retractor
    Army-Navy r.
    Aston nasal r.
    Aston submental r.
    Austin r.
    Bauer r.
    beaver-tail r.
    Bishop r.
    Black r.
    Brinker tissue r.
    cat's paw r.
    cheek r.
    cheek and tongue r.
    Columbia r.
    condylar neck r.
    Converse r.
    corrugated forehead r.
    Cosgrove mitral valve r.
    Cottle nasal r.
    Crowe-Davis mouth r.
    David-Baker eyelid r.
    Deaver r.
    de la Plaza transconjunctival r.
    Desmarres r.
    Dingman r.
    Emory EndoPlastic r.
    endaural r.
    ESI light-weight, narrow mammaplasty r.
    ESI long, narrow mammaplasty r.
    ESI mammary r.
    extraoral sigmoid notch r.
    Gerow-Harrington r., heart-shaped distal end
    Hardy r.
    Hurd pillar r.
    Jannetta r.
    Johnson cheek r.
    LeVasseur-Merrill r.
    Levy articulating r.
    lid r.
    lip r.
    Love r.
    mandibular body r.
    middle fossa r.
    Minnesota r.
    Moorehead r.
    multiprong rake r.
    one-piece lip r.
    orbicular r.
    palate r.
    periareolar r.
    rake r.
    ribbon r.
    Seldin r.
    self-retaining r.
    Senn r.
    Senn-Miller r.
    Shuman r.
    sigmoid notch r.
    spring-loaded self-retaining r.
    Tebbets ribbon r.
    Terino facial implant r.
    tongue r.
    transconjunctival r.
    University of Minnesota r.
    vein hook r.
    Walden-Aufrecht nasal r.
    Weitlaner r.
    Wieder r.
retraining
    neuromuscular r.
retreatment
retrieval
retriever
    Caulfield r.
    silver point r.
retroactive amnesia
retroareolar mass
retroarticular cushion
retroauricular
    r. artery
    r. free flap
    r. hair step
    r. lymph node

r. skin
r. vein
retrobuccal
retrobulbar
r. abscess
r. neuritis
retrocele
retroclination
retrocochlear
r. deafness
retrocuspid papilla
retrocuticular fissure
retrodiscal pad
retrodisplaced maxillae
retrodisplacement
conchal r.
retrofacial
r. air cell
r. cell
retrofill
retrofilling
r. method
retroflex
r. sound
r. vowel
retrogenia
paradoxic r.
retrognathia
inferior r.
mandibular r.
maxillary r.
superior maxillary r.
retrognathic
r. mandible
r. profile
retrognathism
bird-face r.
mandibular r.
retrognathism/retrusion
mandibular r./r.
retrograde
r. amalgam
r. approach
r. dissection
r. filling
r. jugular venography
r. obturation
r. root canal filling method
r. venous drainage
retrogressive
retrojection

retrolabyrinthine
r. approach
r. neurectomy
r. vestibular neurectomy (RVN)
retrolabyrinthine/retrosigmoidal
vestibular neurectomy (RRVN)
retrolingual
retromammary
retromammilar mass
retromandibular
r. fossa
r. point
r. triangle
r. vein
retromandibular/submandibular incision
retromastoid craniotomy
retromaxilla prognathism
retromaxillism
retromolar
r. fossa
r. intubation
r. mucosa
r. pad
r. triangle
r. trigone
r. trigone region
retromylohyoid
r. eminence
r. space
retro-orbicularis fat pad release
retropapillary apex
retroparotid lymph node
retropharyngeal
r. abscess
r. edema
r. lymph node
r. space
Retroplast
R. filling
R. resin composite
retroposition
mandibular r.
maxillary r.
retroprep tip
retropulsion
globe r.
retroseptal transconjunctival approach
retrosigmoid
r. approach
r. vestibular neurectomy
retrosigmoid/internal auditory canal
(RSG/IAC)

R

NOTES

retrosigmoid-transmeatal route
retrospective bronchoscopic telescope
retrosternal esophagocolonic anastomotic
　leak
retrotip
　　ultrasonic r.
retrotuberosity
　　r. intubation
　　r. mucosa
retroversion
retrovirus
retrozygomatic space
retruded
　　r. centric
　　r. contact (RC)
　　r. jaw relation
　　r. mandible
　　r. position
retrusion
　　alveolodental r.
　　mandibular r.
　　maxillary r.
　　midfacial r.
retrusive
　　r. excursion
　　r. movement
　　r. occlusion
return impulse
Retzius
　　calcification lines of R.
　　lines of R.
　　space of R.
　　R. striae
reuniens
　　ductus r.
reusable Sorensen 2000 cc canister
reuse life
revascularization
revascularize
revascularized bone graft
Reveal
　　R. MLR+ camera
　　R. single lens reflex camera
reverberation
　　r. room
　　r. time
Reverdin
　　R. graft
　　R. method
　　R. needle
reversal
　　r. line
　　r. pedicle flap
reverse
　　r. archwire
　　r. bevel
　　r. bevel incision
　　r. condenser

　　r. curve
　　r. digital artery flap
　　r. digital artery island flap
　　r. dorsal digital island flap
　　r. facial osteotomy
　　r. filling
　　r. filling procedure
　　r. flaring
　　r. flow island flap
　　r. flow vascularization
　　r. hyperemia
　　r. Karapandzic flap
　　r. Kingsley splint
　　r. medial arm flap
　　r. phonation
　　r. planning
　　r. plugger
　　r. swallowing
　　r. topographic projection
　　r. U-flap
reverse-action clasp
reversed
　　r. digital artery flap
　　r. extensor digitorum muscle island
　　　flap procedure
　　r. fasciosubcutaneous flap
　　r. first dorsal metatarsal artery flap
　　　procedure
　　r. medialis pedis island flap
　　　procedure
reversibility
reversible
　　r. hydrocolloid
　　r. hydrocolloid impression
　　r. hydrocolloid impression material
　　r. pulpitis
Rēv-Eyes
revised
　　r. Salzburg lag screw system
　　R. Token Test
　　r. Würzburg mandibular
　　　reconstruction system
revision
　　r. stapedectomy
　　r. stapes surgery
Rexed
　　lamina of R.
Reynolds and Horton alar cartilage
　technique
rH (*var. of* rHu)
rhabdomyoma
rhabdomyosarcoma
rhagades
Rhamnus purshiana
rhBMP-2
　　recombinant human bone morphogenetic
　　　protein

RHD
    right hemisphere brain damage
Rhein pick
rheobase
rheostat
rheumatic
    r. arthritis
    r. disease
    r. disorder
    r. fever
    r. heart disease
rheumatica
    polymyalgia r.
rheumatoid
    r. arthritis
    r. sialadenitis
Rheumatrex
rhinalgia
Rhinall Nasal Solution
Rhinatate Tablet
Rhindecon
rhinectomy
    total r.
rhinedema
rhinenchysis
rhinism
rhinitis
    acute r.
    allergic r.
    atopic r.
    atrophic r.
    r. caseosa
    r. cholesteatoma
    chronic r.
    exanthematous r.
    gangrenous r.
    hormonal r.
    hypertrophic r.
    r. medicamentosa
    r. nervosa
    R. Quality of Life Questionnaire
    scrofulous r.
    r. sicca
    r. sicca anterior
    vasomotor r.
rhinoanemometer
rhinocanthectomy
rhinocerebral mucormycosis
rhinocerebrophycomycosis
rhinocheiloplasty
rhinocleisis

Rhinocort
    R. nasal inhaler
rhinodacryolith
rhinodynia
rhinofacial entomophthoramycosis
rhinogenous
rhinogram
rhinokyphectomy
rhinokyphosis
rhinolalia
    r. aperta
    r. clausa
Rhinoline endoscopic sinus surgery system
rhinolite
rhinolith
rhinolithiasis
rhinologic
rhinologist
rhinology
rhinomanometer
    Storz r.
rhinomanometry
    anterior active mask r.
rhinometer
    Hood Laboratories Eccovision acoustic r.
    two-microphone acoustical r.
rhinometry
    acoustic r. (AR)
rhinomucormycosis
rhinomycosis
rhinonecrosis
rhinoorbital mucormycosis
rhinoorbitocerebral mucormycosis
rhinopathy
rhinopharyngolith
rhinophonia
rhinophycomycosis
rhinophyma
rhinoplastic surgeon
rhinoplasty
    Bardach cleft r.
    conservative subtraction-addition r. (CSAR)
    endonasal r.
    English r.
    esthetic r.
    extended open-tip r.
    Indian r.
    Italian r.
    Joseph r.

R

NOTES

rhinoplasty *(continued)*
    open r.
    open sky r.
    open structure r.
    realignment r.
    secondary r.
    tension-control suture technique in open r.
    tip r.
Rhino Rocket dressing
rhinorrhea
    caseous purulent r.
    cerebrospinal fluid r.
    CSF r.
    gustatory r.
    halo test for CSF r.
    paradoxical r.
rhinosalpingitis
rhinoscleroma
rhinoscleromatis
    Klebsiella r.
rhinoscope
rhinoscopic
rhinoscopy
    anterior r.
    median r.
    posterior r.
rhinoseptoplasty
rhinosinusitis
    adult r.
    chronic hypertrophic r.
    hyperplastic r.
    pediatric r.
rhinosporidiosis
rhinostenosis
Rhinosyn
    R.-PD Liquid
    R.-X Liquid
Rhinotec shaver
rhinotomy
    r. procedure
rhinovirus
    r. virus
rhizodontropy
rhizodontrypy
rhizoid
Rhizopus
    R. arrhizus
RHLB
    Right Hemisphere Language Battery
RHN
    Rockwell hardness number
rhodamine
    r. B fluorescent dye
    r. B stain
Rhodotorula
rhombencephalon

rhomboid
    r. aponeurosis
    r. transposition flap
rhomboidal crystal
rhotacism
rhotacized vowel
rHu, rH
    recombinant human
rhubarb
rhythm
    alpha r.
    beta r.
    delta r.
    theta r.
rhytid
    periocular r.
    shoulder of r.
    transverse r.
rhytidectomy
    complex superficial musculoaponeurotic system r.
    composite r.
    deep-plane r.
    extended posterior r.
    platysma r.
    r. procedure
    SMAS r.
    SMILE r.
    subcutaneous r.
    subperiosteal minimally invasive laser endoscopic r.
    sub-SMAS r.
    sub-superficial musculoaponeurotic system r.
    superficial plane r.
rhytidoplasty
    endoscopic forehead-brow r.
rhytidosis
rib
    autologous r.
ribbed sterile tubing
ribbon
    r. arch
    r. arch appliance
    r. arch attachment
    r. arch bracket
    r. arch technique
    r. retractor
ribbon-shaped canal
ribonucleic acid (RNA)
ribosome
rice
    r. bodies
Richards-Rundle syndrome
Richard Wolf nasal epistaxis system
Richey condyle marker
Rich-Mar 510 external ultrasound
Richmond crown

Rickert
    R. formula
    R. formula sealer
Ricketts visualized treatment objective
Rickles test
Rid-A-Pain
Ridell operation
Ridenol
ridge
    alveolar r.
    anatomic r.
    r. augmentation
    basal r.
    bicoronal r.
    buccal r.
    buccal cervical r. (BCR)
    buccal triangular r. (BTR)
    buccocervical r.
    buccogingival r.
    center of r.
    cicatricial r.
    crest of alveolar r.
    cusp r.
    dental r.
    digastric r.
    distal cusp r. (DCR)
    distal marginal r. (DMR)
    distobuccal cusp r. (DBCR)
    distolingual cusp r. (DLCR)
    edentulous r.
    enamel r.
    epithelial r.
    r. extension
    extension r.
    external oblique r.
    filtral r.
    functional r.
    incisal r. (IR)
    internal oblique r.
    key r.
    lap r.
    r. lap pontic
    lingual r. (LR)
    linguocervical r.
    linguogingival r.
    longitudinal r. of hard palate
    mandibular r.
    r. of mandibular neck
    marginal r.
    mental r.
    mesial cusp r. (MCR)
    mesial marginal r. (MMR)

    mesiobuccal cusp r. (MBCR)
    mesiolingual cusp r. (MLCR)
    mylohyoid r.
    oblique r. (OR)
    orbitozygomaticomalar bone r.
    palatine r.
    Passavant r.
    petrosal r.
    petrous r.
    r. relation
    residual r.
    r. resorption
    sublingual r.
    superior petrosal r.
    supplemental r.
    support r.
    supraorbital r.
    transverse r.
    transverse groove of oblique r. (TGOR)
    transverse palatine r.
    triangular r.
    zygomaxillare r.
Riebler resin
Riedel
    R. frontoethmoidectomy procedure
    R. struma
Rieger syndrome
RIF
    rigid internal fixation
rifabutin
Rifadin
    R. Injection
    R. Oral
rifampicin
rifampin
Riga-Fede disease
Riggs disease
right
    r. angle bronchoscopic telescope
    r. frontal sinus
    r. hemisphere brain damage (RHD)
    R. Hemisphere Language Battery (RHLB)
    r. lateral excursion
    r. segmental mandibulectomy
    r. subcostal incision
right-angle
    r.-a. forceps
    r.-a. handpiece
    r.-a. technique

NOTES

521

rigid
    r. connector
    r. external distraction (RED)
    r. internal fixation (RIF)
    r. internal fixation device
    r. lag screw fixation
    r. plate fixation
rigidity
    torsional r.
rim
    alar r.
    bite r.
    fronto-orbital r.
    helical r.
    infraorbital r.
    mandible r.
    r. necrosis
    nostril r.
    occlusal r.
    r. occlusion
    occlusion r.
    orbital r.
    piriform r.
    r. record
    record r.
    superior orbital r.
    supraorbital r.
    surgical occlusion r.
    r. +/-transcolumella incision
rima
    r. glottidis
Rimactane Oral
rimexolone
rimming
    osteoblastic r.
ring
    r. avulsion
    r. avulsion injury
    casting r.
    r. clasp
    coronal r.
    cricoid r.
    r. finger axis
    neonatal r.
    palatopharyngeal r.
    retaining r.
    Schatzki r.
    targetoid r.
    tympanic r.
    Valtrac anastomosis r.
    Waldeyer r.
ring-knife
Rinn
    R. XCP film holder
    R. XCP radiographic paralleling
      device
Rinne test

rinse
    Colgate PerioGard oral r.
    Janar acidulated phosphate
      fluoride r.
    Janar sodium fluoride r.
    Kari r.
    mouth r.
    NaFrinse r.
    oral r.
    Peridex Oral R.
    Phos-Flur daily oral r.
    Phos-Flur oral r. supplement
    Plax anti-plaque pre-brushing r.
    PreviDent Dental R.
    retarDex oral r.
rinsing process
RIP
    respiratory inductive plethysmography
ripple deformity
rippling
    upper pole r.
RIS
    radiographic imaging system
Risdon
    R. approach
    R. pretragal incision
    R. wire
riser
    stress r.
risorius
    r. muscle
    musculus r.
Rispi Micromega reamer
Ritter tester
river birch
rivinian notch
Rivinus
    R. canals
    R. duct
    R. gland
    R. incisure
    R. membrane
    R. notch
RLN
    recurrent laryngeal nerve
RME
    rapid maxillary expansion
RMP
    rapid manual processing
RMS Rectal
RNA
    ribonucleic acid
    EBV-encoded RNA
RND
    radical neck dissection
Roach
    R. attachment
    R. ball precision attachment

R

R. carver
R. clasp
Roaf syndrome
ROAM
roaming optical access multiscope
roaming optical access multiscope (ROAM)
Roane bullet tip
Robafen CF
Robaxin
Robaxisal
Robbins
R. Acrotorque hand engine
R. Speech Sound Discrimination and Verbal Imagery Type Test
Robicillin VK
Robin
R. complex
R. sequence
R. syndrome
Robin-like sequence
Robinow-Sorauf syndrome
Robinson
R. stapes prosthesis
R. vein graft
Robinul
R. Forte
Robitussin
R.-CF
R.-DAC
R.-PE
R. Severe Congestion Liqui-Gels
Robles cutting point cannula
Rocabado 6×6 program
Rocephin
Rochester
R. method
R. oral tissue forceps
R. Russian tissue forceps
Rochette bridge
Roche Z gel kit
Rockwell
R. hardness indenter point
R. hardness number (RHN)
rod
Alta intramedullary r.
analyzing r.
condyle r.
enamel r.
hypocalcified enamel r.
irregular r.
keyhole-shaped r.

Rush r.
r. sheath
Silastic r.
r. tail system
rodent ulcer
rodeo thumb
roentgen (R)
r. absorbed dose (rad)
r. ray
roentgen-equivalent-man (rem)
roentgenogram
cephalometric r.
lateral oblique jaw r.
lateral ramus r.
lateral skull r.
maxillary sinus r.
oblique lateral jaw r.
panoramic r.
periapical r.
submental vertex r.
Towne projection r.
transcranial r.
Waters view r.
roentgenograph
roentgenographic view
roentgenography
Roferon-A
Rogaine
R. for Men
R. for Women
Roger-Anderson
R.-A. pin
R.-A. pin fixation
R.-A. pin fixation appliance
Roger syndrome
Ro intracellular antigen
Rolando
fissure of R.
R. operculum
Rolatuss Plain Liquid
roll
banana r.
cervical-occipital r.
dorsal back r.
flank r.
FLUFTEX gauze r.
lumbar r.
rolled skin tube
roller
Toledo r.
ROM
range of motion

NOTES

Romberg
>R. disease
>R. hemifacial atrophy
>R. quotient
>R. sign
>R. syndrome

Rondamine-DM Drops
Rondec
>R.-DM
>R. Drops
>R. Filmtab
>R. Syrup
>R.-TR

rongeur
>end-biting r.
>end-biting blunt nosed r.
>r. forceps
>Kerrison r.
>Leksell r.
>round-nosed r.
>side-cutting r.

roof
>r. of mouth
>orbital r.

ROOF suspension
room
>dead r.
>free field r.
>International Acoustic Company audiologic assessment r.
>reverberation r.
>r. temperature vulcanized (RTV)

root (R)
>r. abscess
>accessory r.
>accessory buccal r.
>adjacent r.
>r. amputation
>anatomic r.
>r. apex
>r. apex elevator
>artificial r.
>beveling r.
>bicanaled r.
>bifurcation of r. (B1)
>Bolk paramolar r.
>buccal r. (BR)
>r. canal
>r. canal access
>r. canal applicator
>r. canal broach
>r. canal calcification
>r. canal cement
>r. canal debridement
>r. canal disinfection
>r. canal electrosterilization
>r. canal file
>r. canal filling

r. canal filling condenser
r. canal filling spreader
r. canal filling technique obturation
r. canal gun
r. canal instrument
r. canal ionization
r. canal irrigation
r. canal orifice
r. canal plugger
r. canal point
r. canal probe
r. canal restoration
r. canal sealer
r. canal shaping
r. canal spreader
r. canal sterilization
r. canal therapy
r. canal treatment
r. caries
r. caries index
r. cementum
clinical r.
r. curettage
r. cyst
r. dehiscence
distal r. (DR)
distobuccal r. (DBR)
r. end cyst
r. end granuloma
r. end resection
r. exit zone
r. facer
facial r.
facial nerve r.
false unicorn r.
r. foramen
r. formation
r. fracture
r. furcation
r. fusion
r. high-pull face-bow
hypercemented r.
intra-alveolar r.
length of r.
lingual r. (LR)
locked r.
mesial r.
mesiobuccal r. (MBR)
nasal r.
orris r.
palatal r.
palatine r.
r. parallelism
r. perforation
physiological r.
r. pick
r. planing
pleurisy r.

r. prominence
pyramidal r.
r. resorption
r. rest
retained r.
r. rubber dam clamp
r. scaling
sensory r.
r. sheath
r. sheath of Hertwig
supernumerary r.
r. tip
r. of tongue
tongue r.
r. of tooth
vital r.
r. word
R. ZX apex locator
R. ZX ultrasonic unit

root-end
r.-e. filling
r.-e. filling material
r.-e. preparation
r.-e. surface
r.-e. surface area

root-form
r.-f. dental implant
r.-f. device

rootless teeth

root-tip
r.-t. elevator
r.-t. forceps

rope
r. flap
foil r.
gold foil r.

ropy saliva

rosacea
hypertrophic r.

rose
r. cold

rosemary

Rosen
R. incision
R. needle

Rosenberg
R. dissecting cannula
R. dissector tip
R. gynecomastia dissection
instrument

Rosenmüller
fossa of R.

Rosenthal
spiral canal of R.

Rose position

rosin
r. varnish

Rosmarinus officinalis

Rossman fluid

rostrum
sphenoidal r.

rotary
r. cutting instrument
r. instrument
r. mounted point
r. scaling

rotated tooth

rotating
r. condyle
r. spring

rotation
caudal r.
r. flap
r. joint
Mallet scale shoulder external r.
Procrustes r.
pure r.
r. responder
r. test
twin bracket tooth r.

rotational
r. axis
r. chair
r. movement
r. vertigo

rotational-advancement osteotomy

rotationally-induced nystagmus

rotationplasty
hip r.
tibial r.

rote
r. memory

Roth
R. AH 25 sealer
R. arch form
R. 801 Elite Grade sealer
R. sealer
R. setup

Rothermann attachment

roto-osteotome

Rotterdam extended L incision

rotunda
fenestra r.

R

NOTES

rotundum
    foramen r.
rouge
rough
    r. endoplasmic reticulum (RER)
    r. hoarseness
    r. marsh elder
    r. voice
rouleau phenomenon
round
    r. block technique
    r. bur
    r. cell sarcoma
    r. condenser
    r. forceps
    full-jacketed military r.
    r. trough
    r. tumor
    r. window
    r. window niche
    r. window reflex
    r. window rupture
round-cell liposarcoma
rounded
    r. bur
    r. square arch
    r. vowel
rounding
    lip r.
round-nosed rongeur
route
    retrosigmoid-transmeatal r.
Roux-en-Y anastomosis
Roux method
Rowe disimpaction forceps
ROWPVT
    Receptive One Word Picture Vocabulary
    Test
Roxanol
    R. Rescudose
    R. SR Oral
Roxicet
    R. 5/500
    R. Oral Solution
    R. Tablet
Roxicodone
Roxilox
Roxiprin
Royal
    R. alloy
royal mineral succedaneum
Roydent silver point extractor kit
RPA
    recurrent pleomorphic adenoma
RP-I bar
RRVN
    retrolabyrinthine/retrosigmoidal
    vestibular neurectomy

RSC
    rectosigmoid neocolpopoiesis
RSD
    reflex sympathetic dystrophy
RSG/IAC
    retrosigmoid/internal auditory canal
RSP
    rat serum protein
RSTL
    relaxed skin tension line
RT
    reaction time
R-Tannamine Tablet
R-Tannate Tablet
RTLX
    real-time, low-intensity x-ray
RTV
    room temperature vulcanized
R-type rasp
rubber
    r. block
    Brazilian r.
    butadiene-styrene r.
    r. dam
    r. dam apron
    r. dam clamp
    r. dam clamp forceps
    r. dam clamp holder
    r. dam elastic
    r. dam frame
    r. dam inversion
    r. dam pad
    r. dam punch
    r. dam retainer clamp
    r. file
    r. impression
    r. impression material
    r. latex
    r. polisher
    polyether r.
    polysulfide r.
    r. punch dam
    silicone r.
    r. stop
    r. tip
    r. wheel
    r. wheeling
rubber-band extraction
rubber-based impression
rubella
    r. virus
Rubens flap
rubeola
Rubex
Rubin
    R. blade
    R. bone planer
    R. osteotome

Rubinstein-Taybi syndrome
rubor
Rubus strigosus
ruby laser
rudimentary
    r. cilium
    r. inferior turbinate
    r. metacarpal
    r. pinna
Rudmose audiometer
ruffled border
ruga, pl. **rugae**
    palatine r.
    rugae support
rugose frontonasal malformation
rule
    base r.
    buccal object r.
    Clark r.
    morpheme structure r.
    morphographemic r.
    phonological r.
    Price r.
    semantic r.
    sequencing r.
    syntactic r.
ruler
    finger r.
    thumb r.
rum-blossom
Rumex crispus
rum nose
Rungstrom projection
running speech
RUP
    rat urine protein
rupture
    extracapsular r.
    intracapsular r.

    round window r.
    tendon r.
ruptured pexis
Ruschelit polyvinyl chloride
    endotracheal tube
Ruscus aculeatus
Rush rod
Rushton bodies
Russell Periodontal Index
Russian
    R. olive
    R. thistle
rustle
    nasal r.
Rutherford frequency theory
Ru-Tuss
    R.-T. DE
    R.-T. Expectorant
    R.-T. Liquid
Ru-Vert-M
RV
    residual volume
RVG
    radiovisiography
RVN
    retrolabyrinthine vestibular neurectomy
Rx Jeneric dental casting gold
Rybka myocutaneous flap
rye
    r. grass
    r. meal
Rymed
    R.-TR
Ryna
    R.-C Liquid
    R.-CX
Rynatan
    R. Pediatric Suspension
    R. Tablet

R

NOTES

SA
    serratus anterior
sable brush
Sabra OMS 45
sabre
    coup de s.
sac
    dental s.
    enamel s.
    endolymphatic s.
    lacrimal s.
    s. and tack procedure
    tooth s.
saccade
saccadic
    s. pursuit
    s. velocity test
Saccharomyces
saccular
    s. collection
    s. cyst
    s. duct
    s. fossa
    s. nerve
saccule
    Golgi s.
    s. of laryngeal ventricle
sacculus, pl. sacculi
    s. dentis
sacral
    s. ulcer
    s. wound
sacrococcygeal
    s. chordoma
    s. defect
sac-vein decompression
saddle
    s. connector
    s. connector base
    s. curve
    s. defect
    s. deformity
    s. denture base
    denture base s.
    free-end s.
    s. nose
saddlebag
saddle-nose
    s.-n. defect
    s.-n. deformity
Saethre-Chotzen
    S.-C. craniosynostosis
    S.-C. syndrome
safelight
safe-side disk

safe-tipped bur
safety plate
saffron
sage
    coast s.
sagebrush
sagittal
    s. appliance
    s. axis
    s. band
    s. furrow
    s. incisure
    s. mandibular movement
    s. plane
    s. projection
    s. ramus osteotomy
    s. section
    s. sinus
    s. split mandibular osteotomy
    s. split osteotomy (SSO)
    s. split ramus osteotomy (SSRO)
    s. splitting of mandible
    s. synostosis reoperation
sagittovertical
SAI
    Social Adequacy Index
Sainton disease
Saint triad
SAL
    sensorineural acuity level
    suction-assisted lipectomy
    SAL test
Sal-Acid Plaster
Salactic film
Salagen
    S. Oral
    S. tablet
Saleto
Salflex
Salgesic
salicylate
    choline s.
    magnesium s.
    sodium s.
salicylic acid
salience
saline
    s. breast implant
    s. drops
    Grossan nasal irrigator tip with
        Water Pik and s.
    s. implant exchange
    phosphate-buffered s. (PBS)
    physiologic s.
saline-filled expander

saliva
    artificial s.
    s. ejector
    ganglionic s.
    lingual s.
    parotid s.
    s. pump
    ropy s.
    sublingual s.
    submandibular s.
    submaxillary s.
    supersaturated s.
    sympathetic s.
salivant
salivarius
    Streptococcus s.
salivary
    s. calculus
    s. colic
    s. corpuscle
    s. duct
    s. duct carcinoma (SDC)
    s. duct cyst
    s. duct obstruction
    s. fistula
    s. flow
    s. flow test
    s. gland (SG)
    s. gland alveolus
    s. gland antibody
    s. gland aplasia
    s. gland capsule
    s. gland carcinoma (SGC)
    s. gland cyst
    s. gland enlargement
    s. gland neoplasm
    S. Gland Register
    s. gland retention cyst
    s. gland tumor
    s. gland virus disease
    s. immunoglobulin
    s. *Lactobacillus* count
    s. *Lactobacillus* index
    s. leak
    s. lipoma
    s. lithiasis
    s. mucus
    s. neoplasm
    s. peroxidase
    s. pH
    s. protein
    s. stone
    s. tube
salivate
salivation
salivolithiasis
Salman FES stent
salmon

Salmonella
    S. abortus-equi
    S. typhimurium
Salmonine Injection
salmon patch
salpingemphraxis
salpingitic
salpingitis
    chronic interstitial s.
salpingopalatine
    s. fold
    s. membrane
salpingopharyngeal
    s. membrane
    s. muscle
salpingopharyngeus muscle
salpingoplasty
Sal-Plant Gel
salsalate
Salsitab
salt
    calcium s.
    s. cedar
    s. grass
    mineral s.
    s. sterilizer
saltbush
Salter incremental lines
SALT-P
    Slosson Articulation Language Test with
    Phonology
Sal-Tropine
saltwort
salute
    allergic s.
salvage
    knee s.
    s. laryngectomy
    limb s.
    s. rate
Salvisol D
Salzburg
    S. biconcave washer
    S. screw
SAM
    subcutaneous augmentation material
    SAM facial implant
same-day adenotonsillectomy
sample
    language s.
    Parsons Language S.
    random s.
    representative s.
Samter
    S. syndrome
    S. triad
sandblasted
Sanders Venturi injector system

Sandimmune
    S. Injection
    S. Oral
Sandoglobulin
Sandoz nasogastric feeding tube
sandpaper disk
sandwich epicranial flap
sandwich-type splint
Sandwith bald tongue
Sanfilippo
    S. A, B, C syndrome
    mucopolysaccharidosis type III S. A (MPS-IIIA)
    mucopolysaccharidosis type III S. B (MPS-IIIB)
    mucopolysaccharidosis type III S. C (MPS-IIIC)
    S. syndrome
Sanguinaria canadensis
sanguinarine
sanguineous
    s. exudate
    s. inflammation
sanguis
    Streptococcus s.
sanitary pontic
sanitation
Sansert
Santorini
    S. fissures
Santyl
    Collagenase S.
saphenous
    s. bulb
    s. nerve
    s. vein interposition graft
SAPHO
    synovitis, acne, pustulosis, hyperostosis, osteitis
    SAPHO syndrome
sapientiae
    dens s.
Sappey ligament
saprodontia
sarcoidal uveitis
sarcoidosis
sarcoid sialadenitis
sarcoma
    alveolar soft part s. (ASPS)
    ameloblastic s.
    antral s.
    chondrogenic s.

    craniofacial osteogenic s.
    endothelial s.
    epithelial s. (ES)
    epithelioid s.
    Ewing s.
    fibrogenic s.
    idiopathic multiple hemorrhagic s.
    intraoral Kaposi s.
    juxtacortical osteogenic s.
    Kaposi s.
    mesenchymal s.
    neurogenic s.
    osteogenic s.
    parosteal osteogenic s.
    poorly differentiated synovial s.
    pseudo-Kaposi s.
    reticulum cell s.
    round cell s.
    synovial s.
    synovial cell s.
sarcophagization
sardine
Sargenti method
Sargon implant
Sarna
SA-RPE
    surgical assisted-rapid palatal expansion
sarsaparilla
sartorius muscle
SAS
    synthetic absorbable suture
    Ethicon SAS
Saslow solution
Sassouni classification
SAT
    speech awareness threshold
satellite nodule
satin finish
satisfaction
    voice s.
saturation
    low oxyhemoglobin s. (LSAT)
    s. output
    s. recovery sequence
    s. sound pressure level (SSPL)
saucer curve
saucerization
    sequestrectomy and s.
saucerized
saucer-shaped erosion
Sauve Kapandji arthrodesis

NOTES

Save-A-Tooth
    S.-A.-T. kit
    S.-A.-T. preserving system
saver
    anchorage s.
    Catrix lip s.
saw
    Adams s.
    diamond wafering s.
    Gigli wire s.
    gold s.
    Isomet low speed s.
    Isomet Plus precision s.
    Joseph s.
    s. palmetto
    separating s.
saw-tooth noise
SBE
    subacute bacterial endocarditis
S-BP line
SC
    supplementary canal
    SC protein
scabbard trachea
scaffold
    biodegradable polymer s.
scaffolding
    three-dimensional biocompatible s.
scala, pl. **scalae**
    s. media
    s. tympani
    s. vestibuli
scalded-skin syndrome
scale
    Aphasia Language Performance S. (ALPS)
    Arizona Articulation Proficiency S.
    Arthur Adaptation of the Leiter International Performance S.
    Body Dysmorphic Disorder Modification of Yale-Brown Obsessive-Compulsive S., McLean version
    Borg s.
    Brinell s.
    Cattel S.
    Columbia Mental Maturity S.
    developmental s.
    Dos Amigos Verbal Language S.
    FAHI s.
    Glasgow Coma S. (GCS)
    Hearing Threshold Level s.
    Heft-Parker pain s.
    House-Brackman Grading S. (HBGS)
    Howe color s.
    Karnofsky performance status s.
    Knoop hardness s.

    Miller s.
    Minnesota Preschool S.
    modified Mallet s.
    Mohs hardness s.
    Preschool Language S.
    Psycholinguistic Rating S.
    Receptive-Expressive Emergent Language S.
    Receptive-Expressive Observation S.
    REEL s.
    REO s.
    sensory s.
    Sklar Aphasia S.
    Smith-Johnson Nonverbal Performance S.
    sound pressure level s.
    Stanford-Binet Intelligence S.
    Verbal Language Development S.
    Vocabulary Comprehension S.
    Wechsler Adult Intelligence S. (WAIS)
    Wechsler Intelligence S. for Children-Revised (WISC-R)
    Wechsler Preschool and Primary S. of Intelligence (WPPSI)
    Yale-Brown Obsessive-Compulsive S.
scalenus
    s. anterior muscle
    s. medius muscle
    s. posterior muscle
scaler
    anterior s.
    chisel s.
    Columbia s.
    deep s.
    double-ended s.
    s. file
    hoe s.
    Jaquette s.
    McCall s.
    placement s.
    sickle s.
    sonic s.
    superficial s.
    ultrasonic s.
    ultrasonic piezo-electric s.
    wing s.
    Younger-Good s.
scaling
    coronal s.
    deep s.
    electrosurgical s.
    hand s.
    root s.
    rotary s.
    subgingival s.

supragingival s.
ultrasonic s.
scalloped endosseous template
scalloping
s. of lower lid
scalp
s. expansion
locally invasive congenital cellular blue nevus of s.
s. muscle
s. sickle flap
scalpel
s. blade
B.U.S. Endotron-Lipectron ultrasonic s.
electrosurgical s.
Endotron-Lipectron ultrasonic s.
Lipectron ultrasonic s.
Personna Plus disposable Teflon s.
Pre-Cision miniature and microminiature s.
ultrasonic s.
ultrasonic suction s.
scalping
s. flap
s. flap of Converse
postauricular and retroauricular s. (PARAS)
scamping speech
SCAN
Screening Test for Identifying Central Auditory Disorder
scan
CAT s.
^{123}I s.
NMR s.
S. Pattern generator
radioisotope s.
Tc-RBC s.
technetium bone s.
Scandonest
scanner
ATL-HDL color flow Doppler s.
Cencit facial s.
OmniMedia XRS s.
Somatom Plus S whole body s.
Twin Flash s.
scanning
s. communication board
s. electron micrograph (SEM)
s. electron microscope
s. electron microscopy (SEM)

s. electron photomicrograph
radionuclide s.
scintillation s.
s. speech
scanography
scapha
scaphocephalic deformity
scaphocephaly
scaphoid fossa
scaphoid-trapezium-trapezoid (STT)
scapholunate
s. articulation
s. dissociation
s. instability
s. interval
s. motion
scaphomaxillism
scapula, pl. scapulae
s. crest pedicled bone graft
s. free flap
scapular
s. blade
s. flap transfer
s. island flap
s. island flap technique
s. osteocutaneous flap
scar
atrophic s.
atrophic facial acne s.
s. contracture
s. fibroblast
fusiform s.
hypertrophic s.
infra-areolar s.
infrabrow s.
inverted T s.
keloid s.
lateral s.
osteopetrotic s.
parenchymal s.
perioareolar s.
vertical s.
scarabrasion
Scardino vertical flap pyeloplasty
Scar Fx lightweight silicone sheeting
scarification
scarlatinosa
angina s.
Scarpa
S. adipofascial flap
canals of S.
S. fascia

NOTES

S

Scarpa (continued)
  S. foramen
  S. ganglion
scarred deep sinus tract
scarring
  hypertrophic s.
scattered
  s. radiation
  s. x-ray
scavenger
  LySonix Diamond Tip s.
SCC
  squamous cell carcinoma
  oral SCC
    oral squamous cell carcinoma
SCCHN
  squamous cell carcinoma of head and
  neck
scent
scerlosing substance
Schartzmann maneuver
Schatzki ring
Schatzmann attachment
schedule
  continuous reinforcement s.
  fixed interval reinforcement s.
  fixed ratio reinforcement s.
  intermittent reinforcement s.
  reinforcement s.
  variable interval reinforcement s.
  variable ratio reinforcement s.
Scheffe test
Scheibe
  S. deafness
  S. malformation
Scheie
  mucopolysaccharidosis type I S.
  (MPS-IS)
  S. syndrome
Schellong-Strisower phenomenon
schema, pl. schemata
scheme
  occlusal s.
  Topazian classification s.
schenckii
  Sporothrix s.
Schiefelbush-Lindsey Test of Sound
  Discrimination
Schilder
  S. disease
  S. plugger
Schiotz tonometer
Schirmer tear test
schistoglossia
schistometer
schizodontism
schizophrenia
  childhood s.

Schmidt syndrome
Schmincke-Regaud lymphoepithelial
  carcinoma
Schmutz pyorrhea
schneiderian
  s. membrane
  s. papilloma
Schneider technique
Schobinger incision
Schönbein operation
school language
Schour-Massler index
Schreger
  S. band
  S. lines
  S. stria
  S. zone
Schrudde
  S. aspirative lipoplasty
  S. curette technique
Schubiger attachment
Schuchardt procedure
Schuknecht
  S. ablation streptomycin therapy
  S. classification
  S. products
Schüller projection
schwa
Schwabach test
Schwalbe
  S. corpuscle
  S. nucleus
  S. plane
Schwann
  S. cell
  S. cell cytoplasm
  S. tubule
schwannoma
  acoustic s.
  ancient s.
  carotid sheath type
    parapharyngeal s.
  cervical sympathetic s.
  mixed type parapharyngeal s.
  pharyngeal type parapharyngeal s.
  vestibular s. (VS)
Schwartz
  S. plate
  S. sign
Schwartz-Bartter syndrome
Schwarz
  S. activator
  S. appliance
  S. classification
Schwed Flexicut file
Sciatic Function Index
SCID
  severe combined immunodeficiency

science
    Bachelor of Dental S. (BDSc)
    communication s.
    Doctor of Dental S. (DDSc)
    hearing s.
    speech s.
    speech and hearing s.
scientific grammar
scintigram
    technetium s.
scintigraphy
scintillation scanning
scintiscan
scintiscanner
scintography
scissel
scissile
scissors
    angled s.
    AROSupercut s.
    ASSI Super-Cut s.
    Becker s.
    s. bite
    Boettcher tonsil s.
    Castanares face lift s.
    Converse s.
    curved turbinate s.
    curved turbinectomy s.
    Dean s.
    Diamond-Edge Supercut s.
    face-lift s.
    facial plastic surgery s.
    Fomon face lift s.
    Fox s.
    gold and crown s.
    Goldman-Fox s.
    Gorney face lift s.
    Jameson face lift s.
    Kaye face lift s.
    Knight nasal s.
    LaGrange s.
    Laschal s.
    Littauer suture s.
    Lorenz PC/TC s.
    Mayo s.
    micro-mosquito curved s.
    micro-mosquito straight s.
    PowerStar bipolar s.
    Quimby s.
    Rees face lift s.
    sickle s.
    StaySharp face lift Super-Cut s.

    Stevens tenotomy s.
    straight s.
    suture s.
    tenotomy s.
    thin-shaft nasal s.
    tissue s.
    turbinectomy s.
scissors-bite crossbite
sclera
    blue s.
scleral
    s. shell
    s. shield
    s. show
sclerectomy
scleritis
scleroderma
    linear s.
    localized s.
ScleroLaser
    Candela S.
scleroma
    respiratory s.
scleroplasty
ScleroPLUS LongPulse dye laser system
sclerosing
    s. agent
    s. hemangioma
    s. lipogranulomastosis
    s. mastoiditis
    s. osteitis
sclerosis
    amyotrophic lateral s. (ALS)
    dentinal s.
    irregular dentinal s.
    multiple s.
    muscular s.
    pathologic s.
    physiologic s.
    progressive systemic s.
    radiolucency s.
    tubular s.
sclerostosis
sclerotherapy
    tetracycline hydrochloride s.
sclerotic
    s. cemental mass
    s. dentin
    s. mastoiditis
    s. teeth
SCM
    sternocleidomastoid

NOTES

SCM *(continued)*
    synovial chondromatosis
        SCM tumor
        SCM tumor of infancy
scoliosis
Scop
    Transderm S.
Scopace Tablet
scope
    Oral Video S.
scopolamine
    phenylephrine and s.
    s. transdermal
scorbutic gingivitis
score
    Apgar s.
    discrimination s.
    emotional voice handicap s.
    Erb s.
    Hannover Polytrauma S.
    Japan Facial S.
    Klumpke s.
    S. of 10
    OMENS s.
    oral hygiene s.
    orbit, mandible, ear, cranial nerves, and soft tissue s.
    periodontal disease s.
    physical voice handicap s.
    raw s.
    speech discrimination s. (SDS)
    standard s.
    voice handicap s.
    Weber s.
    word discrimination s.
scored alar mucocartilaginous flap
scoring
    Developmental Sentence S. (DSS)
Scotchbond 1 primer
Scott
    S. attachment
    S. chronic wound care system
scout film
SCPL-CHEP
    supracricoid partial laryngectomy with cricohyoidoepiglottopexy
scrap
    s. amalgam
screamer's nodule
screen
    Communication S.
    Communication Abilities Diagnostic Test and S.
    s. film
    intensifying s.
    Joliet 3-Minute Speech and Language S.
    oral s.

    rare earth s.
    vestibular s.
screener
    Smart Screener infant hearing s.
screening
    s. audiometry
    S. Deep Test of Articulation
    S. Kit of Language Development (SKOLD)
    otological s.
    s. RAST
    S. Speech Articulation Test
    s. test
    S. Test of Adolescent Language
    S. Test for Auditory Comprehension of Language
    S. Test for Auditory Perception
    S. Test for Development Apraxia of Speech
    S. Test for Identifying Central Auditory Disorder (SCAN)
screw
    adjustable s.
    Asnis 2 guided s.
    axial anchor s.
    bicortical superior border s.
    Calcitek retaining s.
    Carol Gerard s.
    cortical anchoring s.
    cover s.
    dental implant cover s.
    Dentatus s.
    s. elevator
    expansion s.
    fixation s.
    healing s.
    ImplaMed gold s.
    implant s.
    Implant Innovations titanium s.
    Implant Support Systems titanium s.
    lag s.
    Leibinger Micro Plus s.
    Leibinger Mini Würzburg s.
    Leibinger Würzburg s.
    Luhr vitallium s.
    mandibular angle fracture intraoral open reduction s.
    monocortical s.
    Nobelpharma gold prosthetic retaining s.
    Omega compression hip s.
    orthodontic s.
    Periotest Implant Innovations gold s.
    s. pin
    s. post
    pretapped Synthes lag s.

pull s.
resorbable plate and s.
s. retainer
Salzburg s.
self-tapping Leibinger lag s.
Steinhauser s.
ThreadLoc driver mount s.
ThreadLoc retaining s.
Ti alloy s.
TPS-coated s.
screwdriver
s. instrument
s. teeth
screw-retained prosthesis
screw-type
s.-t. abutment
s.-t. implant
s.-t. implant prosthesis
Screw-Vent
S.-V. implant
S.-V. implant system
scribe
scrofula
scrofulaceum
Mycobacterium s.
scrofulous rhinitis
scroll ear
scrotal
s. elephantiasis
s. hemangioma
s. tongue
s. tourniquet
scrotoplasty
scrotum
scrub
Exidine S.
Techni-Care surgical s.
scrub-brush technique of toothbrushing
SCS
synovial chondrosarcoma
sculpting
body s.
sculpture
sonic s.
Scutellaria lateriflora
scutum
SCV
slow-component velocity
SD
speech discrimination
AlphaNine SD

S/D
Gammagard S/D
Polygam S/D
SDC
salivary duct carcinoma
SDS
speech discrimination score
syringe-driven system
SDS-PAGE
sodium dodecyl sulfate-polyacrylamide
gel electrophoresis
SDT
speech detectability threshold
speech detection threshold
Sea-Bond denture adhesive cream
sea gull tracing
seal
apical s.
border s.
cavity s.
double s.
hermetic s.
oval window s.
palatal s.
peripheral s.
posterior palatal s.
postpalatal s.
velopharyngeal s.
Seal of Acceptance
sealant
amine-accelerated s.
CryoLife light-activated fibrin s.
dental s.
dimethacrylate s.
fibrin s.
fissure s.
light-activated s.
pit and fissure s.
University of Virginia fibrin s.
Sealapex endodontic sealer
sealer
AH-26 silver-free s.
Apexit calcium hydroxide root
canal s.
Calasept s.
Calciobiotic root canal s.
calcium hydroxide root canal s.
(CRCS)
Cavidentin s.
s. cement
chloropercha s.
Diaket s.

S

NOTES

sealer *(continued)*
    endodontic s.
    epoxy resin s.
    Espe Ketac-Endo s.
    excess s.
    s. extrusion
    Grossman formula root canal s.
    histoacryl s.
    Kerr antiseptic root canal s.
    Kerr Pulp Canal s.
    Ketac-Endo glass-ionomer-based s.
    Ketac-Endo glass-ionomer root canal s.
    Ketac-Endo root canal s.
    Nogenol s.
    ProcoSol s.
    pulp canal s. (PCS)
    Pulp Canal Sealer EBT s.
    Rickert formula s.
    root canal s.
    Roth s.
    Roth AH 25 s.
    Roth 801 Elite Grade s.
    Sealapex endodontic s.
    Sealer 26 calcium hydroxide root canal s.
    tear strength eugenol-based s.
    Tubliseal s.
    Tubliseal endodontic s.
    Tubliseal glass-ionomer root canal s.
    Ultra-Fast Araldite s.
    Wach paste s.
    zinc oxide-eugenol s.
    ZOE s.

sealing
    s. perforation

seam
    epithelial s.

seamless band

seasonal antigen

seat
    basal s.
    rest s.

seat-down dentistry

seater
    band s.

sebaceous
    s. adenoma
    s. carcinoma
    s. cyst
    s. gland
    s. gland hyperplasia (SGH)
    s. lymphadenoma
    s. metaplasia
    nevus s.

sebaceum
    adenoma s.

Sebbin
    S. ultrasound-assisted lipoplasty machine
    S. ultrasound device

seborrheic
    s. dermatitis
    s. external otitis
    s. keratosis

secobarbital
    s. sodium

Seconal
    S. Sodium

second
    s. cranial nerve
    cycles per s. (cps)
    s. half-value layer
    s. incisor
    s. messenger system
    s. molar
    s. nerve (N2)
    s. order bend
    s. premolar
    s. premolar alveolus
    second s.
    s. tooth

secondary
    s. abutment
    s. aerodontalgia
    s. articulation
    s. autism
    s. caries
    s. cementum
    s. coping
    s. correction
    s. cuticle
    s. debulking
    s. dentin
    s. dentition
    s. ear reconstruction
    s. expansion
    s. gain
    s. hue
    s. impression
    s. irregular dentin
    s. irritant
    s. lingual bar major connector
    s. occlusal traumatism
    s. palate
    s. periodontitis
    s. radiation
    s. reinforcer
    s. retainer
    s. rhinoplasty
    s. stress
    s. struts implant substructure
    s. stuttering
    s. union

s. varicella-zoster
s. verb

second-look
s.-l. biopsy
s.-l. intervention
s.-l. surgery

second-toe wraparound flap
secretin
secretion
eosinophilic proteinaceous s.'s
glairy s.
nasopharyngeal s.
viscid s.
viscous s.

secretion-clearance pattern
secretomotor fiber
secretory
s. cell
s. component
s. duct
s. granule
s. immunoglobulin
s. otitis media

section
attached cranial s.
dentate s.
detached cranial s.
frozen s.
sagittal s.
tangential s.
vestibular nerve s.

sectional
s. arch wire
s. impression
s. partial denture
s. root canal filling method
s. technique

Secure-on-Touch adhesive
Secur-Its silicon cushion mat
sedative
Seddon classification
sedimentation rate
SEE₂
Signing Exact English
SEE₁
Seeing Essential English
seed
sesame s.
seeding
iodine-125 s.
tumor s.
Seeing Essential English (SEE₁)

seeker
ostium s.

segment
labyrinthine s.
two-tooth s.

segmental
s. alveolar osteotomy
s. analysis
s. bone defect
s. continuity defect
s. demyelination
s. mandibulectomy
s. phoneme
s. surgery

segmentation root canal filling method
segregator
Seidel humeral locking nail
Seiler MC-M900 surgical microscope
seizure
jacksonian s.
psychomotor s.

SELD
slow expressive language development

Seldane
S.-D

Seldin
S. elevator
S. retractor

selective
s. anesthesia
s. grinding
s. listening
s. neck dissection (SND)
s. photothermolysis

selectivity
thermokinetic s. (TKS)

Selenicereus grandiflorus
selenodont
Selenomonas
self-centering prosthesis
self-concept
self-curing
s.-c. pink acrylic
s.-c. resin

self-esteem
self-expandable stent
Self-Help for Hard of Hearing People (SHHH)
self-rectified x-ray tube
self-retaining retractor
self-role concept
self-seal pouch

S

NOTES

self-talk
self-tapping
    s.-t. Leibinger lag screw
    s.-t. screw-type implant
self-threading
    s.-t. pin
    s.-t. post
SELI
   specific expressive language impairment
sella
    dorsum s.
    s. nasion B point
    s. turcica
sella-nasion-subspinale angle (SN_A, S-N-A, SNA)
sella-nasion-supramentale angle (SN_B, S-N-B, SNB)
sellar
    s. tumor
sellion
    orbitale s.
SEM
   scanning electron micrograph
   scanning electron microscopy
semanteme
semantic
    s. aphasia
    behavioral s.'s
    s. constraint
    extension s.'s
    s. feature
    general s.'s
    generative s.'s
    s. implication
    s. integration
    intention s.'s
    referential s.'s
    s. relation
    s. rule
    s. theory of stuttering
    s. use
sememics
semi-adjustable articulator
semiaural hearing protection device
semi-autonomous systems concept of brain function
semicircular
    s. canal
    s. duct
semicohesive gold foil
semi-Fowler position
semihyalinization
semilunar
    s. flap
    s. fold
semilunaris
    hiatus s.
    plica s.

semilunatum
    planum s.
semimalignant tumor
semimembranosus muscle
semimembranous muscle
semiocclusive dressing
semiology
semipermanent retention
semiprecision
    s. attachment
    s. rest
semirecumbent position
semi-rigid fixation
semisolid material
semitone
semivital pulp
semi-vowel
Semken forceps
Semken-Taylor forceps
Semmes-Weinstein
    S.-W. monofilament (SWMF)
    S.-W. monofilament instrument
    S.-W. monofilament test
    S.-W. pressure aesthesiometer filament
Semon
    S. law
    S. symptom
Semon-Rosenbach law
Semprex-D
semustine
seneca snakeroot
senescence
    dental s.
senile
    s. atrophic gingivitis
    s. atrophy
    s. decay
    s. dental caries
    s. hemangioma
    s. keratosis
senilis
    arcus s.
    lentigo s.
senility
senna
Sennheiser electric condenser microphone ME 40-3
Senn-Miller retractor
Senn retractor
sensate
    s. flap
    s. medial plantar free flap
    s. pedicled neoclitoroplasty
sensation
    foreign body s.
    laryngopharyngeal s.
    s. level (SL)

Plax Mint S.
s. unit (SU)
sense
s. of foreign body
sensibility
hand s.
sensitive
s. dentin
s. tooth
sensitivity
periapical s.
postcementation s.
s. prediction from the acoustic
reflex (SPAR)
s. test
s. of tooth
sensitization
sensitometric
s. curve
Sensiv endotracheal tube
Sensodyne
S. F
Senso listening device
Sensonic plaque removal instrument
sensor
ENDEX apex s.
Flexisensor s.
MicroMirror gold s.
s. operation
Oxisensor II adult adhesive s.
position s.
Sensorcaine
sensorimotor
s. act
s. arc
s. intelligence period
sensorineural
s. acuity level (SAL)
s. acuity level technique
s. deafness
s. hearing loss (SNHL)
sensory
s. acuity level bone conduction
s. aphasia
s. impairment
s. integration (SI)
s. nerve
s. nerve fiber bundle
s. neuron
s. organization test (SOT)
s. paralysis
s. receptor

s. root
s. root of trigeminal nerve
s. scale
s. unit
s. and vasomotor impulse
Sentalloy
sentence
S. Articulation Test
s. classification
complex s.
compound s.
compound-complex s.
constituent s.
s. constituent
declarative s.
s. derivation
derived s.
embedded s.
exclamatory s.
first s.
imperative s.
interrogative s.
kernel s.
matrix s.
nonkernel s.
s. recasting
simple s.
sentence-picture matching
sentinel
s. loop
s. lymphatic mapping
s. lymph node (SLN)
s. vein
separated spreader
separating
s. disk
s. medium
s. saw
s. spring
s. strip
s. wire
separation
binaural s.
gradual tooth s.
jaw s.
mechanical tooth s.
s. point
pterygomaxillary s.
s. of teeth
tooth s.
separator
Ferrier s.

S

NOTES

separator *(continued)*
    mechanical s.
    noninterfering s.
    True s.
sepsis, pl. sepses
    joint s.
    oral s.
sept
    fascial s.
septa (*pl. of* septum)
septal
    s. artery
    s. cartilage
    cartilaginous autologous thin s.
      (CATS)
    s. chondromucosal graft
    s. deviation
    s. gingiva
    s. mucoperichondrium
    s. perforation
    s. perforator
    s. reconstruction
    s. resection
    s. space
    s. surgery
septation
    bony s.
    vertical s.
Septa Topical Ointment
septectomy
septi (*gen. of* septum)
septic
    s. arthroses
    s. metastasis
    s. wound
septicemia
Septisol
septocutaneous
    s. island
    s. perforator
septodermoplasty
septofasciocutaneous island
septomeatoplasty
septomuscular perforator
septoplasty
    back-and-forth s.
    endoscopic sphenoethmoidectomy
      with s.
    frontal sinus s.
septorhinoplasty
    esthetic s.
Septra
    S. DS
septum, gen. septi, pl. septa
    alveolar s.
    s. alveoli
    anterior s.
    bony s.

    collagen s.
    depressor septi
    deviated s.
    fibrous connective septa
    gingival s.
    gum s.
    s. interalveolaria maxillae
    interdental s.
    interfrontal s.
    interradicular s.
    s. interradicularia
    intersinus s.
    intersphenoid s.
    Körner s.
    s. linguae
    lingual s.
    mobile s.
    nasal s.
    oblique s.
    s. orbitale
    septa in sinus
    sphenoidal sinus s.
    s. spur
    tethering s.
    s. of tongue
    tracheoesophageal s.
Sep-T-Vac suction canister
sequela, pl. sequelae
    abdominal s.
    poststapedectomy related s.
Sequels
    Diamox S.
sequence
    amniotic band disruption s.
    inversion recovery pulse s.
    isolated Pierre Robin s.
    Pierre Robin s.
    Robin s.
    Robin-like s.
    saturation recovery s.
    spin echo pulse s.
    syllable s.
    word s.
Sequenced Inventory of Communication
   Development
sequencing
    auditory s.
    s. rule
sequential
    s. bilateral breast reconstruction
    s. memory
sequestration
sequestrectomy
    s. and saucerization
sequestrum
    bone s.
    eruption s.

Serena and Serena Mx hand-held
  apnea detection device
Serenoa repens
serial
    s. cephalometric x-ray
    s. content speech
    s. extraction
    s. list learning
    s. scar excision
seriatim speech
seriation
series
    full mouth s.
    lateral jaw panoramic s.
    panoramic s.
    600 s. PDT dye module
    Unitech cannula s.
    Universal cannula s.
serologic test
serology
seroma
Seroma-Cath wound drainage system
seromucinous
seromucous
    s. gland
seropositive
seropositivity
serosanguineous
    s. discharge
serotinus
    dens s.
serotonin
serous
    s. acinus
    s. alveolus
    s. cell
    s. cell cytoplasm
    s. cell nucleus
    s. demilune
    s. demilune cell
    s. exudate
    s. fluid
    s. gland
    s. granule
    s. inflammation
    s. otitis
    s. otitis media (SOM)
serrated
    s. amalgam plugger
    s. pliers
    s. post
serrate suture

Serratia marcescens
serraticus
    stridor s.
serration
serratus
    s. anterior (SA)
    s. anterior muscle
    s. anterior muscle flap
    s. posterior inferior muscle
    s. posterior superior muscle
Serres
    S. pearl
    rests of S.
serum
    fetal bovine s. (FBS)
    s. hepatitis
    s. hyperviscosity syndrome
serumal calculus
Serum-C
    pHaze 15 S.-C.
service
    denture s.
    early intervention s.
    family-centered s.
servomechanistic theory
servosystem
Servox
    S. electronic speech aid
    S. Inton speech aid
SES
    socioeconomic status
sesame seed
sessile
    s. lesion
    s. swelling
    s. vocal nodule
set
    Ciaglia percutaneous tracheostomy
      introducer s.
    insufflation test s.
    Molina mandibular distractor s.
    Novack special
      extraction/injection s.
    preparatory s.
    surgical steel Toomey instrument s.
    Surgimedics/TMP multiperfusion s.
    s. of teeth
    Yudkoff-Okun periodontal
      instrument s.
setback
Set-Op myringotomy kit
setscrew

S

NOTES

setting
- s. expansion
- s. inlay
- s. time

setup, set-up
- diagnostic s.
- Roth s.
- s. wax

seven-pin staple
seventh cranial nerve
severe
- s. combined immunodeficiency (SCID)
- s. hearing impairment
- s. hearing loss

sevoflurane
Sevriton Cavity Seal Primer
Seward technique
sex
- s. conversion
- s. reassignment surgery

sextant
sexual characteristics
sexually transmitted disease (STD)
Sézary syndrome
S-file
- engine S.-f.

S-finder
SFo
- speaking phonation

SFP
- synostotic frontal plagiocephaly

SFS
- superficial fascial system

SG
- salivary gland
- supplemental groove
- SG cell

SGBI
- silicone gel-filled breast implant

SGC
- salivary gland carcinoma

SGH
- sebaceous gland hyperplasia

SGMI
- silicone gel-filled mammary implant
- SGMI explantation surgery

S.H.A.
- Phenchlor S.H.A.

shade
- bioform porcelain s.
- s. guide
- s. verification

shading
shadow
- cloud-like s.
- s. curve

metallic-dense s.
- triple line s.

shadowing
- s. method

shaft prosthesis
shagbark hickory
shampoo
- P&S S.

sham surgery
shank
- bur s.

Shannon
- S. bur
- S. drill

shape
- ear s.
- fleur-de-lis s.
- keyhole s.
- s. memory clamp
- sweet potato s.
- syllable s.

shaped
- s. block-out
- funnel s.
- s. glandular flap
- s. random pattern flap

shaper
- ProFile orifice s.
- rapid body s. (RBS)

shaping
- s. of the breast
- precision fluence s.
- root canal s.

Shapiro syndrome
Shapleigh wax curette
shared nipple
sharing
- nerve s.
- nipple s.

shark-mouth cannula
sharp
- s. dilaceration
- s. dissection
- s. elevator
- s. loop curette

sharpening stone
Sharpey fiber
Sharplan
- S. Erbium SilkLaser
- S. FeatherTouch SilkLaser
- S. laser
- S. Laser 710 Acuspot

SharpLase Nd:YAG laser
sharply falling curve
sharpness
- image s.
- zone of s.

Sharpoint blade

S

sharps
> contaminated s.

Sharptome
> S. crescent blade
> S. microblade

shave
> s. biopsy
> s. excision technique
> superficial upper lateral s.

shaver
> Rhinotec s.

shaving
> s. dentin
> s. stroke

Shea procedure

shear
> s. strength
> s. stress

sheared crown

shearing
> s. cusp
> s. edge
> s. stress

shears

sheath
> carotid s.
> dentinal s.
> epithelial s.
> Hertwig s.
> Hertwig epithelial root s.
> molar s.
> myelin s.
> nerve s.
> Neumann s.
> prism s.
> rod s.
> root s.
> sheath of s.

sheathing

shedding

Sheen postulate

sheep
> s. dander
> s. sorrell

sheet
> Biobrane s.
> polydioxanone s.
> Prolene mesh s.
> Sil-K silicone s.
> in vitro grown palatal mucosa s.

sheeting
> Cica-Care silicone gel s.

> Epi-Derm silicone gel s.
> gel s.
> New Beginnings GelShapes silicone gel s.
> ReJuveness pure silicone s.
> Scar Fx lightweight silicone s.
> silicone gel s.

shelf, pl. **shelves**
> buccal s.
> dental s.
> s. life
> palatal s.
> palatine s.

shell
> s. blaster
> s. crown
> s. earmold
> elastomer s.
> fibrous s.
> implant s.
> implant elastomer s.
> scleral s.
> Terino malar s.
> s. tooth

shellac
> s. base

shelled out

shelves (*pl. of* shelf)

shepherd's purse

Sherer attachment

Sherman plate

SHHH
> Self-Help for Hard of Hearing People

Shick
> S. Sonic-Action denture cleanser
> S. Ultrasonic denture cleanser

shield
> Cox II ocular laser s.
> dental s.
> Durette dental s.
> Durette external laser s.
> gonadal s.
> lead s.
> lingual s.
> metal scleral s.
> oral s.
> radiation s.
> scleral s.
> Stevanovsky metal eye s.
> Surgical Patient Arm s.
> thyroid s.
> Trelles metal scleral s.

NOTES

545

shielding
shield-type graft
shift
  abrupt topic s.
  chemical s.
  Doppler s.
  gradual topic s.
  paradigmatic s.
  permanent threshold s. (PTS)
  pitch s.
  temporary threshold s. (TTS)
  threshold s.
  topic s.
  voice s.
shifter
  suture shape s.
Shikani middle meatal antrostomy stent
Shiley Phonate speaking valve
shimmer
  amplitude s.
shimmer-related measure
shingles
ship
  Fabricius s.
SHL
  sudden hearing loss
SHM
  simple harmonic motion
shock
  anaphylactic s.
  electric s.
shoe
  Neurohr-Williams rest s.
shoeing cusp
shoelace suture
Shofu spherical alloy
Shooshan A carver
short
  s. bowel syndrome
  s. face syndrome
  s. film exposure time
  s. gut syndrome
  s. mandible
  s. ragweed
  s. ragweed antigen
  s. scar technique
  s. tandem repeat polymorphism (STRP)
  S. Test for Use with Cerebral Palsy Children
  s. tooth
short-cone technique
short-scale contrast
Short-Term
  S.-T. Auditory Retrieval and Storage Test (STARS)
short-term
  s.-t. memory

shoulder
  s. dystocia
  s. of furrow
  linguogingival s.
  s. of rhytid
  s. syndrome
  s. with bevel preparation
shoulderless jacket crown
shovel-shaped incisor
show
  conchal s.
  scleral s.
shower collar
Shrapnell membrane
shrimp
shrinkage
  gingival s.
  gold s.
  polymerization s.
  wax s.
shriveled skin envelope
Shuman retractor
shunt
  arteriovenous s.
  capillary bed s.
  endolymphatic-subarachnoid s.
  Gibson inner ear s.
  portacaval s.
  tracheoesophageal s.
  tracheopharyngeal s.
  ventriculoperitoneal s.
shunting
  arteriovenous s.
  electric current s.
shutter flap
Shy-Drager syndrome
SI
  International System of Units
  sensory integration
  SI unit
sialadenitis, sialoadenitis
  acute submandibular s.
  allergic s.
  autoimmune s.
  bacterial s.
  chronic s.
  epithelioid-cell s.
  granulomatous s.
  myoepithelial s.
  obstructive s.
  postirradiation s.
  rheumatoid s.
  sarcoid s.
  submandibular chronic sclerosing s.
  suppurative s.
  viral s.
sialadenography
sialadenoma papilliferum

sialadenoncus
sialadenosis
      metabolic s.
sialadenotropic
sialagogic
sialagogue, sialogogue
sialangiitis
sialectasia
sialectasis
sialemesis
sialism
sialoablation
sialo-acinar reflux
sialoadenectomy
sialoadenitis (*var. of* sialadenitis)
sialoadenotomy
sialoaerophagy
sialoangiectasis
sialoangiitis
sialoangiography
sialocarcinoma
sialocele
sialochemistry
sialocyst
sialodochitis
sialodochoplasty
      parotid s.
sialoductitis
sialoendoscopy
sialogenic pain
sialogenous
sialogogue (*var. of* sialagogue)
sialogram
sialographic
      s. catheter
sialography
      hydrostatic s.
      injection s.
sialolith
sialolithiasis
sialolithotomy
sialometaplasia
      necrotizing s.
sialometry
sialo-odontogenic cyst
sialopathy
      autoimmune s.
sialorrhea
sialoschesis
sialosemiology, sialosemeiology
sialosis
sialostenosis

sialosyrinx
sialozemia
Siamese
      S. twin archwire
      S. twin bracket
Siberian ginseng
sibilant
      s. sound
SiC
    silicon carbide
sicca
      s. caries
      s. complex
      keratoconjunctivitis s.
      laryngitis s.
      pharyngitis s.
      rhinitis s.
      s. syndrome
sickle
      s. blade
      s. flap
      s. knife
      s. scaler
      s. scissors
      s. tooth
sickle-shaped
      s.-s. canal
      s.-s. curve
sickness
      motion s.
side
      balancing s.
      pressure s.
      tension s.
      working s.
side-biting
      s.-b. ostrum punch
      s.-b. Stammberger punch forceps
sideburn
      displaced s.
side-cutting rongeur
side-lip forceps
sideropenic dysphagia
siderosis
      superficial s.
Siegle otoscope
Siemens
      S. Orthoceph 10 x-ray
      S. Somatom Plus S computed
        tomographer
      S. system
sieve graft

S

NOTES

Sievert unit
sieving
    mandibular s.
sigh voice
siglish
sigmatism
Sigma TMB assay kit
sigmoid
    s. notch
    s. notch retractor
    s. sinus
    s. sulcus
sign
    Agee s.
    Aufrecht s.
    Bárány s.
    Battle s.
    Bezold s.
    Biermer s.
    Bozzolo s.
    Brown s.
    Brudzinski s.
    Burton s.
    Ewing s.
    Fay s.
    fistula s.
    Froment s.
    Gerhardt s.
    Griesinger s.
    hair collar s.
    Hennebert s.
    Herying s.
    hilar s.
    Holman-Miller s.
    Horner s.
    Hutchinson s.
    Kernig s.
    s. language
    Leser-Trelat s.
    linguine s.
    lipstick s.
    s. marker
    Nikolsky s.
    Obagi s.
    pantaloon s.
    Pemberton s.
    Phalen s.
    Romberg s.
    Schwartz s.
    soft neurological s.'s
    stepladder s.
    s. system
    thumb s.
    Tinel s.
    Trélat s.
    trumpet s.
    s. word
SignaDRESS dressing

signal
    s. averaging
    bilateral contralateral routing of offside s.'s (BICROS)
    contralateral routing of offside s.'s (CROS)
    front routing of s.'s (FROS)
    high-frequency contralateral routing of offside s.'s (HICROS)
    ipsilateral frontal routing of s.'s (IFROS)
    ipsilateral routing of s.'s (IROS)
    power contralateral routing of s.'s
    s. sound pressure level
    square-wave s.
    therapeutic error s. (TES)
signal-to-noise ratio (S/N)
signed English
significantly subaverage
significative lift
Signing Exact English (SEE$_2$)
SIL
    speech interference level
Siladryl Oral
Silafed Syrup
Silaminic
    S. Cold Syrup
    S. Expectorant
silane
    s. coupling agent
Silapap
    Children's S.
    Infants' S.
Silastic
    S. allograft
    S. foam dressing
    S. implant
    S. rod
    S. strap
Sildicon-E
silex
Silfedrine
    Children's S.
Silhouette
    S. endoscopic laser
    S. therapeutic massage system
silica
silica-carbon layer
silicate
    s. cement
    s. restoration
    s. restorative material
    s. zinc cement
    zirconium s. (ZrSiO$_4$)
siliceous, silicious
    s. dental cement
silicoater

silicon
s. blood level
s. carbide (SiC)
s. carbide abrasive
s. carbide disk
s. dioxide abrasive

silicone
s. adhesive
Biocell textured s.
s. bleed
s. block
s. elastomer
s. epistaxis catheter
extraluminal s.
s. fluid
s. gel
s. gel bleed
s. gel-filled breast implant (SGBI)
s. gel-filled mammary implant (SGMI)
s. gel-filled mammary implant explantation surgery
s. gel prosthesis
s. gel sheeting
s. granuloma
s. impression
s. impression material
s. injection
s. lip augmentation
s. lubricant
s. mastitis
s. microdroplet
s. rubber
s. rubber base
s. rubber impression
s. rubber impression material
s. textured mammary implant
s. tube
vinyl s.

silicone-filled
s.-f. implant
s.-f. mammary implant

silicone-gel
s.-g. breast implant
s.-g. implant

silicone-treated wound
siliconoma
silicophosphate cement
silk
s. dander
floss s.
s. suture

SilkLaser
EpiTouch Ruby S.
FeatherTouch S.
Sharplan Erbium S.
Sharplan FeatherTouch S.

Sil-K silicone sheet
Silktouch laser
Silky-Rock
sill
s. length
nasal s.
nostril s.

silo
Prolene mesh s.
removal mesh s.

Silon-TSR wound dressing
SilqueClenz skin cleanser
Siltussin-CF
Silux Plus
Silvadene
S. cream

silver
s. alloy
s. amalgam
s. amalgam restoration
s. amine sulfate amide hydrate
s. bar
s. cone
s. cone method
electroplated s.
s. fluoride
s. leaf
s. nitrate
s. point
s. point forceps
s. point pliers
s. point retriever
s. point root canal filling method
precipitated s.
s. precipitated crystal
s. protein, mild
s. recovery
s. silver
s. solder
s. sulfadiazine
s. wire

silver-copper
s.-c. alloy
s.-c. system

silverplated
s. cast
s. die

NOTES

S

549

silverplating
 s. apparatus
silver-stained polyacrylamide gel
Silverstein tetracaine base powder anesthetic
silver-tin
 s.-t. alloy
 s.-t. system
Silybum marianum
simile
Simmonds disease
Simonart band
Simons classification of malocclusion
simple
 s. anchorage
 s. apertognathia
 s. aphasia
 s. beam
 s. bone cyst
 s. flaring suture
 s. harmonic motion (SHM)
 s. mandibular distraction
 s. marginal pulpal fiber
 s. periodontal flap
 s. periodontitis
 s. pocket
 s. predentinal nerve fiber
 s. running suture
 s. sentence
 s. sound source
 s. syllabic
 s. syndactyly
 s. tone
 s. wave
 s. word
simplex
 s. bridge
 herpes s.
 periodontitis s.
simplification
Simplified Oral Hygiene Index (OHI-S)
simulator
simultaneous
 s. auditory feedback
 s. latram and mastectomy (SLAM)
 s. method
Sinarest
 S. 12 Hour Nasal Solution
 S., No Drowsiness
Sine-Aid IB
Sine-Aid, Maximum Strength
Sine-Off Maximum Strength No Drowsiness Formula
Sine-U-View endoscope
sine wave
Sinex Long-Acting
Singer-Blom prosthesis

singer's
 s. formant
 s. nodes
 s. nodule
single
 s. cone root canal filling method
 s. denture construction
 s. fracture
 s. lens reflex (SLR)
 s. nutrient vessel
 s. sleeve bar joint
 s. tooth
 s. width bracket
single-beveled cutting instrument
single-chambered
 s.-c. saline Becker prosthesis
 s.-c. saline implant
single-channel cochlear implant
single-hatching undermining
single-lumen cannula
single-paste system
single-pedicle flap
single-plane instrument
single-portal
 s.-p. ECTR
 s.-p. endocarpal tunnel release
single-pour technique
single-rooted tooth
single-stage
 s.-s. castration, vaginal construction, perineoplasty
 s.-s. replacement
 s.-s. screw implant
singleton
 prevocalic s.
single-tooth
 s.-t. macrodontia
 s.-t. microdontia
 s.-t. root form implant
 s.-t. subperiosteal implant
singulare
 foramen s.
singultation
singultous
singultus
sinister
 auris s. (AS)
sinistral
sinistrality
sinodural angle
sinonasal
 s. melanoma
 s. papilloma
 s. tract
sintering
Sinubid
Sinufed Timecelles

Sinupan
sinus, pl. **sinuses**
    accessory s.
    Afrin S.
    alveolar s.
    s. barotrauma
    branchial cleft s.
    cavernous s.
    s. closure
    s. cranialization
    discharging s.
    dura mater venous s.
    s. elevation
    ethmoidal s.
    S. Excedrin Extra Strength
    first branchial cleft s.
    frontal s.
    functional endoscopic s. (FES)
    s. group of air cell
    inferior petrosal s.
    s. irrigation
    lateral s.
    s. lateralis
    lateral venous s. (LVS)
    s. lift osteotome
    s. line
    maxillary s.
    s. of Morgagni
    Motrin IB S.
    s. mucocele
    opacified frontal s.
    paranasal s.
    piriform s.
    posterior s.
    s. radiograph
    right frontal s.
    sagittal s.
    septa in s.
    sigmoid s.
    sphenoidal s.
    straight s.
    s. surgery
    s. thrombophlebitis
    s. thrombosis
    s. tonsillaris
    s. tract
    s. tract cyst
    tympanic s.
    wide sigmoid s.
SinuScope
sinuscopy
    maxillary s.

sinuses (*pl. of* sinus)
sinusitis
    acute frontal s.
    acute maxillary s.
    allergic fungal s. (AFS)
    chronic frontal s.
    chronic maxillary s.
    ethmoidal s.
    frontal s.
    isolated sphenoid s.
    maxillary s.
    osteoblastic s.
    sphenoidal s.
    vacuum s.
sinusoid
sinusoidal
    s. tracking test
    s. vibration
    s. wave
sinusotomy
    endoscopic intranasal frontal s.
SinuSpacer turbinate stent
Sinus-Relief
Sinutab
    S. Tablet
    S. Without Drowsiness
Sipple syndrome
Siremobil
    S. C-arm unit
Sirognathograph
SISI
    small increment sensitivity index
      High Level SISI
      SISI test
Sister Helen mustard table
sister-hook forceps
Sistrunk
    S. operation
    S. procedure
site
    donor s.
    immunocompetent s.
    pedicled enteric donor s.
    pooling s.
    visceral donor s.
situ
    carcinoma in s.
    in s.
    melanoma in s. (MIS)
situs inversus

S

NOTES

six
s. Hertz positive spike
s. Hertz positive spike-wave
six-hole mandibular plate
sixth cranial nerve
sixth-year molar
sixty-cycle hum
size
beam s.
s. of fenestration
parfocal spot s.
sizer
voice prosthesis s.
sizing
ISO s.
Sjögren syndrome
skatole
Skelaxin
skeletal
s. correction
s. deep bite
s. disproportion
s. distraction
s. occlusion
s. open bite
s. pin fixation
skeleton
s. earmold
extralaryngeal s.
hand s.
osseocartilaginous craniofacial s.
skeletonizing
Skelid
skill
auditory s.
basic s.
Differentiation of Auditory
Perception S. (DAPS)
nonverbal communication s.
Test of Auditory-Perceptual S.
skin
ablated s.
biologic creep of s.
s. brassiere
buttonholing of s.
circumferential tearing of s.
s. creep
cycle loading of s.
depigmenting s.
s. edge necrosis
s. envelope invagination
s. expansion technique
flaccid s.
s. flap
glabrous s.
s. graft
s. grafting
harnessing extra s.

heavy s.
hemosiderin staining of the s.
s. hook
inherent extensibility of s.
s. island
juxtabrow s.
s. maceration
mechanical creep of s.
new s.
s. paddle
s. pocket
pseudoptotic s.
S. Repair Oxygen Spray
residual s.
s. resurfacing
retroauricular s.
sliding s.
stress relaxation of s.
suborbicularis s.
s. of teeth
s. test
thick s.
s. undermining
viscoelastic property of s.
s. wheal
Skinlight erbium yttrium-aluminum-garnet laser
skin/muscle flap blepharoplasty
Skinner classification
skin-sparing mastectomy
skin-subcutaneous dissection with SMAS manipulation
Skintech
S. after laser skin product
S. Postoperative Skin Care Kit
S. skin care product
skip
s. lesion
s. metastasis
ski slope curve
Sklar Aphasia Scale
SKOLD
Screening Kit of Language Development
Skoog
S. procedure
S. technique
skull
s. base
s. base chordoma
s. base suture
s. base tumor
s. base tumor resection
cloverleaf s.
s. radiograph
radiolucent s.
radiopaque s.
trilobed s.
skullcap

Skytron surgical table
SL
  sensation level
S/L
  A-Spas S/L
slab
  mixing s.
slag burn
SLAM
  simultaneous latram and mastectomy
slang
slant of occlusal plane
slash pine
sledge hammer
sleep apnea
sleeve
  delivery assistance s.
  s. graft
slender ragweed
SLI
  specific language impairment
slice preparation
slick
  S. stylette endotracheal tube guide
  s. tongue
slide
  s. in centric
  eccentric s.
sliding
  epidermal s.
  s. flap
  s. genioplasty
  s. hook
  s. oblique osteotomy
  s. skin
slight
  s. hearing impairment
  s. hearing loss
sling
  cervicofacial s.
  dynamic s.
  facial s.
  fascia s.
  fascial s.
  s. ligation
  mandibular s.
  muscle s.
  pterygomasseteric s.
  s. ring complex
  static s.
  s. suture, type I, II
  temporalis s.

Slingerland Screening Tests for
  Identifying Children with Specific
  Language Disability
slip
  medial s.
slipped strut
slippery elm
slit
  cholesterol s.'s
  s. fricative
SLN
  sentinel lymph node
  superior laryngeal nerve
slope
  lower ridge s.
  mandibular anteroposterior ridge s.
Slosson
  S. Articulation Language Test with
  Phonology (SALT-P)
  S. Intelligence Test for Children
  and Adults
slot
  Begg s.'s
  bracket s.
  edgewise s.
  gingival s.
  s. preparation
slotted attachment
slot-type preparation
slough
slow
  s. expressive language development
  (SELD)
  s. maxillary expansion
  s. palatal expander
  s. vertex response
slow-component velocity (SCV)
slow-reacting substance of anaphylaxis
  (SRS-A)
slow-twitch fatigue-resistant skeletal
  muscle
SLR
  single lens reflex
SLS Chromos long pulse ruby laser
  system
Sluder
  S. guillotine tonsillectomy
  lower half headache of S.
  S. neuralgia
sludge
sluiceway
slumping

S

NOTES

slurring
   s. speech
Slux resin
Sly
   mucopolysaccharidosis type VII S.
   (MPS-VII)
   S. syndrome
SMA
   spinal muscular atrophy
small
   s. cell carcinoma
   s. cell neuroendocrine carcinoma
   s. cup biopsy forceps
   s. fenestra stapedotomy
   s. incisional biopsy
   s. increment sensitivity index
   (SISI)
   s. increment sensitivity index test
   s. interarch distance
   s. particle composite resin
   s. tooth
small-bore cannula
smallpox
   s. vaccination
small-vessel anastomosis
Smart
   S. Screener infant hearing screener
   S. Trigger Bear 1000 ventilator
Smartdop Doppler
SMAS
   superficial musculoaponeurotic system
   complex SMAS
   SMAS imbrication face-lift
   SMAS lift
   SMAS plication face-lift
   SMAS plication procedure
   SMAS rhytidectomy
   SMAS tissue
smasectomy
   lateral s.
SMAS-platysma flap
smear layer
SMEI
   S. ultrasound-assisted lipoplasty
   machine
   S. ultrasound device
smell
   s. impairment
Smilax officinalis
SMILE
   subperiosteal minimally invasive laser
   endoscopic
   SMILE face-lift
   SMILE rhytidectomy
smile
   canine s.
   corner-of-the-mouth s.
   full-denture s.

   gummy s.
   Mona Lisa s.
   s. reconstruction
SmiLine abutment system
Smith
   S. and Nephew ENT
   nasopharyngoscope
   S. & Nephew Richards bipolar
   forceps
   S. resin cement
   S. zinc cement
Smith-Johnson Nonverbal Performance
   Scale
smoke
   cigarette s.
   s. eater tube
smokeless tobacco
smoker's
   s. cancer
   s. patch
   s. tongue
smooth
   s. broach
   s. muscle antibody
   s. muscle cell
   s. pliers
   s. surface
   s. surface caries
   s. surface cavity
   s. tongue
smooth-pursuit eye movement
smooth-sided post
smotherweed
SMR
   submucous resection
smut
   Bermuda s.
   cultivated barley s.
   cultivated corn s.
   cultivated oat s.
   cultivated rye s.
   cultivated wheat s.
S/N
   signal-to-noise ratio
   S/N ratio
SN$_B$, S-N-B, SNB
   sella-nasion-supramentale angle
SN$_A$, S-N-A, SNA
   sella-nasion-subspinale angle
snaggle tooth
snake
   copperhead s.
   coral s.
   cottonmouth s.
snakeroot
   seneca s.
snap impression
Snaplets-EX

snap-on mandrel
snapping triceps tendon
snare
    dissection s.
    Tydings tonsil s.
snarl
SNB (*var. of* SN$_B$)
S-N-B (*var. of* SN$_B$)
SND
    selective neck dissection
sneeze
Snellen Eye Chart
SNHL
    sensorineural hearing loss
sniffing
sniff method
S-N line
SN-N
    sternal notch-to-nipple
SnO$_2$
    tin oxide
snore
snoring
snort
    nasal s.
snow
    carbon dioxide s.
    s. plow rasp
snow-capped teeth
Snow procedure
snuff
snuffles
Snyder test
SO$_2$
    sulfur dioxide
soap
    PROVON antimicrobial lotion s.
    Psor-a-set S.
soap-bubble appearance
social
    S. Adequacy Index (SAI)
    s. babbling
    s. behavior
    Facial Disability Index S. (FDIS)
    s. gesture speech
    s. interaction
    s. learning theory
socioacusis, sociocusis
socioeconomic status (SES)
sociolect
sociolinguistics

socket
    alveolar s.
    comminution of alveolar s.
    dry s.
    infected s.
    s. joint
    s. joint of tooth
    tooth s.
    s. void
sodium
    s. alginate
    ampicillin s.
    s. ascorbate
    bromfenac s.
    s. caprylate
    s. carbonate
    cefuroxime s.
    s. chloride
    s. citrate
    colistimethate s.
    cromolyn s.
    s. diethyldithiocarbamate
    s. dodecyl sulfate-polyacrylamide
      gel electrophoresis (SDS-PAGE)
    s. fluoride
    s. fluoride dentifrice
    s. fluoride-orthophosphoric acid gel
    s. fluoride-orthophosphoric acid
      solution
    s. fluoride solution
    s. hypochlorite
    Nembutal S.
    pentobarbital s.
    s. perborate (SP)
    piperacillin and tazobactam s.
    s. salicylate
    secobarbital s.
    Seconal S.
    S. Sulamyd Ophthalmic
    sulbactam s.
    sulfacetamide s.
    s. sulfite
    s. tetradecyl
    s. tetradecyl sulfate
sodium-PCA
    lactic acid and s.-P.
sodium-potassium
    s.-p. aluminum silicate abrasive
    s.-p. pump
Sof-Cil

S

NOTES

So-Flo
>S.-F. phosphate topical gel
>S.-F. phosphate topical solution

SOFS
>superior orbital fissure syndrome

soft
>s. biscuit
>s. bisque
>s. bristle
>s. cleft palate
>S. Denture Reline acrylic
>s. liner
>s. mixed odontogenic tumor
>s. mixed odontoma
>s. neurological signs
>s. palate
>s. palate cleft
>s. palate paralysis
>s. tissue
>s. tissue contracture
>s. tissue curettage
>s. tissue cyst
>s. tissue dehiscence
>s. tissue reconstruction
>s. tissue thickness
>s. tissue tumor
>s. tissue undercut
>s. tissue window
>s. whisper
>s. x-ray

Softab
>Bucladin-S S.

softener
>carious dentin s.

Softflo fiber optic probe
SoftLight laser
soft-lined denture
SoftMINT
>Plax S.

Softopac intraoral film
soft-tissue
>s.-t. apposition
>s.-t. calcification
>s.-t. deformity
>s.-t. hypoplasia
>s.-t. mass
>s.-t. nocardiosis

software
>Cafet for Kids s.
>CSL s.
>Dentofacial Planner s.
>Exceltech patient imaging s.
>Jandel Scientific Sigma Image s.
>LySonix ImageFX patient
> imaging s.
>Materialise computer aided
> design s.
>MedMorph III s.

>MirrorOffice s.
>N-terface s.

sol
Solagen Tablet
Solaquin
>S. Forte
>S. Forte cream
>S. Forte gel

Solarcaine
SolarEar hearing aid
solar radiation
solder
>building s.
>gold s.
>hard s.
>silver s.

soldering
sole
soleus muscle
Solfoton
Solfy ZX ultrasonic unit
Solganal
solid
>S. Creation System
>s. dentin
>s. silicone buttock implant

solid-rod rigid telescope
solitarius
>nucleus fasciculus s.

solitary
>s. bone cyst
>s. neurofibroma

Solo-Tach resin
solubility
>s. resistance

Solu-Cortef
Solu-Medrol Injection
Solurex
>S. L.A.

solution
>Adsorbotear Ophthalmic S.
>AK-Dilate Ophthalmic S.
>AK-Nefrin Ophthalmic S.
>AK-Spore Ophthalmic S.
>Akwa Tears S.
>Alconefrin Nasal S.
>Allerest 12 Hour Nasal S.
>AquaSite Ophthalmic S.
>balanced salt s. (BSS)
>Betadine 5% Sterile Ophthalmic
> Prep S.
>Bion Tears S.
>Burow s.
>Chlorphed-LA Nasal S.
>Comfort Tears S.
>Crolom Ophthalmic S.
>Dakin s.
>Dakrina Ophthalmic S.

developer s.
Dey-Drop Ophthalmic S.
dialdehyde s.
disclosing s.
Domeboro s.
Dristan Long Lasting Nasal S.
Dry Eyes S.
Dry Eye Therapy S.
Duration Nasal S.
Dwelle Ophthalmic S.
electrolytic s.
Euro-Collins s.
Eye-Lube-A S.
fixer s.
fluoride s.
Freezone S.
Freon s.
Fungoid S.
glutaraldehyde s.
Hank Balanced Salt S.
hardening s.
Hartman s.
HypoTears PF S.
Intal Nebulizer S.
ion phosphate fluoride topical s.
I-Phrine Ophthalmic S.
Iradicav acidulated phosphate
  fluoride s.
isolyte S multielectrolyte s.
Isopto Plain S.
Isopto Tears S.
Jessner s.
Just Tears S.
Kligman s.
Krebs-Ringer s.
Lacril Ophthalmic S.
Liquifilm Forte S.
Liquifilm Tears S.
Lotrimin AF S.
LubriTears S.
Luride topical s.
Microfil s.
minimal essential s. (MEM)
Murine S.
Murocel Ophthalmic S.
Mycocide NS antimicrobial s.
Mydfrin Ophthalmic S.
NaCl s.
NaFrinse acidulated s.
Nasalcrom Nasal S.
Nature's Tears S.
Neosporin Ophthalmic S.

Neo-Synephrine 12 Hour Nasal S.
Neo-Synephrine Ophthalmic S.
Nostril Nasal S.
NTZ Long Acting Nasal S.
Nu-Tears II S.
OcuCoat PF Ophthalmic S.
ofloxacin otic s.
Pacemaker Nafeen s.
Pacemaker topical fluoride s.
pickling s.
PiercingCare s.
povidone-iodine s.
Prefrin Ophthalmic S.
Puralube Tears S.
Rafluor topical s.
Refresh Plus Ophthalmic S.
Relief Ophthalmic S.
Rhinall Nasal S.
Roxicet Oral S.
Saslow s.
Sinarest 12 Hour Nasal S.
sodium fluoride s.
sodium fluoride-orthophosphoric
  acid s.
So-Flo phosphate topical s.
Span+Aids Homecare S.
St. Joseph Measured Dose
  Nasal S.
surgical marking s.
Tear Drop S.
TearGard Ophthalmic S.
Teargen Ophthalmic S.
Tearisol S.
Tears Naturale Free S.
Tears Naturale II S.
Tears Plus S.
Tears Renewed S.
thrombin s.
trehalose-Euro-Collins s.
Tubulicid Plus root canal
  antibacterial s.
tumescent anesthesia s.
Ultra Tears S.
Verhoeff s.
Vicks Sinex Nasal S.
Viva-Drops S.
4-Way Long Acting Nasal S.
wetting s.
solvent
  s. inhalation
Solvidont

S

NOTES

SOM
serous otitis media
SOMA
System of Multicultural Assessment
Soma
S. Compound
S. Compound w/Codeine
somatic
s. delusion
s. motor nerve
s. swallow
somatization
Somatom Plus S whole body scanner
somatoprosthetics
somatosensory response
somatostatin
somesthetic
s. area
s. dysarthria
somite
mesodermal s.
somitomere
somnoplasty
s. tissue reduction treatment
SOMPA
System of Multicultural Pluralistic
Assessment
sonant
sone
Song and Song method
Sonic
S. Air 1500 device
sonic
s. scaler
s. sculpture
s. wave
Sono-Explorer
sonogram
sonograph
Diasonic DRF 1000 s.
sonographer
Combison 530 3D s.
Sonoline 400 2D s.
Sonoline SL1 2D s.
Sonoline
S. 400 2D sonographer
S. SL1 2D sonographer
sonorant
s. sound
sonority
Sono-stat
S.-s. Plus EMG machine
S.-s. Plus joint sound measuring
and documentation system
S.-s. Plus sound device
sonotrode

Sony
S. professional Walkman WM-D6C
S. video recorder
SOOF
suborbicularis oculi fat
soprano voice
sore
canker s.
ischial pressure s.
Oriental s.
pressure s.
s. throat
Sorensen chisel
sorghum grass
sorption
water s.
sorrel
sheep s.
Sorrin operation
SOT
sensory organization test
squamous odontogenic tumor
Sotradecol
S. Injection
sound
air-blade s.
amphoric voice s.
s. analysis
s. blending
cavernous voice s.
embedded s.
s. field
gross s.
impact s.
s. intensity
s. level
s. level meter
nasal s.
nonnasal s.
nonsonorant s.
nonspeech s.
nonsyllabic speech s.
obstruent s.
Ohio Tests of Articulation and
Perception of S.'s (OTAPS)
perceptually adequate s.
plosive s.
s. power density
s. pressure level (SPL)
s. pressure level range
s. pressure level scale
s. pressure wave
s. quality
s. quantity
retroflex s.
sibilant s.
sonorant s.
s. spectrogram

s. spectrograph
s. spectrum
spirant s.
standard speech s.
syllabic speech s.
velopharyngeal friction s.
s. wave
sound-symbol association
source
ESI fiberoptic light s.
fiberoptic light s.
halogen light s.
simple sound s.
Teclite fiberoptic light s.
xenon light s.
sour dock
South
S. American blastomycosis
S. American trypanosomiasis
soybean
s. grain dust mite
s. meal
SP
sodium perborate
substance P
Cordran SP
Sp6 RNA polymerase
space
air s.
anatomical dead s.
apical s.
arachnoid s.
s. of body of mandible
buccal s.
buccinator s.
buccopharyngeal s.
carotid s.
danger s.
dead s.
deep s.
s. denture
denture s.
digastric s.
s. of Donders
E s.
edentulous s.
embrasure s.
escapement s.'s
extracellular s. (ECS)
extraction s.
fascial s.
fat cell s.

fixed maintainer s.
freeway s.
geniohyoid s.
gingival s.
globular s.'s of Czermak
infraorbital s.
infratemporal s.
interalveolar s.
intercellular s. (ICS)
interdental s.
interglobular s.
interglobular s. of Owen
interocclusal rest s.
interorbital s.
interprismatic s.
interproximal s.
interproximate s.
interradicular s.
interstitial s.
joint s.
lateral pharyngeal s.
lattice s.
leeway s.
s. maintainer
maintainer cast s.
mandibular s.
marrow s.
masseteric s.
masseter-mandibulopterygoid s.
masticator s.
masticatory s.
Nance leeway s.
obtainer s.
orthodontic maintainer s.
paraglottic s.
parapharyngeal s. (PPS)
parotid s.
peridentinoblastic s.
periimplant s.
perineural s.
peripharyngeal s.
periprosthetic s.
peritonsillar s.
pharyngomaxillary s.
posterior airway s. (PAS)
postzygomatic s.
pre-epiglottic s.
pretemporal s.
pretracheal s.
prevertebral s.
proximal s.
proximate s.

S

NOTES

space *(continued)*
    Prussak s.
    pterygoid s.
    pterygomandibular s.
    pterygomaxillary s.
    pterygopalatine s.
    regainer s.
    Reinke s.
    relief s.
    removable maintainer s.
    s. retainer
    s. retaining appliance
    retraction s.
    retromylohyoid s.
    retropharyngeal s.
    retrozygomatic s.
    s. of Retzius
    septal s.
    sphenomaxillary s.
    sphenopalatine s.
    subepicranial s.
    subgingival s.
    sublingual s.
    submandibular s.
    submasseteric s.
    submaxillary s.
    submental s.
    superior joint s.
    suprahyoid s.
    suprasternal s.
    tissue s.
    triangular s.
    visceral s.
    web s.
    zygomaticotemporal s.
space-age wire
spaced teeth
space-maintaining barrier
spacer
    die s.
    Ellipse compact s.
spacial
    s. balance
    s. discrimination
spacing
    excessive s.
    generalized s.
    interdental s.
    unimaxillary s.
spaghetti fat grafting technique
span
    attention s.
    auditory memory s.
    comprehension s.
    condylar s.
    interbracket s.
    memory s.
    visual memory s.

Span+Aids Homecare Solution
Spansule
    Ornade S.
SPAR
    sensitivity prediction from the acoustic
    reflex
sparfloxacin
spasm
    chin s.
    diffuse esophageal s.
    esophageal s.
    facial s.
    glottic s.
    hemifacial s.
    laryngeal s.
    phonic s.
    postparalytic hemifacial s.
    primitive hemifacial s.
spasmodic
    s. croup
    s. dysphonia
    s. laryngeal cough
    s. laryngitis
spasmodica
    dysarthria syllabaris s.
spasmus
    s. glottidis
spastic
    s. contracture
    s. dysarthria
    s. dysphonia
    s. frontalis syndrome
    s. muscle
    s. paralysis
    s. speech
spastica
    dysphonia s.
spasticity
spatial balance
spatium, pl. spatia
    s. interglobulare
    spatia interglobularia
spatula
    cement s.
    metal handle mixing s.
    nonmetallic s.
    No. 7 wax s.
    plaster s.
    plastic s.
    s. tip
spatulate
spatulated
    ASSI breast dissector s.
spatulation
    s. condensation
spatulator
    hand mechanical s.
    power-driven mechanical s.

Spaulding classification
S-2PD
    static two-point discrimination
SPEAK
    spectral peak
    SPEAK cochlear stimulation mode
speaker's nodes
speaking
    choral s.
    s. phonation (SFo)
spear-point drill
special
    s. cell
    s. somatic sensory nerve
specialized mucosa
species
    Proteus s.
specific
    s. expressive language impairment
      (SELI)
    s. granuloma
    s. language impairment (SLI)
specificity theory
specimen
    nontraumatized full-thickness s.
speckled leukoplakia
Spec-T
Spectazole
spectra (*pl. of* spectrum)
spectral peak (SPEAK)
Spectra-System
    S.-S. abutment
    S.-S. implant
Spectrobid
spectrogram
    sound s.
spectrograph
    real-time s.
    sound s.
spectrometer
    liquid scintillation s.
spectrophotometric analysis
spectrophotometry
    atomic absorption s.
    dual wavelength s.
    electrothermal atomic absorption s.
      (EAAS)
spectrum, pl. spectra, spectrums
    acoustic s.
    band s.
    electromagnetic s.

    sound s.
    tonal s.
Spectrum K1 laser
speculum
    Bionix disposable nasal s.
    Cottle nasal s.
    Downes nasal s.
    ear s.
    flat-bladed nasal s.
    s. holder
    Killian nasal s.
    nasal s.
Spee
    curve of S.
speech
    accelerated s.
    acoustically modified s.
    s. act
    alaryngeal s.
    s. apraxia
    s. aspect
    Assessment of Intelligibility of
      Dysarthric S.
    s. audiogram
    s. audiometer
    s. audiometry
    automatic s.
    s. awareness
    s. awareness threshold (SAT)
    babbled s.
    Bell Visible S.
    buccal s.
    s. bulb
    cerebellar s.
    clipped s.
    cold-running s.
    s. community
    compressed s.
    connected s.
    s. conservation
    continuity of s.
    s. correction
    s. correctionist
    cued s.
    dactyl s.
    deaf s.
    s. defect
    delayed s.
    demand s.
    s. detectability threshold (SDT)
    s. detection
    s. detection threshold (SDT)

NOTES

speech *(continued)*
s. development
deviant s.
s. discrimination (SD)
S. Discrimination in Noise
s. discrimination score (SDS)
s. discrimination threshold
s. disorder
displaced s.
s. distortion
echo s.
egocentric s.
esophageal s.
explosive s.
figure of s.
filtered s.
s. fistula
s. frequency
s. gesture
s. and hearing science
helium s.
high-stimulus s.
home-based smooth s.
hot potato s.
hypernasal s.
hyponasal s.
s. impairment
s. impediment
s. improvement
S. Improvement Cards
infantile s.
s. innateness theory
inner s.
s. intelligibility
intensive smooth s.
s. interference level (SIL)
s. and language clinician
s. and language pathologist
s. and language pathology
meaningful s.
s. mechanism
melody of s.
mimic s.
mirror s.
narrative s.
nasal s.
nasalized s.
s. noise
nonpropositional s.
parts of s.
s. pathologist
s. pathology
s. perception
phantom s.
pharyngeal s.
s. production
propositional s.
rate of s.

s. reading
s. reading aphasia
s. reception (SR)
s. reception threshold (SRT)
s. recognition
s. rehabilitation
residual s.
running s.
scamping s.
scanning s.
s. science
Screening Test for Development
  Apraxia of S.
serial content s.
seriatim s.
slurring s.
social gesture s.
s. sound discrimination
s. sound flow
S. Sound Memory Test
spastic s.
spontaneous s.
staccato s.
subvocal s.
syllabic s.
s. therapist
tolerance threshold for s.
tracheoesophageal s.
s. tracking
s. training unit
tremulous s.
unintelligible s.
visible s.
S. with Alternating Masking Index
  (SWAMI)
speech-motor function
speech-noise ratio
SpeechViewer
speed
S. liner
s. quotient
SPELT-P
Structure Photographic Expressive
  Language Test-II
Spence
axillary tail of S.
Speyer dental casting gold alloy
Sphaerophorus fusiformis
S-phase specific drug
sphenoethmoidal
s. recess
s. suture
sphenoethmoidectomy
radical complete s.
sphenofrontal
s. suture
sphenoid
s. bone

greater wing of s.
lateral wall s.
lesser wing of s.
s. process

sphenoidal
s. cyst
s. nasal conchae
s. ostium
s. rostrum
s. sinus
s. sinusitis
s. sinus septum
s. spine
s. turbinated bones

sphenoidale
planum s.

sphenoidotomy
sphenomandibular ligament
sphenomaxillary
s. space
s. suture

sphenooccipital synchondrosis
sphenoorbital encephalocele
sphenopalatine
s. artery
s. canal
s. foramen
s. ganglion
s. neuralgia
s. space

sphenopetroclival region
sphenotemporal
s. suture

sphenozygomatic suture
spherical
s. amalgam
s. amalgam alloy
s. contracture
s. form
s. form of occlusion
s. recess

spherocytosis
spheroiding
sphincter
artificial s.
esophageal s.
eyelid s.
oral s.
s. pharyngoplasty

sphincteroplasty
spiculated
s. lesion

spicule
bone s.
cemental s.

spider
s. nevus
s. varicosity
s. vein

spike
cartilage s.
cemental s.
diphasic s.
enamel s.
fourteen-and-six Hertz positive s.
negative s.
six Hertz positive s.

spike-wave
negative s.-w.
six Hertz positive s.-w.

spillway
axial s.
interdental s.
occlusal s.

spina
s. bifida cystica
s. helicis

spinach
spinal
s. accessory chin lymph node
s. accessory nerve
s. muscular atrophy (SMA)
s. tract of trigeminal nerve
s. vestibular nucleus

spindle
s. cell
s. cell carcinoma
s. cell hemangioendothelioma
s. cell tumor
enamel s.
muscle s.

spindle-cell fibroblast
spine
anterior nasal s. (ANS)
anterior superior iliac s. (ASIS)
Henle s.
mandibular s.
s. of maxilla
mental s.
nasal s.
palatine s.
posterior nasal s. (PNS)
sphenoidal s.

S

NOTES

spine (continued)
    s. of sphenoid bone
    suprameatal s.
spin echo pulse sequence
SpineStat side-directed diskectomy probe
spiney pigweed
spinning
    marginal s.
    s. top test
spinoreticulothalamic
    s. pathway
spinosum
    foramen s.
    stratum s.
spinothalamic
    lateral s.
spinous cell
spiradenoma
    eccrine s.
Spira disease
spiral
    s. archwire
    s. artery
    s. canal of Rosenthal
    s. coil stent
    s. computed tomography
      angiography
    s. effect
    s. endosseous implant
    s. endosteal implant
    s. fluted tungsten carbide bur
    s. ganglion
    s. lamina
    lentula s.
    s. ligament
    S. Mark V portable ultrasonic
      drug inhaler
    s. organ
    s. sulcus
spiralis
    Trichinella s.
spirant
    s. sound
Spirec drill
spirochetal
spirochete
spirometer
    Coach incentive s.
    Spirometrics Micro & s.
    Timeter pocket s.
Spirometrics Micro & spirometer
Spirosense system
spitting
Spitz nevus
SPL
    sound pressure level

splayed
    s. alar cartilage
    s. facial nerve
spleen
Splendore-Hoeppli phenomenon
splenius capitis muscle
splenomegaly
Spline
    S. dental implant system
    S. Twist dental implant
    S. Twist MTX implant
    S. Twist Ti implant
splint
    abutment s.
    acid etch cemented s.
    acrylic ear s.
    acrylic interocclusal s.
    acrylic overlay s.
    acrylic resin bite-guard s.
    anchor s.
    Angle s.
    Aquaplast nasal s.
    Bilson fixable-removable cross arch
      bar s.
    bridge s.
    buccal s.
    canine-to-canine lingual s.
    cap s.
    cast bar s.
    compression s.
    compressive plastic s.
    continuous clasp s.
    copper band-acrylic s.
    crib s.
    cross arch bar s.
    Doyle bi-valved airway s.
    elastic plastic s.
    Elbrecht s.
    Essig s.
    Essig-type s.
    extracoronal s.
    fenestrated s.
    fixed partial denture s.
    folded aluminum ear s.
    fracture s.
    Friedman s.
    functional s.
    Gilmer s.
    Gunning one-piece s.
    Gunning two-piece s.
    Hammond s.
    implant surgical s.
    indexed s.
    inlay s.
    interdental s.
    Kazanjian s.
    Kingsley s.
    labial s.

labiolingual s.
lingual s.
mandibular s.
occlusal s.
onlay s.
oyster s.
permanent s.
plaster of Paris s.
plastic s.
polymethyl methacrylate ear s.
porcelain-fused-to-metal s.
pressure s.
provisional s.
reverse Kingsley s.
sandwich-type s.
Stader s.
surgical s.
temporary s.
thermoplastic s.
Ultraflex ankle dorsiflexion
  dynamic s.
wire s.
splinted abutment
splinter forceps
splinting
cross arch s.
extracoronal s.
intracoronal s.
provisional s.
split
s. acrylic spring
s. acrylic spring space regainer
anterior cricoid s.
s. calvarial graft
s. cast method
s. cast mount
s. cast mounting
cricoid s.
s. half reliability coefficient
s. hand/split foot malformation
mandibular s.
s. papule
s. plate
s. plate appliance
s. tooth
s. uvula
s. word
split-bone technique
split-shank screw post
split-skin graft
splitter
beam s.

split-thickness
s.-t. periodontal flap
s.-t. periodontal graft
s.-t. skin graft (STSG)
splitting
sagittal s. of mandible
SPOA
subperiosteal orbital abscess
spoke-shave
spondaic
spondee
s. word
spondylitis
ankylosing s.
tuberculous s.
Spondylocladium
sponge
absorbable gelatin s.
bronchoscopic s.
Expandacell s.
s. forceps
gelatin s.
s. gold
Ivalon s.
Reston s.
spongiosis
spongiosum
corpus s.
spongiotic lesion
spongy bone
spontaneous
s. conversation
s. emission
s. fracture
s. imitation
s. nystagmus
s. perilymph fistula
s. recovery
s. speech
spoon excavator
spoon-shaped hand
sporadic Burkitt lymphoma
Sporanox
spore
Bacillus stearothermophilus s.
Bacillus subtilis s.
Sporex
sporicidal
Sporicidin
Sporobolomyces
Sporothrix schenckii
sporotrichosis

S

NOTES

Sporotrichum

spot
    aberrant mongolian s.
    Brushfield s.
    café au lait s.
    De Morgan s.
    Filatov s.
    Fordyce s.
    s. grinding
    Koplik s.
    latent image s.
    liver s.
    s. necrosis
    pink s.
    s. welding

sprain
    temporomandibular joint s.

spray
    Astelin nasal s.
    Caldecort Anti-Itch S.
    colored indicator s.
    Fluori-Methane Topical S.
    Hurricaine s.
    Miacalcin Nasal S.
    mometasone furoate monohydrate nasal s.
    Nasarel Nasal S.
    Ony-Clear S.
    Skin Repair Oxygen S.
    titanium plasma s. (TPS)
    triamcinolone acetonide nasal s.

sprayed
    titanium plasma s. (TPS)

spray-wipe-spray disinfection

spread
    droplet s.
    extracapsular s. (ECS)

spread-and-cut technique

spreader
    Endotec s.
    finger s.
    s. graft
    gutta-percha s.
    hand s.
    Mity s.
    root canal s.
    root canal filling s.
    separated s.
    Wakai s.

spring
    auxiliary s.
    bow s.
    s. bridge
    closed s.
    closed-coil nickel titanium s.
    Coffin s.
    coil s.
    finger s.

    free-end s.
    helical s.
    Kesling s.
    open s.
    paddle s.
    perichondrial s.
    s. plate
    rotating s.
    separating s.
    split acrylic s.
    torquing s.
    uprighting s.
    Z s.

springback

spring-loaded self-retaining retractor

Sprinkle
    Deconsal S.

sprouting
    axonal s.

sprouts
    Brussel s.

spruce

sprue
    s. base
    casting s.
    s. former
    s. pin

sprue-former

spruing

9925 SPS ELCOmed100 system

spur
    enamel s.
    nasal s.
    septum s.

sputter
    gold-palladium s.

sputum

squalene oil

squama of temporal bone

squamous
    s. cell carcinoma (SCC)
    s. cell carcinoma of head and neck (SCCHN)
    s. cell carcinoma inhibitory factor (SSCIF)
    s. cell papilloma
    s. cell pseudoepithelioma
    s. epithelial ingrowth
    s. epithelium
    s. odontogenic tumor (SOT)
    s. papilloma

square
    s. arch
    s. bracket
    s. muscle of lower lip
    s. muscle of upper lip
    s. wire

squared

joules per centimeter s. (J/cm^2)

square-wave signal

squash

squaw vine

Squeeze-Mark surgical marker

SR

speech reception

Deconamine SR

Extendryl SR

Indocin SR

Respaire-120 SR

Respaire-60 SR

Sr

Congess Sr

SRC Expectorant

SRS-A

slow-reacting substance of anaphylaxis

SRT

speech reception threshold

S.S.

S. White clamp

S. White J-Notch surgical
handpiece bur

S. White 100 K surgical handpiece
bur

S. White new filling porcelain

S. White pulp tester

S. White punch

SSCIF

squamous cell carcinoma inhibitory
factor

SSD

S. AF

S. Cream

SSL

subtotal supraglottic laryngectomy

SSO

sagittal split osteotomy

SSPL

saturation sound pressure level

SSRO

sagittal split ramus osteotomy

SSW

Staggered Spondaic Word Test

St.

stomion

St. Anthony fire

St. John's wort

St. Joseph Measured Dose Nasal
Solution

St. Joseph Adult Chewable Aspirin

Stabident

S. interosseous local anesthesia
system

S. ultrashort needle

Stabilex attachment

stability

denture s.

dimensional s.

gaze s.

occlusal s.

stabilization

columellar subluxation s.

coronoradicular s.

jaw s.

s. surgery

stabilized

s. base

s. baseplate

stabilizer

endodontic s.

subpectoral s.

stabilizing

s. arm

s. circumferential arm clasp

s. circumferential clasp arm

s. fulcrum line

Stableloc II external fixator system

staccato

s. burst

s. speech

stacked arch

Stader splint

Stadol

S. NS

Stafne

S. bone cyst

S. idiopathic bone cavity

stage

bell s.

bud s.

cap s.

cognitive development s.

desmolytic s.

Dulguerov T s.

eruptive s.

formative s.

S. I appliance

S. I, II, III, IV archwire

interglobular s.

lamina-bud s.

maturative s.

morphogenic s.

NOTES

stage *(continued)*
    organizing s.
    Piaget cognitive development s.
    preeruptive s.
    pre-mycosis fungoides s.
    protective s.
    retiform s.
    stuttering s.
    transitional pulp s.
    ugly duckling s.
    s. whisper
    Wilkes s. I–V
    Wilkes s. V
staged
    s. celiotomy
    s. genioplasty
    s. muscle transfer
    s. procedure
    s. reconstruction
    s. tympanoplasty
Stagesic
staggered
    s. arch
    S. Spondaic Word Test (SSW)
staging
    intraoperative tumor s.
    s. system
    TNM tumor s.
    tumor s.
stagnation
Sta-Guard mouth protector
Stahist
Stahl ear
stain
    Alcian blue s.
    argentaffin s.
    black s.
    brown s.
    Brown and Brenn s.
    dental s.
    elastic s.
    Gomori methenamine silver s.
    Gram s.
    green s.
    hypertrophic port wine s.
    immunoperoxidase s.
    Kernecht red s.
    Masson trichrome s.
    metallic s.
    orange s.
    porcelain s.
    port wine s. (PWS)
    processing s.
    rhodamine B s.
    tobacco s.
    toluidine blue s.
    Verhoeff elastic s.
    Ziehl-Neelsen s.

StainAway Plus denture cleanser
stained crown
staining
    acid-Schiff s.
    custom s.
    extrinsic environmental s.
    Fontana-Masson s.
    H&E s.
    intrinsic s.
stainless
    s. steel AO plate
    s. steel band
    s. steel crown
Stainton-Capdepont syndrome
Stainton syndrome
staller
Stammberger punch forceps
stammer
stammering
stamp
    cusp s.
    s. cusp
stand
    Keeler Lightsource s.
    Mayo s.
    Wilson Mayo s.
Standalloy
standard
    s. deviation
    s. earmold
    s. language
    LySonix TTD Design S.
    s. reference
    s. score
    s. speech sound
    s. word
standardization
    International Organization for S.
standardized
    s. constant bolus
    s. instrument
    s. test
standing
    s. bevel
    s. wave
Standoli technique
Stanford-Binet Intelligence Scale
Stanide stannous fluoride
Stanimax
    S.-Pro
stanine
stannous
    s. fluoride
    s. fluoride dentifrice
Staodyn Insight point locator
stapedectomy
    laser s.
    partial s.

primary s.
revision s.
stapedial
s. acoustic reflex
s. artery
s. fold
s. reflex test
stapediotenotomy
stapedis
plica s.
stapedius
s. muscle
s. reflex
s. tendon
stapedotomy
laser s.
small fenestra s.
YAG laser s.
stapes, pl. **stapes**
s. fenestra
s. footplate
hypomobile s.
s. mobilization
s. mobilization operation
monopodal ankylotic s.
s. subluxation
s. superstructure
s. tendon contraction
Staphcillin
staphylectomy
staphyledema
staphylion
staphylococcal actinophytosis
staphylococci
Staphylococcus
S. *albus*
S. *aureus*
S. *epidermidis*
S. *pyogenes*
staphylococcus
coagulase-negative s.
staphylodialysis
staphyloncus
staphylopharyngorrhaphy
staphyloplasty
staphyloplegia
staphyloptosia
staphyloptosis
staphylorrhaphy
staphyloschisis
staphylotome
staphylotomy

staple
s. bone plate
five-pin s.
seven-pin s.
titanium mandibular s.
stapler
Graftac-S skin s.
Stark classification
Starkey
S. matrix program
S. model ST3 powered stethoscope
Starling hypothesis
Starlite Omni-AT bur
STAR*LOCK
S. multi-purpose submergible
threaded implant
S. Press-Fit cylinder implant
Starret wire gauge
Star root canal file
STARS
Short-Term Auditory Retrieval and
Storage Test
startle
s. reflex
s. technique
Star/Vent
S. one-stage dental screw implant
S. screw implant
stasis
STAT
Suprathreshold Adaptation Test
state
gel s.
gradient recalled acquisition in the
steady s. (GRASS)
hypercoagulable s.
transition s.
transitional pulp s.
static
s. acoustic impedance
s. bone cyst
s. posturography
s. reconstruction
s. relation
s. sling
s. two-point discrimination (S-2PD)
Sta-Tic impression material
Staticin Topical
statin
O-V s.
stationary
s. anchorage

S

NOTES

stationary *(continued)*
    s. bridge
    s. lingual arch
statoacoustic
statoconium, pl. **statoconia**
Stat-Temp II liquid crystal temperature monitor
status
    disease-specific functional s.
    low socioeconomic s. (low-SES)
    socioeconomic s. (SES)
    s. sternuens
    s. thymicolymphaticus
Status-X machine
staurion
StaySharp face lift Super-Cut scissors
stay suture
S-T Cort
STD
    sexually transmitted disease
STE
    subperiosteal tissue expander
steal
    lateral crural s. (LCS)
    vascular s.
steam
    s. autoclave sterilization
    s. heat
    s. heat sterilizer
steatocystoma multiplex
steatopygia
steel
    s. anchorage arch
    s. crown
    s. embolization coil
    s. ligature
Steele
    S. facing
    S. interchangeable tooth
    S. tooth
steel-slotted plastic bracket
steep drop curve
steeple flap
Steiger
    S. attachment
    S. connector
    S. joint
Steiger-Boitel
    S.-B. attachment
    S.-B. bar
Steiglitz pliers
Stein
    S. pontic
    S. test
Steindler flexoplasty
Steiner bracket

Steinhauser
    S. plate
    S. screw
Steinmann pin
stellate
    s. abscess
    s. ganglion block
    s. reticulum
stem
    Howmedica hip fracture s.
    P.C.A. mid s.
    Precision Osteolock s.
Stemphylium
Stenger test
stenion
stenocompressor
stenosis, pl. **stenoses**
    acquired nasopharyngeal s.
    choanal s.
    chronic cicatricial laryngeal s.
    cicatricial s.
    glottic s.
    hypopharyngeal s.
    iatrogenic nasal s.
    laryngeal s.
    laryngotracheal s.
    meatal s.
    nasal s.
    nasopharyngeal s. (NPS)
    nostril s.
    piriform aperture s.
    subglottic s.
    supraglottic s.
    tracheal s.
stenostomia
stenotic cleft
Stensen
    S. duct
    S. duct caruncle
    S. papilla
Stenstrom
    S. alar cartilage technique
    S. otoplasty
    S. rasp
stent
    Aboulker s.
    antihemorrhagic s.
    Doyle II silicone s.
    Dumon silicone s.
    FES s.
    functional endoscopic sinus s.
    Gianturco expanding metallic s.
    S. graft
    s. introducer
    labial s.
    laryngeal s.
    S. mass
    maxillary s.

methyl methacrylate ear s.
Nitinol subglottic stenosis s.
occlusal s.
ostiomeatal s.
Palmaz s.
pedodontic s.
periodontal s.
Salman FES s.
self-expandable s.
Shikani middle meatal
  antrostomy s.
SinuSpacer turbinate s.
spiral coil s.
trismus s.
variable position s.
Wallstent expanding metallic s.

stenting
Stenvers projection
step
branching s.'s
s. deformity
hair s.
s. preparation
retroauricular hair s.

step-back
s.-b. circumferential filing technique
s.-b. filing technique
s.-b. instrumentation technique

stepdown
s. nursery
s. technique

step-down technique
Stephens Oral Language Screening Test
stepladder
s. incision
s. sign

stepping
s. condenser

step-wedge
Sterall
sterculia gum
stereocilia
cochlear s.
vestibular s.

stereognosis
oral s.

stereolithogram
stereomicroscope
stereoscopic
s. extraoral radiography
s. microscope
s. radiography

stereotactic radiation therapy
stereotyped stress
Steri-Dent dry heat sterilizer
sterile
s. field

sterilization
autoclave s.
chemical vapor s.
Cidex liquid chemical s.
cold s.
defined s.
dry heat oven s.
ethylene oxide s.
glutaraldehyde s.
liquid chemical s.
root canal s.
steam autoclave s.
Steris liquid chemical s.
unsaturated chemical vapor s.

Steril-Ize
sterilizer
bead s.
dry heat s.
glass bead s.
Harvey vapor s.
hot oil s.
hot salt s.
salt s.
steam heat s.
Steri-Dent dry heat s.

Steri-Oss
S.-O. dental implant
S.-O. dental prosthesis
S.-O. Hexlock implant
S.-O. implant device

Steris liquid chemical sterilization
Steri-Strip
Stern
S. attachment
S. G/A attachment
S. gingival latch attachment
S. G/L attachment
S. stress-breaker
S. stress-breaker attachment

sternal
s. notch-to-nipple (SN-N)
s. puncture medullogram

Sterngold
S. Bridgette inlay
S. dental casting gold alloy
S. inlay

S

NOTES

571

Sterngold *(continued)*
  S. Supercast dental casting gold
    alloy
sternoclavicularis muscle
sternocleidomastoid (SCM)
  s. fascia
  s. muscle
  s. region
  s. tumor of infancy
sternocleidomastoideus muscle
sternohyoid
  s. muscle
sternohyoideus muscle
sternomastoid muscle
sternothyroid
  s. muscle
  s. muscle flap laryngoplasty
sternothyroideus muscle
sternotomy
sternuens
  status s.
sternutation
sternutatory
steroid
  catabolic s.
  intraregional s.
steroid-impregnated tape
stertor
  hen-cluck s.
stertorous
stethoscope
  Starkey model ST3 powered s.
Stevanovsky metal eye shield
Stevens-Johnson syndrome
Stevens tenotomy scissors
STF
  superficial temporal fascia
stick
  bite s.
  ice s.
  mouth s.
  percutaneous s.
stick-bite test
Stickler syndrome
sticky wax
stiffness
stigma, pl. **stigmas, stigmata**
  nasolabial s.
Stillman
  S. cleft
  S. method
  S. method of toothbrushing
  S. technique
still radiography technique
Stim-U-Dent
stimulability

stimulated
  s. emission
  s. graciloplasty
stimulation
  ampullofugal s.
  calibrated electrical s.
  direct neural s.
  gingival s.
  hypoglossal nerve s.
  osteoblast s.
  thermal s.
stimulator
  Bimler s.
  Butler s.
  electric nerve s.
  Hilger facial nerve s.
  interdental s.
  long-acting thyroid s. (LATS)
  peripheral nerve s.
  pulsed electromagnetic s. (PEMS)
stimulus, pl. **stimuli**
  cognitive evoked potentials to
    speech and tonal s.
  conditioned s.
  s. generalization
  neutral s.
  nociceptive pain s.
  nonpulsed-current s.
  novel s.
  noxious s.
  pulsed-current s.
  s. substitution
  unconditioned s.
stinger
stippled
  s. tongue
  s. zones
stippling
  s. gingiva
  gingival s.
stirrup
stitch
  alar suspension s.
  dermoepidermal Gillies s.
  figure-of-eight s.
  Frost s.
  key s., keystitch
  mattress s.
  Prolene s.
  quilting s.
  subperiosteal pulling s.
S&T Lalonde hook forceps
STO
  surgical treatment objective
stochastic
stock
  s. implant
  s. impression tray

s. and mouth-formed mouth protector

Stoerk blennorrhea

stoma, pl. **stomas, stomata**

   s. blast
   s. button

stomach tooth

stomatalgia

stomatitis

   acute streptococcal s.
   aphthous s.
   catarrhal s.
   contact allergic s.
   denture s.
   fusospirochetal s.
   gangrenous s.
   gonococcal s.
   herpes s.
   herpetic s.
   lead s.
   s. medicamentosa
   membranous s.
   mercurial s.
   mycotic s.
   necrotizing ulcerative s.
   s. nicotina
   nicotine s.
   nonspecific s.
   Plaut-Vincent s.
   primary herpetic s.
   putrid s.
   recurrent aphthous s. (RAS)
   recurrent herpetic s.
   recurrent ulcerative s.
   s. scorbutica
   ulcerative s.
   s. venenata
   vesicular s.
   Vincent s.
   viral vesicular s.
   vulcanite s.

stomatocatharsis

stomatodeum

stomatodynia

stomatodysodia

stomatoglossitis

stomatognathic

   s. system

stomatography

stomatologic

stomatologist

stomatology

stomatomalacia

stomatomenia

stomatomycosis

stomatopathy

stomatoplastic

stomatoplasty

stomatorrhagia

   s. gingivarum

stomatoschisis

stomatoscope

stomatosis

stomatostatin analog

stomion (St.)

stomodeum

Stonadhesive

stone

   Arkansas s.
   black s.
   blue s.
   s. cast impression
   Class I, II s.
   dental s.
   diamond s.
   Die S.
   s. die
   flat s.
   gray s.
   gray green s.
   green s.
   high-strength s.
   improved s.
   intraglandular s.
   mounted s.
   mounted point s.
   pulp s.
   Rapid S.
   red s.
   salivary s.
   sharpening s.
   Vel Mix S.
   wheel s.
   Whip-Mix Die-Rock dental s.
   Whip-Mix Microstone dental s.
   Whip-Mix Quickstone dental s.
   Whip-Mix Silky-Rock dental s.
   white s.

Stop

stop

   Endo s.
   glottal s.
   instrument s.
   Krueger s.

NOTES

S

stop *(continued)*
    Krueger instrument s.
    occlusal s.
    rubber s.
    teardrop s.
    ubiquitous glottal s.
stopcock
Stopko irrigator
stopping
    s. of fricative
    Hill s.
    temporary s.
stop-speculum
storm
    thyroid s.
Story Articulation Test
Storz
    S. 30- and 70-degree endoscope
    S. equipment
    S. miniplate
    S. plate
    S. rhinomanometer
    S. Sine-U-View endoscope
Storz-Hopkins system
Stough punch
Stout continuous wiring
strabismus
straight
    s. ahead bronchoscopic telescope
    s. archwire
    s. burnisher
    s. canal
    s. chisel
    s. enamel
    s. fissure bur
    s. forceps
    s. handpiece
    s. inclined plane elevator
    s. laryngeal mirror
    s. magnifying mirror
    s. mosquito hemostat
    s. scissors
    s. sinus
    s. trough
    s. tympanoplasty knife
    s. wire fixed orthodontic appliance
straight-on radiograph
straight-pin teeth
strain
    Armand Frappier s.
    Connaught s.
    Dutch s.
    eye s.
    s. gauge
    mechanical s.
    nominal s.
    Pasteur s.

    Tice s.
    Tokyo s.
strain-time curve
Straith Z-plasty
strand
    epithelial s.
    lateral enamel s.
strangle
strangulated
strangulation
strap
    API universal foam chin s.
    breast s.
    lingual s.
    s. muscle
    palatal s.
    Press Lift chin s.
    Silastic s.
strata (*pl. of* stratum)
strategic tooth
strategy
    ankle s.
    hip s.
stratified squamous epithelium
stratum, pl. strata
    s. adamantinum
    s. basale
    s. corneum
    s. eboris
    s. granulosum
    s. intermedium
    s. spinosum
    s. superficiale
    superior s.
Strauss syndrome
strawberry
    s. hemangioma
    s. nevus
    s. tongue
    s. tumor
stream
    breath s.
streaming
    acoustical s.
strength
    Acutrim II, Maximum S.
    Allerest Maximum S.
    Anbesol Maximum S.
    Aspirin Free Anacin Maximum S.
    Bayer Low Adult S.
    biting s.
    bond s.
    Clocort Maximum S.
    compressive s.
    Cortaid Maximum S.
    s. deficit
    diametral tensile s.
    s. duration curve

Dynafed, Maximum S.
Ecotrin Low Adult S.
edge s.
Excedrin, Extra S.
grip s.
Orajel Maximum S.
oval window tensile s.
pinch s.
response s.
shear s.
Sine-Aid, Maximum S.
Sinus Excedrin Extra S.
tensile s.
Theraflu Non-Drowsy Formula
  Maximum S.
Tylenol Flu Maximum S.
Tylenol Sinus, Maximum S.
ultimate s.
wet s.
wound tensile s.
yield s.

streptococcal gingivitis

Streptococcus

S. agalactiae
S. anginosus
S. constellatus
S. cremoris
S. faecalis
S. gordonii
S. intermedius
S. mitis
S. morbillorum
S. mutans
S. pneumoniae
S. pyogenes
S. salivarius
S. sanguis
S. viridans

streptococcus, pl. **streptococci**

α-hemolytic s.
anaerobic s.
group A β-hemolytic s. (GABHS)
β-hemolytic s.
hemolytic s.
nonhemolytic s.

streptomycin

stress

axial s.
s. breaker
buccolingual s.
compressive s.
s. divider

dynamic s.
endosseous s.
s. equalizer
force and s.
hydrodynamic shear s.
iambic s.
lateral s.
maximal s.
occlusal s.
oxidative s.
s. pattern
primary s.
s. relaxation of skin
residual s.
s. riser
secondary s.
shear s.
shearing s.
stereotyped s.
tensile s.
tertiary s.
torsive s.
trochaic s.
s. ulcer
weak s.

stress-bearing area

stress-breaker

s.-b. attachment
complete s.-b.
Crismani s.-b.
hinge s.-b.
partial s.-b.
Stern s.-b.

stress-breaking clasp

stress-strain curve

stress-supporting area

stretch

s. receptor
s. reflex

stretcher

Brandy scalp s. II, front closure
Brandy scalp s. I, rear closure

stretching

cochlear nerve s.
s. pliers

stria, gen. and pl. **striae**

acoustic s.
brown striae
striae distensae
striae gravidarum
striae parallelae
Retzius striae

S

NOTES

stria *(continued)*
    Schreger s.
    s. vascularis
striata
    melanonychia s. (MS)
striated
    s. border
    s. duct
    s. muscle fiber
striation
    fatigue s.
stricture
    ductal s.
    esophageal s.
stridency deletion
strident
    s. lisp
stridor
    biphasic s.
    congenital s.
    s. dentium
    expiratory s.
    inspiratory s.
    laryngeal s.
    respiratory s.
    s. serraticus
stridulosa
    laryngitis s.
stridulous
stridulus
    laryngismus s.
string
    s. bean
    initial s.
    intermediate s.
    terminal s.
stringed instrument theory
striola
strip
    abrasive s.
    amalgam s.
    boxing s.
    celluloid s.
    Color Bar Schirmer s.
    demineralized flexible laminar
      bone s.
    fascial s.
    fascia lata s.
    flexible laminar bone s.
    lightning s.
    linen s.
    Mylar s.
    Pacific Coast flexible laminar
      bone s.
    packing s.
    s. perforation
    plastic s.
    polishing s.

    separating s.
    suture s.
    Ultimatics flexible laminar bone s.
stripper
    endonerve s.
    ramus s.
stripping
    pterygomasseteric sling s.
    tooth s.
stroboscope
    Kay rhinolaryngeal s.
stroboscopy
    videolaryngeal s.
strobovideolaryngoscopy
stroke
    brainstem s.
    circumferential s.
    closing s.
    exploratory s.
    glottal s.
    opening s.
    power s.
    shaving s.
stroma, pl. stromata
    glandular s.
    myxochondroid s.
    myxoid s.
stromal desmoplasia
Strombeck technique
strong force
strontium chloride
Stropko air syringe
STRP
    short tandem repeat polymorphism
structural
    s. interface
    s. linguistics
structure
    base s.
    border s.
    cored s.
    deep s.
    denture-supporting s.
    ductlike s. (DLS)
    functional form of supporting s.
    grammatical s.
    implant s.
    intermediate s.
    language s.
    performative pragmatic s.
    S. Photographic Expressive
      Language Test-II (SPELT-P)
    pragmatic s.
    restricted syllable s.
    submicroscopic s.
    supporting s.
    supragingival s.
    surface s.

syllable s.
underlying s.
s. word
structured discourse
struma
s. lymphomatosa
Riedel s.
strut
columellar s.
implant substructure s.
slipped s.
Stryker
S. bed frame
S. drill
STSG
split-thickness skin graft
STT
scaphoid-trapezium-trapezoid
STT fusion
Stuart articulator
stud attachment
Studebaker technique
study
contrast s.
electrodiagnostic s.
electroneurography/nerve
conduction s.
fluorometric s.
immunohistochemical s.
morphometric s.
ultrastructural s.
videofluoroscopic swallow s. (VSS)
stump
nerve s.
Sturge-Weber syndrome
stutter
stuttering
cybernetic theory of s.
exteriorized s.
hysterical s.
implicit s.
incipient s.
interiorized s.
laryngeal s.
laterality theory of s.
neurotic theory of s.
s. pattern
s. phase
phases of s.
primary s.
secondary s.
semantic theory of s.

s. stage
s. theory
transitional s.
two-factor model of s.
style
cognitive s.
Toomey tip s.
stylet
endotracheal s.
styloglossus muscle
stylohyoid
s. ligament
s. muscle
s. syndrome
styloid
s. diaphragm
s. process
ulnar s.
styloidectomy
styloiditis
stylomandibular
s. artery
s. ligament
s. membrane
s. tunnel
stylomastoid
s. artery
s. foramen
stylomaxillary
stylomyloid
stylopharyngeus muscle
stylus tracing
Styrofoam
SU
sensation unit
subacute
s. bacterial endocarditis (SBE)
s. inflammation
s. periapical abscess
s. pulpitis
subantral
s. augmentation
s. region
subapical osteotomy
subarachnoid hemorrhage
subarcuate fossa
subaverage
significantly s.
sub-basilar bulla
subciliary approach
subclass
subclavian triangle

NOTES

577

subclavius muscle
subcondylar oblique osteotomy
subconjunctival hemorrhage
subcoronal hypospadias
subcortical
    s. motor aphasia
    s. supranuclear paralysis
subcostalis muscle
subcrestal pocket
subcultural language
subcutaneous
    s. angiolipoma
    s. augmentation material (SAM)
    s. emphysema
    s. hematoma
    s. implantation
    s. laterodigital reverse flap
    s. leash
    s. lipoma
    s. mastectomy
    s. musculoaponeurotic system
    s. neuroma
    s. pedicled flap
    s. rhytidectomy
    s. suture
    s. temporo-facial face lift
    s. temporo-malar face lift
    s. tissue
    s. turnover flap
subcuticular suture
subcutis
subdental
subdentinoblastic
    s. capillary plexus
    s. zone
subdermal
    deep s.
    s. implant
    s. nasal tissue
subdigastric lymph node
subdural abscess
subepicranial space
subepithelial
    s. connective tissue graft
    s. membrane
    s. nerve plexus
subfascial carpal tunnel decompression
subgaleal
    s. dissection
    s. elevation
    s. emphysema
    s. fascia
    s. flap
    s. plane
subgallate
    bismuth s.
subgingival
    s. apoxesis

s. calculus
s. curettage
s. scaling
s. space
subgingivally
subglandular augmentation
subglossal
subglossitis
subglottic
    s. area
    s. hemangioma
    s. jet ventilation
    s. pressure
    s. resonator
    s. squamous cell carcinoma
    s. stenosis
subimplant membrane
subjacent tissue
subject
    complete s.
subjective
    s. quantity
subjugal
subjunctive mood
sublabial
    s. adhesion
    s. approach
    s. incision
    s. perforation
    s. transsphenoidal approach
sublamina densa fibrils
Sublimaze Injection
sublingual
    s. artery
    s. crescent
    s. cyst
    s. duct
    s. fibrogranuloma
    s. fold
    s. fossa
    s. gland
    s. mucosa
    s. nerve
    s. obstruction
    s. papilla
    s. ridge
    s. saliva
    s. salivary gland
    s. space
    s. space abscess
    s. sulcus
    s. ulcer
sublingualis
    caruncula s.
    plica s.
sublingually
sublinguitis

subluxation
    atlantoaxial s.
    stapes s.
    temporomandibular joint s.
submalar deficiency
submammary
    s. crease
    s. line
    s. neosulcus
submandibular
    s. augmentation
    s. chronic sclerosing sialadenitis
    s. drainage
    s. duct
    s. fossa
    s. ganglion
    s. gland
    s. gland disease
    s. lymph node
    s. node
    s. obstruction
    s. region
    s. saliva
    s. space
    s. space abscess
    s. triangle
    s. trigone
submandibulectomy
submasseteric
    s. space
    s. space abscess
submaxilla
submaxillary
    s. caruncle
    s. cellulitis
    s. duct
    s. fossa
    s. ganglion
    s. lymph node
    s. nerve
    s. region
    s. saliva
    s. salivary gland
    s. space
    s. triangle
submaxillitis
submental
    s. artery
    s. artery flap
    s. fistula
    s. incision
    s. intubation

    s. island flap
    s. liposuction
    s. lymph node
    s. region
    s. space
    s. space abscess
    s. triangle
    s. vertex cephalogram
    s. vertex roentgenogram
submentocervical view
submentonian dermo-fatty flap
submentoplasty
submerge
submerged
    s. tonsil
    s. tooth
submicroscopic structure
submillimetric accuracy
submucosa
submucosal implant
submucous
    s. cleft
    s. cleft palate
    s. fibrosis
    s. layer
    s. membrane
    s. resection (SMR)
submuscular
    s. aponeurotic system
    s. implant
    s. pocket
subnasale
subnasion
subnucleus caudalis
suboccipital
    s. approach
    s. dural defect
    s. plexus
    s. triangle
subocclusal
    s. connector
    s. surface
subodontoblastic
    s. layer
    s. plexus
    s. zone
suborbicularis
    s. oculi fat (SOOF)
    s. skin
subparotid lymph node
subpectoral
    s. augmentation

S

NOTES

subpectoral *(continued)*
    s. implant
    s. reconstruction
    s. stabilizer
subperichondrial dissection
subperiosteal
    s. abscess
    s. brow lift
    s. dissection
    s. elevation
    s. elevator
    s. face lift
    s. frame
    s. implant
    s. implant abutment
    s. implant one-phase technique
    s. malar cheek lift
    s. midfacelift
    s. minimally invasive laser endoscopic (SMILE)
    s. minimally invasive laser endoscopic face-lift
    s. minimally invasive laser endoscopic rhytidectomy
    s. orbital abscess (SPOA)
    s. pickup impression
    s. pulling stitch
    s. tissue expander (STE)
    s. vomerine-ethmoidal plane
subplatysmal
    s. face lift
    s. fat
    s. plane
subpontic hyperostosis
subpulpal
    s. wall
subscapular
    s. artery
    s. axis
    s. system free flap
sub-SMAS rhytidectomy
subsonic
subspinale
substance
    adamantine s.
    caustic s.
    cementing s.
    chemical s.
    corrosive s.
    ground s.
    hydrophilic ground s.
    intercellular s.
    interprismatic s.
    intertubular s.
    scerlosing s.
substance P (SP)
substandard language
substantia, pl. substantiae

    s. adamantina
    s. adamantina dentis
    s. dentalis propria
    s. eburnea
    s. eburnea dentis
    s. gelatinosa
    s. gelatinosa cell
    s. intertubularis dentis
    s. ossea dentis
    s. propria dentis
    s. vitrea
    s. vitrea dentis
substantive
    s. universals
substantivity
substernal colon interposition graft
substitute
    dentin s.
substitution
    s. analysis
    stimulus s.
substitutional lisp
substructure
    abutment implant s.
    auxiliary rest implant s.
    implant denture s.
    interspace implant s.
    neck implant s.
    part implant s.
    peripheral frame implant s.
    post implant s.
    primary struts implant s.
    secondary struts implant s.
sub-superficial musculoaponeurotic system rhytidectomy
subsurface enamel
subterminali
    Clostridium s.
subtotal
    s. cleft palate
    s. glossectomy
    s. laryngectomy
    s. pulp loss
    s. supraglottic laryngectomy (SSL)
    s. thyroidectomy
subtubal air cell
subungual
    s. hematoma
    s. keratoacanthoma (SUKA)
    s. melanoma
    s. squamous cell carcinoma
Sub-Vent implant system
subvocal speech
succedaneous
    s. dentition
    s. teeth
succedaneum
    royal mineral s.

succedaneus
    dens s.
successional
    s. lamina
    s. teeth
successive approximation
succinate
    s. dehydrogenase
    sumatriptan s.
succinic dehydrogenase
succinylcholine drip
suckback
sucking
    s. cushion
    high-amplitude s. (HAS)
    s. pad
Sucquet-Hoyer glomus canal
Sucrets
    S. Sore Throat
suction
    Adson s.
    s. aspiration
    s. aspirator
    s. cannula
    s. drainage
    s. elevator
    s. extraction
    s. forceps
    s. hose
    s. lipectomy
    s. plate
    s. system
    s. tip
    s. tube
    s. tubing
    wound incision and s.
    Yankauer s.
suction-assisted lipectomy (SAL)
suctioning
    malar bag s.
suctorial pad
Sudafed
    S. Cold & Cough Liquid Caps
    S. 12 Hour
    S. Plus Liquid
    S. Plus Tablet
    S. Severe Cold
sudden
    s. drop curve
    s. hearing loss (SHL)
Sufenta Injection
sufentanil

suffocate
suffocation
sugar
    s. beet
    s. maple
Sugita microsurgical table
suit
    total-body compression s.
SUKA
    subungual keratoacanthoma
sulbactam
    ampicillin and s.
    s. sodium
sulcal epithelium
sulcated tongue
sulci (*gen. and pl. of* sulcus)
sulconazole
sulcoplasty
sulcular
    s. epithelium
    s. fluid
sulcus, gen. and pl. **sulci**
    alveolabial s.
    alveolingual s.
    s. anthelicis transversus
    s. auriculae posterior
    buccal s.
    central s.
    s. cruris helicis
    frontal s.
    gingival s.
    s. gingivalis
    gingivobuccal s.
    gingivolabial s.
    implant gingival s.
    intergluteal s.
    internal spiral s.
    labial-buccal s.
    labiodental s.
    labiomarginal s.
    lateral s.
    lingual s.
    mandibular s.
    s. of mandibular neck
    median lingual s.
    mentolabial s.
    mylohyoid s.
    nasolabial s.
    occlusal s.
    palatine s.
    paralingual s.
    petrosal s.

S

NOTES

sulcus *(continued)*
  postcentral s.
  precentral s.
  prejowl s.
  sigmoid s.
  spiral s.
  sublingual s.
  superior petrosal s.
  supratarsal s.
  temporal s.
  terminal s.
  tonsillolingual s.
  s. vocalis
Sulf-10 Ophthalmic
sulfacetamide
  s. sodium
  s. sodium and fluorometholone
  s. sodium and phenylephrine
  s. sodium and prednisolone
sulfacetamide/prednisone
sulfaction
sulfadiazine
  silver s.
sulfamethoxazole
  trimethoprim s.
  trimethoprim and s. (TMP-SMX)
Sulfamylon Topical
sulfanilamide
sulfate
  androsterone s.
  atropine s.
  barium s.
  calcium s.
  chondroitin s.
  chondroitin-4 s.
  chondroitin-6 s.
  copper s.
  dermatan s.
  dermatan-4 s.
  s. hemihydrate
  heparan s.
  morphine s.
  neomycin s.
  potassium indoxyl s.
  pseudoephedrine s.
  sodium tetradecyl s.
  zinc s.
sulfathiazole
Sulfatrim
sulfide
  hydrogen s.
sulfisoxazole
  erythromycin and s.
sulfite
  sodium s.
sulfonamide powder
sulfur
  s. dioxide (SO_2)

  s. granule
  s. and silver point
sulindac
Sullivan nasal VPAP unit
Sultan
  S. Cement UP
  S. Topex 00:60 second topical
    fluoride gel
sumac
  poison s.
sumatriptan succinate
summation
  binaural s.
sump
  Argyle silicone Salem s.
Sumycin
  S. Oral
Sunday bite
Sunderland
  S. classification
  S. type V degree injury
sunken-eye appearance
sunken-in face
sunray appearance
sunscreen
  Esoterica S.
  Porcelana S.
  TI-SILC Moist s.
super
  s. antigen
super-absorptive polymer dressing
Superbond
Supercut
  S. blade
  S. diamond bur
Super-Dent topical fluoride gel
SuperEBA cement
supereruption
superficial
  s. brachial flap
  s. fascial system (SFS)
  s. hemangioma
  s. liposculpture
  s. musculoaponeurotic system
    (SMAS)
  s. palmar arch
  s. parotidectomy
  s. parotid node
  s. petrosal artery
  s. petrosal nerve
  s. plane rhytidectomy
  s. radial nerve
  s. scaler
  s. siderosis
  s. spreading melanoma
  s. suture
  s. temporal artery
  s. temporal crest

s. temporal fascia (STF)
s. temporal vein
s. upper lateral shave
superficiale
    stratum s.
superficialis
    fascia penis s.
    s. tendon
superfine disk
superflap
superimposition
superinfection
superior
    s. alveolar artery
    ankyloglossia s.
    arcus dentalis s.
    s. auricular artery
    s. border plate
    s. cantholysis
    s. cervical ganglion
    s. constrictor muscle
    s. constrictor pharyngeal muscle
    s. crus of antihelix
    s. deep cervical node
    s. dental arch
    s. dermal pedicle
    s. incudal fold
    s. incudal ligament
    s. joint space
    s. laryngeal artery
    s. laryngeal nerve (SLN)
    s. laryngeal vein
    s. laryngotomy
    s. lip
    s. longitudinal muscle of tongue
    s. mallear fold
    s. mallear ligament
    s. malposition
    s. marginotomy
    s. maxillary bone
    s. maxillary foramen
    s. maxillary nerve
    s. maxillary retrognathia
    s. meatus
    s. nasal concha
    s. nasal nerve
    nucleus salivatorius s.
    s. olivary complex
    s. ophthalmic vein
    s. orbital fissure
    s. orbital fissure syndrome (SOFS)
    s. orbital rim

s. petrosal ridge
s. petrosal sulcus
s. pharyngeal artery
s. pharyngeal constrictor
s. stratum
s. surface of horizontal plate of
    palatine bone
s. teeth
s. thyroid artery
s. thyroid vein
s. turbinate
s. turbinated bone
s. tympanic artery
s. vena cava syndrome
s. vestibular nucleus
superioris
    caput angulare quadratus labii s.
    labrale s.
    levator palpebrae s.
    musculus levator labii s.
superiorly
    s. based Dardour lateral flap
    s. based Nataf lateral flap
superius
    interdentale s. (IdS)
    labrale s.
    orbitale s. (OS)
superlative
supermarket vertigo
supernumerary
    s. auricle
    s. limb
    s. molar
    s. nipple
    s. nostril
    s. root
    s. tooth
superolateral surface of maxilla
superomedial
Superoxyl
Superpaste
Super punctum plug
supersaturated saliva
supersonic
    s. ray
    s. wave
superstructure
    attaching material implant s.
    s. attachment
    attachment implant s.
    s. casting
    s. connector

S

NOTES

superstructure *(continued)*
    connector implant s.
    denture implant s.
    s. frame
    frame implant s.
    implant denture s.
    implant surgical splint s.
    stapes s.
    temporary s.
    s. tooth

superwet
    s. preoperative subcutaneous
      infiltration
    s. technique

supination

supinator muscle

supplement
    Fluor-A-Day S.'s
    Osteogen vitamin and mineral s.
    Phos-Flur oral rinse s.
    Poly-Vi-Flor multivitamin mineral
      and fluoride s.
    Tri-Vi-Flor multivitamin mineral
      and fluoride s.

supplemental
    s. air
    s. groove (SG)
    s. lobe
    s. ridge
    s. tooth

supplementary
    s. canal (SC)
    s. gesture
    s. marginotomy

suppletion

supplied tooth

supply
    gingival blood s.

support
    abutment s.
    alveolar s.
    breath s.
    cast s.
    chin s.
    Dale oxygen cannula s.
    Dale ventilator tubing s.
    excessive lip s.
    facial s.
    fixed s.
    free s.
    insufficient lip s.
    multiple abutment s.
    neck s.
    orbital s.
    periodontal s.
    postoperative mammary s.
    restrained s.
    s. ridge

    rugae s.
    tooth s.

supporting
    s. area
    s. bone
    s. cell
    s. cell of olfactory epithelium
    s. cusp
    s. structure
    s. tissue
    s. vessel

supportive mechanisms of teeth

support-load ratio

suppository
    AVC S.

suppression
    failure of fixation s. (FFS)
    tinnitus s.

Supprettes
    B&O S.

suppuration
    alveodental s.

suppurativa
    axillary hidradenitis s.
    hidradenitis s.

suppurative
    s. apical periodontitis
    s. core
    s. exudate
    s. gingivitis
    s. inflammation
    s. labyrinthitis
    s. osteomyelitis
    s. otitis media
    s. parotitis
    s. periodontitis
    s. periostitis
    s. pulpitis
    s. sialadenitis
    s. tenosynovitis

supraalar pinching

supraalveolar
    s. fiber

suprabasilar bulla

suprabony pocket

suprabuccal

suprabulge

supracarotid air cell

supraclavicular
    s. lymph node

supraclusion

supracochlear air cell

supracrestal pocket

supracricoid
    s. laryngectomy
    s. laryngectomy with
      cricohyoidoepiglottopexy

s. partial laryngectomy with cricohyoidoepiglottopexy (SCPL-CHEP)

supraerupted
s. molar

supraeruption

supragingival
s. calculus
s. scaling
s. structure

supragingivally

supraglottic
s. carcinoma
s. closure
s. jet ventilation
s. laryngectomy
s. larynx
s. resonator
s. squamous cell carcinoma
s. stenosis

supraglottitis

supraglottoplasty

suprahyoid
s. epiglottis
s. muscle
s. neck dissection
s. node
s. space

supralaryngeal tension

supramandibular
s. node

supramarginal
s. angular gyri
s. gyrus

supramaxilla

supramaxillary

suprameatal
s. spine
s. triangle

supramental

supramentale
s. mandibular alveolus

supramicrosurgery

Supramid
S. polyamide mesh
S. suture

supramodal perception

supranuclear
s. paralysis
s. pathway

supraocclusion

supraomohyoid
s. neck dissection

supraorbital
s. air cell
s. canal
s. ethmoid
s. nerve
s. notch
s. plate
s. ridge
s. rim
s. rim of frontal bone

supra-perichondrial dissection

supraperiosteal
s. flap
s. implant

Suprarenin

suprasegmental
s. analysis
s. phoneme

suprasellar

suprasternal
s. fascia
s. space

suprastructure

supratarsal sulcus

supratemporal

supratentorial approach

Suprathreshold Adaptation Test (STAT)

supratip
s. deformity
s. fullness

supratonsillar fossa

supratragal notch

supratrochlear
s. artery
s. nerve

supraversion

Suprax

supreme
s. nasal concha
s. turbinate
s. turbinated bone

suprofen

Suprol

sural
s. height
s. island flap for foot and ankle reconstruction
s. nerve
s. nerve cable graft

surd

NOTES

Sure-Closure
 S.-C. device
 S.-C. skin closure system
SureFlex nickel-titanium file
SureScan
 S. scanning handpiece
 S. system
surface
 alveolar s.
 anterior s.
 axial s.
 balancing occlusal s.
 basal s.
 buccal s.
 s. cell layer
 contact s. of tooth
 s. cover
 s. cracking
 decayed, missing, filled deciduous
  teeth s.'s (dmfs)
 decayed, missing, filled permanent
  teeth s.'s (DMFS)
 dentin s.
 denture basal s.
 denture foundation s.
 denture impression s.
 denture occlusal s.
 s. disinfectant
 s. disinfection
 distal s.
 facial s.
 foundation s.
 gingival s.
 grinding s.
 implant-bearing s.
 impression s.
 s. impression
 incisal s.
 inferior s.
 labial s.
 lingual s.
 masticating s.
 masticatory s.
 maxillary s.
 medial s.
 mesial s.
 occlusal s.
 oral s.
 osteophilic s.
 palatine s.
 polished s.
 proximal s.
 proximate s.
 ratio of decayed and filled s.'s
  (RDFS)
 s. rest
 root-end s.
 s. root resorption

 smooth s.
 s. structure
 subocclusal s.
 temporal s.
 s. tension
 UHMWPE articulating s.
 vestibular s. of tooth
 working occlusal s.
surface-coil MRI
Surf-A-Cide
Surgamid polyamide suture material
surgeon
 dental s.
 nonoculoplastic s.
 oculoplastic s.
 oral s.
 reconstructive hand s.
 rhinoplastic s.
surgery
 access flap in osseous s.
 apically repositioned flap in
  mucogingival s.
 Bachelor of Dental S. (BDS)
 body-contour s.
 Bosker TMI s.
 combination s.
 conchal s.
 conservation s.
 cosmetic s.
 craniofacial s.
 craniomaxillofacial s.
 dental s.
 dentofacial s.
 destabilization s.
 Doctor of Dental S. (DDS)
 double jaw s.
 ear s.
 endodontic s.
 endolymphatic decompression s.
 endolymphatic sac s. (ELS)
 endolymphatic sac/shunt s.
 endoscopic sinus s. (ESS)
 esthetic s.
 esthetic s.
 featural s.
 full flap in mucogingival s.
 functional endoscopic sinus s.
  (FESS)
 helical s.
 InstaTrak System image-guided s.
 laryngeal framework s.
 laser s.
 levator aponeurosis s.
 Licentiate in Dental S. (LDS)
 mandibular s.
 Marzola hair restoration s.
 Master of Dental S. (MDS)
 maxillary s.

antrostomy

maxillofacial s.
microlaryngeal s.
microvascular s.
minimally invasive sinus s.
Mohs s.
Mohs micrographic s. (MMS)
mucogingival s.
nonendoscopic sinus s.
oblique flap in mucogingival s.
oral s.
oral and maxillofacial s. (OMS)
orthognathic s.
osseous s.
pedicle flap in mucogingival s.
periapical s.
pharyngeal flap s.
plastic s.
powered endoscopic sinus s.
 (PESS)
preprosthetic s.
radical s.
reconstructive preprosthetic s.
revision stapes s.
second-look s.
segmental s.
septal s.
sex reassignment s.
SGMI explantation s.
sham s.
silicone gel-filled mammary implant
 explantation s.
sinus s.
stabilization s.
suspension microlaryngeal s.
transsexual s.

Surgica K6 laser
surgical
s. appliance
s. aspirator
s. assisted-rapid palatal expansion
 (SA-RPE)
s. bone impression
s. bur
s. ciliated cyst
s. compression garment
s. crown lengthening
s. curette
s. debulking
s. endodontics
s. eruption
s. extirpation
s. hoe

s. ligation
s. marking solution
s. neck of tooth
s. needle
s. occlusion rim
s. oncologist
s. orthodontia
s. orthodontics
S. Patient Arm shield
s. positioning
s. prediction imaging
s. preparation
s. prosthesis
s. pulp exposure
s. rejuvenation
s. retention
S. Simplex P bone cement
s. splint
s. steel Toomey instrument set
s. syndactyly
s. synovectomy
s. template
s. tongue reduction
s. treatment objective (STO)
s. wound

surgically
s. assisted mandibular arch
 lengthening
s. denervated area

Surgicel
S. absorbable hemostat for dental
 use

Surgident
Surgi-Fine reusable cannula tip
Surgilase ECS.01 smoke evacuator
Surgilube
Surgimedics/TMP multiperfusion set
Surgipulse XJ 150 CO_2 laser
Surgitek handpiece
Surgitron
S. ultrasound-assisted lipoplasty
 machine
S. 3000 ultrasound device

surrounding wall
survey
intraoral s.
lateral jaw and occlusal s.
s. line
panoramic s.
periapical radiographic s.
radiation s.

surveying

NOTES

S

surveyor
  dental s.
  Jelenko s.
  Ney s.
  Williams s.
survival
  neuronal s.
Susac syndrome
susceptibility
suspending suture
suspension
  AK-Spore H.C. Ophthalmic S.
  s. anastomosis
  Children's Advil Oral S.
  Children's Motrin Oral S.
  Cipro HC Otic s.
  Cortisporin Ophthalmic S.
  FML-S Ophthalmic S.
  frontalis s.
  Fungizone oral s.
  s. laryngoscopy
  s. microlaryngeal surgery
  s. microlaryngoscopy
  nasal valve s.
  Poly-Pred Ophthalmic S.
  ROOF s.
  Rynatan Pediatric S.
  Terra-Cortril Ophthalmic S.
  Vexol Ophthalmic S.
suspensory ligament
Sustain
  S. dental implant system
  S. HA-coated screw implant
sustentacular cell
susurrus
  s. aurium
Sutcliffe laser shield and retracting instrument
Suteraloy alloy
Sutton disease
suture
  absorbable s.
  adjustable external s.
  anchor s.
  anterior palatine s.
  approximation s.
  autoplastic s.
  basal bunching s.
  basting s.
  bolster s.
  Bondek absorbable s.
  Bunnell s.
  button s.
  catgut s.
  chromic s.
  cinch s.
  coated Vicryl Rapide s.
  continuous running s.

  continuous sling s.
  Cottony-Dacron hollow s.
  cranial vault s.
  deep suspension s.
  dentate s.
  epineurial s.
  epiperineurial s.
  Ethibond extra polyester s.
  Ethicon s.
  Ethilon s.
  ethmoidomaxillary s.
  eyelid crease s.
  s. forceps
  frontal s.
  frontomalar s.
  frontomaxillary s.
  frontozygomatic s.
  harelip s.
  horizontal mattress s.
  Hu-Friedy PermaSharp s.
  incisive s.
  interendognathic s.
  interfascicular guide s.
  intermaxillary s.
  interrupted s.
  intracuticular running s.
  intradermal s.
  intrafascicular s.
  lambdoidal s.
  large-caliber nonabsorbable s.
  longitudinal s.
  malar periosteum-SMAS flap fixation s.
  malomaxillary s.
  mastoid-conchal s.
  mattress s.
  Maxon s.
  median palatine s.
  modified Frost s.
  Monocryl s.
  monofilament s.
  monofilament nylon s.
  Mustardé s.
  nasofrontal s.
  nonabsorbable mattress s.
  nonresorbable s.
  Nurolon s.
  palatine s.
  palatomaxillary s.
  Pancoast s.
  patent s.
  PDS II s.
  perineurial s.
  PermaSharp PGA s.
  petroclival s.
  petrotympanic s.
  poliglecaprone 25 s.
  Polydek s.

polydioxanone s. (PDS)
polyglactin 910 s.
polyglycolic acid s.
premaxillary s.
presphenoethmoid s.
Prolene s.
pull-out s.
purse-string s.
pursestring s.
s. scissors
serrate s.
s. shape shifter
shoelace s.
silk s.
simple flaring s.
simple running s.
skull base s.
sling s., type I, II
sphenoethmoidal s.
sphenofrontal s.
sphenomaxillary s.
sphenotemporal s.
sphenozygomatic s.
stay s.
s. strip
subcutaneous s.
subcuticular s.
superficial s.
Supramid s.
suspending s.
synthetic absorbable s. (SAS)
temporomalar s.
temporozygomatic s.
tension-requiring s.
Tevdek s.
through-and-through reabsorbable s.
traction s.
tympanomastoid s.
tympanosquamosal s.
vertical mattress s.
Vicryl Rapide s.
zygomaticofrontal s.
zygomaticomaxillary s.
zygomaticotemporal s.
sutured in place, shield-shaped tip graft
SutureStrip Plus wound closure
suturing
SUVAG
system universal verbotonol audition Guberina
Suzanne gland

swab
Hurricaine s.
swage
swaged needle
swager
wax s.
swaging graft
swallow
s. method
somatic s.
visceral s.
swallowing
s. center
deviant s.
infantile s.
s. reflex
reverse s.
s. threshold
visceral s.
SWAMI
Speech with Alternating Masking Index
swan neck deformity
sway
aphysiologic s.
sweat bee
sweating
gustatory s.
Swede-Vent
S.-V. taper-lock
S.-V. TL implant
S.-V. TL self-tapping external hex implant
sweep-check test
sweet
s. potato
s. potato shape
s. vernal grass
sweetgum
swell body
swelling
prenodular s.
sessile s.
swimmer's ear
swine dander
swing
epiglottis s.
swinging
s. door technique
Swinging Story Test
swing-lock
s.-l. denture
s.-l. prosthesis

S

NOTES

Swiss
S. blue
S. chard
S. cheese
S. Precision cannula system
S. Therapy eye mask
switch
compression s.
s. flap
nasal tube s.
SWMF
Semmes-Weinstein monofilament
Swyrls swim mold
Sybraloy high-copper alloy
syllabic
s. aphonia
complex s.
s. consonant
simple s.
s. speech
s. speech sound
syllabication, syllabification
syllable
closed s.
s. deletion
deletion of unstressed s.
s. duplication
nonsense s.
open s.
paired s.'s
s. reduction
s. sequence
s. shape
s. structure
syllable-stumbling
Syllamalt
sylvian
s. fissure
s. vein
Sylvius
fissure of S.
symbiotic
symbol
PIC s.
picture s.'s (PICSYMS)
s. set system
Wing s.
symbolic play
symbolism
symbolization
Visual-Tactile System of
Phonetic S.
symbrachydactyly
Syme amputation level
symmetric syndactyly
symmetry
Detailed Evaluation of Facial S.
(DEFS)

facial s.
Facial Grading System Resting s.
(FGSR)
tooth arch s.
sympathectomy
cervical s.
sympathetic
s. nerve
s. root of submandibular ganglion
s. saliva
s. vibration
sympatholytic
sympathomimetic
symphalangism
symphysial, symphyseal
s. fracture
s. height of mandible
symphysis
mandibular s.
os s.
Symphytum officinale
symptom
Bezold s.
complex of s.'s
s. concept
cushingoid s.
Demarquay s.
extralabyrinthine s.
Griesinger s.
Semon s.
vertiginous s.
symptomatic
s. laryngocele
s. therapy
symptomatology
cerebral palsy s.
Synacort
Synalar
S.-HP
Synalgos-DC
synapse, pl. synapses
ectopic s.
excitatory s.
inhibitory s.
synaptic
s. terminal
s. vesicle
synaptophysin
syncheilia, synchilia
synchondrosis
occipitosphenoidal s.
sphenooccipital s.
synchronic linguistics
synchronous
s. lingual granular cell tumor
s. metastasis
syncope
laryngeal s.

syncretism
syncytial
syndactyly
    complete s.
    incomplete s.
    s. release
    simple s.
    surgical s.
    symmetric s.
syndesmoplasty
syndrome
    abnormal airway resistance s.
    acquired immunodeficiency s.
     (AIDS)
    acute radiation s.
    aglossia-adactylia s.
    Aicardi s.
    Albrecht s.
    Albright s.
    Alezzandrini s.
    Alport s.
    Alström s.
    amelo-onychohypohidrotic s.
    amniotic band s.
    Andemann s.
    androgen insensitivity s.
    ankyloglossia superior s.
    Apert s.
    Ascher s.
    auriculotemporal s.
    Avellis s.
    baby bottle s.
    Baillarger s.
    basal cell nevus s.
    Bassen-Kornzweig s.
    battered buttock s.
    Bazex s.
    Beckwith-Wiedemann s.
    Behçet s.
    Berry s.
    Beuren s.
    Binder s.
    Birt-Hogg-Dube s.
    Björnstad s.
    blepharochalasis s.
    blepharophimosis s.
    Bloch-Sulzberger s.
    Boerhaave s.
    Böök s.
    branchial arch s.
    Briquet s.
    Brissaud-Marie s.

    callosal disconnection s.
    Capdepont s.
    Capdepont-Hodge s.
    carpal tunnel s. (CTS)
    Carpenter s.
    cat cry s.
    celiac s.
    cephalopolysyndactyly s.
    cerebellopontine angle s.
    cerebrocostomandibular s. (CCMS)
    cervico-oculo-acoustic s.
    Charlie-M s.
    Charlin s.
    cheilitis-glossitis-gingivitis s.
    chromosome 21-trisomy s.
    chronic fatigue s.
    chronic mononucleosis s.
    cleft lip/palate s.
    cleft palate and lateral synechia s.
     (CPLS)
    clostridial s.
    Cogan s.
    Cohen s.
    Collet-Sicard s.
    compartment s.
    congenital alveolar synechia s.
    congenital ectodermic dysplasia s.
    Costen s.
    Cowden s.
    cracked-tooth synergistic s.
    Crandall s.
    cri du chat s.
    Crouzon s.
    cryptophthalmus s.
    Cushing s.
    Dejerine s.
    dentinal crack s.
    dentopulmonary s.
    de Quervain s.
    Down s.
    dry-eye s.
    dry socket s.
    Dubreuil-Chambardel s.
    Eagle s.
    Eaton-Lambert s.
    Ellis-van Creveld s.
    eosinophilia-myalgia s. (EMS)
    exploding head s.
    Fargin-Fayolle s.
    fat embolus s.
    fetal alcohol s.
    fetal valproate s.

S

NOTES

syndrome *(continued)*
    fragile X s.
    Franceschetti s.
    Fraser s.
    Frey s.
    Gardner s.
    gay bowel s.
    gender dysphoria s.
    Gerstmann s.
    Gilles de la Tourette s.
    gingivostomatitis s.
    Goldenhar s.
    Goldscheider s.
    Goltz s.
    Gorlin s.
    Gougerot-Sjögren s.
    Gradenigo s.
    Greig s.
    Grisel s.
    Guillain-Barré s.
    Hallermann-Streiff s.
    Hallgren s.
    Hanhart s.
    Hecht-Beals-Wilson s.
    Heerfordt s.
    Helweg-Larssen s.
    Herrmann s.
    Horner s.
    Hunt s.
    Hunter s.
    Hurler s.
    Hurler-Scheie s.
    Hutchinson-Gilford s.
    Hutchison s.
    hyoid s.
    hypereosinophilic s. (HES)
    hyperkinetic s.
    hypoglossia-hypodactylia s.
    immotile cilia s.
    Jackson s.
    Jadassohn-Lewandowski s.
    Juberg-Marsidi s.
    jugular foramen s.
    juvenile periodontitis s.
    Kallmann s.
    Kanner s.
    Kartagener s.
    kleeblattschädel s.
    Klinefelter s.
    Klippel-Trénaunay s.
    Laband s.
    lacrimoauriculodentodigital s.
    Lambert-Eaton myasthenic s.
    Landry-Guillain-Barré s.
    Larsen s.
    lateral medullary s.
    lateral synechia s.
    Laurence-Moon-Biedl s.

    Leigh s.
    Lermoyez s.
    long face s.
    MacKenzie s.
    Maffucci s.
    Mallory-Weiss s.
    Marfan s.
    Marshall s.
    Mayer-Rokitansky s.
    Mayer-Rokitansky-Küster-Hauser s.
      (MRKHS)
    McCune-Albright s.
    median cleft face s.
    Meige s.
    Melkersson s.
    Melkersson-Rosenthal s.
    Ménière s.
    Meyenburg-Altherr-Uehlinger s.
    middle fossa s.
    Miege s.
    Mikulicz s.
    Miller-Fisher variant of Guillain-
      Barré s.
    minimal brain dysfunction s.
      (MBD)
    Möbius s.
    Mohr-Tranebjaerg s.
    mole melanoma s.
    Morquio s.
    MPD s.
    mucocutaneous lymph node s.
    multiple hamartoma s.
    myofacial pain-dysfunction s.
    myofascial pain s. (MPS)
    Nager s.
    nerve compression s.
    neuropolyendocrine s.
    Noonan s.
    numb chin s. (NCS)
    obstructive sleep apnea s. (OSAS)
    occipital condyle s.
    occuloglandular s.
    ocular-mucous membrane s.
    oculo-auriculo-vertebral s.
    oculopharyngeal s.
    oculovestibulo-auditory s.
    oral-facial-digital s.
    orbital apex s. (OAS)
    orbital compartment s.
    organophosphate toxicity s.
    orofacial dysfunction s.
    otodental s.
    otopalatodigital s.
    pain s.
    Papillon-Lefèvre s.
    parasellar s.
    parasellar and orbital apex s.
    paratrigeminal s.

Parinaud s.
Parkes-Weber s.
Paterson-Kelly s.
Pendred s.
petrosphenoidal s.
Peutz-Jeghers s.
Pfeiffer s.
pharyngeal pouch s.
Pierre Robin s.
Plummer-Vinson s.
Poland s.
Pospischill-Feyrter s.
postconcussion s.
postpoliomyelitis s.
Prader-Willi s.
Psaume s.
Raeder s.
Ramsay Hunt s.
Reiter s.
Richards-Rundle s.
Rieger s.
Roaf s.
Robin s.
Robinow-Sorauf s.
Roger s.
Romberg s.
Rubinstein-Taybi s.
Saethre-Chotzen s.
Samter s.
Sanfilippo s.
Sanfilippo A, B, C s.
SAPHO s.
scalded-skin s.
Scheie s.
Schmidt s.
Schwartz-Bartter s.
serum hyperviscosity s.
Sézary s.
Shapiro s.
short bowel s.
short face s.
short gut s.
shoulder s.
Shy-Drager s.
sicca s.
Sipple s.
Sjögren s.
Sly s.
spastic frontalis s.
Stainton s.
Stainton-Capdepont s.
Stevens-Johnson s.

Stickler s.
Strauss s.
Sturge-Weber s.
stylohyoid s.
superior orbital fissure s. (SOFS)
superior vena cava s.
Susac s.
Tapia s.
Teebi s.
temporal s.
temporomandibular dysfunction s.
temporomandibular joint s.
temporomandibular joint pain-
 dysfunction s.
thalamic s.
Thiebierge-Weissenbach s.
TMJ s.
tooth-and-nail s.
Tornwaldt s.
Tourette s.
toxic shock s.
Treacher Collins s. (TCS)
trichodento-osseous s.
trigeminal trophic s. (TTS)
trismus-pseudocamptodactyly s.
Trotter s.
Turner s.
Ullrich-Feichtiger s.
Urbach-Wiethe s.
Usher s.
Vail s.
van der Hoeve s.
Van der Woude s.
vascular loop compression s.
Veeneklaas s.
velocardiofacial s.
Vernet s.
voice fatigue s.
Waardenburg s.
Waardenburg-Klein s.
Wallenberg s.
Weber-Cockayne s.
Weyers s.
Weyers-Fülling s.
Wildervanck s.
Wildervanck-Smith s.
Witkop-von Sallman s.
Wolf-Hirschhorn s. (WHS)
Zinsser-Engman-Cole s.

synechia
 nasal s.
synechial band

S

NOTES

Synemol
synergistic
    s. necrotizing cellulitis
    s. system
syngeneic
    s. bone marrow transplant
    s. graft
syngenesioplasty
syngenesiotransplantation
syngnathia
syngraft
synkinesis
    facial s.
    Facial Grading System S. (FGSS)
synostosis
    coronal s.
    cranial suture s.
    metopic s.
    plagiocephaly without s.
    unicoronal s.
    unilambdoid s.
    unilateral coronal s.
synostotic frontal plagiocephaly (SFP)
synotia
synovectomy
    radical s.
    surgical s.
synovial
    s. cell sarcoma
    s. chondromatosis (SCM)
    s. chondrosarcoma (SCS)
    s. dissector
    s. membrane
    s. sarcoma
    s. villus
synovitis
    s., acne, pustulosis, hyperostosis, osteitis (SAPHO)
    pigmented villonodular s.
synovium
synpolydactyly
syntactic
    s. aphasia
    s. element
    s. parsing
    s. rule
    s. violation
syntagmatic
    s. response
    s. word
syntax
Synthes
    S. AO reconstruction plate
    S. carbon rod external fixation system
    S. lengthener
    S. maxillofacial titanium plate
    S. mini-depth gauge

    S. stainless steel minifragment plate
    S. titanium minifragment plate
synthesis, pl. syntheses
    auditory s.
    collagen s.
    phonemic s.
synthetic
    s. absorbable suture (SAS)
    s. bone
    s. bone graft
    s. cell
    s. implant
    s. mesh
    s. method
    s. porcelain
    s. sapphire tip
    S. Sentence Identification Test
    s. zipper
Synthodont dental implant
syphilis
    congenital s.
    meningovascular s.
    tertiary s.
syphilitic teeth
syrigmus
syringe
    air s.
    Arnold-Bruening s.
    B-D Luer s.
    Centrix-type s.
    chip s.
    C-R s.
    dental s.
    endodontic irrigating s.
    Endovage s.
    Henke-Ject intraligamental s.
    hypodermic s.'s
    irrigation s.
    Irrivac s.
    laryngeal s.
    Ligmajet s.
    s. liposculpture
    Luer-Lok B-D s.
    Max-I-Probe endodontic irrigation s.
    pressure s.
    probe s.
    Pulpdent s.
    Stropko air s.
    water s.
syringe-assisted liposuction
syringe-driven system (SDS)
syringitis
syringoma
syringomyelia
    Chiari type I malformation with s.
syrup
    Actagen S.

Allerfrin S.
Allerphed S.
Ambenyl Cough S.
Amgenal Cough S.
Anamine S.
Aprodine S.
Bromanyl Cough S.
Bromfed S.
Bromotuss w/Codeine Cough S.
Carbodec S.
Cardec-S S.
Dallergy-D S.
Decofed S.
Deconamine S.
Demazin S.
Drixoral S.
Genamin Cold S.
Histalet S.
Histor-D S.
hydrocodone PA S.
Naldecon-EX Children's S.
Phenergan VC S.
Promethazine VC S.
Promethazine VC Plain S.
Rondec S.
Silafed S.
Silaminic Cold S.
Temazin Cold S.
Thera-Hist S.
Triaminic S.
Triaminicol Multi-Symptom Cold S.
Triofed S.
Triphenyl S.
Triposed S.
Tussar SF S.

system
ABL520 blood gas measurement s.
ACUSTAR I neurosurgical
  localization s.
adhesive s.
Adolph Gasser camera s.
Algipore Picasso visual
  transmission s.
All Access laser s.
Allen traction s.
Anspach 65K instrument s.
AO/ASIF titanium craniofacial s.
AO mandibular s.
Aston cartilage reduction s.
augmentative communication s.
autonomic nervous s.
Autovac autotransfusion s.

Barry Five Slate S.
Becker vibrating cannula s.
Benzaquen-Chajchir
  extraction/reinjection s.
Beta Glucan skin care s.
BiliBlanket phototherapy s.
BioBarrier membrane guided tissue
  regeneration s.
BioDIMENSIONAL s.
Bio-Esthetic abutment s.
Bioplate screw fixation s.
Bioquant histomorphometry s.
Blade-Vent implant s.
Boehringer Autovac
  autotransfusion s.
bone tack s.
Bosker TMI Reconstruction s.
Bosker transmandibular
  reconstructive surgical s.
Brånemark implant s.
Cafet s.
Calasept medicament delivery s.
Calcitek implant s.
Canal Finder s.
canalicular s.
carpal tunnel release s. (CTRS)
Cavi-Endo ultrasonic s.
Cavitron ultrasonic s.
Celay s.
Cencit imaging s.
central auditory nervous s. (CANS)
central nervous s. (CNS)
Centrax bipolar s.
CeraOne implant s.
CEREC s.
chairside economical restorations of
  esthetic ceramics s.
Champy miniplate, rigid fixation s.
chemically activated s.
CIS-2 s.
clotting s.
CMS AccuProbe 450 s.
cochleovestibular s.
Coleman microinfiltration s.
Coltene inlay s.
COM/MAND mandibular fixation s.
complement s.
computer assisted neurosurgical
  navigational s. (CANS)
computerized morphometric s.
CoreVent Implant s.
Cusp-Lok cuspid traction s.

S

NOTES

system *(continued)*

Dall-Miles cable grip s.
deep muscular aponeurotic s.
  (DMAS)
DentiCAD s.
dentinal s.
Dentsply implant s.
Diolite 532 laser s.
direct motor s.
2D linear plating s.
dorsalis pedis-FDMA s.
3D plating s.
drainage s.
Dumbach mandibular
  reconstruction s.
Dunlap cold compression wrap s.
Duoloid impression s.
Dur-A-Sil silicone impression s.
Durette s.
DUX s.
Easy Introduction s. (EIS)
Eccovision acoustic reflection
  imaging s.
Eccovision acoustic rhinometry s.
Ellman press-form s.
Emergence Profile implant s.
ENAC ultrasonic instrument s.
Endermologie adipose destruction s.
endocrine s.
Endopore dental implant s.
endosteal implant s.
Endotrac endoscopic carpal tunnel
  release s.
EpiLaser s.
EpiLight hair removal s.
EpiTouch Alex laser hair
  removal s.
EpiTouch ruby SilkLaser hair
  removal s.
erbium:YAG laser s.
esthetic laser s.
etch s.
ethmoidal infundibular s.
EXAKT cutting/grinding s.
Extra Oral S. (EOS)
extrapyramidal s.
E-Z Flap cranial flap fixation s.
Facial Grading S. (FGS)
fibrinolytic s.
Five Slate S.
fluid colloidal s.
Fonix 6500-CX hearing aid test s.
FRIALITE-2 dental implant s.
front recess drainage s.
GelShapes scar management s.
GlyMed Camouflage S.
GlyMed Plus post-surgical skin
  care s.

gold-copper s.
Goldenberg implant s.
Gold Series bone drilling s.
Golgi s.
haptic s.
haversian s.
Heliomolar s.
Herculite XRV Lab s.
Hertel eye position evaluation s.
Hoffman external fixation s.
Hopkins angle-view 30-degree
  optical s.
Hopkins rod lens s.
Hopkins straight-view optical s.
Horizon nasal CPAP s.
Howmedica HNR s.
Hunsaker Mon-Jet tube
  anesthesia s.
hydrodynamic s.
3i Implant Innovations implant s.
IMCOR No-Touch implant
  placement s.
Immediate Implant Impression s.
immune s.
ImplaMed implant s.
implant s.
Implatome dental tomography s.
IMZ implant s.
indirect motor s.
Innovation implant s.
international two-digit tooth-
  recording s.
Interpore IMZ implant s.
interprobe s.
Irri-Cath suction s.
irrigation s.
ITI dental implant s.
3i wide-diameter dental implant s.
JS Quick-fill s.
Karl Storz pediatric
  bronchoscopy s.
KaVo oral surgery s.
K-Fix Fixator s.
kinin s.
Kleen-Needle s.
KLS-Martin modular
  osteosynthesis s.
Kramer-Rhodes periodontal
  collection s.
KTP/Nd:YAG XP surgical laser s.
Kulzer inlay s.
Kurer anchor s.
LactoSorb resorbable fixation s.
LaminOss Implant S.
LaseAway ruby laser s.
laser s.
Leibinger plating s.

Leibinger titanium Würzburg mandibular reconstruction s.
Lekholm-Zarb classification s.
Level Anchorage s.
Lifecore Restore wide diameter implant s.
Lorenz Micro-Power dense bone drilling and cutting s.
Lorenz plating s.
Luhr maxillofacial fixation s.
Luhr microfixation s.
Luhr pan fixation s.
Luminex post s.
LySonix 2000 complete ultrasonic surgical s.
LySonix 2000 Micro ultrasonic surgical s.
LySonix Post-Operative patient s.
LySonix Series 250 operative s.
LySonix 2000 Standard ultrasonic surgical s.
LySonix TTD Cannula S.'s
LySonix 2000 ultrasonic surgical s.
Magna-Site locating s.
masticatory s.
M.D. Forté glycolic acid-based skin care s.
Mectra irrigation/aspiration s.
Medical Research Council muscle strength scale s.
Medtronics Sequestra 1000 autotransfusion s.
Mentor Contour Genesis ultrasonic assisted lipoplasty s.
MicroLux video camera s.
Micro Plus plating s.
Microsponge delivery s.
Micro-Vent implant s.
mini Würzburg Flexplates craniomaxillofacial plating s.
mini Würzburg standard craniomaxillofacial plating s.
Modulus CD anesthesia s.
Montgomery thyroplasty implant s.
S. of Multicultural Assessment (SOMA)
S. of Multicultural Pluralistic Assessment (SOMPA)
musculoaponeurotic s.
Natural Profile abutment s.
Nd:YAG laser s.

neodymium:yttrium-aluminum-garnet laser s.
Neosonic (P-5) SPM super powered mini retroprep/endo s.
NeoStrata skin rejuvenation s.
nervous s.
New Vision magnification s.
Niamtu Video Imaging S.
Nobelpharma implant s.
Norwegian s.
No-Touch delivery and mounting s.
NovaPulse laser s.
Nu-Trake Weiss emergency airway s.
Obagi Nu-Derm s.
occlusal scheme s.
Opmilas laser s.
Oral Scan computer imaging s.
Oral Scan video imaging s.
Orascoptic acuity s.
Osseous Coagulum Trap collecting s.
oxalate s.
oxylate dentin bonding s.
Paragon single-stage dental implant s.
Paragon single-stage implant s.
Park-O-Tron drill s.
Paulus trocar s.
P-700 Color Velocity Imaging s.
pediatric circle s.
Pegasus Airwave pressure relief s.
periodontal hydrodynamic s.
periodontal pitch s.
periodontal resilient s.
periodontal vascular s.
periotemp s.
Periotest s.
peripheral nervous s. (PNS)
Permark micropigmentation s.
permucosal implant s.
Perspective dental imaging s.
PGA-PLLA plating s.
phosphonated dimethacrylate/phosphated bis-GMA s.
PhotoDerm VL/PL hair removal s.
PhotoGenica T laser s.
PhotoGenica T^{10} tattoo removal s.
pitch s.
Plastic Endosurgical S. (P.E.S.)
platinum-silver s.

S

NOTES

system *(continued)*

PlumeSafe Whisper 602 smoke evacuation s.
PowerProxi Sonic interdental toothbrush s.
Procera s.
Pro-Post S.
ProSeries laparoscopic laser s.
Pruzansky classification s.
PulseDose portable compressed oxygen s.
pyramidal s.
Quantrex Sweep 650 ultrasonic cleansing s.
radiographic image processing s.
radiographic imaging s. (RIS)
Rekow s.
Renaissance Crown s.
Renaissance spirometry s.
Replace implant s.
resorbable copolymer PGA/PLLA-Lactosorb miniplate fixation s.
respiratory s.
response s.
Restore close tolerance dental implant s.
revised Salzburg lag screw s.
revised Würzburg mandibular reconstruction s.
Rhinoline endoscopic sinus surgery s.
Richard Wolf nasal epistaxis s.
rod tail s.
Sanders Venturi injector s.
Save-A-Tooth preserving s.
ScleroPLUS LongPulse dye laser s.
Scott chronic wound care s.
Screw-Vent implant s.
second messenger s.
Seroma-Cath wound drainage s.
Siemens s.
sign s.
Silhouette therapeutic massage s.
silver-copper s.
silver-tin s.
single-paste s.
SLS Chromos long pulse ruby laser s.
SmiLine abutment s.
Solid Creation S.
Sono-stat Plus joint sound measuring and documentation s.
Spirosense s.
Spline dental implant s.
9925 SPS ELCOmed100 s.
Stabident interosseous local anesthesia s.
Stableloc II external fixator s.

staging s.
stomatognathic s.
Storz-Hopkins s.
subcutaneous musculoaponeurotic s.
submuscular aponeurotic s.
Sub-Vent implant s.
suction s.
superficial fascial s. (SFS)
superficial musculoaponeurotic s. (SMAS)
Sure-Closure skin closure s.
SureScan s.
Sustain dental implant s.
Swiss Precision cannula s.
symbol set s.
synergistic s.
Synthes carbon rod external fixation s.
syringe-driven s. (SDS)
tail s.
Tebbets EndoPlastic instrument s.
Tessier craniofacial cleft classification s.
THORP s.
thread mate s. (TMS)
three-dimensional plating s.
TiMesh 1.0/1.5/2.2 combination s.
TiMesh craniomaxillofacial plating s.
TiMesh 2.2-mm craniofacial s.
TiMesh 1.0-mm Micro S.
TiMesh 1.5-mm midface and cranial s.
TiMesh rigid fixation bone plating s.
Toomey tip s.
TRAKE-fit s.
Tulip syringe s.
two-dimensional linear plating s.
two-paste s.
Ultra Image.db computer imaging s.
UltraLite headlight s.
ultrasonic retroprep s.
Ultra-X external fixation s.
UniFile Imaging and Archiving s.
UniPlast Imaging and Archiving s.
Unitrax unipolar s.
Universal F breathing s.
Universal Numbering s.
s. universal verbotonol audition Guberina (SUVAG)
Venodyne compression s.
VID 1 color micro camera s.
video imaging s. (VIS)
visceral nervous s.
visible light-activated s.

Vitek-Kent hemi TMJ
  replacement s.
Vitek-Kent total TMJ
  replacement s.
Voice restoration s.
W&H surgical s.
Würzburg fracture s.
Würzburg maxillofacial plating s.
Würzburg reconstruction s.

Xerox dental radiographic
  imaging s.
systematic method
systemic
  s. chondromalacia
  s. lesion
  s. lupus erythematosus
  s. mycosis
s/z ratio

NOTES

S

T

T bar of Kazanjian
T cell
T cell count
T clasp arm
T cytotoxic/suppressor lymphocyte
T helper/inducer lymphocyte
T loop archwire
T lymphocyte
T protein

T₃

triiodothyronine

T-helper

T.-h. cell
T.-h. lymphocyte

T12 nerve division
T3 RNA polymerase
T-4 Gel
T4/Leu2a marker
T4/Leu3a marker
T4/T8 ratio
TA

terminal arteriole

T&A

tonsillectomy and adenoidectomy

tabes dorsalis
table

Andrews spinal surgery t.
back t.
Cutler-Ederer prediction t.
Hixon-Oldfather prediction t.
occlusal t.
t. occlusion
Sister Helen mustard t.
Skytron surgical t.
Sugita microsurgical t.

tablet

Actagen T.
Actifed Allergy T. (Night)
Afrin T.
Allercon T.
Allerfrin T.
Aprodine T.
Benadryl Decongestant Allergy T.
Bromfed T.
Bromphen T.
Carbiset T.
Carbiset-TR T.
Carbodec TR T.
Ceftin t.
Cenafed Plus T.
Chlor-Rest T.
Chlor-Trimeton 4 Hour Relief T.
D.A.II T.
Deconamine T.

Dimaphen T.
Dimetapp T.
Disophrol T.
Dispertab T.
Dynabac t.
E-Mycin Delayed-Release T.
Fedahist T.
Genac T.
Histalet Forte T.
Histatab Plus T.
Hista-Vadrin T.
Klerist-D T.
Lortab T.
PCE T.
Pseudo-Gest Plus T.
Rhinatate T.
Roxicet T.
R-Tannamine T.
R-Tannate T.
Rynatan T.
Salagen t.
Scopace T.
Sinutab T.
Solagen T.
3Space t.
Sudafed Plus T.
Tanoral T.
Triaminic Allergy T.
Triaminic Cold T.
Tri-Nefrin Extra Strength T.
Triotann T.
Triposed T.
Tri-Tannate T.
Tylenol Cold Effervescent
Medication T.
Vicks DayQuil Allergy Relief 4
Hour T.

tabulation
Tac-3
Tac-40
Tach-E-Z

T.-E.-Z. attachment
T.-E.-Z. retainer

tachistoscope
tachycardia
tachylalia
tachyphemia
tack

Ace Bone Screw t.
Graftac absorbable skin t.
titanium t.

tacking
TACL-R

Tests for Auditory Comprehension of
Language-R

tacrolimus
Tactaid hearing aid
tactile
> t. agnosia
> t. corpuscles
> t. exteroception
> t. feedback
> t. kinesthetic perception

tact operant
Taebuia impetiginosa
tag
> Gore-Tex t.
> t. question

Tagamet
> T. HB

tagliacotian operation
tail
> t. system
> velar t.

tainting
Takahara disease
Takahashi forceps
take
> good t.
> poor t.

takedown
> fistula t.

TAL
> total autogenous latissimus
> TAL breast reconstruction

Talacen
talc
> t. poudrage
> zinc oxide, cod liver oil, and t.

talk
> baby t.
> cross t.
> parallel t.

tall
> t. dock
> Lumex Tub Guard T.

talon cusp
Talwin
> T. Compound
> T. NX

Tamine
tamoxifen
tamponade
> balloon t.
> esophageal balloon t.
> nasal t.
> postnasal balloon t.

tamponage
> vaselinized nasal t.

Tanac
Tanacetum parthenium

tang
tangential
> t. excision
> t. projection
> t. section

tangible
> t. reinforcement of operant
> conditioned audiometry (TROCA)
> t. reinforcement of operant
> conditioning

tank
> processing t.

tannic acid
Tanoral Tablet
Tan otoplasty
tantalum
tanyphonia
TAP-D
> Test of Articulation Performance-
> Diagnostic

tape
> dental t.
> floss t.
> Hy-Tape surgical t.
> Medipore H surgical t.
> Micropore t.
> steroid-impregnated t.

taper
> funnelform t.
> t. hand file

tapered
> t. crown
> t. fissure bur
> t. post

tapering arch
taper-lock (TL)
> Swede-Vent t.-l.

tapetum, pl. tapeta
> t. alveoli

Tapia syndrome
tapir
> bouche de t.

tapping
TAP-S
> Test of Articulation Performance-Screen

Taraxacum officinale
tarda
> dentia t.

Targa+ image capture board
target
> t. response
> t. tissue

targetoid ring
tarnish
tarsorrhaphy
tartar

tartrate
> belladonna, phenobarbital, and
> ergotamine t.
> ergotamine t.

**tartrate-resistant acid phosphatase
(TRAP)**

task
> across-speech t.
> t. analysis
> nonspeech respiratory t.
> offline cloze t.
> online t.
> respiratory control t.

Tasserit shoulder attachment

taste
> t. bud
> t. cell
> t. center
> t. corpuscle
> franklinic t.
> t. pore
> t. test
> voltaic t.

TAT
> triple advancement transposition
> TAT procedure

Tatagiba line

tattoo
> amalgam t.
> decorative t.
> graphite t.
> pencil-point t.
> t. removal
> traumatic t.

Taub minute stain kit

Tauredon

taurodontism

tautologous

Tavist
> T.-1
> T.-D

Taxol

Tazicef

Tazidime

T-band matrix

T-bar elevator

TBG
> thyroxine-binding globulin

T-breast reduction

TBSA
> total body surface area

TC
> tungsten carbide

Tc
> technetium
> Tc cell

^{99m}Tc
> technetium-99m

TCA
> trichloroacetic acid
> TCA peel

TCB
> transconjunctival blepharoplasty

TCB/TCA
> transconjunctival
> blepharoplasty/trichloroacetic acid
> combination
> TCB/TCA combination

TCL
> transverse carpal ligament

TCN
> terminal capillary network

Tc-RBC scan

TCS
> Treacher Collins syndrome

TD
> threshold of discomfort

T.D.
> Diamine T.D.

Td
> tetanus-diphtheria

TDD
> telecommunication device for the deaf

TDL
> temporal difference limen

TDMAC
> tridodecylmethylammonium chloride
> graft coating material

TDP
> tenderness to digital palpation

TDSP
> time domain signal processor

TDTH cell

TE
> tonsillectomy

TE$_{mic}$
> tonsillectomy with operating microscope

tea

teachers' nodes

teaching
> diagnostic t.

team
> craniofacial multidisciplinary t.

NOTES

tear
cemental t.
cementum t.
T. Drop Solution
retinal t.
t. strength eugenol-based sealer
t. test

teardrop
t. foramen
inverted t.
t. stop

TearGard Ophthalmic Solution
Teargen Ophthalmic Solution
tearing
gustatory t.

Tearisol Solution
tearout
enamel t.

tears
artificial t.
crocodile t.
T. Naturale Free Solution
T. Naturale II Solution
T. Plus Solution
T. Renewed Solution

Teaser
Tebbets
T. EndoPlastic instrument system
T. ribbon retractor

Techmedica prosthesis
technetium (Tc)
t.-99m (^{99m}Tc)
t.-99m phosphate
t. bone scan
t. scintigram

Techni-Care surgical scrub
technician
Certified Dental T. (CDT)
dental t.
dental laboratory t.

technique
acid etch bonding t.
advance cochlear echo t.
Aiache t.
airbrasive t.
angle bisection t.
anterior scoring t.
ascending t.
aseptic t.
aural-oral t.
Azzolini t.
Baek musculocutaneous pedicle t.
balanced force t.
balanced-force instrumentation t.
Barkann t.
barrier t.
Bass t.

Begg light wire differential force t.
Benelli t.
Bernard-Burow t.
bioprogressive t.
bisecting angle t.
bisecting-the-angle t.
bitewing t.
Blaskovics eyelid shortening t.
blepharoplasty, modified Loeb and de la Plaza t.
Bowles t.
Box t.
Bramante t.
bulk pack t.
Canal Master instrumentation t.
canal-wall-up t.
cap t.
capping t.
cerclage wire t.
channel shoulder pin t.
Charters t.
chevron marking t.
chew-in t.
Class V Multiple Step Build-up t.
communicative t.
compensation t.
continuous gum t.
controlled water added t.
Converse t.
cross-facial t.
cross-section t.
crown down t.
culturing t.
Delerm and Elbaz t.
Dental Exposure Normalization T. (DENT)
dermal brassiere t.
dermal orbicular pennant t.
dermal pedicle t.
dermofat t.
descending t.
Dibbell cartilage strut t.
differential force t.
direct t.
direct/indirect t.
distal pedicle flap t.
dome-sectioning t.
double pedicle t.
double-sealant t.
dry field t.
dual impression t.
Eames t.
edgewise t.
elliptical excision t.
endodontic t.
epithelialization t.
ESP face lift t.

extended mesh t.
extended supraplatysmal plane face lift t.
fallopian bridge t.
fascial staple t.
fast exposure t.
fenestration t.
filling first t.
film exposure t.
Fischer curette t.
fixed-tissue t.
flow t.
folding t.
Fones t.
four-flap Webster-Bernard t.
Frank t.
gel t.
Giampapa t.
glanular triangular flap t.
Goldman-Ponti t.
gold plate t.
gradient echo t.
half-mouth t.
Hamas and Rohrich t.
HAS t.
head turn t.
heat-sear t.
hemostat t.
high-amplitude sucking t.
high heat casting t.
histochemical t.
Holmstrom t.
Hood t.
House wire and Gelfoam t.
hydroflow t.
hygroscopic t.
Ilizarov t.
Illouz liposuction t.
immediate extension t.
impression t.
incision-halving t.
indirect t.
intact canal wall t.
isolation t.
Karapandzic t.
Kawamoto t.
Kazanjian vestibuloplasty t.
Kesselring curette t.
Kessler suture t.
kinesthetic t.
Kuhnt-Szymanowski t.
labiolingual t.

language expansion t.
laser dissection t.
Lassus t.
Lejour t.
lid-loading t.
lid-sharing t.
light around wire t.
Lightspeed canal preparation t.
lingual split-bone t.
lipoinjection t.
lipo layering t.
liposuction t.
localization t.
Loeb sliding pad t.
long-axis t.
long cone t.
lost wax pattern t.
mammaplasty reduction t.
masking t.
maxillary sinus Foley catheter balloon placement t.
McCraw t.
McGoon t.
McIndoe t.
McSpadden endodontic t.
Merendino t.
Messerklinger t.
microetching t.
micrograft punctiform t.
Millard forked flap t.
modified anterior scoring t.
modified Bernard-Burow t.
modified Skoog t.
Mohs micrographic surgery by fixed-tissue t.
mucoperiosteal flap t.
mucosal relaxing incision t.
multiplanar endoscopic facial rejuvenation t.
multiplanar upper facial rejuvenation t.
Mustardé t.
Muti t.
nasal Fraser suction t.
Nealon t.
N2-Sargenti t.
Obtura injectable t.
Ochterlony gel diffusion t.
one-phase subperiosteal implant t.
one-pour t.
onlay t.
open flap t.

T

NOTES

technique *(continued)*
    Orticochea scalping t.
    oval window seal t.
    parallel t.
    paralleling t.
    Pardue t.
    Parodi t.
    periareolar t.
    Perko t.
    pinch t.
    plastic matrix t.
    pollicization t.
    polysomnographic t.
    porcelain cervical contact and
      single bake t.
    porcelain cervical ditching t.
    postresection filling t.
    pressure t.
    presuturing t.
    Proetz displacement t.
    projective t.
    pull-through t.
    Pulvertaft weave suture t.
    pushback t.
    quick angulation t.
    Rainville t.
    regional blocking anesthesia t.
    retained papilla t.
    Reynolds and Horton alar
      cartilage t.
    ribbon arch t.
    right-angle t.
    round block t.
    scapular island flap t.
    Schneider t.
    Schrudde curette t.
    sectional t.
    sensorineural acuity level t.
    Seward t.
    shave excision t.
    short-cone t.
    short scar t.
    single-pour t.
    skin expansion t.
    Skoog t.
    spaghetti fat grafting t.
    split-bone t.
    spread-and-cut t.
    Standoli t.
    startle t.
    Stenstrom alar cartilage t.
    step-back circumferential filing t.
    step-back filing t.
    step-back instrumentation t.
    stepdown t.
    step-down t.
    Stillman t.

    still radiography t.
    Strombeck t.
    Studebaker t.
    subperiosteal implant one-phase t.
    superwet t.
    swinging door t.
    Teimourian and Adhan t.
    Teimourian curette t.
    Terzis t.
    thermal expansion t.
    thermocatalytic t.
    thermo-photocatalytic t.
    tissue-expansion t.
    Todd-Evans stepladder tracheal
      dilatation t.
    total etch t.
    Trifecta obturation t.
    Tsuge suture t.
    tubeless spontaneous respiration t.
    tube-shift t.
    tube switch t.
    tumescent local anesthesia t.
    twist-off t.
    two-portal open carpal tunnel
      release t.
    two-pour t.
    two-step t.
    underlay fascia t.
    Van Beek-Zook t.
    vertical-cut t.
    vertical scar with lipoaspiration t.
    vest-over-pants t.
    Wagner-Baldwin t.
    Walsh-Ogura t.
    Wardill t.
    wash t.
    washed-field t.
    wax pattern thermal expansion t.
    Weine t.
    Weir t.
    wet t.
    Willi glass crown t.
    window t.
    wire-gelatin t.
    wire loop/gelatin sponge t.
    Zocchi ultrasound-assisted
      lipoplasty t.
    Z-plasty t.
    Zuker and Manktelow t.
technologist
    dental t.
    dental laboratory t.
technology
    CE-3000 video t.
    Cogent Micro Illumination t.
    Lifecore cutting advance t.

Oxismart advanced signal
processing and alarm
management t.
ultrapulse t.

Teclite
T. fiberoptic light source

tectonic

tectorial membrane

Teebi syndrome

teeth (*pl. of* tooth)

teething
Babee T.
Numzit T.

TEF
tracheoesophageal fistula

TefGen-FD
T.-F. guided tissue regeneration
membrane
T.-F. plastic membrane

Teflon
T. granuloma
T. injection
T. material
T. mold
T. paste
T. piston

Tegaderm dressing

tegmen
low-lying t.
t. mastoideum
t. plate

tegmental encephalocele

Tegopen

Tegretol

Tegrin-HC

Teimourian
T. and Adhan technique
T. aspirative lipoplasty
T. curette technique

Telachlor

telangiectasia
hemorrhagic t.

telangiectasis
hereditary hemorrhagic t.

telangiectatic cell

telangiectaticum
granuloma t.

TELD
Tests of Early Language Development

Teldrin

telecanthus

telecobalt irradiation

telecoil

**telecommunication device for the deaf
(TDD)**

telegraphic utterance

telemetry
intraoral t.

telephone
t. booster circuit
t. ear
text t. (TT)
t. theory

telephone-place theory

telescope
angled t.
bronchoscopic t.
0-degree t.
30-degree t.
70-degree t.
Foroblique bronchoscopic t.
retrospective bronchoscopic t.
right angle bronchoscopic t.
solid-rod rigid t.
straight ahead bronchoscopic t.

telescoped word

telescopic
t. coping
t. crown
t. denture
t. prosthesis

telescoping
t. crossbite

teletactor

Telfa
T. dressing
T. gauze
T. sterile adhesive pad

telorbitism

telorism

TEM
transmission electron microscope
transmission electron microscopy
transverse electromagnetic mode

Temazin Cold Syrup

Temovate

**Tempa-DOT single-use clinical
thermometer**

Tempak
Ward T.

temper

temperature
maturing t.
molding t.

T

NOTES

tempering
> gold t.

template
> implant t.
> Jacobsen t.
> occlusal t.
> postablative t.
> scalloped endosseous t.
> surgical t.
> tissue expander t.
> tissue sizer t.
> wax t.

Temple University Short Syntax Inventory (TUSSI)

Templin-Darley Tests of Articulation

Templin Phoneme Discrimination Test

tempo

temporal
> t. arteritis
> t. artery
> t. bone
> t. bone anomaly
> t. bone fracture
> t. diameter
> t. difference limen (TDL)
> t. fascia proper
> t. fossa
> t. fossa abscess
> t. gyrus
> t. island pedicle scalp flap
> t. line
> t. line of fusion
> t. lobe
> t. lobe abscess
> t. lobe epilepsy
> t. margin
> t. muscle
> t. nerve
> t. plane
> t. process of mandible
> t. process of zygomatic bone
> t. region
> t. sulcus
> t. surface
> t. surface of frontal bone
> t. surface   of great wing
> t. surface of zygomatic bone
> t. syndrome
> t. vein
> t. vessel

temporalis
> t. fascia
> t. fascia graft
> t. fascia proper (TFP)
> t. flap
> linea t.
> t. muscle
> t. muscle-fascia transfer
> t. muscle flap
> t. muscle transposition
> t. sling
> t. superficialis fascia

temporal-pterygomaxillary fossa

temporary
> t. acrylic crown
> t. base
> cavit t.
> t. cement
> t. crown
> t. dentition
> t. endodontic restorative material (TERM)
> t. entropion
> t. filling
> t. lip augmentation
> t. master apical file (TMAF)
> t. material
> t. partial denture
> t. prosthesis
> t. restoration
> t. splint
> t. stopping
> t. superstructure
> t. teeth
> t. threshold shift (TTS)
> t. tooth

temporization
> t. kit

temporodiskal

temporofacial
> t. nerve

temporofrontal

temporohyoid

temporomalar
> t. endoscopic lift
> t. nerve
> t. suture

temporomandibular
> t. arthralgia
> t. arthroscopy
> t. arthrosis
> t. disorder (TMD)
> t. dysfunction syndrome
> t. extraoral radiography
> t. joint (TMJ)
> t. joint ankylosis
> t. joint articular eminence
> t. joint articulation
> t. joint capsule
> t. joint click
> t. joint dislocation
> t. joint dysfunction (TMD, TMJ)
> t. joint fossa
> t. joint hypermobility
> t. joint osteoarthritis (TMJ-OA)
> t. joint pain-dysfunction syndrome

t. joint radiograph
t. joint sprain
t. joint subluxation
t. joint syndrome
t. joint synovial fluid (TMJ-SF)
t. ligament
t. luxation
t. neuralgia
t. pain dysfunction (TMPD)
t. pain-dysfunction disorder

temporomaxillary
temporoparietal
t. fascia
t. fascial flap (TPFF)
t. fascial flap interposition

temporoparietalis
t. fascia
t. fascia flap

temporoparieto-occipital
t.-o. Juri flap

temporozygomatic
t. suture

Tempra
Temrex zinc oxide-eugenol cement
Tenacin zinc phosphate cement
tenaculum
Coakley t.
t. forceps
White t.

tendency
bleeding t.
central t.

tenderness
t. to digital palpation (TDP)
rebound t.

tendinitis
tendinoplasty (*var. of* tenontoplasty)
tendinous
t. inscription
t. intersection

tendon
Achilles t.
extensor digiti minimi t.
extensor digitorum communis t.
extensor indicis proprius t.
flexor carpi radialis t.
flexor carpi ulnaris t.
t. graft
inferior crus of lateral canthal t.
intermediate t.
masseter t.
palmaris longus t.

plantaris t.
t. plasty
t. rupture
snapping triceps t.
stapedius t.
superficialis t.
tensor tympani t.
t. transfer
t. transplantation

tendoplasty (*var. of* tenontoplasty)
teniposide
Tennison
T. repair
T. triangular flap

Tennison-Randall triangular flap
tenolysis
tenomyoplasty
tenontomyoplasty
tenontoplastic, tenoplastic
tenontoplasty, tendinoplasty, tendoplasty,
   tenoplasty
tenosynovitis
coccidioidomycosis t.
fulminant t.
granulomatous t.
suppurative t.
tuberculosis t.
tuberculous t.

tenotomy scissors
tenovagosynovitis
pigmented villonodular t. (PVNS)

tensa
pars t.

tense
t. pause
t. phoneme
t. vowel

tensile
t. force
t. strength
t. stress

Tensilon
T. myasthenia gravis test

tension
t. headache
interfacial surface t.
laryngeal t.
peak t.
t. pneumocephalus
t. side
supralaryngeal t.
surface t.

T

NOTES

tension-control suture technique in open rhinoplasty
tension-free
    t.-f. repair
    t.-f. scalp fixation
tensionless
tension-requiring suture
tensor
    t. fasciae latae
    t. fasciae latae flap
    t. fold
    t. tympani
    t. tympani muscle
    t. tympani nerve
    t. tympani tendon
    t. veli palatini muscle
tensoris
    incisura t.
tent
    croup t.
tenth cranial nerve
tentorium
tenuis
    Alternaria t.
TENVAD
    Tests of Nonverbal Auditory Discrimination
Tenzel elevator
TEOAE
    transient evoked otoacoustic emission
TEP
    tracheoesophageal prosthesis
    tracheoesophageal puncture
    transesophageal puncture
Terak Ophthalmic Ointment
teratodermoid
teratoid cyst
teratoma, pl. **teratomata**
    benign cystic t.
    congenital oral t.
    mature t.
Terazol Vaginal
terbinafine, topical
terconazole
teres
    t. major muscle
    t. major skin island
    t. minor
    t. minor muscle
terfenadine
    t. and pseudoephedrine
Terino
    T. facial implant retractor
    T. implant
    T. malar shell
TERM
    temporary endodontic restorative material

terminal
    t. abutment
    t. arteriole (TA)
    axon t.
    t. bar
    t. behavior
    t. capillary loop
    t. capillary network (TCN)
    clause t.
    t. contour
    t. dentition
    t. duct carcinoma
    t. hinge position
    t. jaw relation record
    t. juncture
    t. lag
    t. nerve
    t. occlusion
    t. plane
    presynaptic t.
    t. retention
    t. string
    t. sulcus
    t. sulcus of tongue
    synaptic t.
    t. web
terra alba
Terra-Cortril
    T.-C. Ophthalmic Suspension
terrae
    Mycobacterium t.
Terramycin
    T. I.M. Injection
    T. Oral
    T. w/Polymyxin B Ophthalmic Ointment
tertiary
    t. dentin
    t. stress
    t. syphilis
Terzis technique
TES
    therapeutic error signal
Tessier
    T. classification
    T. cleft
    T. cleft axis
    T. craniofacial cleft classification system
    T. craniofacial instrument
    T. osteomicrotome
test
    ability t.
    acoustic impedance t.
    acuity t.
    adaptation t.
    T. of Adolescent Language
    Adolescent Language Screening T.

albumin t.
alcohol sniff t. (AST)
alkaline phosphatase t.
Allen t.
alternate binaural loudness
  balance t.
Ammons Full Range Picture
  Vocabulary T.
aptitude t.
Armitage-Cochran t.
articulation t.
T. of Articulation Performance-
  Diagnostic (TAP-D)
T. of Articulation Performance-
  Screen (TAP-S)
audiometric t.
Auditory Analysis T.
auditory brainstem response t.
T.'s for Auditory Comprehension
  of Language-R (TACL-R)
auditory discrimination t.
T. of Auditory-Perceptual Skill
Auditory Pointing T.
Austin Spanish Articulation T.
BALB t.
Bankson Language Screening T.
Bárány caloric t.
Basic Language Concepts T.
t. battery
Bellugi-Klima Language
  Comprehension T.
Berko T.
Bernstein t.
Berry-Talbott Language T.
binaural alternate loudness
  balance t.
Bing T.
bithermal-caloric t.
Boston University Speech Sound
  Discrimination T.
Brinell hardness t.
Brown t.
California Consonant T.
caloric t.
carbon dioxide snow t.
Carrell Discrimination T.
Carrow Auditory-Visual Abilities T.
cavity t.
centrifuge t.
chi-square t.
coagulation t.
coin t.

cold t.
cold bend t.
Cold-Running Speech T.
colorimetric caries susceptibility t.
Completing Sentence T. (CST)
Complex Speech Sound
  Discrimination T.
CO_2-snow t.
could not t. (CNT)
coupling fitness t.
criterion-referenced t.
culture t.
Culture Fair Intelligence T.
deep articulation t.
dental aptitude t. (DAT)
Developmental Articulation T.
  (DAT)
diagnostic t.
diagnostic articulation t.
dichotic consonant-vowel t.
Discourse Comprehension T.
Doerfler-Stewart t.
D-S t.
Duncan multiple range t.
T.'s of Early Language
  Development (TELD)
edrophonium chloride t.
electric pulp t.
ELISA t.
EquiTest motor coordination t.
EquiTest sensory organization t.
evoked visual potential t.
T. for Examining Expressive
  Morphology (EEM)
Expressive One-Word Picture
  Vocabulary T.
Fein Articulation Screening T.
  (FAST)
t. file gauge
Fisher exact t.
fistula t.
FIT t.
Flowers Auditory Screening T.
  (FAST)
Fluharty Speech and Language
  Screening T.
forced duction t.
Fosdick-Hansen-Epple t.
fusion-inferred threshold t.
gaze t.
Gellé t.
glycerol t.

T

NOTES

test *(continued)*

Goodenough draw-a-man t.
Hallpike t.
t. handle
t. handle instrument
heterophile antibody t.
hot t.
ice t.
Illinois Children's Language
Assessment T.
immittance t.
Iowa Pressure Articulation T.
James Language Dominance T.
Jebsen t.
Kappa t.
Kindergarten Auditory Screening T.
Kindergarten Language
Screening T. (KLST)
Knoop hardness t.
Kolmogorov-Sirnov Two Sample T.
Kruskal-Wallis t.
lacrimation t.
T. of Language Competence (TLC)
T. of Language Competence for
Children (TLC-C)
T. of Language Development-
Intermediate (TOLD-I)
T. of Language Development-
Primary (TOLD-P)
Language Processing T.
Language Proficiency T. (LPT)
lateral excursion t.
Lillie-Crow t.
Lindamood Auditory
Conceptualization T.
Lombard voice-reflex t.
maximum stimulation t. (MST)
median nerve compression t.
Merrill Language Screening T.
Metz recruitment t.
Miller-Yoder Comprehension T.
T.'s of Minimal Articulation
Competence
Minimum Auditory Capabilities T.
(MAC)
Moberg pickup t.
Mohs hardness t.
Monaural Loudness Balance T.
(MLB)
monofilament t.
monothermal caloric t.
motor control t.
motor coordination t. (MCT)
Mueller t.
nerve excitability t. (NET)
nonverbal t.
T.'s of Nonverbal Auditory
Discrimination (TENVAD)

T. of Nonverbal Intelligence
(TONI)
norm-referenced t.
Northwestern Syntax Screening T.
(NSST)
Northwestern University Children's
Perception of Speech T.
NU Auditory T. Lists 4 and 6
nystagmus t.
objective t.
ocular dysmetria t.
optokinetic t.
Oral Language Sentence Imitation
Screening T. (ORSIST)
oral mucosal transudate t.
t. patch
Patterned Elicitation Syntax
Screening T. (PESST)
Paul-Bunnell t.
Peabody Picture Vocabulary T.
Pediatric Speech Intelligibility T.
(PSI)
penetration t.
percussion t.
performance t.
performance-intensity function t.
phenylephrine t.
Photo Articulation T. (PAT)
Picture Articulation and Language
Screening T.
Picture Speech Discrimination T.
pinch t.
platform posture t.
Plomp t.
position t.
positional t.
Pragmatic Screening T.
Preschool Language Screening T.
Preschool Speech and Language
Screening T.
processor-machine performance t.
Prognostic Value of Imitative and
Auditory Discrimination T.
promontory stimulation t. (PST)
provocative t.
pulmonary function t.
pulp t.
pulp vitality t.
Queckenstedt t.
Quick T.
Quickscreen t.
radioactive iodine uptake t.
radioallergosorbent t. (RAST)
rapidly alternating speech
perception t.
RASP t.
Receptive One Word Picture
Vocabulary T. (ROWPVT)

recruitment t.
Revised Token T.
Rickles t.
Rinne t.
Robbins Speech Sound
  Discrimination and Verbal
  Imagery Type T.
rotation t.
saccadic velocity t.
SAL t.
salivary flow t.
Scheffe t.
Schirmer tear t.
Schwabach t.
screening t.
Screening Speech Articulation T.
Semmes-Weinstein monofilament t.
sensitivity t.
sensory organization t. (SOT)
Sentence Articulation T.
serologic t.
Short-Term Auditory Retrieval and
  Storage T. (STARS)
sinusoidal tracking t.
SISI t.
skin t.
small increment sensitivity index t.
Snyder t.
Speech Sound Memory T.
spinning top t.
Staggered Spondaic Word T.
  (SSW)
standardized t.
stapedial reflex t.
Stein t.
Stenger t.
Stephens Oral Language
  Screening T.
stick-bite t.
Story Articulation T.
Structure Photographic Expressive
  Language T.-II (SPELT-P)
Suprathreshold Adaptation T.
  (STAT)
sweep-check t.
Swinging Story T.
Synthetic Sentence Identification T.
taste t.
tear t.
Templin Phoneme Discrimination T.
Tensilon myasthenia gravis t.
thermal pulp vitality t.

thyroid suppression t.
thyrotropin stimulation t.
Time Compressed Speech T.
Tobey-Ayer t.
token t.
tone decay t.
topagnostic t.
torsion-chair t.
Tri-County Contextual
  Articulation T.
Trieger psychomotor function dot t.
tuning fork t.
Tzanck t.
University of Pennsylvania Smell
  Identification T. (UPSIT)
vestibular autorotation t. (VAT)
vestibular function t.
vestibulo-ocular reflex rotational
  chair t.
Vickers hardness t.
viscosity of saliva t.
Visual Aural Digit Span T.
  (VADS)
vitality t.
Washington Speech Sound
  Discrimination T.
Watson scaphoid shift t.
W-22 Auditory T.
Weber t.
Weiss Comprehensive
  Articulation T.
Weiss Intelligibility T.
Western blot t.
Word T.
T. of Word Finding (TWF)
W-1/W-2 Auditory T.

tester

Accu-Measure personal body fat t.
Analytic Technology pulp t.
Crane Vitapulp pulp t.
electric pulp t.
Green Endo-Ice pulp t.
high-frequency pulp t.
low-frequency pulp t.
Neosono Ultima apex
  locator/pulp t.
Olsen stiffness t.
pulp t.
Ritter t.
S.S. White pulp t.
Tinius Olsen stiffness t.
Vitapulp pulp t.

NOTES

testes (*pl. of* testis)
testing
    electric pulp t.
    electrodiagnostic t.
    electrometric t.
Testing-Teaching Module of Auditory Discrimination (TTMAD)
testis, pl. testes
testosterone
    t. analog
test-retest reliability coefficient
tetani
    Clostridium t.
tetanus
    t. immune globulin human
    t. prophylaxis
tetanus-diphtheria (Td)
tetany
    t. neonatorum
tethering
    t. effect
    t. septum
tetism
tetracaine
tetracuspid
tetracycline
    Actisite periodontal fiber t.
    t. discoloration
    t. hydrochloride sclerotherapy
tetradecyl
    sodium t.
tetrahydrozoline
tetramethylbenzidine (TMB)
Tetrasine
    T. Extra Ophthalmic
    T. Ophthalmic
Tevdek suture
Texas
    T. Goodstein sharp tip
    T. tip
text
    mathetic t.
    nonobtrusive t.
    obtrusive t.
    pragmatic t.
    t. telephone (TT)
textlinguisitcs
textual operant
texture
    gingival surface t.
textured saline breast implant
texturing
TFCC
    triangular fibrocartilage complex
T-file
    engine T.-f.
    Mity engine T.-f.

TFP
    temporalis fascia proper
Tgb
    thyroglobulin
T-Gesic
TGF-β
    transforming growth factor-β
    transforming growth factor beta
TGOR
    transverse groove of oblique ridge
TG Osseotite single-stage procedure implant
Thal
    thalassemia
    α-Thal-1-trait
    α-Thal-2-trait
thalamic syndrome
thalamocortical area
thalamus
thalassemia (Thal)
    t. intermedia
    t. major
thallium imaging
the
    t. oronasal acoustic ratio (TONAR)
    T. Pacific Coast Tissue Bank
    t. Treaser surgical instrument
thecodont
theleplasty
thenar
    t. eminence
    t. flap
theophylline
theoretical linguistics
theory
    acidogenic t.
    anticipatory and struggle behavior t.'s
    approach-avoidance t.
    Begg t.
    biolinguistic t.
    Brännström hydrodynamics t.
    breakdown t.
    cementogenic t.
    cerebral dominance and handedness t.
    chemicoparasitic t.
    communication failure t.
    conditioned disintegration t.
    convergence t.
    diagnosogenic t.
    direct conduction t.
    dysphemia and biochemical t.
    ecological t.
    empiricist t.
    frequency t.
    frequency-place t.
    gate control t.

Helmholtz place t.
hydrodynamics t.
innateness t.
instrumental avoidance act t.
language t.
learning t.
markedness t.
mendelian t.
Miller t.
Miller chemicoparasitic t.
mixture t.
modular t.
myoelastic t.
nativist t.
neurochronaxic t.
operant behavior t.
orthodontic t.
pattern t.
periodontal t.
perseveration t.
phylogenetic t.
place t.
proteolysis-chelation t.
proteolytic t.
rationalist language t.
reed instrument t.
repressed need t.
Rutherford frequency t.
servomechanistic t.
social learning t.
specificity t.
speech innateness t.
stringed instrument t.
stuttering t.
telephone t.
telephone-place t.
transduction t.
traveling wave t.
volley t.

Theraflu Non-Drowsy Formula Maximum Strength
Thera-Flur
    T.-F. Gel-Drops
    T.-F.-N Gel-Drops
Thera-Hist Syrup
Theramin Expectorant
therapeutic
    Accepted Dental T.'s (ADT)
    t. appliance
    t. error signal (TES)
    t. mouthwash

provisionally accepted dental t.
unaccepted dental t.
therapist
    language t.
    speech t.
    voice t.
therapy
    activator t.
    active appliance t.
    antihormonal t.
    antirejection drug t.
    antiretroviral t.
    bite plane t.
    cold t.
    corrective t. (CT)
    Crozat t.
    diagnostic t. (Dx)
    drug t.
    endodontic t.
    expansion and activator t.
    functional orthodontic t.
    habituation t.
    HBO t.
    hyperbaric oxygen t.
    immunosuppressive t.
    incremental t.
    indirect pulpal t.
    interstitial radiation t.
    intramuscular streptomycin
      titration t.
    intravesical t.
    Intron A t.
    myofunctional t.
    nasopharyngoscopy biofeedback t.
    neutron beam t.
    nonbiofeedback t.
    occlusal t.
    occlusal appliance t.
    operant t.
    orthodontic t.
    oxygen t.
    periodontal t.
    photodynamic t. (PDT)
    photoradiation t.
    physical t.
    play t.
    precision t.
    programmed t.
    pulp canal t.
    radiation t.
    root canal t.
    Schuknecht ablation streptomycin t.

T

NOTES

therapy *(continued)*
    stereotactic radiation t.
    symptomatic t.
    titration streptomycin t.
    tongue thrust t.
    tumoricidal radiation t.
    vascular lesion t.
    voice t.
    x-ray t. (XRT)
Thermafil
    T. plastic carrier
    T. Plus obturator
thermal
    t. burn
    t. coefficient expansion
    t. conductivity
    t. dimensional change
    t. expansion technique
    t. imaging
    t. injury
    t. irritation
    t. noise
    t. pulp vitality test
    t. stimulation
Thermazene
thermesthesiometer
thermocatalytic technique
thermocouple
    Chromel-Alumel t.
Thermodent
thermography
    recovery-enhanced t.
thermokinetic selectivity (TKS)
thermoluminescence
thermoluminescent dosimetry
thermometer
    Tempa-DOT single-use clinical t.
thermo-photocatalytic
    t.-p. bleaching
    t.-p. technique
thermoplast
thermoplastic
    t. gutta-percha
    t. impression material
    t. polymer
    t. splint
Thermoprep heating oven
thermoset
theta
    t. rhythm
    t. wave
thick
    t. description
    t. skin
thickened bone
thickness
    Breslow t.
    dentin t.

    half-value t.
    soft tissue t.
thick-walled Dacron-backed implant
Thiebierge-Weissenbach syndrome
Thielemann principle
Thiersch
    T. graft operation
    T. method
    T. skin graft
thigh lift
thimble crown
thimerosal
thin filament
thinking
thin-shaft nasal scissors
thiobarbiturate
thiocyanate ion
thioglycolate
6-thioguanine
Thiokol rubber impression
thiomalate
    gold sodium t.
thiourea
third
    t. branchial anomaly
    t. cranial nerve
    t. dentition
    gingival t.
    t. molar
    t. octave filter
    t. order bend
    t. projection of Chausse
thistle
    milk t.
    Russian t.
thixotropic
    t. fluoride gel
Thomas post extractor
Thom facing
Thompson
    T. dowel
    T. line
thoraces (*pl. of* thorax)
thoracic
    t. duct
    t. nerve
    t. respiration
thoracoacromial
    t. artery
    t. flap
thoracodorsal
    t. artery
    t. fascia flap
    t. nerve
thoracoplasty
thoracopneumoplasty
thorax, pl. **thoraces**
Thorazine

Thornwaldt (*var. of* Tornwaldt)
THORP
    titanium hollow osseointegrating
      reconstruction plate
      THORP system
THORP-type mandibular reconstruction
  plate
thread
    A-Lastic t.
    elastic t.
    t. mate system (TMS)
    t. mate system pin
threaded post
ThreadLoc
    T. driver mount screw
    T. implant
    T. non-cast-to abutment
    T. retaining screw
three-armed stellate incision
three-buttress defect
three-day measles
three-dimensional (3D)
    t.-d. biocompatible scaffolding
    t.-d. computed tomography (3D CT)
    t.-d. plating system
    t.-d. record
    t.-d. ultrasound (3D US)
three-paddle tensor fasciae latae free
  flap
three-point fixation
three-quarter crown
three-sitting treatment
three-unit bridge
three-wall orbital decompression
threshold
    absolute t.
    acoustic reflex t.
    air t.
    audibility t.
    t. audiometry
    auditory t.
    bone t.
    bone conduction t.
    detectability t.
    detection t.
    differential t.
    t. of discomfort (TD)
    t. dose
    equivalent speech reception t.
    false t.
    feeling t.
    t. force

    fusion-inferred t. (FIT)
    t. hearing level
    intelligibility t.
    t. kneepoint potentiometer
    noise detection t. (NDT)
    pain t.
    pressure t.
    pressure pain t. (PPT)
    pure-tone t. (PTT)
    pure tone air-conduction t.
    pure tone bone-conduction t.
    t. shift
    t. shift method
    speech awareness t. (SAT)
    speech detectability t. (SDT)
    speech detection t. (SDT)
    speech discrimination t.
    speech reception t. (SRT)
    swallowing t.
    tickle t.
    vibrotactile t.
thrill
throat
    ears, nose, and t. (ENT)
    eye, ear, nose, and t. (EENT)
    frog in the t.
    sore t.
    Sucrets Sore T.
    Vicks Chloraseptic Sore T.
thrombin
    t. solution
    t. topical
Thrombinar
thromboangiitis obliterans
thrombocytopenia
Thrombogen
thrombophlebitis
    lateral sinus t. (LST)
    sinus t.
thrombosed renal dialysis fistula
thrombosis
    cavernous sinus t.
    coronary t.
    inferior dental vessel t.
    lateral sinus t.
    microvascular t.
    sinus t.
Thrombostat
thromboxane
through-and-through
    t.-a.-t. buttonhole fashion excision

T

NOTES

through-and-through *(continued)*
    t.-a.-t. defect
    t.-a.-t. drainage
    t.-a.-t. reabsorbable suture
thrush
thrust
    tongue t.
thrusting
    tongue t.
thumb
    biphalangeal t.
    Blauth type II hypoplastic t.
    cerebral t.
    t. forceps
    t. polydactyly
    rodeo t.
    t. ruler
    t. sign
    triphalangeal t.
thumb-sucking appliance
thyme
thymicolymphaticus
    status t.
thymidine
thymol iodide
thymoma
thymus
    cervical t.
Thymus vulgaris
thyration indicator
thyroarytenoid muscle
thyrocervical trunk
thyroepiglottic
    t. ligament
    t. muscle
thyrofissure
thyroglobulin (Tgb)
    t. antibody
thyroglossal
    t. duct
    t. duct cyst
    t. fistula
    t. tract cyst
thyrohyoid
    t. fold
    t. ligament
    t. membrane
    t. muscle
thyroid
    t. adenoma
    t. ala
    t. artery
    t. bed
    t. carcinoma
    t. cartilage
    t. C cell
    t. collar
    t. exposure guideline

    t. gland
    t. hormone
    t. ima artery
    t. ima vein
    lingual t.
    t. lobectomy
    t. malignoma
    t. nodule
    t. notch
    t. plexus
    t. shield
    t. storm
    t. suppression test
    t. tissue
thyroidectomy
    completion t.
    provocative food t.
    subtotal t.
    total t.
thyroiditis
    de Quervain granulomatous t.
thyroidotomy
thyroid-stimulating hormone (TSH)
thyroplasty
    Isshiki t.
    Isshiki t. type I
thyrotomy
thyrotoxic myopathy
thyrotoxicosis
    juvenile t.
thyrotropin
    t. stimulation test
thyrotropin-releasing hormone (TRH)
thyroxine
thyroxine-binding globulin (TBG)
Ti
    T. alloy screw
TIA
    transient ischemic attack
tibialis
    t. anterior muscle
    t. posterior muscle
tibial rotationplasty
tic
    t. douloureux
    facial t.
    glossopharyngeal t.
Ticar
ticarcillin
    t. and clavulanate potassium
Tice strain
tickle threshold
Ticonium
    T. 44, 50, 100 alloy
    T. dental casting gold alloy
    T. denture
    T. hidden-lock denture

T. 44, 50, 100 nickel-chromium base metal crown and bridge

tidal
t. air
t. volume (TV, V_T)

tie
cable t.
circumferential suture t.
elastometric t.
Kobayashi t.

tie-back loop archwire
tie-over
t.-o. bolster
t.-o. dressing

tightening
eyelid t.
t. wrench

tight-to-shaft (TTS)
t.-t.-s. Aire-Cuf tracheostomy tube

tile
K-type t.

tilt responder
tiludronate
timbre
time
cold ischemic t.
T. Compressed Speech Test
developing t.
t. domain signal processor (TDSP)
echo t.
exposure t.
fixing t.
t. out (TO)
phonation t.
t. pressure
reaction t. (RT)
reflex t.
relaxation t.
resin hardening t.
response t.
reverberation t.
setting t.
short film exposure t.
voice onset t. (VOT)
voice termination t. (VTT)

Timecelles
Cebid T.
Histor-D T.
Sinufed T.

time/frequency domain
Timentin
time-of-flight imaging

timer
t. accuracy
exposure t.
interval t.
x-ray t.

TiMesh
T. burrhole cover
T. 1.0/1.5/2.2 combination system
T. cranial mesh
T. craniomaxillofacial plating system
T. mandibular crib
T. 2.2-mm craniofacial system
T. 1.0-mm Micro System
T. 1.5-mm midface and cranial system
T. orbital mesh
T. orthognathic strap plate
T. patient configured titanium craniomaxillofacial implant
T. rigid fixation bone plating system
T. titanium mesh

timetable
endodontic t.

Timeter pocket spirometer
timolol
Timoptic
T. Ophthalmic
T.-XE Ophthalmic

timothy
t. grass
t. grass antigen

TIN
tone in noise

tin
t. ear
t. foil
t. oxide (SnO_2)

Tinactin
T. for Jock Itch

tincture
Fungoid T.
opium t.

tine
Tinel sign
tinfoil
Ting
Tinius Olsen stiffness tester
tinnitus
t. aurium
t. cerebri

T

NOTES

tinnitus *(continued)*
    clicking t.
    explosive t.
    Leudet t.
    t. masker
    pulsatile t.
    t. suppression
    transitory t.
tinted denture base
tioconazole
tip
    accelerator t.
    Batt t.
    Becker flat dissector t.
    Becker round dissector t.
    Becker twist dissector t.
    t. bossing
    buccal fat extractor t.
    buccal tooth t.
    bulbous nasal t.
    cannula t.
    chisel t.
    Cobra + t.
    Cobra K t.
    Cobra K+ t.
    Colorado electrocautery t.
    coned heparin t.
    CUSA laparoscopic t.
    custom t.
    disposable cannula t.
    eel cobra t.
    exit t.
    fiberoptic t.
    flap t.
    Flexoreamer Batt t.
    Fournier t.
    Gasparotti bevel t.
    Hetter pyramid t.
    2-hole standard t.
    3-hole standard t.
    Illouz modified t.
    Illouz standard t.
    Implantech SE-100 smoke
     aspiration t.
    interdental t.
    Keel t.
    K-Flexofile Batt t.
    Klein cannula t.
    Klein 1-hole infiltrator t.
    Klein multihole infiltrator t.
    Leon cobra t.
    mastoid t.
    Mercedes t.
    modified submental retractor,
     flared t.
    nasal t.
    Omni laser t.
    overprojecting nasal t.

    petrous t.
    Pinto dissector t.
    2-port radial t.
    3-port radial t.
    t. projection
    pyramid Toomey t.
    retroprep t.
    t. rhinoplasty
    Roane bullet t.
    root t.
    Rosenberg dissector t.
    rubber t.
    spatula t.
    suction t.
    Surgi-Fine reusable cannula t.
    synthetic sapphire t.
    Texas t.
    Texas Goodstein sharp t.
    Toledo flap dissector t.
    Toledo standard dissector t.
    Toledo V dissector t.
    Trevisani t.
    TriEye t.
    triport t.
    TT t.
    tungsten t.
    Unitri t.
    uvula t.
    Yankauer tonsil suction t.
tip-lifting procedure
tip-off
tip-of-the-tongue phenomenon
tipped tooth
tipping
    t. of cusp
    t. movement
    t. movement of tooth
tip-plasty
    nasal t.-p.
Ti-Screen
TI-SILC Moist sunscreen
Tisseel
    T. biologic fibrogen adhesive
    T. fibrin glue
tissue
    abdominal adipose t.
    aberrant breast t.
    t. ablation
    accessory mammary t.
    adipose t.
    angiomatous neoplastic t.
    Antoni A, B t.
    t. architecture
    areolar t.
    autogenous composite t.
    axillary breast t.
    border t.
    brown adipose t.

cavernous t.
cementoid t.
cervical soft t.
collagenous t.
t. compression
t. conditioner
connective t.
coronal pulp t.
denuded t.
dermoadipose t.
t. displaceability
earlobe adipose t.
endoscopically harvested t.
t. engineering
t. expander
t. expander template
t. expansion
extracapsular t.
fibrofatty t.
fibromxyomatous connective t.
fibrous t.
t. forceps
gingival t.
t. glue
granulation t.
granulomatous t.
hard t.
hard and soft t.
t. hyperplasia
hyperplastic t.
incorporated t.
t. injury factor
interdental t.
interstitial t.
keratinized t.
t. macrophage
mineralized t.
t. molding
nasion soft t.
necrotic hyalinized t.
non-weight-bearing t.
oral t.
orbit, mandible, ear, cranial nerves, and soft t. (OMENS)
orbitonasal t.
paraoral t.
paratransplantal t.
periapical t.
perichondrial-periosteal t.
periimplant t.
peripheral lymphoid t.

peritendinous soft t.
periungual t.
phantom t.
radionecrotic t.
redundant t.
t. registration
t. scissors
t. sizer template
SMAS t.
soft t.
t. space
subcutaneous t.
subdermal nasal t.
subjacent t.
supporting t.
target t.
thyroid t.
t. tolerance
t. transglutaminase
t. trimming
weight-bearing t.
tissue-base relationship
tissue-bearing area
tissue-borne
　　t.-b. macrophage
　　t.-b. partial denture
tissue-engineered construct
tissue-equivalent material
tissue-expansion technique
tissue-spreading forceps
tissue-supported base
tissue-tissue-supported base
tissue-trimming
titanium
　　t. AO plate
　　commercially pure t.
　　CP t.
　　t. fixation device
　　t. hollow osseointegrating reconstruction plate (THORP)
　　t. mandibular staple
　　t. mesh tray
　　t. miniplate
　　t. plasma spray (TPS)
　　t. plasma sprayed (TPS)
　　t. plasma sprayed dental implant
　　t. rigid fixation
　　t. tack
titanium-sprayed IMZ implant
Titan slow-speed handpiece
titration streptomycin therapy

NOTES

TKS
    thermokinetic selectivity
        TKS laser
TL
    taper-lock
TLC
    Test of Language Competence
    total lung capacity
TLC-C
    Test of Language Competence for
    Children
TLP
    total laryngopharyngectomy
TLS surgical drain
TMAF
    temporary master apical file
TMB
    tetramethylbenzidine
TMD
    temporomandibular disorder
    temporomandibular joint dysfunction
TMH
    trainable mentally handicapped
TMI
    transmandibular implant
        TMI implant
TMJ
    temporomandibular joint
    temporomandibular joint dysfunction
        TMJ ankylosis
        lateral condylar pole of the TMJ
        TMJ syndrome
TMJ-OA
    temporomandibular joint osteoarthritis
TMJ-SF
    temporomandibular joint synovial fluid
TMPD
    temporomandibular pain dysfunction
        TMPD disorder
TMP-SMX
    trimethoprim and sulfamethoxazole
TMS
    thread mate system
T-Naf
TNF
    tumor necrosis factor
        TNF-α
            tumor necrosis factor-α
TNM tumor staging
TO
    time out
toaster oven
tobacco
    t. abrasion
    smokeless t.
    wild t.
Tobey-Ayer test
TobraDex Ophthalmic

tobramycin
    t. and dexamethasone
Tobrex Ophthalmic
Todd-Evans stepladder tracheal
    dilatation technique
toddler language delay
toe fillet flap procedure
toe-to-hand transfer
toe-to-thumb
    t.-t.-t. microvascular transplant
    t.-t.-t. transfer
Tofflemire amalgam matrix retainer
toilet
    cavity t.
    t. of cavity
token
    t. test
    T. Test for Children
    T. Test for Receptive Disturbances
    in Aphasia
Tokyo strain
TOLD-I
    Test of Language Development-
    Intermediate
TOLD-P
    Test of Language Development-Primary
Tolectin
    T. DS
Toledo
    T. dissector
    T. flap dissector tip
    T. roller
    T. standard dissector tip
    T. V-dissector cannula
    T. V dissector tip
tolerance
    acoustic t.
    frustration t.
    t. level
    t. range
    t. threshold for speech
    tissue t.
    vibration t.
tolmetin
tolnaftate
toluidine
    t. blue
    t. blue stain
tomato
Tomes
    T. fiber
    T. granular layer
    T. process of ameloblast
tomodensitometry
tomographer
    Siemens Somatom Plus S
    computed t.

tomography
    computed t. (CT)
    computed axial t. (CAT)
    computerized axial t. (CAT)
    curved layer t.
    dynamic computed t.
    high-resolution computed t. (HRCT)
    Ortho Trans Linear t.
    pluridirectional t.
    three-dimensional computed t. (3D
        CT)
tonal spectrum
TONAR
    the oronasal acoustic ratio
tone
    Ambi Skin T.
    cheek t.
    t. color
    complex t.
    t. control
    t. deafness
    t. decay
    t. decay test
    difference t.
    t. focus
    fundamental t.
    glottal t.
    modal t.
    t. in noise (TIN)
    Ora T.
    partial t.
    pure t.
    simple t.
    warble t.
toner
    color t.
tongue
    amyloid t.
    antibiotic t.
    bald t.
    base of t. (BOT)
    beefy t.
    beet t.
    bifid t.
    t. biting
    black t.
    black hairy t.
    t. blade
    blade of t.
    body of t.
    burning t.
    cardinal t.

cerebriform t.
cleft t.
coated t.
cobblestone t.
corolliform papillae of t.
crenation of t.
t. crib
crocodile t.
t. depressor
dotted t.
enamel t.
extrinsic muscle of t.
fissured t.
t. flap
flat t.
fluted t.
foramen cecum of t.
t. forceps
forked t.
frenulum of t.
frenum of t.
furred t.
furrowed t.
geographic t.
gland of t.
grooved t.
hairy t.
t. height
hemiatrophy of the t.
hemihypertrophy of the t.
hobnail t.
inferior longitudinal muscle of t.
inferior surface of t.
intrinsic muscle of t.
lobulated t.
long t.
longitudinal muscle of t.
longitudinal raphe of t.
lymphatic follicles of t.
lymphatic vessels of t.
magenta t.
mappy t.
margin of t.
motor nerve of t.
mucoepidermoid carcinoma of
    the t.
mucous membrane of t.
opium smoker's t.
papillae of t.
parrot t.
plicated t.
t. plication

T

NOTES

tongue *(continued)*
    t. press
    t. pressure
    t. retractor
    root of t.
    t. root
    Sandwith bald t.
    scrotal t.
    septum of t.
    slick t.
    smoker's t.
    smooth t.
    stippled t.
    strawberry t.
    sulcated t.
    superior longitudinal muscle of t.
    terminal sulcus of t.
    t. thrust
    t. thrust classification
    t. thrusting
    t. thrust therapy
    t. traction
    transverse muscle of t.
    trombone tremor of t.
    undersurface of t.
    varnished t.
    vertical muscle of t.
    villous papillae of t.
    white hairy t.
    wrinkled t.
tongue-jaw-neck dissection
tongue-retaining device (TRD)
tongue-swallowing
tongue-thrust appliance
tongue-tie
TONI
    Test of Nonverbal Intelligence
tonic
    t. bite
    t. block
    t. vibration reflex (TVR)
tonofibril
tonofilament
tonometer
    Schiotz t.
tonometry
    applanation t.
tonophant
tonotopic
tonsil
    faucial t.
    t. forceps
    Gerlach t.
    t. guillotine
    kissing t.'s
    lingual t.
    Luschka t.
    palatine t.

    pharyngeal t.
    t. pole
    t. position
    submerged t.
    tubal t.
tonsillar
    t. artery
    t. calculus
    t. carcinoma
    t. fossa
    t. pillar
tonsillaris
    sinus t.
tonsillar-subdigastric node
tonsillectomy (TE)
    t. and adenoidectomy (T&A)
    bipolar cautery dissection t.
    outpatient suction cautery t.
    quinsy t.
    Sluder guillotine t.
    t. with operating microscope
        (TE$_{mic}$)
tonsillith, tonsillolith
tonsillitis
    chronic fibrotic t.
    follicular t.
    hyperplastic t.
    hypertrophic t.
    lacunar t.
    ulcerative t.
    Vincent t.
tonsillolingual sulcus
tonsillolith *(var. of* tonsillith*)*
tonsillopathy
tonsillotome
tonsillotomy
tonus
    muscle t.
Toomey
    T. angled cannula
    T. G-bevel cannula
    T. standard cannula
    T. tip style
    T. tip system
tooth, pl. teeth
    t. abrasion
    absent t.
    abutment t.
    accessional teeth
    accessory t.
    acrylic resin t.
    t. adnexa
    aged t.
    t. alignment
    amputated t.
    anatomic teeth
    anchor t.
    t. angle

ankylosed t.
ankylosis of t.
anterior teeth
anterior flared t.
anterior surface of premolar and
  molar teeth
t. arch symmetry
t. arrangement
artificial t.
t. attachment fiber
auditory teeth
avulsed t.
t. avulsion
t. of axis
baby t.
back teeth
t. banding
barred t.
bicuspid t.
biscuspidized t.
blue t.
bodily movement of t.
t. bonding
broken-down t.
t. brush
t. brushing
buccal teeth
buck t.
t. bud
canine t.
carious t.
carnassial t.
cavity of t.
t. cement
central incisor t.
cervical zone of t.
cheek t.
cheoplastic t.
Chiaie t.
chipped t.
cingulum of t.
t. conditioner
conical t.
connate t.
contact surface of t.
t. contour
t. coolant
corner t.
crossbite teeth
cross-pin t.
crowded t.
crowding of teeth

crown of t.
C-shaped t.
cuspid t.
cuspidate t.
cuspless t.
cutting t.
dead t.
t. decay
decayed, extracted, filled deciduous
  teeth (def)
decayed, extracted, filled permanent
  teeth (DEF)
decayed and filled teeth
decayed and filled deciduous teeth
  (df)
decayed and filled permanent teeth
  (DF)
decayed, missing, filled deciduous
  teeth (dmf)
decayed, missing, filled permanent
  teeth (DMF)
decayed, missing, filled surfaces
  deciduous teeth (dmfs)
decayed, missing, filled surfaces
  permanent teeth (DMFS)
deciduous t.
denture teeth
t. depression
devitalized t.
diatoric teeth
dilacerated t.
displaced t.
drifting t.
early t.
t. elevator
t. elongation
embedded t.
endosseous dental implant
  placement for replacement of
  missing teeth
t. eruption
etched t.
evulsed t.
t. evulsion
exaggerated feminine t.
exaggerated masculine t.
extracted t.
t. extraction
extruded teeth
extrusion of a t.
eye t.
first teeth

T

NOTES

tooth *(continued)*
first deciduous molar t.
first premolar t.
floating t.
fluoridated teeth
t. form
Fournier teeth
t. fracture
fractured t.
fulcrum of t.
fulcrum t.
fused teeth
geminated teeth
t. germ
ghost t.
golden t.
Goslee t.
green t.
grinding t.
hag teeth
hair t.
t. hemisection
hereditary brown opalescent teeth
hereditary dark teeth
hereditary opalescent teeth
t. hood
Horner teeth
hot t.
Huschke auditory teeth
Hutchinson teeth
hypersensitive t.
t. hypersensitivity
hypoplasia of t.
t. immobilization
impacted t.
incisive t.
incisor t.
inclination of t.
inferior teeth
intruded t.
irreplaceable t.
kinked t.
labial teeth
late t.
lateral incisor t.
t. ligation
teeth ligation
lingual surface of t.
long t.
lower teeth
malacotic teeth
malaligned t.
malformed t.
teeth malocclusion
malposed t.
teeth malposition
malpositioned t.
mandibular teeth

maxillary teeth
maxillary anterior t.
maxillary posterior t.
t. measurement
metal insert t.
migrated t.
migrating teeth
migration of t.
t. migration
milk teeth
missing t.
mobile t.
t. mobility
mobility of t.
molar t.
molar teeth
Moon teeth
t. morphology
morsal teeth
mottled teeth
t. movement
t. movement appliance
t. and mucosa-borne denture
mulberry t.
multicanaled t.
multicuspid t.
multirooted t.
narrow t.
natal teeth
neck of t.
neonatal teeth
nonanatomic teeth
nonrestorable t.
nonstrategic t.
nonvital t.
normally posed t.
notched teeth
oral teeth
overinstrumented t.
t. paste
peg t.
pegged t.
peg-shaped t.
t. perforation
permanent teeth
perpetually growing t.
persistently growing t.
t. pick
pink t. of Mummery
pinless teeth
t. plane
plastic teeth
t. polyp
t. position
t. positioner
t. positioning
posterior teeth
postpermanent teeth

predeciduous teeth
premature teeth
premilk teeth
premolar t.
primary teeth
t. primordium
protruded t.
protruding teeth
t. pulp
pulpless t.
rake teeth
ratio of decayed and filled teeth
  (RDFT)
replaced t.
t. resorption
retention area of t.
root of t.
rootless teeth
rotated t.
t. sac
sclerotic teeth
screwdriver teeth
second t.
sensitive t.
sensitivity of t.
t. separation
separation of teeth
set of teeth
shell t.
short t.
sickle t.
single t.
single-rooted t.
t. size analysis
t. size discrepancy
skin of teeth
small t.
snaggle t.
snow-capped teeth
t. socket
socket joint of t.
spaced teeth
split t.
Steele t.
Steele interchangeable t.
stomach t.
straight-pin teeth
strategic t.
t. stripping
submerged t.
succedaneous teeth
successional teeth

superior teeth
supernumerary t.
superstructure t.
supplemental t.
supplied t.
t. support
supportive mechanisms of teeth
surgical neck of t.
syphilitic teeth
temporary t.
temporary teeth
tipped t.
tipping movement of t.
tooth within a t.
t. torsion
torsion of a t.
t. transplantation
t. trauma
treated t.
tricanaled t.
tricuspid t.
trirooted t.
tube teeth
t. tube
tubercle of crown of t.
Turner t.
twin teeth
typodont teeth
unerupted t.
upper teeth
upper single t. (UST)
vestibular surface of t.
vital t.
vital staining of teeth
wandering t.
t. wasting
t. wear
wide t.
wisdom t.
wolf t.
zero-degree teeth
toothache
tooth-and-nail syndrome
tooth-borne
  t.-b. base
  t.-b. denture
  t.-b. partial denture
tooth-borne/tissue-borne partial denture
toothbrush
  Bass t.
  electric t.
  interproximal t.

T

NOTES

toothbrush *(continued)*
    Oral-B t.
    powered t.
    t. trauma
    Wisdom t.
toothbrushing, tooth brushing
    Bass method of t.
    Charters method of t.
    crevicular method of t.
    Fones method of t.
    maxillofacial and facioproximal
      surface t.
    maxillopalatal and palatoproximal
      surface t.
    occlusal surface t.
    physiologic method of t.
    scrub-brush technique of t.
    Stillman method of t.
Toothkeeper
tooth-moving force
toothpaste
    retarDent t.
toothpick
toothpowder
tooth-to-tooth position
TOP
    total ossicular prosthesis
topagnostic test
Topazian classification scheme
toper's nose
tophus, pl. tophi
    dental t.
topical
    Achromycin T.
    Aclovate T.
    Actinex T.
    Akne-Mycin T.
    amphotericin B t.
    t. anesthesia
    t. application
    Aquacare T.
    A/T/S T.
    Baciguent T.
    BactoShield T.
    Baker P&S T.
    Carmol T.
    Carmol-HC T.
    Cloderm T.
    Cyclocort T.
    t. decongestant
    Del-Mycin T.
    DesOwen T.
    Dyna-Hex T.
    Elase T.
    Elase-Chloromycetin T.
    Elocon T.
    Emgel T.
    Eryderm T.

    Erygel T.
    Erymax T.
    erythromycin, t.
    E-Solve-2 T.
    ETS-2% T.
    Exelderm T.
    Furacin T.
    Garamycin T.
    Gelfoam T.
    G-myticin T.
    Hibiclens T.
    Hibistat T.
    Lanaphilic T.
    Lida-Mantle HC T.
    MetroGel T.
    Micatin T.
    Monistat-Derm T.
    Mycifradin Sulfate T.
    Mycitracin T.
    Mycogen II T.
    Mycolog-II T.
    Myconel T.
    Mytrex F T.
    NeoDecadron T.
    Neomixin T.
    N.G.T. T.
    Nutraplus T.
    t. otic preparation
    Oxistat T.
    Polysporin T.
    Staticin T.
    Sulfamylon T.
    terbinafine, t.
    thrombin t.
    Tridesilon T.
    Tri-Statin II T.
    Ultra Mide T.
    Ureacin T.
    Vytone T.
Topicale liquid
Topicort
    T.-LP
topic shift
TopiFoam gel-backed self-adhering foam pad
topographic projection
topography
    gingival t.
Toradol
    T. Injection
    T. Oral
Toraloy dental amalgam
torch
tori *(pl. of* torus)
Tornwaldt, Thornwaldt
    T. abscess
    T. bursa
    T. cyst

T. disease
T. syndrome
Toronto
T. Tests of Receptive Vocabulary, English/Spanish
T. two-stage mammaplasty
T. wide rectus plication
torque
t. arch
edgewise t.
labial t.
light wire t.
t. ratchet wrench
t. wire
t. wrench
torqued slot bracket
torque-twist rate
torquing
t. auxiliary
Begg t.
t. key
t. spring
torsion
clasp t.
neck t.
penile t.
t. of a tooth
tooth t.
torsional
t. loading
t. rigidity
t. wave
torsion-chair test
torsive
t. occlusion
t. stress
torsiversion
torsoclusion
torticollis
congenital t.
labyrinthine t.
muscular t.
ocular t.
Torulopsis
torus, pl. **tori**
mandibular t.
t. mandibularis
palatine t.
t. palatinus
t. tubarius
Totacillin
T.-N

total
t. alloplastic TMJ reconstruction prosthesis
t. autogenous latissimus (TAL)
t. autogenous latissimus breast reconstruction
t. biopsy
t. body surface area (TBSA)
t. cleft palate
t. communication
t. ear obliteration
t. etch technique
t. ethmoidectomy
t. glossectomy
t. ipsilateral lobectomy
t. laryngectomy
t. laryngopharyngectomy (TLP)
t. lung capacity (TLC)
t. midface osteotomy
t. ossicular prosthesis (TOP)
t. ossicular replacement prosthesis
t. parotidectomy
t. pelvic exenteration
t. pulpitis
t. pulp loss
t. pulpotomy
t. rhinectomy
t. space analysis
t. thyroidectomy
t. unilateral vestibular deafferentation
t. upper lip resection
total-body compression suit
Toti operation
Touch
touch-up
t.-u. procedure
toughness
Tourette syndrome
tourniquet
t. band
pneumatic t.
scrotal t.
Touro LA
Tourtual canal
towelette
Towne
T. projection
T. projection radiograph
T. projection roentgenogram
toxic
t. deafness

NOTES

toxic *(continued)*
    t. shock syndrome
    t. waste
toxicity
toxin
    botulinum t.
    botulinum t. type A
    lyophilized botulinum t. A
Toxoplasma
    T. gondii
toxoplasma lymphadenitis
toxoplasmosis
Toynbee tube
TPB
    transpalatal bar
T-Perio
TPFF
    temporoparietal fascial flap
TPI
    Treatment Priority Index
TPS
    titanium plasma spray
    titanium plasma sprayed
        TPS dental implant
TPS-coated
    T.-c. cylinder
    T.-c. screw
TPWM
    tympanoplasty with mastoidectomy
TPWOM
    tympanoplasty without mastoidectomy
trabecula, pl. trabeculae
    bone t.
trabecular bone
trabeculation
    arachnoid t.
tracer
    arrow-point t.
    Gothic arch t.
    needle-point t.
TrachCare
    Neonatal Y T.
trachea, pl. tracheae
    scabbard t.
tracheal
    t. adenoma
    t. agenesis
    t. atresia
    t. chondroma
    t. compression
    t. diverticulum
    t. fenestration
    t. fistula
    t. osteochondroma
    t. papilloma
    t. reconstruction
    t. stenosis
    t. tube

    t. tug
    t. ulcer
    t. ulceration
    t. web
    t. window resection
trachealgia
trachealis muscle
tracheitis, trachitis
trachelocele
trachelodynia
tracheloplasty
tracheoaerocele
tracheobronchial
    t. foreign body
    t. tree
tracheobronchitis
    necrotizing t. (NTB)
tracheobronchomalacia
tracheobronchopathia osteoplastica
tracheobronchoscopy
tracheocele
tracheocutaneous fistula
tracheoesophageal
    t. cleft
    t. fistula (TEF)
    t. prosthesis (TEP)
    t. puncture (TEP)
    t. puncture dilator
    t. septum
    t. shunt
    t. speech
tracheomalacia
tracheomegaly
tracheopathia
    t. chondro-osteoplastica
    t. osteoplastica
tracheopharyngeal shunt
tracheophony
tracheoplasty
    pericardial patch t.
tracheorrhagia
tracheoschisis
tracheoscope
tracheoscopic
tracheoscopy
tracheostenosis
tracheostoma
    t. valve
tracheostomy
    Bjork flap t.
    percutaneous dilational t.
    t. tube
tracheotome
tracheotomy
    t. hook
    laryngofissure with t.
    percutaneous t.
    t. tube

trachitis (*var. of* tracheitis)
trachomatis
    Chlamydia t.
trachyphonia
tracing
    arrow-point t.
    Békésy Forward-Reverse T.
    cephalometric t.
    extraoral t.
    Gothic arch t.
    I t.
    interrupted t.
    intraoral t.
    needle-point t.
    panographic t.
    sea gull t.
    stylus t.
tracking
    speech t.
tract
    aerodigestive t.
    atretic outflow t.
    dead t.
    extrapyramidal t.
    iliotibial t.
    lateral spinothalamic t.
    nasal t.
    olfactory t.
    pyramidal t.
    respiratory t.
    scarred deep sinus t.
    sinonasal t.
    sinus t.
    upper aerodigestive t.
    upper respiratory t.
    vocal t.
traction
    t. diverticulum
    elastic t.
    external t.
    t. headache
    intermaxillary t.
    internal t.
    maxillomandibular t.
    t. suture
    tongue t.
traditional
    t. analysis
    t. grammar
    t. lipoplasty
tragacanth

tragal
    t. border
    t. cartilage
    t. notch
    t. pointer
tragi (*pl. of* tragus)
tragion
tragophonia
tragus, pl. **tragi**
    distorted t.
trainable mentally handicapped (TMH)
trainer
    computer-aided fluency
      establishment t. (CAFET)
    desk-type auditory t.
    frequency modulation auditory t.
    hard-wire auditory t.
    Look and Say Articulation T.
training
    auditory t.
    discrimination t.
    ear t.
    Language Sampling, Analysis,
      and T.
    visual t.
TRAKE-fit system
TRAM
    transverse rectus abdominis muscle
    transverse rectus abdominis
      musculocutaneous
    transverse rectus abdominis
      myocutaneous
      distraction TRAM
      TRAM flap
tramadol
TRAMP
    transverse rectus abdominis
      musculoperitoneal
    transversus and rectus abdominis
      musculoperitoneal
      TRAMP flap
tranexamic acid
Tranquility Quest continuous positive airway pressure
tranquilizer
transantral
    t. approach
    t. ethmoidectomy
    t. orbital decompression
transareolar
    t. mastectomy
    t. mastocele

T

NOTES

transarterial embolization
transaudient
transaxillary
    t. breast augmentation
transblepharoplasty
    t. approach
    t. forehead lift
    t. procedure
    t. subperiosteal midface elevation
transbuccal trocar
transcalvarial suture fixation
transcanine approach
transcartilaginous incision
transcatheter
    t. embolization of AVF
    t. embolization of AVM
transcervical approach
transcochlear
    t. approach
    t. cochleovestibular neurectomy
    t. vestibular neurectomy
transcolumella
transconjunctival
    t. approach
    t. blepharoplasty (TCB)
    t. blepharoplasty/trichloroacetic acid
      combination (TCB/TCA)
    t. endoscopic orbital decompression
    t. lower lid blepharoplasty
    t. retractor
transcortical sensory aphasia
transcranial
    t. facial bipartition
    t. monobloc frontofacial
      advancement
    t. radiograph
    t. roentgenogram
    t. temporomandibular joint
      radiograph
transcription
    broad t.
    close t.
    narrow t.
    phonemic t.
    phonetic t.
transcutaneous
Transderm
    T. Scop
    T. Scop Patch
transdermal
    Duragesic T.
    scopolamine t.
transducer
    bite force t.
    7.5 MHz linear array B-mode
      ultrasound t.
transducing

transduction
    t. theory
transection
transendoscopic procedure
transepiglottic laryngotomy
transesophageal
    t. puncture (TEP)
    t. varix ligation
transfemoral balloon occlusion
transfer
    buried free forearm flap t.
    t. coping
    dermal fat free tissue t.
    fascia lata t.
    t. fork
    free colon t.
    free muscle t.
    free tissue t.
    hypoglossal-to-facial nerve t.
    ilium microvascular t.
    impedance t.
    intermodal t.
    intersensory t.
    island frontalis muscle t.
    linear energy t. (LET)
    masseter muscle t.
    microvascular bone t.
    microvascular free flap t.
    microvascular free tissue t.
    muscle t.
    nerve t.
    pedicled colon t.
    regional muscle t.
    scapular flap t.
    staged muscle t.
    temporalis muscle-fascia t.
    tendon t.
    toe-to-hand t.
    toe-to-thumb t.
transference
transferred
    t. meaning
    t. mesenteric vascular pedicle
transferring enzyme
transfixation incision
transformation
    malignant t.
transformational
    t. generative grammar
    t. grammar
transformer
transforming
    t. growth factor-β (TGF-β)
    t. growth factor beta (TGF-β)
transglottic squamous cell carcinoma
transglutaminase
    tissue t.
transhyoid pharyngotomy

transient
    t. bacteremia
    t. blindness
    t. distortion
    t. evoked otoacoustic emission
      (TEOAE)
    t. ischemic attack (TIA)
    rest t.
    t. vibration
transillumination
transistor
transition
    normal t.
    t. state
transitional
    t. cell carcinoma
    t. dentition
    t. denture
    t. papilloma
    t. pulp
    t. pulp stage
    t. pulp state
    t. stuttering
transitive verb type
transitory tinnitus
transit-time flowmeter
transjunctival lipectomy
translabial access
translabyrinthine
    t. approach
translation
    condylar t.
    pure t.
translatory movement
translocation
    facial t.
    preeruptive t.
translucency
    coronal t.
transmandibular
    t. approach
    t. implant (TMI)
    t. reconstruction
transmastoid approach
transmaxillary approach
transmeatal
    t. approach
    t. tympanoplasty incision
transmission
    t. cell
    cross-talk t.
    t. electron micrograph

    t. electron microscope (TEM)
    t. electron microscopy (TEM)
    ephaptic t.
    hepatitis B t.
    HIV t.
    nonpercutaneous dental t.
    percutaneous t.
    vertical t.
    virus t.
transmitter
transmutation
transnasal
    t. ligation of internal maxillary
      artery
Transonic
    T. flowmeter
    T. laser Doppler perfusion monitor
transoral
    t. catheter
    t. coronoidectomy
    t. open biopsy
    t. resection
transorbital projection
transosseous implant
transosteal
    t. implant
    t. implant jig
transpalatal
    t. approach
    t. bar (TPB)
transpalpebral
    t. approach
    t. corrugator muscle
transparency
    Broadbent-Bolton t.
transparent
    t. dentin
**transpharyngeal temporomandibular
joint radiograph**
transplant
    alloplastic t.
    bone marrow t. (BMT)
    laser hair t.
    renal t.
    syngeneic bone marrow t.
    toe-to-thumb microvascular t.
transplantation
    autogenous tooth t.
    bone marrow t.
    hair t.
    homogenous tooth t.
    laser hair t.

NOTES

T

transplantation *(continued)*
    tendon t.
    tooth t.
transport
    t. disk
    mucociliary t. (MCT)
transportation
    apical t.
transpose
transposed
    t. crevicular cuticle
    t. omentum
transposition
    bilateral advancement t. (BAT)
    bilateral gluteus maximus t.
    t. flap
    t. of graft
    muscle t.
    nonstimulated gracilis t.
    omental t.
    parotid duct t.
    penoscrotal t.
    temporalis muscle t.
    tripartite frontalis muscle flap t.
    triple advancement t. (TAT)
    ulnar nerve t.
    Z-plasty t.
transseptal
    t. approach
    t. fiber
    t. ligament
transsexual
    female-to-male t.
    male-to-female t.
    t. surgery
    t. voice
transsexualism
transsigmoid
transsphenoidal approach
transtentorial
transtrusion
transtympanic neurectomy
transubstantiation
transudate
    mucosal t.
    oral mucosal t.
transumbilical plane
Trans-Ver-Sal
    T.-V.-S. AdultPatch
    T.-V.-S. PediaPatch
    T.-V.-S. PlantarPatch
transversalis
    crista t.
    t. fascia
transverse
    t. arytenoid muscle
    t. carpal ligament (TCL)
    t. cervical artery
    t. cervical node
    t. cervical pedicle
    t. crest
    t. discrepancy
    t. electromagnetic mode (TEM)
    t. facial artery
    t. facial fracture
    t. facial vein
    t. groove of oblique ridge (TGOR)
    t. horizontal axis
    t. maxillary fracture
    t. mid abdominal incision
    t. muscle of tongue
    t. palatine ridge
    t. pedicled flap
    t. plane
    t. projection
    t. rectus abdominis muscle (TRAM)
    t. rectus abdominis muscle flap
    t. rectus abdominis musculocutaneous (TRAM)
    t. rectus abdominis musculoperitoneal (TRAMP)
    t. rectus abdominis myocutaneous (TRAM)
    t. rhytid
    t. ridge
    t. temporal gyri
    t. wave
transversion
transversus
    t. abdominis aponeurosis
    t. abdominis muscle
    t. linguae
    t. linguae muscle
    t. linguae musculus
    t. perinei profundus muscle
    t. and rectus abdominis musculoperitoneal (TRAMP)
    t. and rectus abdominis musculoperitoneal flap
    sulcus anthelicis t.
    t. thoracis muscle
TRAP
    tartrate-resistant acid phosphatase
trap
    collection t.
    extraction t.
    in-line t.
    Lukens t.
    osseous coagulum t.
trapezius
    t. flap
    t. muscle
trapezoid
    t. body
    t. incision

trapezoidal
  t. arch
  t. flap
Trasylol
trauma, pl. **traumata, traumas**
  auricular t.
  blast energy induced t.
  dental t.
  t. from occlusion
  iatrogenic t.
  t. induced saddle bag
  laryngotracheal t.
  midface t.
  occlusal t.
  occult t.
  oral t.
  perinatal t.
  potential t.
  tooth t.
  toothbrush t.
traumagram
  facial t.
traumatic
  t. alopecia
  t. bone cyst
  t. brain injury
  t. carotid-cavernous sinus fistula
  t. crescent
  t. cyst
  t. dentin
  t. discoloration
  t. eosinophilic granuloma
  t. exorbitism
  t. fibroma
  t. fracture
  t. granuloma
  t. incontinence
  t. injury
  t. laryngitis
  t. luxation
  t. neuroma
  t. occlusion
  t. osteoclasia
  t. peri-implantoclasia
  t. pseudolipoma
  t. tattoo
  t. ulatrophy
  t. ulcer
  t. ulcerative granuloma
traumatism
  periodontal t.

  primary occlusal t.
  secondary occlusal t.
traumatogenic
  t. occlusion
Trautmann
  T. angle
  T. triangle
traveling wave theory
tray
  acrylic resin t.
  annealing t.
  t. compound
  compound heater t.
  flap t.
  impaction t.
  impression t.
  orthodontic impression t.
  ProTech instrument protection t.
  stock impression t.
  titanium mesh t.
  vacuum-formed resin impression t.
TRD
  tongue-retaining device
Treacher
  T. Collins deformity
  T. Collins syndrome (TCS)
treated tooth
treatment
  Abdopatch Gel Z self-adhesive
    scar t.
  antiandrogen t.
  antioxidant eye t.
  Baxter method of burn t.
  Emdogain t.
  endodontic t.
  t. filling
  hardening heat t.
  heat t.
  homogenizing heat t.
  Mammopatch gel self-adhesive
    scar t.
  Marx protocol for ORN t.
  neurodevelopmental t. (NDT)
  Obagi Blue Peel skin peel t.
  oxygen recovery skin t.
  Pads Médipatch Gel Z self-
    adhesive scar t.
  t. partial denture
  postburn scar contracture t.
  post-op soothing skin t.
  Reach ACT fluoride anti-cavity t.
  ReJuveness scar t.

T

NOTES

treatment *(continued)*
    root canal t.
    somnoplasty tissue reduction t.
    three-sitting t.
    Tweed edgewise t.
    ultrasound t.
Treatment Priority Index (TPI)
tree
    t. diagram
    tracheobronchial t.
**Tree/Bee Test of Auditory
  Discrimination**
trehalose-Euro-Collins solution
Treitz ligament
Trélat sign
Trelles metal scleral shield
tremolo
tremor
    essential t.
    intentional t.
    t. linguae
    vocal t.
tremulousness
tremulous speech
trench
    t. gum
    t. mouth
trenching
Trendelenburg position
trepanation, trephination
    circular t.
    dental t.
trephine
    mini t.
Treponema
    T. buccale
    T. denticola
    T. microdentium
    T. mucosum
    T. pallidum
    T. vincentii
tretinoin
    t. emollient cream
Trevisani tip
TRH
    thyrotropin-releasing hormone
Triacet
Triacin-C
triad
    Bezold t.
    Hutchinson t.
    Kartagener t.
    Saint t.
    Samter t.
triage
trial
    t. base
    t. cementation

    t. denture
    t. lesson
    Multicenter Selective
      Lymphadenectomy t.
    t. point
Triam-A
triamcinolone
    t. acetonide
    t. acetonide nasal spray
    intralesional t.
    nystatin and t.
Triam Forte
Triaminic
    T. Allergy Tablet
    T. AM Decongestant Formula
    T. Cold Tablet
    T. Expectorant
    T. Oral Infant Drops
    T. Syrup
Triaminicol Multi-Symptom Cold Syrup
triangle
    Assézat t.
    Bolton t.
    Bonwill t.
    Burow t.
    digastric t.
    facial t.
    Kiesselbach t.
    Macewen t.
    retromandibular t.
    retromolar t.
    subclavian t.
    submandibular t.
    submaxillary t.
    submental t.
    suboccipital t.
    suprameatal t.
    Trautmann t.
    Tweed diagnostic t.
    Wilde t.
triangular
    t. blank file
    t. crest
    t. eminence
    t. fibrocartilage complex (TFCC)
    t. fold
    t. fossa
    t. muscle
    t. ridge
    t. skin flap
    t. space
    t. vestibular nucleus
    t. wave
triangularis
    crista t.
    eminentia t.
    fossa t.
    plica t.

triangulation
β-tricalcium
    β-t. phosphate-300
    β-t. phosphate-40
tricanaled tooth
trichiasis
trichilemmoma
Trichinella spiralis
trichinosis
trichion
Trichlor Fresh Pac
trichloroacetic
    t. acid (TCA)
    t. acid peel
trichloromonofluoromethane
    dichlorodifluoromethane and t.
trichodento-osseous syndrome
Trichoderma
trichoepithelioma
trichofolliculoma
trichoglossia
trichophytic
Trichophyton
trichrome
Tri-Clear Expectorant
triconodont
Tri-County Contextual Articulation Test
tricuspal
tricuspid
    t. tooth
tricuspidal
tricuspidate
trident
tridentate
Triderm
Tridesilon Topical
tridodecylmethylammonium chloride
    graft coating material (TDMAC)
tridymite
Trieger psychomotor function dot test
triethanolamine polypeptide oleate-
    condensate
triethiodide
    gallamine t.
TriEye
    T. cannula
    T. tip
trifacial neuralgia
Trifecta obturation technique
Trifed-C
triflupromazine
trifluridine

Trifolium pratense
trifurcation
    t. involvement
trigeminal
    t. artery
    t. hypesthesia
    t. impression of temporal bone
    t. nerve
    t. nerve artifact
    t. neuralgia
    t. notch
    t. nuclear complex
    t. paralysis
    t. trophic syndrome (TTS)
trigeminal-facial nerve reflex
trigeminal-vagal reflex
trigger
    t. point
    t. zone
trigone
    t. region
    retromolar t.
    submandibular t.
trigonid
trigonocephaly
triiodothyronine (T₃)
Tri-Kort
Trilisate
trill
trilobed
    t.-l. flap
    t.-l. skull
Trilog
Trilogy I hearing aid
Trilone
trim
    freeze t.
trimalar fracture
trimethoprim
    t. and polymyxin B
    t. and sulfamethoxazole (TMP-
    SMX)
    t. sulfamethoxazole
trimetrexate glucuronate
trimmer
    gingival margin t. (GMT)
    margin t.
    model t.
    plaster t.
    proximal t.
    wax t.

T

NOTES

trimming
    muscle t.
    tissue t.
Trimox
Trimpex
Trinalin
Tri-Nefrin Extra Strength Tablet
Triocut
Triofed Syrup
Triotann Tablet
tripartite frontalis muscle flap
  transposition
Tri-Pax
tripelennamine
triphalangeal thumb
Tri-Phen-Chlor
Triphenyl
    T. Expectorant
    T. Syrup
triphosphatase
    adenosine t.
triphosphate
    adenosine t. (ATP)
triphthong
Tripier
    T. bipedicle skin and muscle flap
triplant
    t. implant
triple
    t. advancement transposition (TAT)
    t. buccal tube
    t. line shadow
    t. lumen implant
triple-angle
triplegia
triple-paddle flap
tripod fracture
tripoli
triport tip
Triposed
    T. Syrup
    T. Tablet
triprolidine and pseudoephedrine
triprolidine, pseudoephedrine, and
  codeine
Tripton
TripTone Caplets
trirooted tooth
trisalicylate
    choline magnesium t.
trismus
    cancrum oris (noma) noma t.
    conversion t.
    t. stent
trismus-pseudocamptodactyly syndrome
Tri-Statin II Topical
Tristoject
Tri-Tannate Tablet

trite
triticea
    cartilago t.
Tritin
    Dr Scholl's Maximum Strength T.
tritubercular
triturate
trituration
triturator
    Dentomat t.
    mechanical t.
trivalent botulinum antiserum
Tri-Vi-Flor multivitamin mineral and
  fluoride supplement
TROCA
    tangible reinforcement of operant
    conditioned audiometry
Trocaine
trocar
    t. cystostomy
    Hasson laparoscopic t.
    transbuccal t.
trochaic stress
trochanteric depression
trochanterplasty
troche
    Cēpacol Anesthetic T.
    Mycelex T.
trochlear nerve
Trolard
    vein of T.
trombone tremor of tongue
tromethamine
    ketorolac t.
    lodoxamide t.
trophoneurosis
    lingual t.
Tropicacyl
tropicamide
    hydroxyamphetamine and t.
tropocollagen
    t. molecule
Trotter syndrome
trough
    t. curve
    focal t.
    gingival t.
    infraorbital tear t.
    round t.
    straight t.
Troyer Patient Education Series chart
Truarch wire
Tru-Canal hearing aid
true
    t. cementoma
    t. chondroma
    t. cyst
    t. denticle

t. dermatochalasis
t. generalized macrodontia
t. generalized microdontia
t. language
t. occlusal topographic intraoral radiography
T. separator
t. vocal cord (TVC)
t. vocal fold

trumpet
nasal t.
t. sign
truncal
truncated
t. cone effect
t. tetrahedral pyramid
truncation
predicate t.
trunk
central t.
cervicofacial t.
nerve t.
thyrocervical t.
trunk-to-trunk repair
Tru-Pulse
T.-P. carbon dioxide laser
T.-P. CO$_2$ skin resurfacing laser
trusion
bimaxillary t.
bodily t.
coronal t.
mandibular t.
maxillary t.
Trusopt
TruStone
try-in
t.-i. wax
trypanosomiasis
South American t.
trypsin, balsam peru, and castor oil
tryptophane
t. deamination
t. decarboxylation
T-scar
TSH
thyroid-stimulating hormone
T-shaped graft
TSTI
tumor-specific transplantation immunity
Tsuge suture technique
T-suppressor lymphocyte

TT
text telephone
TT tip
T-technique
TTMAD
Testing-Teaching Module of Auditory Discrimination
TTS
temporary threshold shift
tight-to-shaft
trigeminal trophic syndrome
T-type reamer
tubal
t. catarrh
t. tonsil
tubarius
torus t.
tube
Aire-Cuf tracheostomy t.
angulated buccal t.
aspiration t.
auditory t.
Baker self-sumping t.
Benjamin t.
Ben-Jet t.
bicanalicular silicone t.'s
Bouchut t.
buccal t.
Carden bronchoscopy t.
cast buccal t.
Celestin t.
Clearcut II with smoke eater t.
Cole uncuffed endotracheal t.
Donaldson t.
double-cannula tracheostomy t.
double-lumen suction irrigation t.
t. drain
Durham t.
edgewise buccal t.
end t.
endoneurial t.
endotracheal t. (ETT)
eustachian t.
t. extrusion
feeding t.
Fome-Cuf tracheostomy t.
gastrostomy feeding t.
Har-el pharyngeal t.
Heimlich t.
horizontal t.
Hyperflex tracheostomy t.
Inconel t.

NOTES

tube *(continued)*
    intratracheal t.
    Jiffy t.
    Kangaroo gastrostomy feeding t.
    Laryngoflex reinforced
      endotracheal t.
    Laser-Shield XII wrapped
      endotracheal t.
    Laser Trach wrapped
      endotracheal t.
    Lukens collecting t.
    molar t.
    Montgomery T t.
    Moss balloon triple-lumen
      gastrostomy t.
    nasogastric t.
    nasotracheal t. (NTT)
    neural t.
    O'Dwyer t.
    orotracheal t.
    PE t.
    polyvinyl chloride endotracheal t.
    Portex Blue Line tracheostomy t.
    Portex F29 Blue Line tracheal t.
    pressure equalization t.
    red rubber endotracheal t.
    resistant t.
    rolled skin t.
    Ruschelit polyvinyl chloride
      endotracheal t.
    salivary t.
    Sandoz nasogastric feeding t.
    self-rectified x-ray t.
    Sensiv endotracheal t.
    silicone t.
    smoke eater t.
    suction t.
    t. switch technique
    t. teeth
    tight-to-shaft Aire-Cuf
      tracheostomy t.
    tooth t.
    Toynbee t.
    tracheal t.
    tracheostomy t.
    tracheotomy t.
    triple buccal t.
    tympanostomy t.
    tympanotomy t.
    ventilation t.
    vertical t.
    Wolf suction t.
    Xomed plastic and rubber
      endotracheal t.
    x-ray t.
**TubeCheck esophageal intubation
detector**

tubed
    t. flap
    t. pedicle flap
tubehead
tubeless
    t. spontaneous respiration technique
tube-patient distance
tubercle
    articular t.
    auricular t.
    t. bacillus
    Carabelli t.
    corniculate t.
    crown t.
    t. of crown of tooth
    cuneiform t.
    darwinian t.
    dental t.
    epiglottic t.
    genial t.
    geniohyoid t.
    genioid t.
    labial t.
    marginal t.
    mental t.
    molar t.
    Montgomery t.'s
    paramolar t.
    postglenoid t.
    pubic t.
    t. of root of zygoma
    t. of upper lip
    Whitnall t.
    t. of zygoma
    zygomatic t.
tubercula (*pl. of* tuberculum)
tubercular
tuberculocidal
tuberculoid granuloma
tuberculoma
tuberculosis
    cutaneous t.
    laryngeal t.
    Mycobacterium t.
    t. prophylaxis
    t. tenosynovitis
tuberculous
    t. adenitis
    t. aneurysm
    t. gingivitis
    t. infection
    t. otitis media
    t. spondylitis
    t. tenosynovitis
tuberculum, pl. tubercula
    t. coronae
    t. coronae dentis

t. dentis
t. mentale mandibulae
tuberosa
chorditis t.
tuberosity
fractured t.
malar t.
maxillary t.
pterygoid t.
pyramidal t.
reduction t.
t. reduction
tuberosum
xanthoma t.
tube-shift technique
Tubi-Grip circumferential elastic bandage
tubing
air/water syringe t.
clear sterile t.
clear sterile premium t.
coiled t.
fabric covered t.
handpiece t.
ribbed sterile t.
suction t.
Tygon t.
Tubliseal
T. endodontic sealer
T. EWT
T. glass-ionomer root canal sealer
T. sealer
tuboplasty
tubotympanic recess
tubular
t. reconstruction
t. sclerosis
tubule
dentinal t.
endoneurial t.
mucous t.
Schwann t.
Tubulicid Plus root canal antibacterial solution
tubulin
tuck
chin t.
Tucker
T. bougie
T. mediastinoscope
T. staple forceps
T. tack and pin forceps

tuft
enamel t.
tug
tracheal t.
tugback
tularemia
tularensis
Francisella t.
Tulip syringe system
Tullio phenomenon
tumbleweed
tumefaction
gingival t.
tumefactive cartilage proliferation
tumesce
tumescence
tumescent
t. anesthesia
t. anesthesia solution
t. liposuction
t. local anesthesia technique
tumofactive asymmetry
tumor
t. ablation
acinic cell t.
acoustic t.
adenoid cystic t.
adenomatoid odontogenic t. (AOT)
adnexal skin t.
aerodigestive t.
ameloblastic adenomatoid t.
anterior pillar t.
atypical carcinoid t.
basaloid t.
benign epithelial odontogenic t.
benign mesenchymal t.
benign mixed t.
benign triton t.
brain t.
Brooke t.
t. burden
calcifying epithelial odontogenic t.
t. capsule
carcinoid t.
carotid body t.
central giant cell t.
central granular cell odontogenic t. (CGCOT)
cerebellopontine angle collision t.
clear cell odontogenic t. (CCOT)
collision t.
CPA collision t.

NOTES

tumor *(continued)*
deep-lobe parotid t.
de novo t.
denture injury t.
dermal analogue t.
desmoid t.
ectodermal t.
eighth nerve t.
en plaque t.
epidermoid t.
extra-axial t.
extraosseous plasma cell t.
extraskeletal osseous t.
fibrofatty t.
giant cell t. (GCT)
gigantic benign facial t.
glial t.
glomus jugulare t.
glomus tympanicum t.
glomus vagale t.
granular cell t. (GCT)
t. imaging
intracranial t.
intraparotid mesenchymal t.
jugular foramen t.
keloid t.
keratinizing epithelial odontogenic t.
Küttner t.
lipogenic t.
lymphoreticular t.
malignant odontogenic t.
t. marker
melanotic neuroectodermal t.
mesenchymal t.
mesodermal t.
metachronous t.
mixed t.
mucoepidermoid t.
multicentric glomus t.
t. necrosis factor (TNF)
t. necrosis factor-α (TNF-α)
nerve sheath t.
neural sheath t.
neuroendocrine t.
neurogenic t.
odontogenic t.
odontogenic adenomatoid t.
parapharyngeal t.
pearl t.
peripheral giant cell t.
peripheral neuroectodermal t.
peripheral odontogenic t.
petrous apex t.
phosphaturic mesenchymal t.
Pindborg t.
pituitary t.
pleomorphic t.
Pott puffy t.

pregnancy t.
primary t.
pseudomalignant osseous t.
ranine t.
retinal anlage t.
round t.
salivary gland t.
SCM t.
t. seeding
sellar t.
semimalignant t.
skull base t.
soft mixed odontogenic t.
soft tissue t.
spindle cell t.
squamous odontogenic t. (SOT)
t. stage grouping
t. staging
strawberry t.
synchronous lingual granular cell t.
turban t.
typical carcinoid t.
vascular t.
vasoformative t.
Warthin t.
tumoral exophthalmos
tumorectomy
tumoricidal
t. dose
t. radiation
t. radiation therapy
tumor-induced osteomalacia
tumor-like
t.-l. gingival enlargement
t.-l. necrosis
tumor-specific
t.-s. antigen
t.-s. transplantation immunity (TSTI)
tumor-to-tumor metastasis
tunable
t. dye laser
t. laser with hexascan
t. notch filter
t. tinnitus masker
tuna fish
tungsten
t. carbide (TC)
t. carbide bur
t. tip
tunic
Bichat t.
tunica
t. adventitia
t. albuginea
t. intima
t. media

t. propria
t. vaginalis
tuning
cochlear t.
t. curve
t. fork
t. fork test
tunnel
Corti t.
double t.
resorption t.
stylomandibular t.
tunnelized dermic flap
turban tumor
turbinal crest
turbinate
inferior t.
middle t.
neck of middle t.
paradoxic t.
rudimentary inferior t.
superior t.
supreme t.
turbinated bones
turbinectomy
concomitant t.
t. scissors
turbinoplasty
turbinotome
turbinotomy
turbo file
turbulence
nasal t.
turcica
sella t.
turgidity
turgor
turkey feather dander
turmeric
turmschädel
turned down forearm flap
Turner
T. hypoplasia
T. syndrome
T. tooth
Turnera diffusa
turnip
turnover flap
turret
five-position t.
turribrachycephaly
turricephaly

Tussafed Drops
Tussafin Expectorant
tussal
Tuss-Allergine Modified T.D. Capsule
Tussar SF Syrup
TUSSI
Temple University Short Syntax
Inventory
tussicular
tussiculation
Tussilago farfara
tussis
tussive
Tuss-LA
Tussogest Extended Release Capsule
TV
tidal volume
TVC
true vocal cord
TVR
tonic vibration reflex
twang
nasal t.
Tweed
T. diagnostic triangle
T. edgewise treatment
T. method
T. method of dentofacial analysis
twelfth
t. cranial nerve
t. nerve paralysis
twelfth-year molar
TWF
Test of Word Finding
Twice-A-Day Nasal
twig
nerve t.
twin
t. bracket tooth rotation
conjoined t.'s
t. edgewise bracket
T. Flash scanner
t. formation
t. language
t. teeth
t. wire
twin-barreled fibular graft
twinning
twin-wire
t.-w. attachment
t.-w. fixed orthodontic appliance

T

NOTES

twist
    t. drill
    T. MTX implant
    octave t.
    T. Ti implant
twisted archwire
twisting closure
twist-off technique
two-buttress defect
two-dimensional (2D)
    t.-d. linear plating system
    t.-d. ultrasound (2D US)
two-factor model of stuttering
two-holed miniplate
two-joule Erbium laser
two-microphone acoustical rhinometer
two open ends
two-paste
    t.-p. polysulfide rubber impression material
    t.-p. system
two-piece implant
two-plane occlusion
two-point discrimination (2 PD)
two-pointed premolar
two-portal open carpal tunnel release technique
two-pour technique
two-step technique
two-team dissection
two-tiered genioplasty
two-toned voice
two-tooth segment
two-word utterance
Tycos
    T. gauge
    T. pressure infusion line
Tydings tonsil snare
Tygon tubing
Tylenol
    T. Cold Effervescent Medication Tablet
    T. Cold No Drowsiness
    T. Extended Release Caplets
    T. Extended Relief
    T. Flu Maximum Strength
    T. Sinus, Maximum Strength
    T. With Codeine
tylosis, pl. tyloses
    t. linguae
Tylox
tympanal
tympanectomy
tympani
    canaliculus of chorda t.
    cavum t.
    chorda t.

    scala t.
    tensor t.
tympanic
    t. annulus
    t. artery
    t. cavity
    t. cell
    t. fold
    t. homograft
    t. membrane
    t. muscle
    t. nerve
    t. neurectomy
    t. plexus
    t. ring
    t. sinus
tympanica
    incisura t.
tympanicity
tympanicus
    annulus t.
tympanitis
tympanocentesis
tympanogram
    t. classification Feldman model
    t. classification Jerger model
tympanomastoid
    t. abnormality
    t. fissure
    t. suture
tympanomastoidectomy
tympanomastoiditis
tympanomeatal flap
tympanomeatomastoidectomy
tympanometry
tympanophonia
tympanoplasty
    canal wall-down t.
    closed t.
    crowncork t.
    t. knife
    t. mastoidectomy
    t. ossiculoplasty
    staged t.
    t. with mastoidectomy (TPWM)
    t. without mastoidectomy (TPWOM)
tympanosclerosis
tympanosclerotic
tympanosquamosal suture
tympanostomy
    t. tube
tympanotomy
    t. tube
type
    addition t.
    Békésy tracing t.
    t. C fasciocutaneous flap

collagen t. IV
condensation t.
ditransitive verb t.
t. II earlobe cleft
t. I, II, III frontal plagiocephaly
T. I, II, III, IV canal
t. I vascular pattern
transitive verb t.
undifferentiated carcinoma of
nasopharyngeal t.
voice signal t.
typhimurium
Salmonella t.
Typhoon cutter blade

typical carcinoid tumor
typodont
t. teeth
tyrosine crystal
tyrothricin
Tytin
T. high-copper alloy
T. high copper amalgam
Tyzine Nasal
Tzanck
T. cell
T. test
T-Z-plasty

NOTES

T

UAD Otic
UAL
    ultrasound-assisted lipectomy
UAM universal fixation driver
UAO
    upper airway obstruction
ubiquitous glottal stop
ubm Erbium Renaissance laser
UCE
    upper completely edentulous
UCL
    uncomfortable level
UCLA-type-retained prosthesis
UCLL
    uncomfortable listening level
    uncomfortable loudness level
UDMA
    urethane dimethacrylate
U-flap
    reverse U.-f.
ugly duckling stage
UHMWPE
    ultra-high molecular weight polyethylene
    UHMWPE articulating surface
UICC
    Union Internationale Contre Cancrum
UJV AMS 1000 high frequency jet
  ventilator
ulaganactesis
ulalgia
ulatrophy
    afunctional u.
    atrophic u.
    calcic u.
    ischemic u.
    traumatic u.
  ulcer
    aphthous u.
    Barrett u.
    contact u.
    Crombie u.
    Cushing u.
    decubitus u.
    dental u.
    denture u.
    duodenal u.
    eosinophilic u.
    herpetic u.
    Marjolin u.
    moorean u.
    oropharyngeal u.
    peptic u.
    Plaut u.
    recurrent aphthous u. (RAU)
    rodent u.

    sacral u.
    stress u.
    sublingual u.
    tracheal u.
    traumatic u.
ulcerated granuloma
ulceration
    agranulocytic u.
    corneal u.
    crescentic u.
    nasogastric tube retrocricoid u.
    tracheal u.
ulcerative
    u. eosinophilic granuloma
    u. gingivitis
    u. inflammation
    u. peri-implantoclasia
    u. pharyngitis
    u. pulpitis
    u. stomatitis
    u. tonsillitis
ulceromembranous
    u. gingivitis
    u. pharyngitis
ulectomy
ulemorrhagia
Ulex europaeus **antigen**
ulitis
    aphthous u.
    interstitial u.
Ullrich-Feichtiger syndrome
Ulmus fulva
ulnar
    u. club hand
    u. nerve transposition
    u. styloid
ulocace
ulocarcinoma
uloglossitis
uloncus
ulorrhagia
ulorrhea
ulotomy
ulotripsis
ULR-LA
ultimate strength
Ultimatics
    U. demineralized cortical bone
      powder
    U. flexible laminar bone strip
Ultiva
ULTRA
    U. ultrasonic aspirator
Ultra
    U. Brite

U

Ultra *(continued)*
  Grisactin U.
  U. Image.db computer imaging
    system
  U. Low resistance voice prosthesis
  U. Mide Topical
  U. Tears Solution
  U. Voice speech aid
Ultrabond
Ultra-Fast Araldite sealer
Ultrafill
Ultrafine
  Command U.
**Ultraflex ankle dorsiflexion dynamic
  splint**
ultragonography
**ultra-high molecular weight polyethylene
  (UHMWPE)**
ultra-high-speed handpiece
UltraLine Nd:YAG laser fiber
UltraLite headlight system
Ultram
ultramicrotome
Ultra-Precision ultrasonic probe
ultraprognathous
UltraPulse
  U. carbon dioxide laser
  U. CO$_2$ laser
  U. surgical laser
ultrapulse
  u. carbon dioxide laserbrasion
  u. technology
ultrapulsed laser
ultrasonic (US)
  u. cleaning
  u. curettage
  u. frequency
  u. handpiece
  u. lancet
  u. liposculpturing
  u. liposuction
  u. piezo-electric scaler
  u. preparation
  u. ray
  u. retroprep system
  u. retrotip
  u. scaler
  u. scaling
  u. scalpel
  u. suction scalpel
  u. surgical aspirator
  u. unit
ultrasonics
ultrasonography
  Voluvision three dimensional u.
ultrasound (US)
  Belgium u. (B.U.S.)
  duplex u.

  u. generator
  high-resolution u.
  u. liposuction
  7.5 MHz linear array B-mode u.
    transducer
  Rich-Mar 510 external u.
  three-dimensional u. (3D US)
  u. treatment
  two-dimensional u. (2D US)
ultrasound-assisted
  u.-a. lipectomy (UAL)
  u.-a. liposuction
ultrasound-guided biopsy
ultrastructural study
ultraterminal excementosis
Ultravate
ultraviolet
  u. light
  u. light-polymerized resin
Ultra-X external fixation system
umbilicoplasty
umbilicus
umbo, pl. **umbones**
umbrella
  u. graft
Umbrella punctum plug
unacceptable
  u. device
  u. material
unaccepted dental therapeutic
unaesthetic
  u. contour deformity
  u. incision
unaffected crystal
unaided augmentative communication
Unasyn
unattached gingiva
unbonded resin
uncalcified
  u. cementum
  u. dentin
uncinate process
uncinectomy
uncomfortable
  u. level (UCL)
  u. listening level (UCLL)
  u. loudness level (UCLL)
unconditioned
  u. reinforcer
  u. response
  u. stimulus
uncoupling
  nasal u.
undemineralized
  u. bone graft
underangulation
underbite

undercut
> u. gauge
> gauge u.
> retentive u.
> soft tissue u.
> unusable u.

underexpose
underextension
underhung bite
underlayer cantilever bone graft
underlay fascia technique
underlying structure
undermasking
undermine
undermining
> cross-hatching u.
> u. resorption
> single-hatching u.
> skin u.

undermix
undersurface of tongue
undifferentiated
> u. carcinoma
> u. carcinoma of nasopharyngeal
>   type
> u. cell
> u. mesenchymal cell

undisplaced fracture
undulant fever
unerupted
> u. tooth
> u. tooth resorption

uneruption
unexposed
> u. crystal
> u. intraoral film

unfilled
> u. acrylic plastic
> u. acrylic polymer
> u. resin

Uni-Ace
unibevel chisel
unicameral
> u. bone cyst
> u. cyst

unicoronal synostosis
unicuspid
unicuspidate
unicystic ameloblastoma
Uni-Decon
unification

Uni-File
> Burns U.-F.

UniFile Imaging and Archiving system
Unigauge handle
unilambdoid synostosis
Unilase CO$_2$ laser
unilateral
> u. abductor paralysis
> u. adductor paralysis
> u. cleft lip
> u. cleft lip nose deformity
> u. cleft lip and palate
> u. coronal synostosis
> u. distocclusion
> u. facial hypertrophy
> u. glossitis
> u. hearing loss
> u. isometric bite force
> u. macroglossia
> u. mesiocclusion
> u. neck pain
> u. partial denture
> u. plagiocephaly
> u. turbinate volume reduction
> u. vocal cord paralysis (UVCP)
> u. weakness

unilocular
unimaxillary spacing
UniMax 2000 laser micromanipulator
unimodal
unintelligible speech
union
> autogenous u.
> U. Internationale Contre Cancrum
>   (UICC)
> primary u.
> secondary u.

unipedicle flap
Unipen
> U. Injection
> U. Oral

UniPlast
> U. Imaging and Archiving system
> U. video imaging

unipolar neuron
Unipost implant
unisensory
unit
> Ångström u. (Å)
> auditory training u.'s
> Baird Electric System 5000 Power
>   Plus electrosurgical u.

U

NOTES

unit *(continued)*
 bipolar electrosurgical u.
 Celay milling u.
 Dalbo extracoronal u.
 Dalbo stud u.
 dental u.
 dentoperiodontal u.
 Dolder bar u.
 EIE MiniEndo piezoelectric
 ultrasonic u.
 EXAKT cutting/grinding u.
 exposure u.
 fiberoptic u.
 gingival u.
 Hounsfield u.
 intraoral light-curing u.
 loudness u.
 u. membrane
 Neosonic piezo ultrasonic u.
 Neuropulse u.
 Ocoee scalp cleansing u.
 Ohmeda intermittent suction u.
 Orthoceph x-ray u.
 ostiomeatal u. (OMU)
 partial denture u.
 piezoelectric ultrasonic u.
 pilosebaceous u.'s
 Pulsatron u.
 Root ZX ultrasonic u.
 sensation u. (SU)
 sensory u.
 SI u.
 Sievert u.
 Siremobil C-arm u.
 Solfy ZX ultrasonic u.
 speech training u.
 Sullivan nasal VPAP u.
 ultrasonic u.
 vacuum former u.
 vacuum polymerization u.
 Varistim u.
 Visio Beta vacuum
 polymerization u.
Unitech
 U. cannula series
 U. Instruments
 U. Toomey cannula
Unitek appliance
uni-tip deformity
Unitrax unipolar system
Unitri
 U. cannula
 U. tip
Unitrol
Unitron Esteem CIC hearing aid
universal
 u. bracket
 U. cannula series

 u. curette
 U. F breathing system
 u. fixed orthodontic appliance
 u. forceps
 u. grammar
 u. Luer lock
 U. Numbering system
 u. orthodontic attachment
 u. subperiosteal implant
universality
universals
 formal u.
 linguistic u.
 substantive u.
University
 U. of Minnesota retractor
 U. of Pennsylvania Smell
 Identification Test (UPSIT)
 U. of Virginia fibrin sealant
 U. of Washington rubber dam
 clamp forceps
unmeshed
 u. split-thickness skin graft
unmitigated echolalia
unmodified zinc oxide-eugenol cement
unmyelinated
 u. nerve fiber
unoperated cleft
unpedicled flap
unrepositioned flap
unresectable squamous cell carcinoma
unrestored
unrounded vowel
unsaturated chemical vapor sterilization
unstrained jaw relation
unstressed
 u. vowel
unsustained bite
unusable undercut
unwaxed regular dental floss
upbiting forceps
UPE
 upper partially edentulous
UPP
 uvulopalatoplasty
upper
 u. aerodigestive tract
 u. airway
 u. airway obstruction (UAO)
 u. arch
 u. bound
 u. cervical nerve
 u. completely edentulous (UCE)
 u. face rejuvenation
 u. impression
 u. incisor angulation
 u. jaw
 u. lateral nasal cartilage

u. lip
u. lip length
u. partial
u. partially edentulous (UPE)
u. pole
u. pole fullness
u. pole rippling
u. respiratory infection (URI)
u. respiratory obstruction (URO)
u. respiratory tract
u. respiratory tract infection
u. reticular dermal peel
u. reticular dermal penetration
u. single tooth (UST)
u. teeth
u. tooth to upper lip relationship
u. trapezius flap
u. universal forceps

UPPP
uvulopalatopharyngoplasty

uprighting
u. spring

UPSIT
University of Pennsylvania Smell Identification Test

upturned forceps

upward
u. bent forceps
u. masking

Uracel

uraniscochasm

uraniscochasma

uranisconitis

uraniscoplasty

uraniscorrhaphy

uraniscus

uranoplasty
Wardill-Kilner four-flap u.

uranorrhaphy

uranoschisis

uranoschism

uranostaphyloplasty

uranostaphylorrhaphy

uranostaphyloschisis

uranoveloschisis

Urbach-Wiethe syndrome

urea
u. and hydrocortisone
u. peroxide

Ureacin Topical

Ureaphil Injection

urease

Urecholine

uremia

uremic gingivitis

ureteroplasty

ureteropyeloplasty

urethane
u. dimethacrylate (UDMA)
u. dimethacrylate luting composite resin

urethrae
neomeatus u.

urethral
u. epithelium
u. reconstruction

urethroplasty
mesh graft u.

URI
upper respiratory infection

uric acid

urine
extravasation of mouse u.

URO
upper respiratory obstruction

Urobak

urokinase
intra-arterial u.

Uroplastique material

Urtica dioica

US
ultrasonic
ultrasound
2D US
two-dimensional ultrasound
3D US
three-dimensional ultrasound

usage doctrine

USASI

use
intravenous drug u. (IVDU)
u. life
semantic u.
Surgicel absorbable hemostat for dental u.

useful
u. radiation
u. ray

U-shaped
U.-s. arch
U.-s. curve
U.-s. incision
U.-s. interdigitated muscle flap
U.-s. skin excision

U

NOTES

Usher syndrome
Usnea spp.
UST
    upper single tooth
Ustilago
Utah Test of Language Development
uteroplasty
uterque
    auris u. (AU)
utility
    u. arch
    u. glove
    u. wax
Utilization
    Dental Auxiliary U.
utricle
utricular duct
utriculitis
utriculoendolymphatic valve
utriculosaccular duct
utriculus
utterance
    holophrastic u.
    mean length of u. (MLU)
    mean relational u. (MRU)
    polymorphemic u.
    telegraphic u.
    two-word u.
uva-ursi
UVCP
    unilateral vocal cord paralysis

uveitis
    sarcoidal u.
uveoparotid fever
UV photo-oxidation
uvula, gen. and pl. uvuli
    bifid u.
    cleft u.
    forked u.
    palatine u.
    pendulous u.
    split u.
    u. tip
uvulaptosis
uvular
    u. muscle
uvulatome
uvulectomy
uvuli (*gen. and pl. of* uvula)
uvulitis
uvulopalatopharyngoplasty (UPPP)
uvulopalatoplasty (UPP)
    laser-assisted u. (LAUP)
    u. procedure
uvulopharyngeal
uvuloptosis
uvulotome
uvulotomy
U X-Acto gouge

V
    venule
    volt
    voltage
        V bend
        V flap
        V motor paralysis
        V to Y fashion closure
V_T

V_T
    tidal volume
V2 nerve distribution
vaccination
        smallpox v.
        variola v.
vaccine
        Bacille Calmette-Guérin v.
        plasma-derived hepatitis B v.
        recombinant DNA v.
vaccinia
Vaccinium myrtillus
Vacudent
Vacu-Irrigator
        Lap V.-I.
vacuolated Hurler cell
vacuolation
vacuole
        intracytoplasmic v.
vacutome
Vacutron suction regulator
vacuum
        v. casting
        v. former unit
        v. investing
        v. polymerization unit
        v. sinusitis
        v. type former
vacuum-formed resin impression tray
VADS
        Visual Aural Digit Span Test
vagale
        glomus v.
vagal paraganglioma
vagina
        artificial v.
vaginal
        v. agenesis
        v. atresia
        v. dimple
        v. epithelialization
        v. malformation
        Monistat V.
        v. process of the sphenoid bone
        Terazol V.
        Vagistat-1 V.

vaginalis
        tunica v.
vaginoperineal reconstruction
vaginoperineoplasty
vaginoplasty
        colon interposition v.
        free flap v.
        intestinal v.
        penile skin inversion v.
        v. procedure
Vagistat-1 Vaginal
Vagitrol
vagotomy
vagus
        v. nerve
        v. nerve imaging
Vail syndrome
Valacon
valacyclovir
valerate
        hydrocortisone v.
valgus
        hallux v.
validity
        concurrent v.
        construct v.
        content v.
        criterion related v.
        face v.
        predictive v.
Valisone
Valium
vallate papilla
vallecula, pl. valleculae
vallecular dysphagia
Valmid
Valsalva-induced cervical thymic cyst
Valsalva maneuver
Valtrac anastomosis ring
value
        Hertel v.
        Periotest v.
Valux
valve
        anterior nasal v.
        Argyle anti-reflux v.
        Blom-Singer v.
        dysfunctional nasal v.
        v.'s of Kerckring
        Montgomery speaking v.
        nasal v.
        Passe Muir v.
        Provox tracheoesophageal
            speaking v.
        Shiley Phonate speaking v.

valve *(continued)*
    tracheostoma v.
    utriculoendolymphatic v.
    velopharyngeal v.
valvoplasty
valvuloplasty
Van
    V. Beek-Zook technique
    V. der Woude syndrome
    V. Nes procedure
van
    v. Buchem disease
    v. der Hoeve syndrome
Vancenase
    V. AQ
    V. AQ Inhaler
    V. Nasal Inhaler
    V. Pockethaler
Vanceril Oral Inhaler
Vancocin
    V. HCl
Vancoled
vancomycin
    v. HCl
vanilla
vanillism
vanishing bone disease
Vantin
vaporization
vapotherapy
variable
    v. compression potentiometer
    v. high cut potentiometer
    v. interval reinforcement schedule
    v. low cut potentiometer
    v. position stent
    v. positive airway pressure (VPAP)
    v. ratio reinforcement schedule
    v. release compression
variance
    analysis of v. (ANOVA)
variant
    v. nerve
    orthokeratinized v.
    parakeratinized v.
variation
    episodic v.
    free v.
    linguistic v.
    noise-related v.
    phonetic v.
varicella
varicella-zoster
    v.-z. encephalitis
    primary v.-z.
    secondary v.-z.
    v.-z. virus
varicelliform rash

varices (*pl. of* varix)
varicosity
    spider v.
variegated pattern
variola
    v. vaccination
variotii
    Paecilomyces v.
Varistim unit
varix, pl. **varices**
    esophageal v.
varnish
    Caulk v.
    Cavi-Line cavity v.
    cavity v.
    copal v.
    Copalite cavity v.
    dental v.
    Duraflor sodium fluoride v.
    Handi-Liner cavity v.
    mastic v.
    periodontal v.
    rosin v.
varnished tongue
vascular
    v. birthmark
    v. bulldog
    v. bundle
    v. bundle implantation
    v. bundle implantation into bone
    v. carrier
    v. dentin
    v. disorder
    v. endothelial growth factor (VEGF)
    v. endothelium
    v. headache
    v. hyperpermeability
    v. lesion therapy
    v. loop
    v. loop compression syndrome
    v. malformation
    v. neoplasm
    v. nidus
    v. occlusive disease
    v. pedicle
    v. pericyte of Zimmerman
    v. pressure
    v. steal
    v. tumor
vascularis
    stria v.
vascularity
    flap v.
vascularization
    reverse flow v.
vascularized
    v. bone graft (VBG)

v. calvarial flap
v. double-sided preputial island flap and W flap glanuloplasty hypospadias repair
v. fascial patch
v. island bone flap
v. preputial flap
v. sensate neoclitoris
v. spare part
v. tendon graft
v. tibial bone flap

vasculature
pulpal v.

vasculitis
Churg-Strauss v.

Vaseline

Vaseline-coated gauze

vaselinized nasal tamponage

vaselinoma

vasoactive
v. agglutinate
v. intestinal peptide

Vasocidin Ophthalmic

VasoClear Ophthalmic

Vasocon-A Ophthalmic

Vasocon Regular Ophthalmic

vasoconstriction

vasoconstrictive agent

vasoconstrictor

vasodentin

vasodilating agent

vasodilation
local v.

vasodilator

vasoformative tumor

vasomotor
v. rhinitis

vasonervorum

vasopressin

vasospasm

Vasosulf Ophthalmic

vastus medialis

VAT
vestibular autorotation test

Vater
papilla of V.

vault
nasal v.

V-bend

VBG
vascularized bone graft
vertical banded gastroplasty

VC
vital capacity

V-C
vowel-consonant

V-Cillin K

V-Dec-M

Veau
V. classification
cleft muscle of V.

Veau-Wardill-Kilner
V.-W.-K. pushback operation
V.-W.-K. repair

vector
v. of aging
v. analysis
force v.
v. of skin pull

Vectrin

Veeneklaas syndrome

Veetids

vegetable wax

vegetans
pemphigus v.

vegetative bacteria

VEGF
vascular endothelial growth factor

Vehe carver

Veillonella
V. alcalescens
V. parvula

vein
angular facial v.
anterior condylar v.
anterior facial v.
auditory v.
axillary v.
cerebellar v.
cochlear v.
collecting v. (CV)
common facial v.
condylar emissary v.
cortical v.
deep inferior epigastric v.
emissary v.
external jugular v.
facial v.
v. hook retractor
inferior thyroid v.
internal auditory v.
internal jugular v.
jugular v.
Labbé v.

V

NOTES

vein *(continued)*
    laryngeal v.
    mastoid emissary v.
    maxillary v.
    middle thyroid v.
    pharyngeal v.
    posterior facial v.
    ranine v.
    retroauricular v.
    retromandibular v.
    sentinel v.
    spider v.
    superficial temporal v.
    superior laryngeal v.
    superior ophthalmic v.
    superior thyroid v.
    sylvian v.
    temporal v.
    thyroid ima v.
    transverse facial v.
    v. of Trolard
vela (*pl. of* velum)
velar
    v. area
    v. assimilation
    backing to v.
    v. consonant
    v. fronting
    v. insufficiency
    v. tail
velarized consonant
Velcro binder
Vel Mix Stone
velocardiofacial syndrome
velocimeter
    optical Doppler v.
velocity
    conduction v.
    particle v.
    slow-component v. (SCV)
velopharyngeal
    v. closure
    v. competence (VPC)
    v. competency
    v. friction sound
    v. function
    v. incompetence (VPI)
    v. insufficiency (VPI)
    v. isthmus
    v. part
    v. port
    v. portal
    v. seal
    v. valve
velopharynx
veloplasty
    functional v.
    intravelar v.

Velosef
velosynthesis
velum, pl. vela
    artificial v.
    Baker v.
    v. palati
Velvalloy amalgam alloy
velvet grass
vena comitans, pl. venae comitantes
veneer
    ceramic v.
    direct labial v.
    laminate v.
    laminated esthetic v.
    v. metal crown
    porcelain laminate v.
veneered crown
venenata
    dermatitis v.
    stomatitis v.
venereal warts
Venn diagram
Venodyne compression system
Venoglobulin-I, -S
venography
    jugular v.
    retrograde jugular v.
venom
    bee v.
    flea v.
venous
    v. flap
    v. hemorrhage
    v. lake
    v. loop
    v. malformation
venous-to-venous
    v.-t.-v. anastomosis (VVA)
vent
    v. implant
vented
    v. earmold
    v. post
venter frontalis musculi occipitofrontalis
ventilation
    CPAP v.
    cuirass v.
    high-frequency jet v. (HFJV)
    jet v.
    subglottic jet v.
    supraglottic jet v.
    v. tube
    v. tube inserter
    Venturi jet v.
ventilator
    Acutronic AMS 1000 automatic
      jet v.
    Smart Trigger Bear 1000 v.

UJV AMS 1000 high frequency
jet v.
ventplant
vent-plate implant
ventral
ventricle
appendix of laryngeal v.
Galen v.
laryngeal v.
Morgagni v.
saccule of laryngeal v.
ventricular
v. dysphonia
v. fold
v. fold dysphonia
v. phonation
ventricularis
dysphonia plicae v.
ventriculocordectomy
ventriculoperitoneal shunt
ventriculoplasty
ventriculus laryngis
ventroposteroinferior nucleus
Venturi jet ventilation
venule (V)
collecting v.
main v. (MV)
postcapillary v. (PCV)
vera
neuralgia facialis v.
verb
auxiliary v.
GAP v.
general all purpose v.
helping v.
v. lexicon
linking v.
secondary v.
verbal
v. aphasia
v. apraxia
v. fluency
V. Language Development Scale
v. mediation
v. operant
v. paraphasia
v. play
verbigeration
verbotonal method
verge
anal v.
Vergon

Verhoeff
V. elastic stain
V. solution
Veribest 22 K inlay
verification
v. radiograph
shade v.
vermilion
v. Abbe flap
v. border
v. border of lip
central v.
dry v.
v. notching
projection of v.
wet v.
vermilionectomy
vermilion-white line malalignment
vernacular
Vernet syndrome
Vernier caliper
Verocay bodies
Verrex-C&M
verruca
v. plana
recalcitrant v.
v. vulgaris
verruciform
v. leukoplakia
v. xanthoma
verruciformis
epidermodysplasia v.
verrucous
v. carcinoma
v. hyperplasia
v. lesion
v. leukoplakia
v. xanthoma
Versacaps
VersaLight laser
versatile flap
Versed
version
vertebra
cervical v.
vertebral
v. artery
v. chordoma
vertebral-basilar artery disease
vertex potential
vertical
v. angulation

V

NOTES

vertical *(continued)*
    v. axis
    v. banded gastroplasty (VBG)
    v. bone loss
    v. bony height
    v. condensation root canal filling
    method
    v. corrugator line
    v. crest
    v. dimension
    v. displacement on opening
    v. dysplasia
    v. elastic
    v. extension radiolucency
    v. face-lift
    v. fracture
    v. glabellar crease
    v. impaction
    v. lip biopsy
    v. loop
    v. mammaplasty
    v. mandibular posturing
    v. mattress suture
    v. maxillary excess (VME)
    v. midline approach
    v. muscle of tongue
    v. opening
    v. osteotomy
    v. osteotomy of ramus of
    mandible
    v. overbite
    v. overlap
    v. plane
    v. plate of palatine
    v. position
    v. preputial vascularized flap
    v. relation
    v. resorption
    v. rhomboid de-epithelialization
    v. scar
    v. scar with lipoaspiration
    technique
    v. septation
    v. skin excision
    v. slot Lewis bracket
    v. tooth fracture
    v. transmission
    v. tube
    v. vs. horizontal preparation
vertical-cut
    v.-c. method
    v.-c. technique
verticalis linguae muscle
Verticillium
verticomental
vertiginous
    v. symptom

vertigo
    v. ab aure laeso
    auditory v.
    aural v.
    benign paroxysmal positional v.
    (BPPV)
    benign paroxysmal postural v.
    benign positional v. (BPV)
    central v.
    cervical v.
    Charcot v.
    episodic v.
    labyrinthine v.
    laryngeal v.
    paroxysmal positional v.
    postural v.
    rotational v.
    supermarket v.
vesicle
    olfactory v.
    otic v.
    synaptic v.
vesicular stomatitis
vesiculated ending
vesiculobullous lesion
vespid
    Hymenopterous v.
Vesprin
vessel
    blood v.
    v. caliber mismatch
    cervical v.
    choke v.
    circumflex scapular v.
    fasciocutaneous v.
    friable v.
    intercostal v.
    lymphatic v.
    mucosal blood v.
    palatine v.
    perforator v.
    periosteal v.
    peroneal v.
    receipt v.
    recipient v.
    single nutrient v.
    supporting v.
    temporal v.
vessel-nerve conflict
vest
    gynecomastia v.
vestibula (*pl. of* vestibulum)
vestibular
    v. abscess
    v. adaptation
    v. apparatus
    v. aqueduct
    v. autorotation test (VAT)

v. canal
v. cecum
v. depth
v. dysfunction
v. epithelium
v. fold
v. fornix
v. fossa
v. function test
v. ganglion
v. hydrops
v. hyperreactivity (VH)
v. labyrinth
v. lamina
v. ligament
v. membrane
v. mucosa
v. nerve
v. nerve section
v. neurectomy (VN)
v. neuritis
v. neuronitis
v. neurotomy
v. nucleus
v. nystagmus
v. oral plate
v. paresis
v. pathway
v. reflex
v. rehabilitation
v. response
v. schwannoma (VS)
v. screen
v. stereocilia
v. surface of tooth
v. system disorder
v. web
v. window
vestibule
buccal v.
v. of cheek
labial v.
laryngeal v.
mandibular v.
v. of mouth
nasal v.
vestibuli (*gen. of* vestibulum)
vestibulitis
nasal v.
vestibulocerebellar connection
vestibulocerebellum

vestibulocochlear
v. artery
v. nerve
vestibulofibrosis
vestibulo-infraglottic duct
vestibulometry
vestibulo-ocular
v.-o. reflex (VOR)
v.-o. reflex rotational chair test
vestibulo-oculomotor reflex
vestibuloplasty
Kazanjian v.
vestibulospinal disorder
vestibulotomy
Edlan v.
Kazanjian v.
vestibulotoxic
v. drug
v. effect
vestibulum, gen. **vestibuli**, pl. **vestibula**
fenestra vestibuli
v. oris
scala vestibuli
vest-male
compression v.-m.
vest-over-pants technique
Vexol Ophthalmic Suspension
V-flap
VH
vestibular hyperreactivity
VHI
Voice Handicap Index
Viadent
Viaspan
Vibramycin
V. Injection
V. Oral
vibrant consonant
Vibra-Tabs
vibrating line
vibration
v. condensation
forced v.
free v.
glottal v.
v. meter
sinusoidal v.
sympathetic v.
v. tolerance
transient v.
vibrato

V

NOTES

vibrator
  automatic v.
  bone-conduction v.
vibratory cycle
vibrissa, pl. **vibrissae**
  nasal v.
vibrometer
vibrotactile
  v. hearing aid
  v. response
  v. threshold
Viburnum opulus
Vicat needle
Vickers
  V. hardness indenter point
  V. hardness number
  V. hardness test
  V. ring tip forceps
Vicks
  V. Children's Chloraseptic
  V. Chloraseptic Sore Throat
  V. DayQuil Allergy Relief 4 Hour
  Tablet
  V. DayQuil Sinus Pressure &
  Congestion Relief
  V. 44D Cough & Head
  Congestion
  V. 44 Non-Drowsy Cold & Cough
  Liqui-Caps
  V. Sinex Nasal Solution
Vicodin
  V. ES
  V. HP
Vicoprofen
Vicryl
  V. mesh
  V. Rapide suture
Victoreen Digital Densitometer
vidarabine
VID 1 color micro camera system
vide infra
video
  v. fluoroscopic imaging chair
  v. imaging system (VIS)
  v. monitoring
videoendoscopy
videofluoroscope
videofluoroscopic swallow study (VSS)
videofluoroscopy
videolaryngeal stroboscopy
videomicroscopy
videonasopharyngoscopy
videostrobe
**videostroboscopic diagnostic
  determination**
videostroboscopy (VS)
vidian
  v. artery

  v. canal
  v. nerve
  v. neuralgia
view
  anterior v.
  bird's-eye v.
  buccal v.
  Caldwell v.
  chin-nose v.
  frontal v.
  incisal quadrant v.
  intaglio v.
  jug-handle v.
  laryngoscopic v.
  lateral oblique transcranial v.
  mandibular occlusal v.
  maxillary occlusal v.
  Mayer v.
  occipitomeatal v.
  occlusal quadrant v.
  orthopantographic v.
  Owen v.
  panoramic v.
  Panorex v.
  roentgenographic v.
  submentocervical v.
  Waters v.
  worm's-eye v.
Vigilon dressing
Viking II EMG system electromyograph
Vilex plastic surgery instrument
Vilkki procedure
Villaumite sodium fluoride
villous
  v. papillae of tongue
villus, pl. **villi**
  arachnoid villi
  synovial v.
vimentin
  v. filament
vinblastine
Vincent
  V. angina
  V. disease
  V. gingivitis
  V. infection
  V. organism
  V. stomatitis
  V. tonsillitis
vincentii
  Borrelia v.
  Treponema v.
vincristine
vine
  squaw v.
vinyl
  v. ethyl methacrylate
  v. palatal appliance

v. plastic
v. plastisol
v. polysiloxane impression material
v. silicone

violation
syntactic v.

violet
Gentian v.

Viquin Forte cream
Vira-A Ophthalmic
Viractin Cream
viral
v. hepatitis
v. infection
v. labyrinthitis
v. sialadenitis
v. vesicular stomatitis

viridans
Streptococcus v.

virilization
Viroptic Ophthalmic
Virtual Model 330 distortion-product otoacoustic emission device
virucidal
virulence
virus
adenovirus v.
AIDS-related v. (ARV)
coronavirus v.
coxsackie v.
ECHO v.
enterocytopathogenic human orphan v.
Epstein-Barr v. (EBV)
functional assessment of human immunodeficiency v. (FAHI)
hepatitis A v. (HAV)
hepatitis B v. (HBV)
hepatitis C v. (HCV)
hepatitis delta v. (HDV)
herpes v.
herpes simplex v., type 1, 2
human immunodeficiency v. (HIV)
human T cell lymphotrophic v. (HTLV)
hydrophilic v.
influenza A and B, A, A2 v.
lipophilic v.
lymphadenopathy-associated v. (LAV)
measles v.
mumps v.

non-A-G hepatitis v.
non-A hepatitis v.
non-B hepatitis v.
parainfluenza v.
poliomyelitis v.
poliovirus v.
poliovirus type 2 v.
respiratory syncytial v.
rhinovirus v.
rubella v.
v. transmission
varicella-zoster v.

VIS
video imaging system

VISA multi-patient monitor
Visarfil
viscera (*pl. of* viscus)
visceral
v. arch
v. compartment
v. deglutition appliance
v. donor site
v. fascia
v. nervous system
v. pouch
v. space
v. swallow
v. swallowing
v. swallowing appliance

viscid
v. secretion

viscoelastic property of skin
viscosity
v. of saliva test

viscosus
Actinomyces v.

viscous
v. secretion

viscus, pl. viscera
visibility
visible
v. calculus
v. light-activated system
v. light-polymerizing composite
v. speech

Visine
V. Extra Ophthalmic
V. L.R. Ophthalmic

Visio
V. Beta vacuum polymerization unit
V. Dispers

V

NOTES

Visiofil
Visioform light-curing resin
Visio-Gem
Visiomolar
Visipitch TM digital tape recorder
Vismark skin marker
visor
    v. angle
    v. flap
    v. osteotomy
Vistacon
Vistaject-25
Vistaject-50
Vistaquel
Vistaril
Vistazine
Vistide
Visual
visual
    v. acuity
    v. agnosia
    v. alexia
    v. area
    V. Aural Digit Span Test (VADS)
    v. biofeedback
    v. closure
    v. cue
    v. discrimination
    v. figure-ground
    v. figure-ground discrimination
    v. hearing
    v. light-polymerized adhesive
    v. listening
    v. memory
    v. memory span
    v. method
    v. perception
    v. probe
    V. Reinforcement Audiometry
    v. training
visualized treatment objective (VTO)
visual-motor
    v.-m. coordination
    v.-m. function
visual-spatial impairment
Visual-Tactile System of Phonetic
  Symbolization
visual-verbal agnosia
Vita-C
Vitacide
vitae
    arbor v.
vital
    v. capacity (VC)
    v. pulp
    v. root
    v. staining of teeth
    v. tooth

vitality
    pulp v.
    v. test
Vitallium
    V. alloy
    V. device
vitalometer
    Burton v.
vitalometry
vitamin
    v. A, B deficiency
    v. A and vitamin D
    v. C facial lotion
    v. E
    v. K
Vitapulp pulp tester
Vitec
Vite E Creme
Vitek interpositional implant
Vitek-Kent
    V.-K. hemi TMJ replacement
    system
    V.-K. total TMJ replacement
    system
Vitex agnus-castus
vitiligo
Vitrasert
vitrea
    substantia v.
Vitrebond cement
Vitremer glass-ionomer restorative
  material
vitreodentin
vitreous cavity
vitrification
Viva-Drops Solution
VK
    Robicillin VK
V-LACE real-time digital video
  enhancement
V-Lok disposable blood pressure cuff
VME
    vertical maxillary excess
V-MI
    Volpe-Manhold Index
VN
    vestibular neurectomy
VNO
    vomeronasal organ
vocabulary
    core v.
    expressive v.
    receptive v.
Vocabulary Comprehension Scale
vocal
    v. abuse
    v. attack
    v. band

v. capability battery
v. constriction
v. cord
v. cord bowing
v. cord injection
v. cord medialization
v. cord nodule
v. cord paralysis
v. efficiency
v. effort
v. fatigue
v. focus
v. fold
v. fold approximation
v. fold augmentation
v. fold paralysis
v. fry
v. ligament
v. misuse
v. mode
v. muscle
v. nodule
v. organ
v. phonics
v. play
v. polyp
v. polyposis
V. Profiles Analysis (VPA)
v. range
v. register
v. rehabilitation
v. resonance
v. tract
v. tremor

vocalic
v. glide

vocalis
v. muscle
sulcus v.

vocalization
prelinguistic v.

vocalized pause

voice
active v.
adolescent v.
alaryngeal v.
breathy v.
v. building
chest v.
v. clinician
v. disorder
v. disorders of phonation

v. disorders of resonance
v. dysfunction
epigastric v.
esophageal v.
eunuchoid v.
falsetto v.
v. fatigue
v. fatigue syndrome
gravel v.
guttural v.
v. handicap
V. Handicap Index (VHI)
v. handicap score
hot potato v.
hyperfunctional v.
inspiratory v.
light v.
male soprano v.
modal v.
muffled v.
mutation v.
myxedema v.
v. onset time (VOT)
passive v.
v. pathologist
v. prosthesis
v. prosthesis sizer
pulsated v.
v. register
v. rehabilitation
V. restoration system
rough v.
v. satisfaction
v. shift
sigh v.
v. signal type
soprano v.
v. termination time (VTT)
v. therapist
v. therapy
v. tone focus
transsexual v.
two-toned v.

voiced consonant
voiceless
v. consonant

voicelessness
degree of v. (DUV)

voice-preserving procedure
voicing
consonant v.
v. distinction

NOTES

void
> socket v.

volar
> v. flap advancement
> v. tissue flap

volition
> v. oral movement

Volkmann ischemic contracture
volley theory
Volpe-Manhold Index (V-MI)
volt (V)
voltage (V)
> v. peak (Vp)

voltaic taste
voltaism
Voltaren
> V. Ophthalmic
> V. Oral
> V.-XR Oral

Voltolini disease
volume
> v. control
> v. deficient face
> expiratory reserve v. (ERV)
> forced expiratory v. (FEV)
> inspiratory reserve v. (IRV)
> lung v.
> nasal v.
> residual v. (RV)
> respiratory v.
> tidal v. (TV, V$_T$)
> v. unit meter (VU meter)

volumetric dimensional change
voluntary
> v. interincisal opening
> v. mutism

Voluvision three dimensional ultrasonography
vomer
> v. flap
> v. mucosa

vomeronasal
> v. cartilage
> v. organ (VNO)

vomeropremaxillary crest
vomerosphenoidal articulation
vomiting reflex
von
> v. Ebner line
> v. Frisch bacillus
> V. Ihring plane
> v. Kossa-positive zone
> v. Kossa reaction
> v. Koss method
> v. Langenbeck bipedicle mucoperiosteal flap
> v. Langenbeck palatal closure
> v. Langenbeck palatal flap
> v. Langenbeck pedicle flap
> v. Langenbeck repair
> v. Meyenburg disease
> v. Recklinghausen disease
> v. Recklinghausen neurofibromatosis
> v. Spee curve

von Ebner (*var. of* Ebner)
von Frey (*var. of* Frey)
Vontrol
VOR
> vestibulo-ocular reflex

VōSol HC Otic
VOT
> voice onset time

vowel
> back v.
> cardinal v.
> central v.
> close v.
> v. error
> front v.
> high v.
> indefinite v.
> interconsonantal v.
> lax v.
> light v.
> low v.
> mid v.
> narrow v.
> nasal v.
> nasalization of v.
> neutral v.
> v. neutralization
> obscure v.
> open v.
> postconsonantal v.
> preconsonantal v.
> pure v.
> v. quadrilateral
> retroflex v.
> rhotacized v.
> rounded v.
> tense v.
> unrounded v.
> unstressed v.

vowel-consonant (V-C)
vowelization
vowel-to-consonant babble
vox
VP16-213
Vp
> voltage peak

VPA
> Vocal Profiles Analysis
> VPA protocol

VPAP
> variable positive airway pressure

VPC
    velopharyngeal competence
VPI
    velopharyngeal incompetence
    velopharyngeal insufficiency
VS
    vestibular schwannoma
    videostroboscopy
V-shaped
    V.-s. arch
    V.-s. erosion
    V.-s. skin excision
V̄ol Otic
VSS
    videofluoroscopic swallow study
VTO
    visualized treatment objective
VTT
    voice termination time
V-tunnel
    V.-t. drill procedure
    V.-t. guide
vu
    déjà v.
vulcanite
    v. file
    v. stomatitis
vulcanize
vulcanized
    heat temperature v. (HTV)
    room temperature v. (RTV)

vulgaris
    lupus v.
    pemphigus v.
    Proteus v.
    verruca v.
vulneris
    Escherichia v.
vulvovaginal reconstruction
vulvovaginoplasty
VU meter
Vumon Injection
VVA
    venous-to-venous anastomosis
V-Y
    V.-Y. advancement
    V.-Y. advancement for columellar
    lengthening
    V.-Y. closure
    V.-Y. lip roll mucosal advancement
    V.-Y. mucosal flap
    V.-Y. plasty
    V.-Y. procedure
    V.-Y. pushback
    V.-Y. pushback procedure
    V.-Y. repair
    V.-Y. transposition flap
Vytone Topical

NOTES

V

W

W arch
W procedure
W-1/W-2 Auditory Test
W-22 Auditory Test
Waardenburg-Klein syndrome
Waardenburg syndrome
WAB

Western Aphasia Battery
W-abdominoplasty
Wach

W. paste
W. paste sealer
wafer

acrylic bite w.
Wagner-Baldwin technique
WAIS

Wechsler Adult Intelligence Scale
Wakai spreader
Walden-Aufrecht nasal retractor
Waldenström macroglobulinemia
Waldeyer ring
Walker

W. appliance
W. articulator
walking bleach
Walkman

Sony professional W. WM-D6C
wall

axial w.
axial w. of the pulp chambers
cavity w.
chest w.
dentinal w.
enamel w.
gingival cavity w.
incisal w.
infratemporal w.
w. ledging
peripheral cavity w.
perpendicular anterior w.
pharyngeal w.
pocket w.
pulpal w.
subpulpal w.
surrounding w.
Wallenberg syndrome
wallerian degeneration
Wallstent expanding metallic stent
walnut

black w.
Walsh-Ogura

W.-O. technique
W.-O. transantral approach

waltzed flap
wand

ISG Viewing w.
wandering

pathologic tooth w.
w. rash
w. tooth
warble tone
Wardill

W. pharyngoplasty
W. technique
Wardill-Kilner

W.-K. four-flap uranoplasty
W.-K. procedure
W.-K. V-Y palatal repair
Ward Tempak
warfarin

w.-induced necrosis
w. ingestion
warm

w. condensation
w. gutta-percha
warm-wire anemometer
warp

lateral w.
wart

venereal w.'s
Warthin

W. area
W. tumor
Warthin-Starry staining method
Wart-Off
warty dyskeratoma
wash

w. impression
w. impression material
pHisoHex facial w.
w. technique
washed-field

w.-f. dentistry
w.-f. technique
washer

anchor w.
biconcave w.
Salzburg biconcave w.
washing process
Washington Speech Sound Discrimination Test
Washio flap
washout

abdominal w.
wasp

paper w.
Wassmund procedure

wastage
    air w.

waste
    contaminated w.
    hazardous w.
    infectious w.
    medical w.
    regulated w.
    toxic w.

wasting
    tooth w.

water
    w. moccasin
    w. sorption
    w. sorption/desorption method
    w. syringe

water-based disinfectant

waterfall curve

watermelon

water-powder ratio

Waters
    W. extraoral radiography
    W. view
    W. view radiograph
    W. view roentgenogram

watertight
    w. closure
    w. skin closure

water-turbine handpiece

Watson
    W. duckbill forceps
    W. scaphoid shift test

watt

wave
    alpha w.
    aperiodic w.
    beta w.
    complex w.
    cosine w.
    damped w.
    delta w.
    diffracted w.
    electromagnetic w.
    w. filter
    incident w.
    Jewett w.
    longitudinal w.
    nonperiodic w.
    notched w.
    periodic w.
    pure w.
    reflected w.
    refracted w.
    simple w.
    sine w.
    sinusoidal w.
    sonic w.
    sound w.

    sound pressure w.
    standing w.
    supersonic w.
    theta w.
    torsional w.
    transverse w.
    triangular w.

waveform
    w. distortion
    glottal w.

wavelength

waveshape

Wavicide-01

wax
    adhesive w.
    barnsdahl w.
    baseplate w.
    w. bite
    bite registration w.
    block-out w.
    bone w.
    boxing w.
    Brazil w.
    burnout w.
    w. burnout
    candelilla w.
    carding w.
    carnauba w.
    w. carver
    casting w.
    corrective impression w.
    w. curette
    dental w.
    dental inlay w.
    dental inlay casting w.
    ear w.
    earth w.
    w. elimination
    elimination w.
    w. expansion
    fluid w.
    fluxed w.
    w. form
    Horsley bone w.
    hydrocarbon w.
    impression w.
    w. impression
    inlay casting w.
    inlay pattern w.
    Kerr hard w.
    Kerr regular w.
    lignite w.
    lost w.
    microcrystalline w.
    mineral w.
    model denture w.
    w. model denture
    montan w.

mouth denture w.
w. myrlte
w. out
w. pack
paraffin w.
pattern w.
w. pattern
w. pattern thermal expansion
  technique
Peck purple hard w.
plant w.
processing w.
setup w.
w. shrinkage
sticky w.
w. swager
w. template
w. trimmer
try-in w.
utility w.
vegetable w.
white w.
yellow w.

WaxBuster wax remover
waxing, waxing up
w. die

w/C
Aprodine w/C

WCB
Workers' Compensation Board

w/Codeine
Allerfrin w.
Bromphen DC w.
Soma Compound w.

WCS-90
Clorpactin WCS-90

WDRC
wide dynamic range compression

weak
w. contact
w. stress
w. syllable deletion

weakness
w. of pressure consonant
unilateral w.

wear
abnormal occlusal w.
compensatory w.
Design Veronique compression w.
interproximal w.
occlusal w.
w. pattern

physiologic w.
Rainey Ultra-Flex compression w.
tooth w.

weaver's cough
web
esophageal w.
laryngeal w.
myringeal w.
w. space
w. space deepening
w. space flap
terminal w.
tracheal w.
vestibular w.

webbing
Weber
W. audiometry
W. gland
W. lateralizing
W. score
W. test
W. test for hearing

Weber-Cockayne syndrome
Weber-Ferguson
W.-F. incision
W.-F. method
W.-F. procedure

Webster needle holder
Wechsler
W. Adult Intelligence Scale
  (WAIS)
W. Intelligence Scale for Children-
  Revised (WISC-R)
W. Preschool and Primary Scale
  of Intelligence (WPPSI)

Wedelstaedt chisel
wedge
dental w.
w. elevator
light-reflecting w.
Medpor Biomaterial w.
plastic w.
w. and post forceps
step-w.
wooden w.

wedge-shaped erosion
wedging
w. effect

weed
careless w.
poverty w.
Western water hemp w.

NOTES

W

weeping
    w. case
    w. fig
    w. willow
Weerda distending operating laryngoscope
Wegener granulomatosis
weight-bearing tissue
weight loss
Weil
    W. basal layer
    W. basal zone
Weimert epistaxis packing
Weine technique
Weir technique
Weiss
    W. Comprehensive Articulation Test
    W. Intelligibility Test
Weitlaner retractor
Welch
    W. Allyn LumiView portable binocular microscope
    W. Allyn Solarc headlight
weld
welded inlay impression
welding
    arc w.
    cold w.
    fusion w.
    gas w.
    laser w.
    pressure w.
    resistance w.
    spot w.
well-differentiated carcinoma
wellness
    Ayurvedic total w.
wen
Werdnig-Hoffman disease
Wernicke
    W. aphasia
    W. area
Westcort
Western
    W. Aphasia Battery (WAB)
    W. blot test
    W. juniper
    W. ragweed
    W. water hemp weed
Westmore model
Weston crown
wet
    w. hoarseness
    w. strength
    w. technique
    w. vermilion
wettability
wetting
    w. agent
    w. solution

wet-to-dry dressing
Wever-Bray
    W.-B. effect
    W.-B. phenomenon
Weyers-Fülling syndrome
Weyers syndrome
W&H
    W&H Endodontic Contra Angle
    W&H handpiece
    W&H surgical system
Whaledent Parapost
Wharton duct
wheal
    skin w.
wheat
    w. grain dust mite
    whole w.
wheel
    bristle w.
    w. bur
    Burlew w.
    carborundum w.
    color w.
    diamond w.
    dry felt w.
    felt w.
    grinding w.
    leather w.
    rag w.
    rubber w.
    w. stone
    wire w.
wheeling
    rubber w.
wheeze
    asthmatoid w.
Whip-Mix
    W.-M. articulator
    W.-M. Die-Rock dental stone
    W.-M. Microstone dental stone
    W.-M. Quickstone dental stone
    W.-M. Silky-Rock dental stone
whipping condensation
Whirl-a-Dent denture cleanser
whirlybird
whisper
    buccal w.
    forced w.
    soft w.
    stage w.
whispering
    involuntary w.
whistle
    Galton w.
whistling
    w. deformity

White
    W. tenaculum
white
    w. ash
    w. burrobrush
    w. dural fold
    egg w.
    w. enamel
    w. folded gingivostomatitis
    w. gold
    w. gold alloy
    w. graft
    w. hairy tongue
    w. mouth
    w. mulberry
    w. noise
    w. oak antigen
    w. pine
    w. point
    w. poplar
    w. potato
    w. sponge lesion of Cannon
    w. sponge nevus
    w. stone
    w. wax
white-faced hornet
whitegraft reaction
white-spot lesion
whiting
Whitlockite crystal
whitlow
    W. and Constable alar cartilage
      correction
    herpetic w.
    melanotic w.
Whitnall tubercle
whole
    w. body radiation
    w. wheat
whoop
WHO probe
Whorf hypothesis
whorfian hypothesis
whorled
    w. cellular pattern
    w. enamel
WHS
    Wolf-Hirschhorn syndrome
WIC
    Women, Infants, and Children
wick
    Pope w.

wide
    w. decompression
    w. dynamic range compression
      (WDRC)
    w. excision
    w. jaw
    w. range audiometer
    w. resection biopsy
    w. sigmoid sinus
    w. tooth
wide-band noise
wide-field total laryngectomy
widener
    orifice w.
Widex listening device
Widman flap
width
    anterior arch w.
    apical w.
    arch w.
    bicanine w.
    bimolar w.
    biologic w.
    bitemporal w.
    buccopalatal w.
    mesiodistal w.
    physiognomic w.
    posterior arch w.
Wieder retractor
Wigraine
wild
    w. cherry
    W. operating microscope
    w. rye grass
    w. tobacco
Wildcat wire
Wilde
    W. ethmoid forceps
    W. triangle
Wildermuth ear
Wildervanck-Smith syndrome
Wildervanck syndrome
Wilkes
    W. stage I–V
Wilkinson dental casting gold alloy
Williams
    W. gold wire alloy
    W. periodontal probe
    W. surveyor
Willi glass crown technique

NOTES

W

Willis
    circle of W.
    W. paracusis
willisiana
willow
    weeping w.
Wilson
    W. bimetric arch
    W. curve
    W. Mayo stand
window
    bone w.
    cochlear w.
    w. crown
    epineural w.
    lung w.
    nasoantral w.
    neo-round w.
    oval w.
    round w.
    soft tissue w.
    w. technique
    vestibular w.
windpipe
wing
    maxillary surface of great w.
    nasal w.
    w. plate
    w. scaler
    temporal surface of great w.
winged incisor
Wing symbol
Winkler disease
Winter
    W. arch bar
    W. classification
WIPI
    Word Intelligibility by Picture
    Identification
wire
    arch w.
    w. arch
    Australian Special Plus w.
    auxiliary w.
    braided w.
    brass w.
    circumdentinal w.
    Coffin-type transpalatal w.
    continuous loop w.
    w. cutter
    diagnostic w.
    double keyhole loop w.
    w. fixation
    flexible spiral w. (FSW)
    Force w.
    Gilmer w.
    House w.

    interdental w.
    interosseous w.
    intraoral w.
    Ivy w.
    J w.
    Jelenko super w.
    Kirschner w.
    labial w.
    ligature tie w.
    lingual w.
    w. loop/gelatin sponge technique
    measuring w.
    Mowrey 12% w.
    Mowrey No. 1 w.
    w. nipper
    orthodontic w.
    w. osteosynthesis
    Quadcat w.
    rectangular w.
    w. removal
    Respond w.
    Risdon w.
    sectional arch w.
    separating w.
    silver w.
    space-age w.
    w. splint
    square w.
    torque w.
    Truarch w.
    twin w.
    w. wheel
    Wildcat w.
    wrought w.
wire-bending pliers
wire-gelatin technique
wire-Gelfoam prosthesis
wireloop/Gelfoam construction
wire-vein prosthesis
wiring
    Baudens w.
    Black w.
    circumferential w.
    circummandibular w.
    circumzygomatic w.
    continuous loop w.
    craniofacial suspension w.
    Gilmer w.
    interosseous w.
    Ivy loop w.
    mandibular w.
    multiple loop w.
    perialveolar w.
    pyriform aperture w.
    Stout continuous w.
Wironium casting alloy
Wiron S crown and bridge alloy

WISC-R
> Wechsler Intelligence Scale for Children-Revised

wisdom
> w. tooth
> W. toothbrush

Wise
> W. pattern
> W. pattern mastopexy

witch's
> w. chin
> w. chin deformity

Witkop-von Sallman syndrome
Wits appraisal
Wizard frame
Wohlfart-Kugelberg-Welander disease
Wolf
> W. equipment
> W. suction tube

Wolfe
> W. graft
> W. method

Wolfe-Krause graft
Wolf-Hirschhorn syndrome (WHS)
wolf tooth
Wolinella recta
women
> Rogaine for W.

Women, Infants, and Children (WIC)
wood
> w. block
> orange w.
> w. point

Woodcock Language Proficiency Battery, English Form
wooden wedge
Woodson No. 1 elevator
Wookey flap
wool
word
> ambiguous w.
> w. approximation
> base w.
> w. blindness
> w. calling
> class w.
> w. class
> clipped w.
> complex w.
> compound w.
> w. configuration
> content w.

contentive w.
w. count
w. deafness
w. discrimination score
feared w.
first w.
form w.
function w.
giant w.
heterogeneous w.
homogenous w.
W. Intelligibility by Picture Identification (WIPI)
interstitial w.
Jonah w.
lexical w.
monosyllabic w.
nonsense w.
open w.
paradigmatic w.
PB w.
phonetically balanced w.
pivot w.
polysyllabic w.
portmanteau w.
probe w.
relational w.
root w.
w. sequence
sign w.
simple w.
split w.
spondee w.
standard w.
structure w.
syntagmatic w.
telescoped w.
W. Test

word-finding
> w.-f. difficulty
> w.-f. problem

worker's compensation
Workers' Compensation Board (WCB)
working
> w. bite
> w. bite relation
> w. cast
> w. contact
> w. memory
> w. occlusal surface
> w. occlusion
> w. path

NOTES

W

working *(continued)*
    w. radiograph
    w. side
    w. side condyle
workstation
    Endoplan w.
    LySonix 250 operative w.
worm
    blood w.
worm-eaten appearance
worm's-eye
    w.-e. view
wormwood
wort
    St. John's w.
wound
    w. approximation
    w. botulism
    w. care
    w. dehiscence
    w. excision
    factitious w.
    w. fibroblast
    full-jacketed bullet w.
    gunshot w. (GSW)
    high-energy gunshot w.
    high-velocity gunshot w.
    w. incision and suction
    w. infection
    lacerated w.
    w. matrix contraction
    missile-caused w.
    Mohs w.
    w. necrosis
    nonhealing w.
    penetrating w.
    puncture w.
    sacral w.
    septic w.
    silicone-treated w.
    surgical w.
    w. tensile strength
woven bone
W-plasty
WPPSI
    Wechsler Preschool and Primary Scale of
    Intelligence

W-P ratio
wrap
    Ace w.
    Coban w.
wraparound
    w. periapical lesion
wrap-around flap
wrapper
    opaque waterproof w.
wrench
    DynaTorq w.
    tightening w.
    torque w.
    torque ratchet w.
Wrightington wrist radiograph stage 1, 2, 3, 4
wrinkle
    frontoglabella w.
    glabellar w.
    periorbital w.
    radial w.
wrinkled tongue
wrinkling
    forehead w.
    perioral w.
Wrisberg
    W. cartilage
    cuneiform cartilage of W.
wrist ganglionectomy
wristlet
writer
    cusp w.
written language
written-like language form
wrought
    w. clasp
    w. metal
    w. wire
Würzburg
    W. fracture system
    W. maxillofacial plating system
    W. reconstruction system
Wyamine
Wycillin
Wydase Injection
Wygesic
Wymox

X
X paralysis
X-12 alloy
X-act cutaneous x-ray marker
X-Acto
X.-A. blade
X.-A. gouge
Xalatan
Xanax
xanthelasma
xanthine
x. oxidase
xanthodont
xanthodontus
xanthogranuloma
juvenile x.
xanthoma
x. tuberosum
verruciform x.
verrucous x.
xanthomatosis
Xantopren impression material
X-bite
xenogeneic bone
xenograft
porcine x.
x. wound covering
xenon light source
xenophonia
xerochilia
xeroderma
x. pigmentosum
Xeroform gauze
xerogram
xerography
xeromammogram
xeromycteria
xeronosus
xerophthalmia
xeroradiogram
xeroradiography
xerosis
xerostomia
postradiation x.
xerostomic mucositis
xerotic
x. keratitis

Xerox dental radiographic imaging system
xiphisternum
xiphoid
XL
Lodine XL
X-linked
X.-l. albinism and sensorineural hearing loss
X.-l. deafness
X.-l. progressive mixed deafness with perilymphatic gusher (DFNX3)
Xomed plastic and rubber endotracheal tube
XP
Cophene XP
XP peritympanic hearing instrument
x radiation
x-ray
x.-r. absorption
x.-r. beam
x.-r. exposure guideline
x.-r. film
hard x.-r.
x.-r. image
x.-r. mount
real-time, low-intensity x.-r. (RTLX)
scattered x.-r.
serial cephalometric x.-r.
Siemens Orthoceph 10 x.-r.
soft x.-r.
x.-r. therapy (XRT)
x.-r. timer
x.-r. tube
XR primer
XRT
x-ray therapy
XT
Contuss XT
XX fine disk
xylene
Xylocaine
xylol
xylometazoline

675

Y

Y clasp arm
Y flap
Y incision
Yaeger plate
YAG

yttrium-aluminum-garnet
YAG laser
YAG laser stapedotomy
Yale-Brown Obsessive-Compulsive Scale
Yankauer

Y. suction
Y. tonsil suction tip
yarrow
Yashica Dental Eye II camera
yawn
yawning
yawn-sigh approach
yaws
Y-cord hearing aid
yeast
yellow

y. dock

y. hornet
y. jacket
y. mustard
y. wax
yes-no question
yield strength
yolk

egg y.
Youlten nasal inspiratory peak flow
meter
Young

Y. frame
Y. rubber dam holder
Youngblood natural mineral powder
Younger-Good

Y.-G. curette
Y.-G. scaler
Y-port connector
Y-shaped skin paddle
yttrium-aluminum-garnet (YAG)
Yudkoff-Okun periodontal instrument
set
Y-V flap

Z
 Z angle
 Z flap
 Z procedure
 Z spring
ZAAG
 Zest Anchor Advanced Generation
 ZAAG abutment
 ZAAG guide and pin
 ZAAG implant anchor
Zagam
Zantac
 Z. 75
Zapit
 Z. cement
 Z. resin
Zeasorb-AF Powder
Zefazone
Zeiss
 Z. index
 Z. microscope
 Z. operating microscope
 Z. osteotome
Zeiss/Jena surgical microscope
Zelco Flexlite
Zellballen
 Z. pattern
Zenker diverticulum
Zephiran
Zephrex
 Z. LA
Z-epicanthoplasty
zero
 z. amplitude
 audiometric z.
 z. hearing level
 z. morpheme
zero-degree teeth
Zest
 Z. Anchor Advanced Generation
  (ZAAG)
 Z. anchor system attachment
 Z. implant
 Z. implant anchor
Ziehl-Neelsen stain
zigzag
 z. incision
 z. method
Zilactin
 Z.-B
 Z.-B Medicated
 Z.-L
ZilaDent
Zimany bilobed flap

Zimmer
 Z. clip
 Z. Micro-E fixation drill
Zimmerman
 vascular pericyte of Z.
Zinacef
 Z. Injection
zinc
 z. acetate crystal
 z. carbonate
 z. eugenolate
 z. oxide
 z. oxide cement
 z. oxide, cod liver oil, and talc
 z. oxide-eugenol (ZOE, ZnOE)
 z. oxide-eugenol cement
 z. oxide-eugenol cement Type IV
 z. oxide-eugenol dental cement
 z. oxide-eugenol impression
  material
 z. oxide-eugenol impression paste
 z. oxide-eugenol sealer
 z. oxyphosphate cement
 z. phosphate cement
 z. polyacrylate cement
 z. polycarboxylate cement
 z. silicophosphate cement
 z. sulfate
zinc-free alloy
Zingiber officinalis
Zinsser-Engman-Cole syndrome
zip
 apical z.
 avoiding z.
 elbow z.
 z. foramen
 z. formation
zipped
 z. canal
zipper
 abdominal z.
 z. amalgam implant
 z. phenomenon
 synthetic z.
Zipperer finger plugger
zipping
Zircate paste
zirconium
 z. silicate ($ZrSiO_4$)
 z. silicate abrasive
Ziroxide prophylactic paste
**Zisser-Madden method upper lip
 reconstruction**
Zitelli bilobed nasal flap
Zithromax

679

Z-mammaplasty
ZMC
    zygomatic malar complex
    zygomatic maxillary complex
    zygomaticomaxillary complex
    ZMC fracture
Zocchi ultrasound-assisted lipoplasty technique
ZOE, ZnOE
    zinc oxide-eugenol
    ZOE sealer
Zolicef
Zomax
zomepirac
zona
    z. arcuata
    z. pellucida
Zonalon Topical Cream
zone
    apical z.
    basement membrane z.
    bilaminar z.
    calcification z.
    ceil-free z.
    cell-poor z.
    cell-rich z.
    central z.
    cervical z.
    clear z.
    contact area z.
    coronal z.
    degenerative z.
    dentinoblastic z.
    dentofacial z.
    exudative z.
    fatty z.
    gingival z.
    glandular z.
    granulomatous z.
    hyalinized z.
    inflammatory z.
    z. of injury
    intermediate z.
    intertubular z.
    marginal z.
    middle z.
    necrotic z.
    neutral z.
    pericemental z.
    Z. Periodontal Pak
    peritubular z.
    predentinal z.
    proliferation z.
    proliferative inflammatory z.
    z. of Ranvier
    reserve cell z.
    root exit z.
    Schreger z.

    z. of sharpness
    stippled z.'s
    subdentinoblastic z.
    subodontoblastic z.
    trigger z.
    von Kossa-positive z.
    Weil basal z.
zonula
    z. adherens
    z. occludens
zoograft
zoografting
zooplastic graft
zooplasty
ZORprin
zoster
    geniculate z.
    herpes z.
Zosyn
Zovirax
Zoysia grass
Z-pac
Z-plasty
    double opposing Z-p.
    Z-p. effect
    Furlow double opposing Z-p.
    Furlow double reversing Z-p.
    Z-p. procedure
    Straith Z-p.
    Z-p. technique
    Z-p. transposition
$ZrSiO_4$
    zirconium silicate
Zuckerkandl perforating canal
Zuker and Manktelow technique
Zydone
zygion
zygofrontal
zygoma
    tubercle of z.
    tubercle of root of z.
zygomal cell
zygomatic
    z. arch
    z. arch fracture
    z. arch radiograph
    z. bone
    z. branch
    z. breadth
    z. buttress
    z. complex fracture
    z. crest
    z. fissure
    z. foramen
    z. frontal nerve
    z. malar complex (ZMC)
    z. margin
    z. maxillary complex (ZMC)

z. maxillary complex fracture
z. muscle
z. osteomyelitis
z. process
z. process of frontal bone
z. process of maxilla
z. process of temporal bone
z. recess
z. tubercle
zygomatic-coronoid ankylosis
zygomatic maxillary complex (ZMC)
zygomaticofacial
z. canal
z. nerve
zygomaticofrontal
z. region
z. suture
zygomaticomandibular muscle
zygomaticomaxillary
z. buttress
z. complex (ZMC)
z. hypoplasia

z. osteotomy
z. region
z. suture
zygomatico-orbital
zygomaticotemporal
z. canal
z. nerve
z. space
z. suture
zygomaticus
arcus z.
z. major muscle
z. minor muscle
z. muscle
zygomaxillare
z. ridge
zygomaxillary
Zygomycetes
Zymafluor fluoride
Zymogen granule
Zyplast injectable collagen
Zyrtec

NOTES

Z

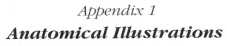

Appendix 1

Anatomical Illustrations

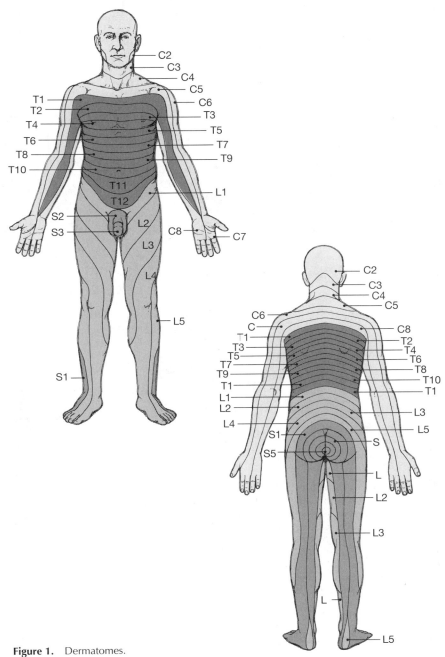

Figure 1. Dermatomes.

Anatomical Illustrations

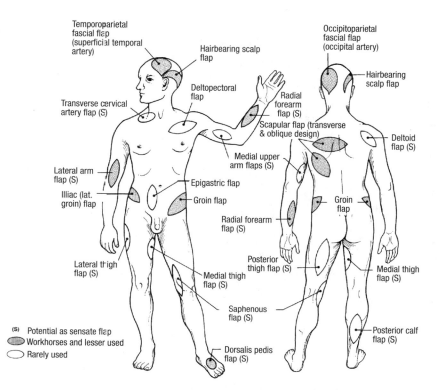

Figure 2. Cutaneous free flap donor site territories.

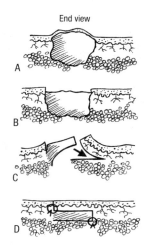

Figure 3. Buried dermal flap technique. **A,** A wide hypertrophic scar extends below the skin surface. **B,** Scar is deepithelialized, with removal of epidermis and a small amount of contiguous scar. **C,** Flap of scar "dermis" is elevated; opposing skin flap is elevated to accept the dermal flap. Deeper scar may be left, should be excised if too bulky. **D,** Flap of dermis (actually scar) is advanced under the skin. It is anchored at both sides with absorbable sutures. A running subcuticular suture can be used for the final skin layer.

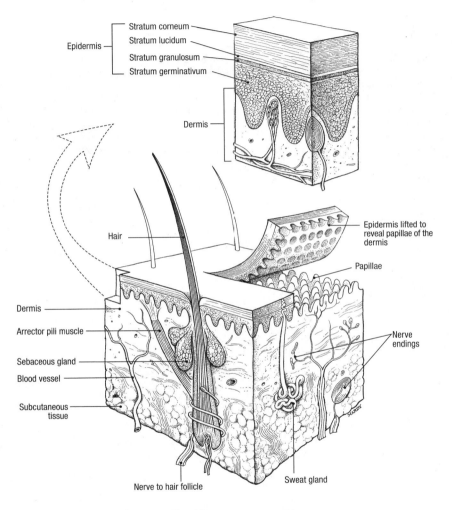

Figure 4. The skin components and layers.

Anatomical Illustrations

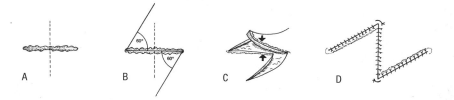

Figure 5. The classic Z-plasty. **A,** A thick, contracted scar crosses a skin fold. Design is begun by drawing a perpendicular line at the midpoint of the scar; this line helps establish flap incisions, but it is not itself incised. **B,** Completing the design, the limbs of flaps are equal to each other and to the length of the scar. Angles of the flaps are 60%. **C,** Flaps are elevated, preserving the subdermal plexus. Undermining is accomplished around flap bases. The scar is excised unless it is too wide; here a portion of scar is left for clarity in showing flap transposition. **D,** Flaps are transposed and sutured. A 3-corner suture (half- buried horizontal mattress) is used to anchor narrow tips, avoiding necrosis that could result from simple sutures near tips.

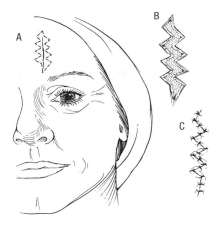

Figure 6. The W-plasty. **A,** Dotted lines show the design for the excision of the scar. **B,** Flaps have now been developed and are ready for interdigitation. The W-flaps are in position.

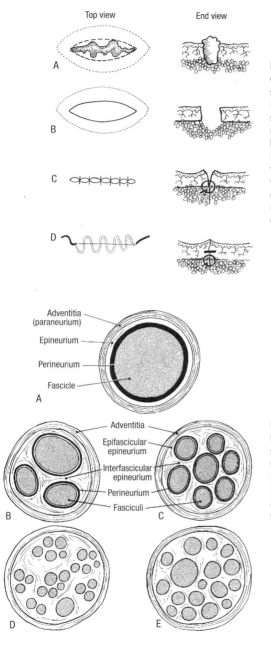

Top view   End view

A

B

C

D

Figure 7. Linear scar revision. **A,** Outline for planned repair. **B,** Excision and undermining. **C,** Deep layer closure. The end view (right) shows that the wound should be almost fully closed. **D,** Final closure, buried running subcuticular Prolene. The top view left shows suture weaving back and forth across wound in dermis, piercing the epidermis only at each end. The thickness of the suture is exaggerated for clarity.

Adventitia (paraneurium)

Epineurium

Perineurium

Fascicle

A

Adventitia

Epifascicular epineurium

Interfascicular epineurium

Perineurium

Fasciculi

B

C

D

E

Figure 8. Nerve repair, cross-section anatomy. **A,** Monofascicular structure. **B,** Oligofascicular structure, 2–5 fascicles. **C,** Oligofascicular structure, 6 or more fascicles. **D,** Polyfascicular structure, group arrangement. **E,** Polyfascicular structure, without group arrangement.

Anatomical Illustrations

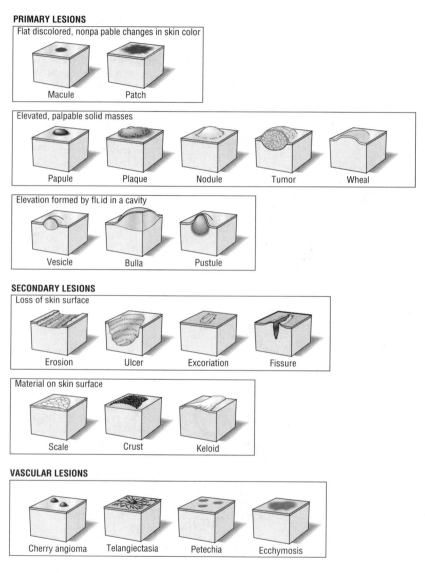

Figure 9. Lesions: types of primary, secondary, and vascular lesions.

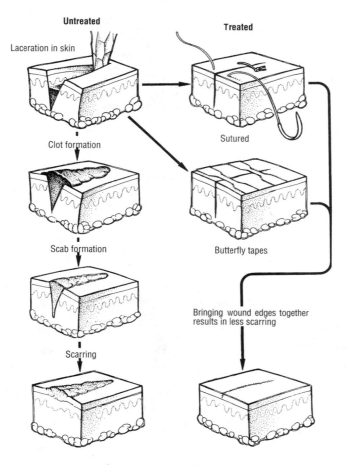

Figure 10. Wound healing.

Anatomical Illustrations

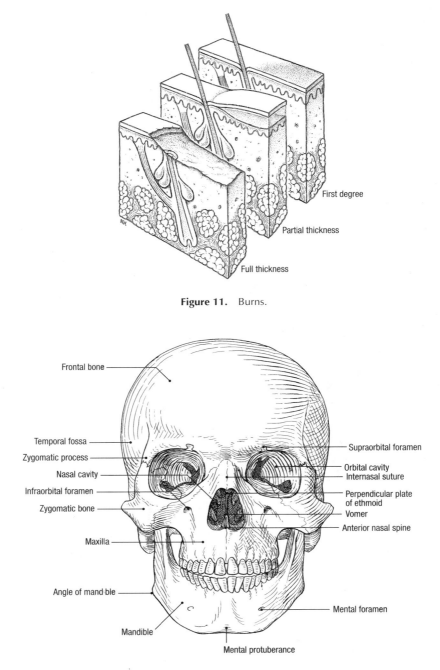

Figure 11. Burns.

First degree

Partial thickness

Full thickness

Frontal bone

Temporal fossa

Zygomatic process

Nasal cavity

Infraorbital foramen

Zygomatic bone

Maxilla

Angle of mand ble

Mandible

Mental protuberance

Supraorbital foramen

Orbital cavity
Internasal suture

Perpendicular plate
of ethmoid

Vomer

Anterior nasal spine

Mental foramen

Figure 12. Frontal view of skull.

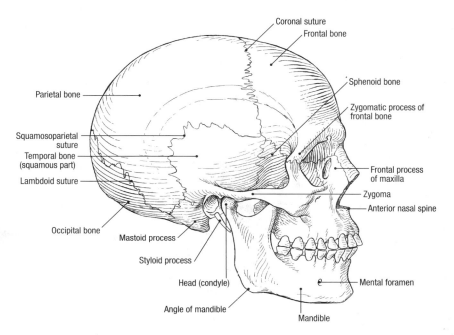

Figure 13. Lateral view of the skull.

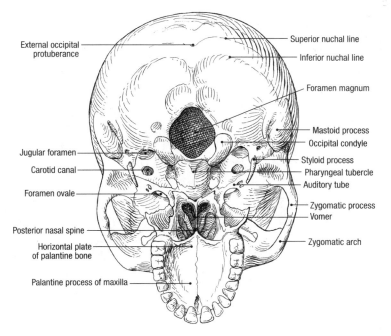

Figure 14. Base of the skull.

Anatomical Illustrations

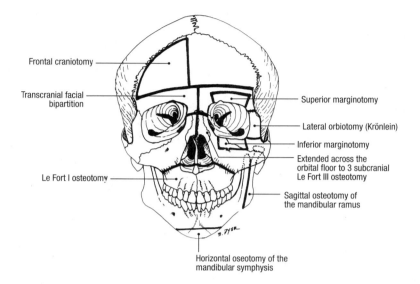

Figure 15. Commonly used access osteotomies: frontal craniotomy; superior marginotomy; lateral orbitotomy (Krönlein); inferior marginotomy; extended across the orbital floor to 3-subcranial Le Fort III osteotomy; Le Fort I osteotomy; sagittal osteotomy of the mandibular ramus; horizontal osteotomy of the mandibular symphysis; transcranial facial bipartition.

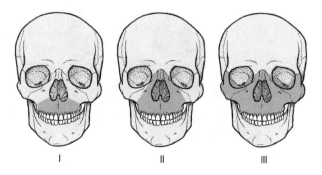

Figure 16. Le Fort fractures.

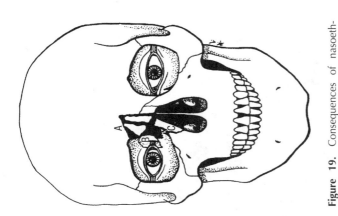

Figure 19. Consequences of nasoethmoidal fracture. **A,** Nasal dorsum, displacement into skull. **B,** Central segment, displacement into orbital rim. **C,** Circumscribed portion affecting lacrimal fossa and nasolacrimal duct.

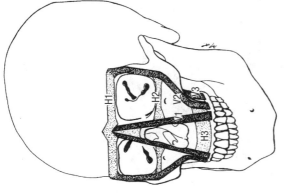

Figure 18. Facial fracture stabilization with buttresses. **V,** vertical buttress; **H,** horizontal buttress; **V₁,** nasomaxillary; **V₂,** zygomaticomaxillary; **V₃,** pterygomaxillary; **H₁,** supraorbital rim; **H₂,** infraorbital rim; **H₃,** nasal floor and palate.

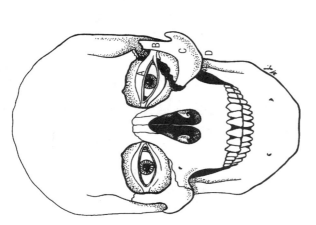

Figure 17. Fracture of zygoma. **A,** Globe of eye. **B,** Palpebral fissure. **C,** Malar prominence. **D,** Coronoid process.

Anatomical Illustrations

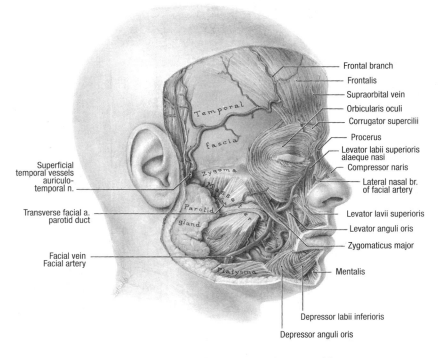

Figure 20.   Muscles of expression and arteries of face.

Frontal branch

Frontalis

Supraorbital vein

Orbicularis oculi

Corrugator supercilii

Procerus

Levator labii superioris alaeque nasi

Compressor naris

Lateral nasal br. of facial artery

Levator lavii superioris

Levator anguli oris

Zygomaticus major

Mentalis

Depressor labii inferioris

Depressor anguli oris

Superficial temporal vessels auriculo-temporal n.

Transverse facial a. parotid duct

Facial vein Facial artery

Temporal

fascia

Zygoma

Masseter

Parotid gland

Platysma

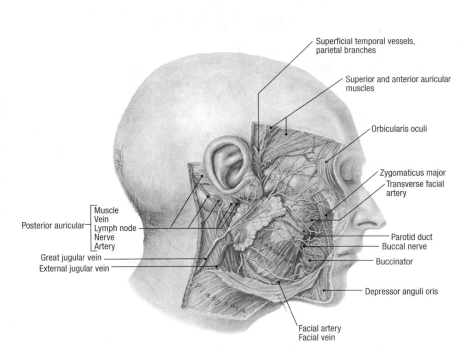

Superficial temporal vessels, parietal branches

Superior and anterior auricular muscles

Orbicularis oculi

Zygomaticus major
Transverse facial artery

Muscle
Vein
Posterior auricular — Lymph node
Nerve
Artery

Parotid duct
Buccal nerve

Great jugular vein
External jugular vein

Buccinator

Depressor anguli oris

Facial artery
Facial vein

Figure 21. Face: terminal branches of the facial nerve.

Anatomical Illustrations

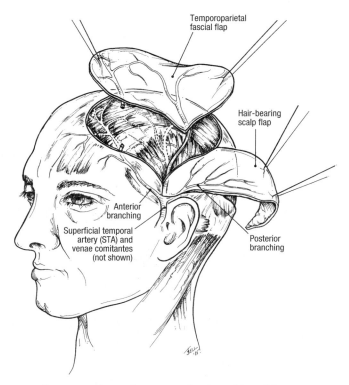

Figure 22. Surgical anatomy of scalp and fascial flap.

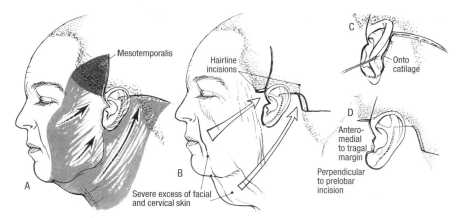

Figure 23. Classic face-lift incisions. **A,** Areas of incision. **B,** Hairline incisions. **C,** Postauricular incisions for redrape. **D,** Retrotragal approach for redrape.

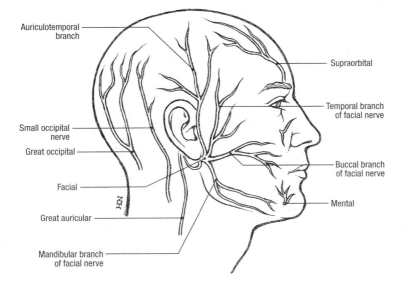

Figure 24. Nerve supply to the head and neck.

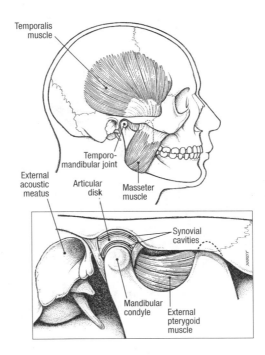

Figure 25. Temporomandibular joint.

Anatomical Illustrations

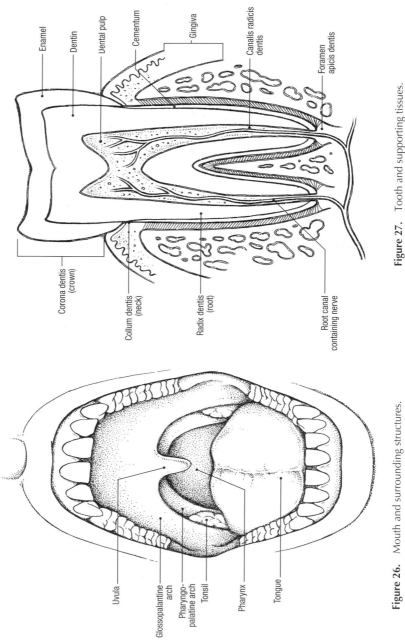

Enamel

Dentin

Dental pulp

Cementum

Gingiva

Canalis radicis dentis

Foramen apicis dentis

Corona dentis (crown)

Collum dentis (neck)

Radix dentis (root)

Root canal containing nerve

Figure 27. Tooth and supporting tissues.

Uvula

Glossopalantine arch

Pharyngo-palatine arch

Tonsil

Pharynx

Tongue

Figure 26. Mouth and surrounding structures.

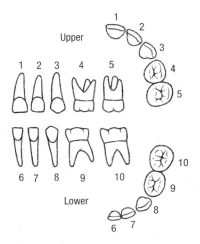

Figure 28. Deciduous dentition: (1, 6) central incisor; (2, 7) lateral incisor; (3, 8) canine; (4, 9) first molar; (5, 10) second molar.

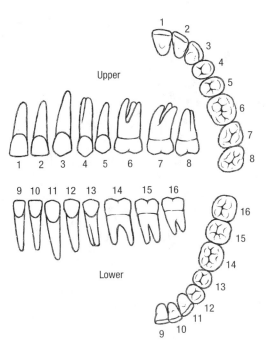

Figure 29. Permanent dentition: (1, 9) central incisor; (2, 10) lateral incisor; (3, 11) canine; (4, 12) first bicuspid; (5, 13) second bicuspid; (6, 14) first molar; (7, 15) second molar; (8, 16) third molar.

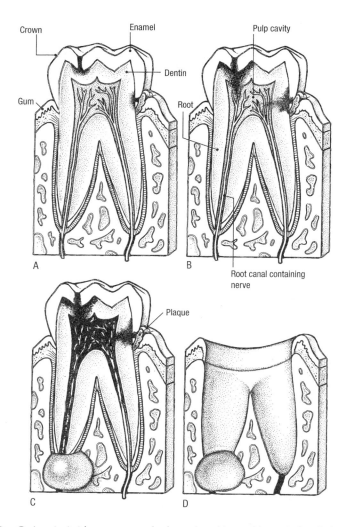

Figure 30. Caries: **A,** Acid, enzymes, or both produced by oral bacteria break down enamel to form cavities. **B,** Bacteria penetrate dentin to invade pulp cavity. **C,** Infection destroys pulp and extends through left root canal to cause periapical disease. **D,** Tooth has been lost, leaving periapical cyst on the left.

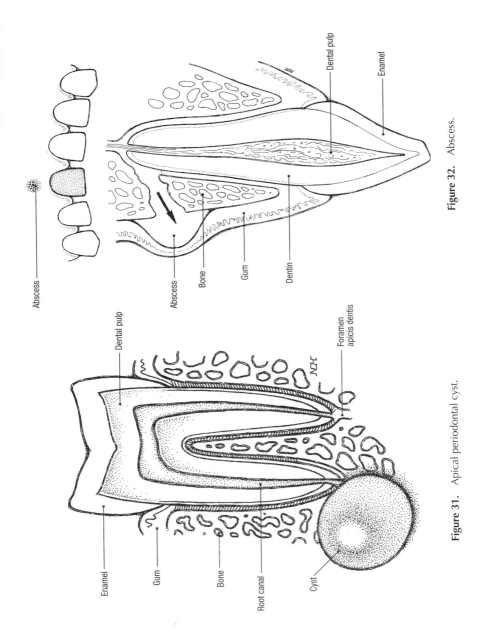

Abscess

Dental pulp

Enamel

Abscess

Bone

Gum

Dentin

Figure 32. Abscess.

Dental pulp

Foramen
apicis dentis

Enamel

Gum

Bone

Root canal

Cyst

Figure 31. Apical periodontal cyst.

Anatomical Illustrations

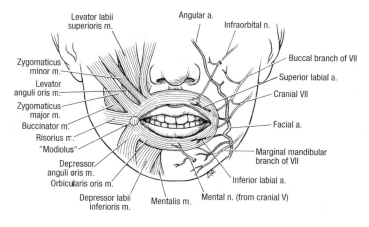

Figure 33. Anatomy of the lip.

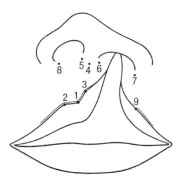

Figure 34. Anatomy of the normal and unrepaired unilateral cleft lip indicating key points used for planning repair: **1,** lowest point in arch of Cupid's bow, midline of the lip; **2,** peak of Cupid's bow on the noncleft side; **3,** proposed peak of Cupid's bow; **4,** midpoint of the columella; **5, 6,** base of columella laterally; **7, 8,** inset of alar base into nostril sill; **9,** a point on the well developed vermilion cutaneous roll of the lateral lip and the same horizontal plane as the peak of Cupid's bow on the noncleft side.

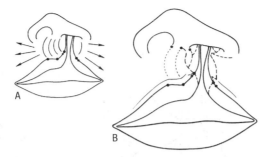

Figure 35. Cleft lip repair. **A,** Unrepaired cleft lip stresses. **B,** Incorporating stresses into repair.

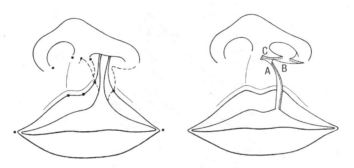

Figure 36. Rotation advancement flap technique. **A,** Medial lip element. **B,** Lateral lip element. **C,** Small medial flap.

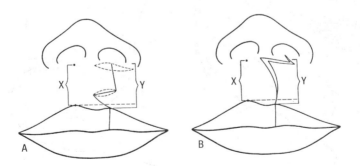

Figure 37. Cleft lip redo surgery. **A,** Previous triangular or quadrangular repair flap. **B,** rotation advancement flap redo technique.

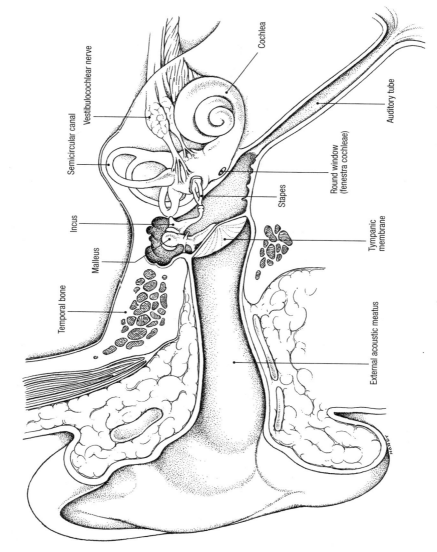

Figure 38. Ear.

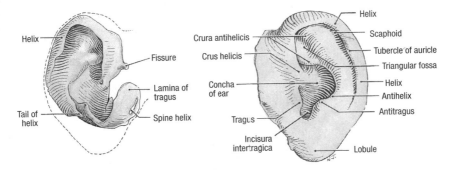

Figure 39. The auricle.

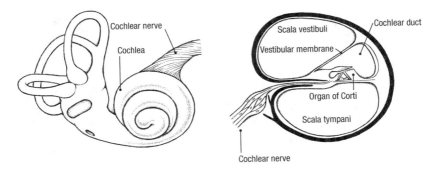

Figure 40. Cochlea, with cross section.

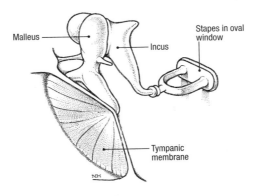

Figure 41. Auditory ossicles.

Anatomical Illustrations

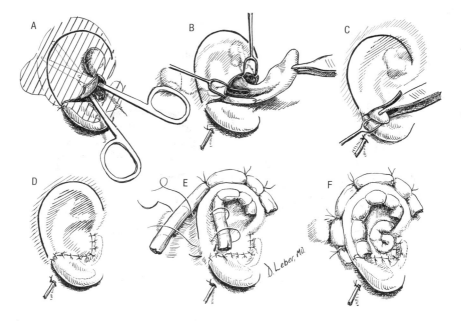

Figure 42. Otoplasty techniques. **A,** Preparing subcutaneous pocket. **B,** Placing cartilage graft material. **C,** Incorporating helix. **D,** Separate placement of tragal material. External sutures. **E,** Stent placement for external shaping. **F,** Conchal floor pressure dressing.

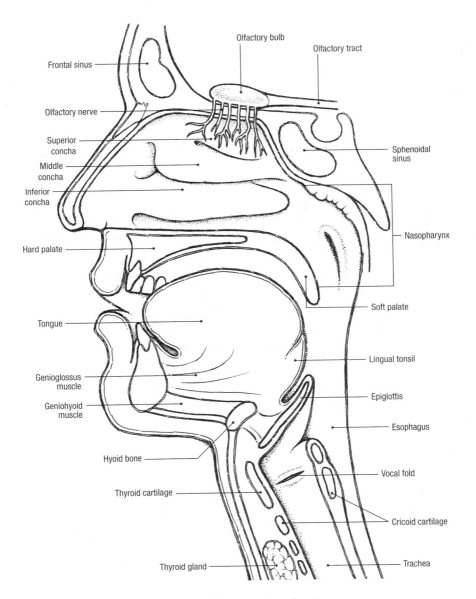

Figure 43. Pharynx and nasal cavity.

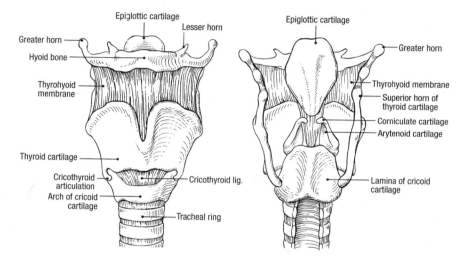

Figure 44. Anatomy of the larynx, anterior view (left) and posterior view (right).

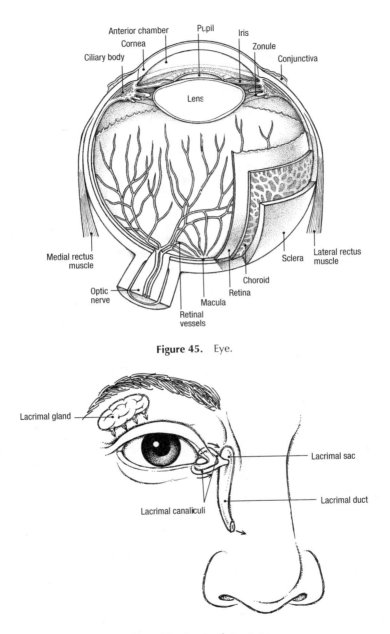

Figure 45. Eye.

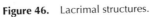

Figure 46. Lacrimal structures.

Anatomical Illustrations

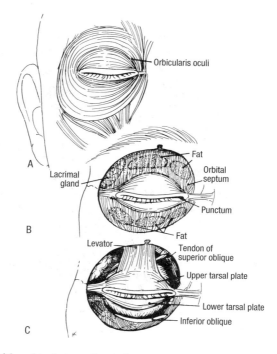

Figure 47. **A,** Extent of the orbicularis oculi muscle (eyelid sphincter). **B,** The fat compartments and the relationship of the lacrimal gland. **C,** The orbit, with only the superficial fat removed, reveals the superior oblique and inferior oblique tendons.

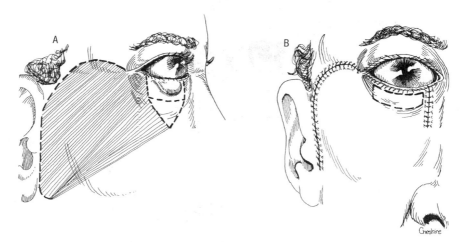

Figure 48. A Mustardé cheek flap may be used with a chondromucosal graft for reconstruction of large defects.

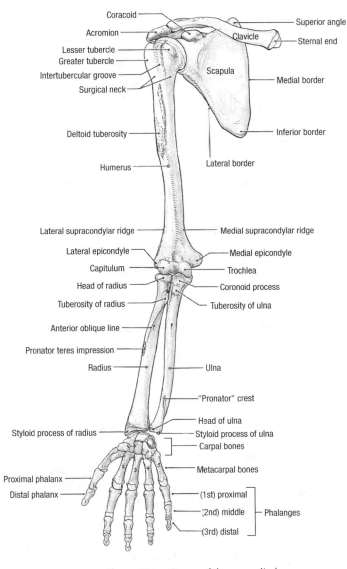

Figure 49A. Bones of the upper limb.

Anatomical Illustrations

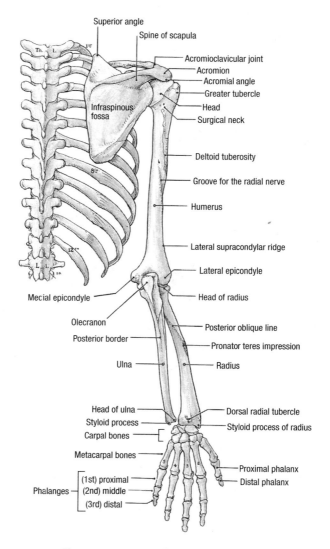

Figure 49B. Bones of the upper limb.

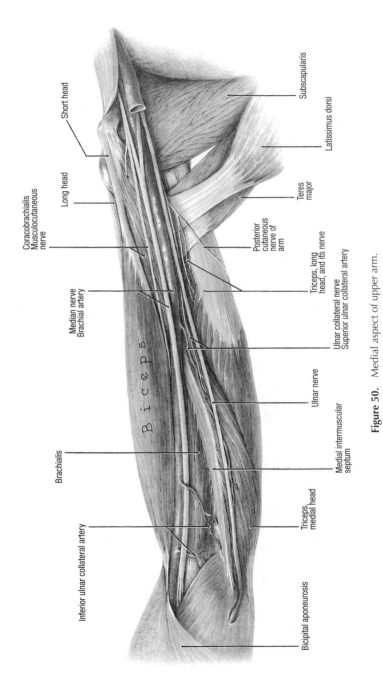

Short head

Long head

Coracobrachialis
Musculocutaneous
nerve

Median nerve
Brachial artery

Brachialis

Inferior ulnar collateral artery

Subscapularis

Latissimus dorsi

Teres
major

Posterior
cutaneous
nerve of
arm

Triceps, long
head, and its nerve

Ulnar collateral nerve
Superior ulnar collateral artery

Ulnar nerve

Medial intermuscular
septum

Triceps,
medial head

Bicipital aponeurosis

B i c e p s

Figure 50. Medial aspect of upper arm.

A31

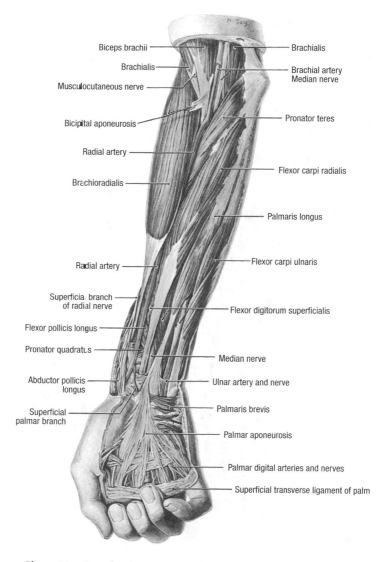

Biceps brachii

Brachialis

Musculocutaneous nerve

Bicipital aponeurosis

Radial artery

Brachioradialis

Radial artery

Superficial branch
of radial nerve

Flexor pollicis longus

Pronator quadratus

Abductor pollicis
longus

Superficial
palmar branch

Brachialis

Brachial artery
Median nerve

Pronator teres

Flexor carpi radialis

Palmaris longus

Flexor carpi ulnaris

Flexor digitorum superficialis

Median nerve

Ulnar artery and nerve

Palmaris brevis

Palmar aponeurosis

Palmar digital arteries and nerves

Superficial transverse ligament of palm

Figure 51. Superficial muscles of the forearm and palmar aponeurosis.

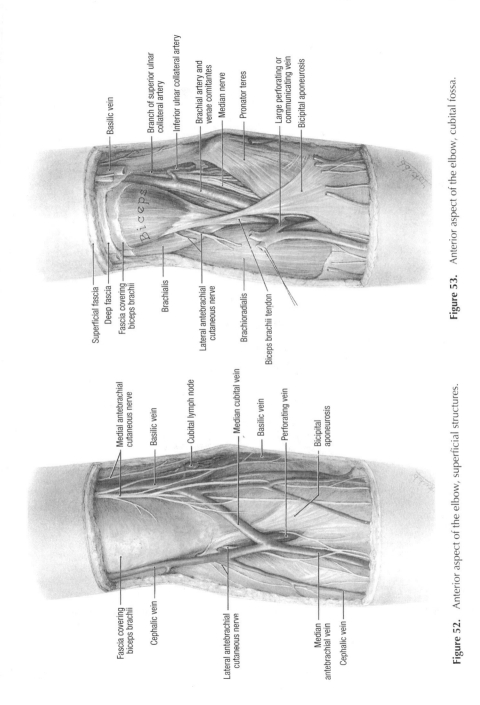

Figure 53. Anterior aspect of the elbow, cubital fossa.

Figure 52. Anterior aspect of the elbow, superficial structures.

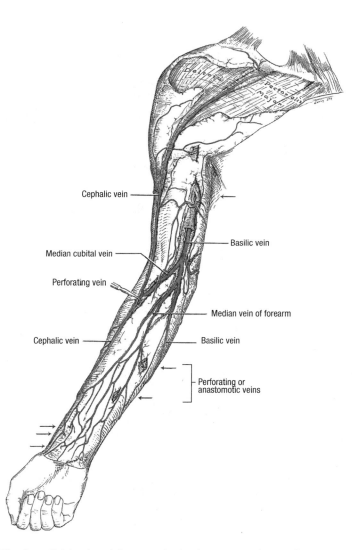

Cephalic vein

Median cubital vein

Perforating vein

Cephalic vein

Basilic vein

Median vein of forearm

Basilic vein

Perforating or anastomotic veins

Figure 54. Superficial veins of the upper limb. The arrows indicate where perforating veins pierce the deep fascia and bring the superficial and deep veins of the limb into communication with each other.

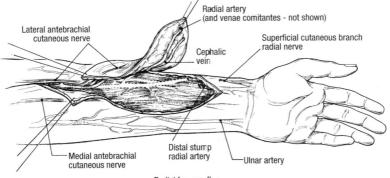

Radial artery
(and venae comitantes - not shown)

Lateral antebrachial
cutaneous nerve

Cephalic
vein

Superficial cutaneous branch
radial nerve

Medial antebrachial
cutaneous nerve

Distal stump
radial artery

Ulnar artery

Radial forearm flap

Figure 55. Surgical anatomy of the radial forearm flap.

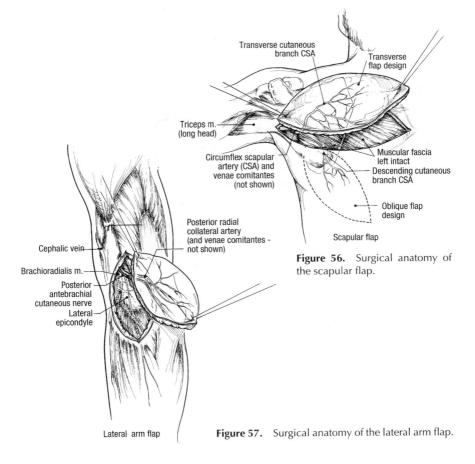

Transverse cutaneous
branch CSA

Transverse
flap design

Triceps m.
(long head)

Circumflex scapular
artery (CSA) and
venae comitantes
(not shown)

Muscular fascia
left intact

Descending cutaneous
branch CSA

Oblique flap
design

Scapular flap

Figure 56. Surgical anatomy of
the scapular flap.

Cephalic vein

Brachioradialis m.

Posterior
antebrachial
cutaneous nerve

Lateral
epicondyle

Posterior radial
collateral artery
(and venae comitantes -
not shown)

Lateral arm flap

Figure 57. Surgical anatomy of the lateral arm flap.

A35

Anatomical Illustrations

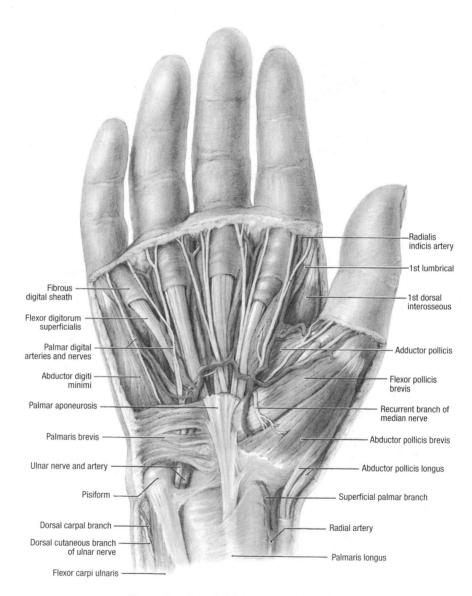

Radialis indicis artery

1st lumbrical

1st dorsal interosseous

Adductor pollicis

Flexor pollicis brevis

Recurrent branch of median nerve

Abductor pollicis brevis

Abductor pollicis longus

Superficial palmar branch

Radial artery

Palmaris longus

Fibrous digital sheath

Flexor digitorum superficialis

Palmar digital arteries and nerves

Abductor digiti minimi

Palmar aponeurosis

Palmaris brevis

Ulnar nerve and artery

Pisiform

Dorsal carpal branch

Dorsal cutaneous branch of ulnar nerve

Flexor carpi ulnaris

Figure 58. Superficial dissection of the palm.

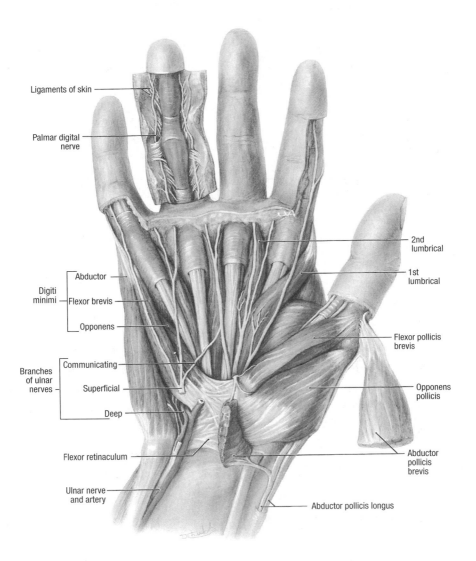

Ligaments of skin

Palmar digital
nerve

Abductor

Digiti
minimi — Flexor brevis

Opponens

Branches
of ulnar
nerves — Communicating

Superficial

Deep

Flexor retinaculum

Ulnar nerve
and artery

2nd
lumbrical

1st
lumbrical

Flexor pollicis
brevis

Opponens
pollicis

Abductor
pollicis
brevis

Abductor pollicis longus

Figure 59. Superficial dissection of the palm, ulnar and median nerves.

Anatomical Illustrations

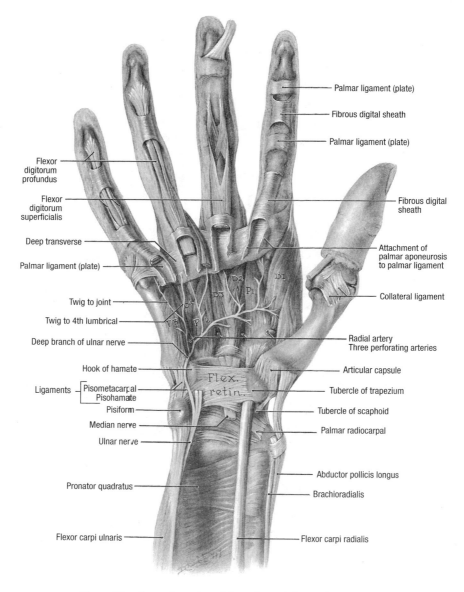

Palmar ligament (plate)

Fibrous digital sheath

Palmar ligament (plate)

Flexor digitorum profundus

Flexor digitorum superficialis

Deep transverse

Palmar ligament (plate)

Fibrous digital sheath

Attachment of palmar aponeurosis to palmar ligament

Twig to joint

Twig to 4th lumbrical

Deep branch of ulnar nerve

Collateral ligament

Radial artery
Three perforating arteries

Hook of hamate

Ligaments — Pisometacarpal
            Pisohamate

Pisiform

Median nerve

Ulnar nerve

Articular capsule

Tubercle of trapezium

Tubercle of scaphoid

Palmar radiocarpal

Pronator quadratus

Abductor pollicis longus

Brachioradialis

Flexor carpi ulnaris

Flexor carpi radialis

Figure 60. Deep dissection of the palm and digits, ulnar nerve.

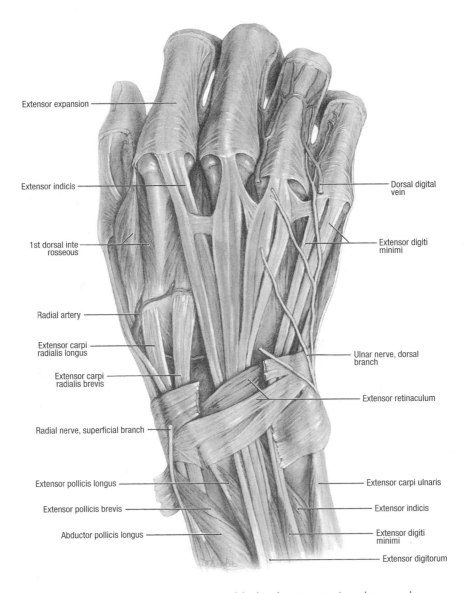

Extensor expansion

Extensor indicis

1st dorsal inte
rosseous

Radial artery

Extensor carpi
radialis longus

Extensor carpi
radialis brevis

Radial nerve, superficial branch

Extensor pollicis longus

Extensor pollicis brevis

Abductor pollicis longus

Dorsal digital
vein

Extensor digiti
minimi

Ulnar nerve, dorsal
branch

Extensor retinaculum

Extensor carpi ulnaris

Extensor indicis

Extensor digiti
minimi

Extensor digitorum

Figure 61. Tendons on the dorsum of the hand, extensor retinaculum muscle.

Anatomical Illustrations

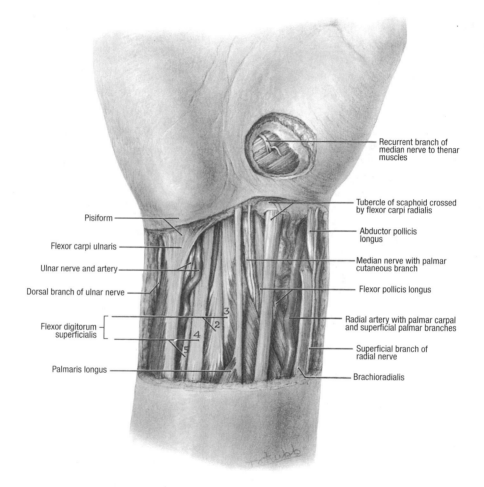

Figure 62. Structures of the anterior aspect of the wrist.

Recurrent branch of median nerve to thenar muscles

Tubercle of scaphoid crossed by flexor carpi radialis

Abductor pollicis longus

Median nerve with palmar cutaneous branch

Flexor pollicis longus

Radial artery with palmar carpal and superficial palmar branches

Superficial branch of radial nerve

Brachioradialis

Pisiform

Flexor carpi ulnaris

Ulnar nerve and artery

Dorsal branch of ulnar nerve

Flexor digitorum superficialis

Palmaris longus

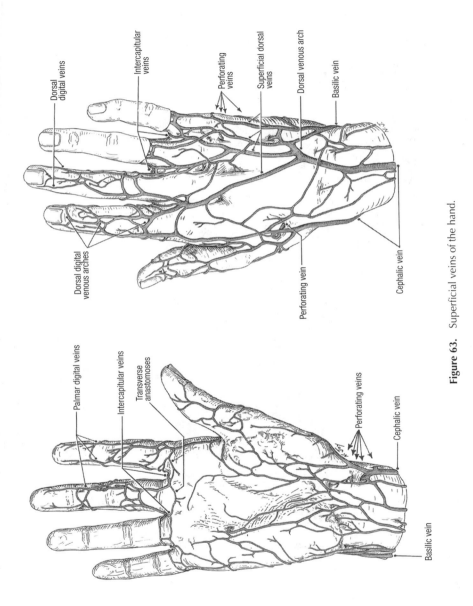

Figure 63. Superficial veins of the hand.

Anatomical Illustrations

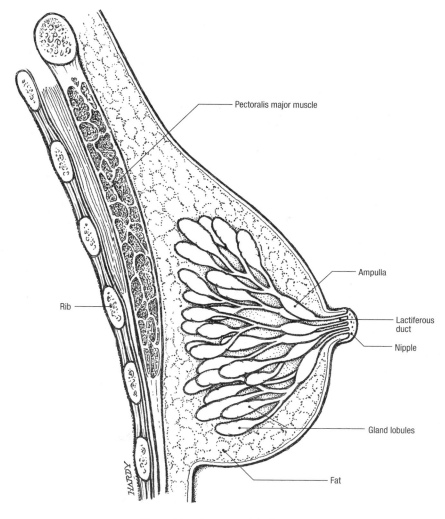

Figure 64. Anatomy of the breast.

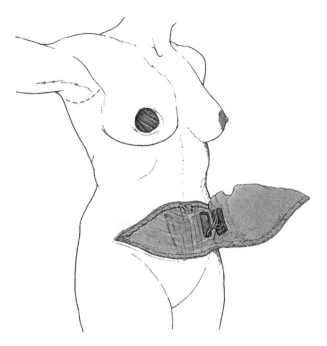

Figure 65. Concept of the skin-sparing mastectomy by using the periareolar approach. In this case, the depicted free TRAM flap is based on the deep inferior epigastric artery and vein.

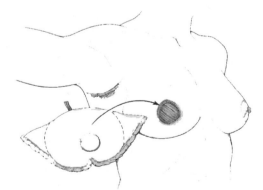

Figure 66. The flap is then passed through the periareolar incision, with the microvascular anastomoses performed through a small separate axillary incision.

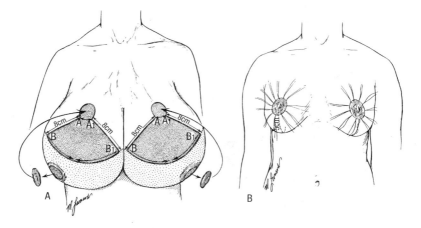

Figure 67. **A,** The width of the breast amputation and dermal pedicle may vary depending on the size of each breast. The nipple-areolas are excised from the breast tissue specimen. **B,** The position of the new nipple-areola site is determined with the patient in a semi-upright position and the nipple-areola specimen placed on the dermal base as a free graft.

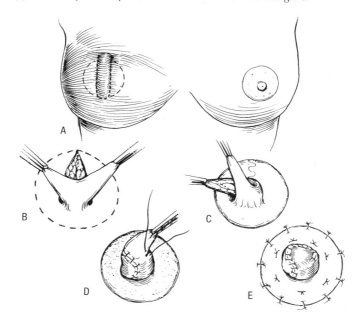

Figure 68. **A,** The redundant area of a TRAM flap is marked for the position of a new areola. **B,** Flaps 1 and 2 are elevated utilizing the redundant TRAM flap tissue. **C,** Flaps 1 and 2 are now interpolated. **D,** The position of new flaps 1 and 2. The surrounding area of areola is deepithelialized. **E,** The newly reconstructed nipple and full-thickness skin graft.

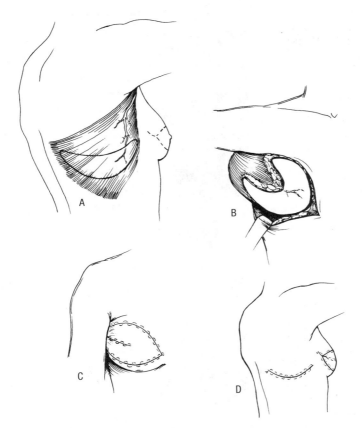

Figure 69. **A,** The latissimus myocutaneous flap outline. **B,** Myocutaneous flap being transferred beneath a lateral axillary skin bridge. **C,** Transferred flap in its new position. **D,** Location of the final incisions.

Anatomical Illustrations

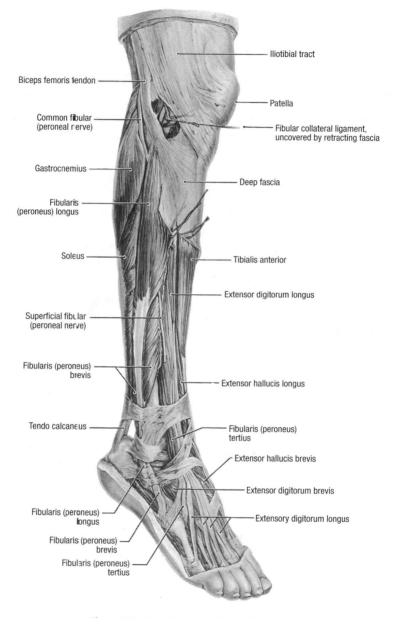

Iliotibial tract

Biceps femoris tendon

Patella

Common fibular (peroneal nerve)

Fibular collateral ligament, uncovered by retracting fascia

Gastrocnemius

Deep fascia

Fibularis (peroneus) longus

Soleus

Tibialis anterior

Extensor digitorum longus

Superficial fibular (peroneal nerve)

Fibularis (peroneus) brevis

Extensor hallucis longus

Tendo calcaneus

Fibularis (peroneus) tertius

Extensor hallucis brevis

Extensor digitorum brevis

Fibularis (peroneus) longus

Extensory digitorum longus

Fibularis (peroneus) brevis

Fibularis (peroneus) tertius

Figure 70. Muscles of the leg and foot.

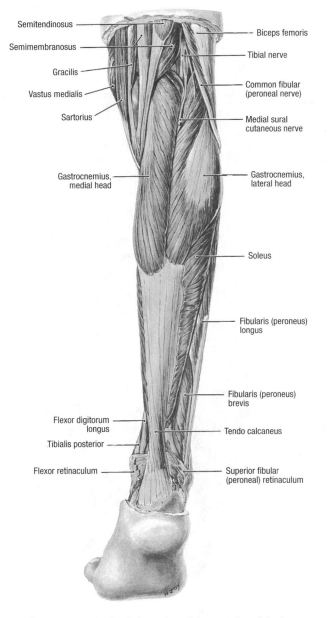

Semitendinosus

Semimembranosus

Gracilis

Vastus medialis

Sartorius

Gastrocnemius, medial head

Flexor digitorum longus

Tibialis posterior

Flexor retinaculum

Biceps femoris

Tibial nerve

Common fibular (peroneal nerve)

Medial sural cutaneous nerve

Gastrocnemius, lateral head

Soleus

Fibularis (peroneus) longus

Fibularis (peroneus) brevis

Tendo calcaneus

Superior fibular (peroneal) retinaculum

Figure 71. Superficial dissection of the muscles of the leg.

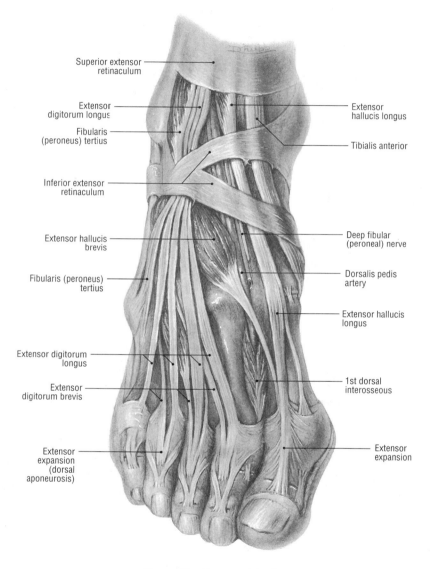

Superior extensor retinaculum

Extensor digitorum longus

Fibularis (peroneus) tertius

Inferior extensor retinaculum

Extensor hallucis brevis

Fibularis (peroneus) tertius

Extensor digitorum longus

Extensor digitorum brevis

Extensor expansion (dorsal aponeurosis)

Extensor hallucis longus

Tibialis anterior

Deep fibular (peroneal) nerve

Dorsalis pedis artery

Extensor hallucis longus

1st dorsal interosseous

Extensor expansion

Figure 72. Dorsum of the foot.

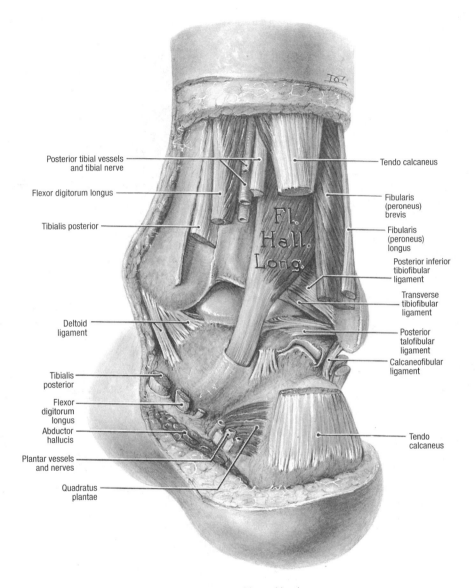

Posterior tibial vessels and tibial nerve

Flexor digitorum longus

Tibialis posterior

Tendo calcaneus

Fibularis (peroneus) brevis

Fibularis (peroneus) longus

Posterior inferior tibiofibular ligament

Transverse tibiofibular ligament

Posterior talofibular ligament

Calcaneofibular ligament

Deltoid ligament

Tibialis posterior

Flexor digitorum longus

Abductor hallucis

Plantar vessels and nerves

Quadratus plantae

Tendo calcaneus

Fl. Hall. Long.

Figure 73. Ankle and heel.

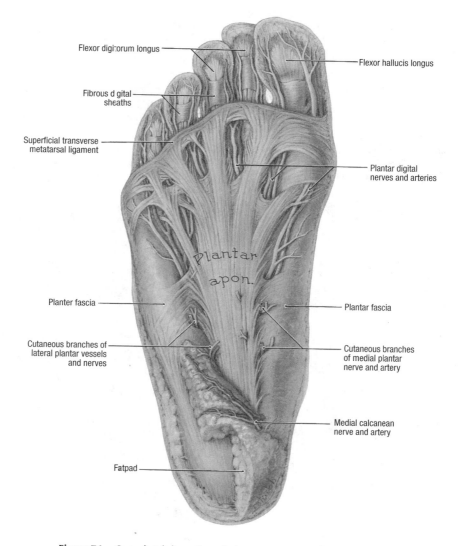

Flexor digitorum longus

Flexor hallucis longus

Fibrous digital sheaths

Superficial transverse metatarsal ligament

Plantar digital nerves and arteries

Planter fascia

Plantar fascia

Cutaneous branches of lateral plantar vessels and nerves

Cutaneous branches of medial plantar nerve and artery

Medial calcanean nerve and artery

Fatpad

Figure 74. Superficial dissection of plantar aspect, or sole, of the foot.

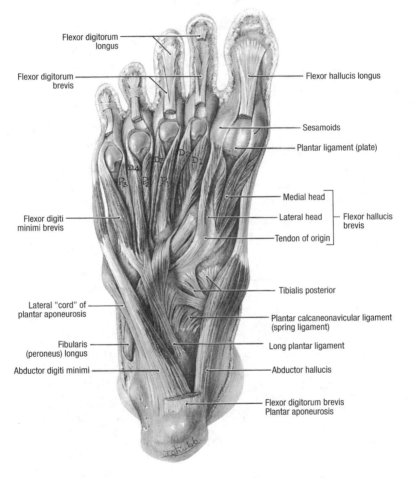

Flexor digitorum longus

Flexor digitorum brevis

Flexor hallucis longus

Sesamoids

Plantar ligament (plate)

Medial head

Lateral head

Tendon of origin

Flexor hallucis brevis

Flexor digiti minimi brevis

Tibialis posterior

Lateral "cord" of plantar aponeurosis

Plantar calcaneonavicular ligament (spring ligament)

Fibularis (peroneus) longus

Long plantar ligament

Abductor digiti minimi

Abductor hallucis

Flexor digitorum brevis Plantar aponeurosis

Figure 75. Fourth layer of plantar muscles.

Anatomical Illustrations

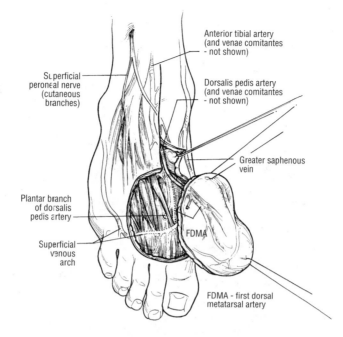

Figure 76. Surgical anatomy of the dorsalis pedis flap.

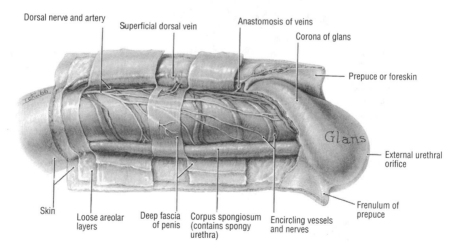

Figure 77. Penis.

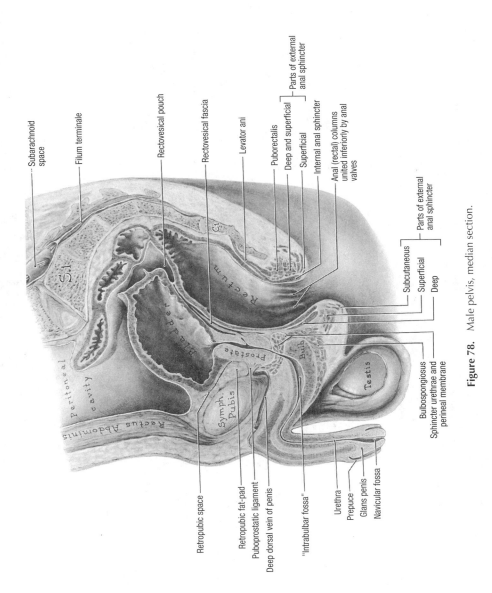

Figure 78. Male pelvis, median section.

Anatomical Illustrations

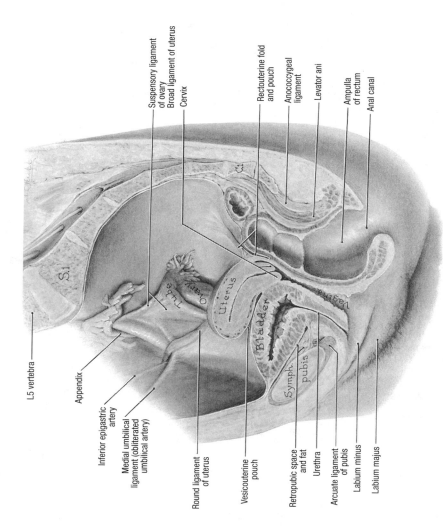

Figure 79. Female pelvis, median section.

Sample Reports

SAMPLE BLEPHAROPLASTY WITH RETRO-ORBICULARIS OCULI FAT PAD RESECTION AND ORBICULOPEXY

TITLE OF OPERATION: Bilateral upper lid blepharoplasty with resection of retro-orbicularis oculi fat pads and bilateral orbiculopexy and bilateral transconjunctival lower lid blepharoplasty.

PREOPERATIVE DIAGNOSIS: Bilateral upper skin excess with extensive retro-orbicularis oculi fat pad and bilateral extensive pseudoherniation of lower lid orbital fat pads.

POSTOPERATIVE DIAGNOSIS: Bilateral upper skin excess with extensive retro-orbicularis oculi fat pad and bilateral extensive pseudoherniation of lower lid orbital fat pads.

INDICATION FOR OPERATION: The patient is a 52-year-old woman well-known to me for previous stages of left breast reconstruction. She had previously indicated interest in possible upper and lower lid blepharoplasty. Examination confirms significant bilateral upper lid skin excess with heavy lateral upper lids consistent with thickened retro-orbicularis oculi fat pad. The patient also has significant pseudoherniation of lower lid orbital fat pads with lower eyelid bulging. The patient has a mild degree of brow ptosis. Correction by bilateral upper lid blepharoplasty with resection of retro-orbicularis oculi fat and bilateral orbiculopexy and bilateral lower lid transconjunctival blepharoplasty for removal of fat pads was recommended. The nature of the procedure and risks, including bleeding, hematoma, infection, poor wound healing, scarring, asymmetry, lid dysfunction, prolonged eye irritation, globe injury, and remote risk of vision loss were all discussed. The patient understands and wishes to proceed as outlined.

PROCEDURE IN DETAIL: After successful general laryngeal mask anesthesia was obtained, the patient was oriented supine on the operating table with the head supported on the doughnut, back raised, and neck slightly extended. Appropriate anatomic landmarks were marked preoperatively. Skin resection was estimated with skin removal resulting in a slight opening of the eyelids on closure. Upper and lower eyelids were then infiltrated with 1% lidocaine with epinephrine. The CO_2 laser in continuous-wave mode 5 watts was used to make upper lid skin incisions along the skin markings. Upper lid skin and orbicularis muscle were then excised together using the carbon dioxide (CO_2) laser. Retro-orbicularis oculi fat pad resection was then initiated with the laser medially. Laterally, resection was completed with electrocautery. The orbital septum was identified and opened over a moistened cotton swab. Upper lid fat pads were then resected over a moist swab. Hemostasis was assured. The lateral orbicularis muscle was sutured to the arcus marginalis of the lateral orbital rim with three 5-0 Vicryl sutures. Closure was then carried out using running 6-0 Prolene.

Attention was then turned to the lower lid, which was distracted from the globe, and the conjunctiva was incised with the cautery at 6 watts continuous-wave, protecting the globe with a Yaeger lid retractor.

Dissection was carried down through the lower lid retractors to the level of the orbital fat. However, fat pockets were entered with immediate bulging of the orbital fat pads. These were resected over a Desmarres retractor external to the inferior orbital rim. The medial, middle, and lateral orbital fat pads were identified and resected, taking the fat back to the level of the orbital rim. Hemostasis was assured. The lower lid was redraped and the ocular shield that had been placed prior to the surgical procedure was removed.

Attention was then turned to the left-hand side. This had been marked for the same amount of skin excision as the right-hand side. The upper lid skin incision was excised with a cautery at 5 watts and the skin and muscle flap removed. Orbital septum was identified, opened, and the orbital fat pads were excised over a moistened cotton swab. The retro-orbicularis oculi fat pad was identified and resected with laser and electrocautery as on the right-hand side. Hemostasis was assured and closure was carried out using running 6-0 Prolene following lateral orbiculopexy as on the right-hand side.

Attention was turned to the lower lid. The conjunctiva was incised with the laser at 6 watts continuous-wave. Orbital fat pads were identified, opened, and resected anterior to the orbital rim using the laser. Hemostasis was achieved with defocusing of the laser beam. Upper and lower lids were compared for amount of fat resection and correction of the lower lid bulge. Lower lid was redraped. Ocular shields were removed. Ophthalmic solution was placed in both eyes. The patient was awakened, extubated, and returned to the recovery room in stable condition. Blood loss was minimal. The procedure was well-tolerated.

SAMPLE RHINOPLASTY

TITLE OF OPERATION: Aesthetic rhinoplasty.

PREOPERATIVE DIAGNOSIS: Congenital external nasal deformity.

POSTOPERATIVE DIAGNOSIS: Congenital external nasal deformity.

INDICATION FOR OPERATION: The patient is a 26-year-old male who presented with concerns for nasal airway obstruction and discontent with the external appearance of his nose. He feels that his nose is excessively long, has excessive projection, has a visible dorsal hump, and bony and cartilage irregularities, and there is excess columellar show, with overly wide and effaced columellar labial angle. Examination confirms the above-noted concerns with a widened nasal base, palpable and visible dorsal cartilage and nasal bones. The patient also had airway complaints, to be addressed with a turbinectomy and septoplasty.

Correction of the external deformity by open rhinoplasty with osteotomy, lowering of the dorsum, lowering of the cartilaginous dorsum, narrowing of the nasal bones, resection and narrowing of the nasal tip, excision of caudal septum and nasal spine were discussed. The patient also wished for shave excision of a benign mole on the right side of the nose. The nature of the procedures and risks, including bleeding, hematoma, infection, poor wound healing, scarring, asymmetry, airway difficulties, palpable or visible nasal structures and possible need for secondary procedures were all discussed. The patient understands and wishes to proceed as outlined.

PROCEDURE IN DETAIL: The patient initially underwent bilateral turbinectomy and septoplasty, which was dictated as a separate procedure. After this was completed, open rhinoplasty was carried out through a columellar chevron incision. The nose was copiously infiltrated with 1% lidocaine with epinephrine prior to incision. The chevron incision was incised and carried to bilateral rim incisions. The nasal skin was then degloved using sharp dissecting scissors. This was opened over the nose up to the root of the nose to allow full exposure. The irregular nasal bones were initially smoothed with a rasp. Excision of the dorsal nasal bone was then carried out using a straight guarded osteotome. Approximately one millimeter thickness of bone was removed. Medial osteotomies were then carried out with a guarded straight osteotome. Lateral osteotomies were then carried out through a lateral broach with a 2-mm osteotome. After osteotomy was completed from a low to high position, infracture of the nasal bones was carried out. This provided good narrowing of the nasal base. The cartilaginous nasal dorsum was then smoothed and brought down, using direct shave excision with a #15 blade under direct vision. Portions of the upper lateral cartilage are also excised. When the dorsum was fully straightened, the upper lateral cartilage was resutured to the septum, using interrupted 6-0 PDS. The nasal fibro-fatty tissue between the lower lateral cartilage was excised. The nasal tip was narrowed, using interrupted 6-0 PDS sutures. The alar domes were also sharpened with narrowing sutures of 6-0 PDS. Dissection was then carried down through the inferior columellar base. The caudal septum was identified, which protruded to the level and to the right of the medial crura. Approximately 3 mm of caudal septum was excised. Dissection was carried down to the anterior nasal spine, which was removed using a bone biter. The medial crura were allowed to drop down and the nose was examined with the skin redraped. The position of the medial crura was identified with the skin redraped and providing a good nasal contour. The degree of overlap was marked and a segment of the medial crura was excised bilaterally. The medial crura were reestablished using interrupted 6-0 PDS sutures to suture the upper elements to the lower and footplate elements of the medial crura. A small piece of septal cartilage was crushed and flattened using the cartilage crusher and this was placed over the nasal dorsum. Contour was again checked and confirmed. Hemostasis was assured. The skin was redraped and closure was carried out using interrupted 6-0 Prolene for the columellar and stab incisions. Interrupted 5-0 plain gut sutures were used to close the rim incisions and the septal transfixion incision. Xeroform packs were removed and nasal splints were placed. A second set of Xeroform packs was placed lateral to the nasal splints. The dorsum of the nose was taped and a dorsal thermoplast splint was also placed. The procedure was well-tolerated. The posterior throat was suctioned and a throat pack that had been placed at the beginning of the procedure was removed. The patient was awakened and extubated and discharged to the recovery room in stable condition.

SAMPLE SEPTOPLASTY AND BILATERAL TURBINECTOMY

TITLE OF OPERATION: Septoplasty and bilateral turbinectomy.

PREOPERATIVE DIAGNOSIS: Nasal airway obstruction, secondary to urbinate hypertrophy and deviated septum.

POSTOPERATIVE DIAGNOSIS: Nasal airway obstruction, secondary to turbinate hypertrophy and deviated septum.

INDICATION FOR OPERATION: The patient is a 26-year-old male who presented for evaluation of a nasal airway obstruction. This has been a long-standing problem and unresponsive to medical therapy. He has been seen by his primary care physician who referred him to plastic surgery for possible evaluation and surgical treatment of his nasal airway obstruction.

Examination revealed a thin male with a relatively long narrow nose. Intranasal exam confirmed a significantly deviated septum with the septum protruding significantly into the left nasal airway with a large septal spur inferiorly. The left turbinate was moderately enlarged. This resulted in a near-complete airway obstruction on the left-hand side. On the right-hand side, the turbinate was very significantly enlarged, producing almost complete obstruction on the right-hand side. Correction of the airway problem by septoplasty, removal of nasal septal spur, probable submucous resection, and bilateral turbinectomy was recommended. The nature of the procedure and risks, including bleeding, hematoma, infection, septal perforation, and persistent airway problems were discussed. The patient understands and wishes to proceed as outlined.

PROCEDURE IN DETAIL: After successful general orolaryngeal anesthesia was achieved, the patient was oriented supine on the operating table with the head supported on the doughnut and the back and shoulders slightly elevated. The facial area was sterilely prepped and draped. Examination with the headlight confirmed deviated septum and enlarged turbinates. The septum and turbinates were copiously infiltrated with 1% lidocaine with epinephrine. A left hemitransfixion incision was carried out approximately 1.5 cm above the end of the caudal septum. This was made with a #15 scalpel blade. The septal mucosa was then elevated to the superior conchae with a Freer elevator. The mucosal elevation was carried down inferiorly and over and around the septal spur. The transfixion incision was carried through the cartilage to the right-hand side below the level of the mucosa. Mucosal elevation was carried out on the left-hand side using the Freer elevator. A swivel knife was then used to excise the most deviated central inferior portion of the cartilage. This was saved. Further removal of the deviated bony septum was carried out using a bone-biting instrument. The inferior cartilaginous spur was also removed. This produced significant improvement in the left nasal airway. A partial excision of the left turbinate was then carried out. A large straight scissors was placed over the protruding half of the turbinate. The turbinate mucosa was excised by straight excision. The raw surface was cauterized.

Attention was turned to the right airway, where the large turbinate was again identified. There was no significant protrusion of the septum on this side. An approximately 3/4 excision of the right turbinate was then carried out using straight scissors. These were placed over the turbinate and straight excision was performed. The mucosal surface was electrocauterized. Xeroform packs were then placed within each naris.

Attention was then turned to the external nose for external rhinoplasty which is dictated as a separate procedure.

SAMPLE OSSEOINTEGRATED DENTAL IMPLANT

TITLE OF OPERATION: Osseointegrated dental implant.

PROCEDURE IN DETAIL: The patient was brought into the operating room and the anesthesiologist started an intravenous anesthesia line. After the patient was inducted the surgeon placed a moistened gauze pack in the patient's throat to prevent povidone-iodine from entering the patient's throat. The patient's face and oral cavity were prepped. Sterile drapes, suction and irrigation tubing, and the dental drill were placed.

The surgeon applied lidocaine and epinephrine to the surgical site then made bilateral incisions on the buccal side of the alveolar processes. Once the incisions were completed to the crest of bone the labial and lingual gingiva were reflected with a periosteal elevator using a #7 wax spatula.

The mucoperiosteal flaps were raised and the incisions were extended to the maxillary frenulum.

The surgeon used a small round bur to mark the site first and then used a 15-mm long 2-mm twist drill with external irrigation. A second guide-pin was placed to check the direction. The final tapping was done by hand. In this case the bone was quite dense so the surgeon tapped 10 mm into the bone. The 15-mm 3.75-diameter implant was a titanium alloy with a treated surface. The implant was then completely seated with profuse irrigation. Cover screws were placed over each implant to prevent tissue from growing into the cylinders of the implants and then the incisions were sutured.

The surgeon removed the throat pack and placed gauze packing between the patient's cheeks and gums. The patient was extubated and moved to the postanesthesia care

SAMPLE AUGMENTATION MAMMOPLASTY

TITLE OF OPERATION: Augmentation mammoplasty.

PREOPERATIVE DIAGNOSIS: Postpartum breast involution.

POSTOPERATIVE DIAGNOSIS: Postpartum breast involution.

INDICATION FOR OPERATION: The patient is a 29-year-old woman who presented for consideration for augmentation mammoplasty. She complained of marked postpartum breast involution. She had been a B-cup prior to pregnancy, and wishes to be in the C-cup range, following augmentation. Examination confirmed marked breast tissue involution, with minimal breast tissue. Patient wishes to have as natural appearing augmentation as possible, without appearing to be over-augmented. After a thorough discussion, McGhan style 468 implant of volume 300 cc was selected. The nature of the procedure and risks, including bleeding, hematoma, infection, poor wound healing, scarring, asymmetry, capsular contracture, implant deflation, visible or palpable implant, and possible need for secondary procedures were all discussed. The patient understands and wishes to proceed as outlined.

PROCEDURE IN DETAIL: The patient was marked preoperatively and brought into the operating room and placed on the operating room table in the supine position. General laryngeal mask anesthesia was then instituted. The chest area was sterilely prepped and draped. The procedure started on the right-hand side where a 4-cm inframammary incision was made just lateral of the mid-nipple line. Dissection was carried down to the subcutaneous tissue using electrocautery. Inferior border of the pectoralis major muscle was identified. The pectoralis major muscle was then elevated off the chest wall using electrocautery. Medial pectoralis attachments were divided. Hemostasis was assured. The pocket was irrigated with bacitracin, saline, and a sterile lap sponge was placed within the pocket.

Attention was then turned to the left-hand side where a similar inframammary incision was made. Dissection was carried out with electrocautery to develop a corresponding submuscular pocket. Attention was then turned back to the right-hand side, where hemostasis was assured and the pocket was then irrigated. A 300-cc McGhan style 468 implant was then selected. This was emptied of all air and checked for leaks. The implant was then rolled and placed through the inframammary incision and unfurled. The implant was then inflated to 310 cc. The implant was appropriately positioned and attention was turned to the right-hand side. Lap sponge was removed. Attention was then turned back to left-hand side. Hemostasis was assured and a pocket appropriately configured. A 300-cc McGhan implant was chosen, checked for leaks, and deflated. This was then rolled, placed within the pocket, unfurled and inflated to 310 cc. Some further modification of the left-side pocket appeared necessary. Therefore, the implant was removed and placed in a bacitracin solution. Further dissection was carried out with electrocautery and the pocket was irrigated with bacitracin saline. The implant was again emptied, unfurled, placed in the inframammary incision, opened and reinflated with total 310 cc of injectable saline.

The patient was then placed in a semi-sitting position and implant positioning was assessed. Appropriate repositioning was carried out to maximize symmetry. Patient was then placed supine and an additional 5 cc was added to each implant for a total volume of 315 cc. Fill tubes were removed. Valve position was checked. Closure was carried out using interrupted 3-0 Vicryl for the fascia, interrupted 3-0 Vicryl for deep dermis, and running 4-0 Prolene subcuticular for each breast incision. The wounds were dressed with Steri-Strips and gauze. The patient was then placed in a supportive Ace wrap. She was awakened, extubated and discharged to the recovery room in stable condition.

Sample Reports

SAMPLE TUMESCENT LIPOSUCTION AND ABDOMINOPLASTY (TUMMY TUCK)

TITLE OF OPERATION:	1. Tumescent liposuction, bilateral hips. 2. Full abdominoplasty.
PREOPERATIVE DIAGNOSIS:	Lower abdominal adipose excess, skin excess, and abdominal wall laxity and adipose excess hips.
POSTOPERATIVE DIAGNOSIS:	Lower abdominal adipose excess, skin excess, and abdominal wall laxity and adipose excess hips.

INDICATION FOR OPERATION: The patient is a 36-year-old woman who presented with concerns of lower abdominal fullness, skin laxity, and fullness in her hip area. She has had prior pregnancies. Examination confirms adipose excess and skin laxity of her lower abdomen with bulging of the abdominal wall, and adipose excess of the hip area. Striae are also present across the lower abdomen and anterior hip area. Correction of these areas by hip liposuction and full contouring was discussed. The nature of the procedure and risks, including bleeding, hematoma, infection, poor wound healing, scarring, asymmetry, umbilical loss, tissue loss, skin rippling, sensory changes, pigmentary changes, and possible need for secondary procedures were all discussed. The patient's incision was planned to lie within the line of a high-cut bathing suit, although she was advised that necessary contouring might result in some extension outside of the bathing suit lines. The patient understands these issues and wishes to proceed as outlined.

PROCEDURE IN DETAIL: The patient was prepped in the standing position and then placed supine on a sterile operating room table. Laryngeal mask anesthesia was obtained. The patient's abdomen and hip area were marked preoperatively. The patient was then placed in the left lateral decubitus position. Tumescent liposuction was then carried out in the right hip area. Dilute lidocaine, epinephrine, and lactated Ringer's solution, 500 cc, was infiltrated into the outlined area. Suction was then carried out using a 3.7-mm cannula, Mercedes-type tip, using multiple passes from multiple directions. Adequate subcutaneous adipose layer was maintained. When good contouring was achieved, the incisions were closed using a single 5-0 nylon suture. A total of 600 cc was aspirated from the right hip.

The patient was then placed in the right lateral decubitus position and the left hip area was approached. Stab incisions were made and the left hip was infiltrated with 550 cc of dilute tumescent fluid. Suctioning was carried out on the right side with a 3.7-mm cannula from multiple directions using cross-tunneling. Appropri-

A64

ate contouring was carried out. Total volume of 600 cc aspirate was removed. The incisions were closed with 5-0 nylon.

The patient was then placed in the supine position with the table flexed and back elevated. The abdominal area was then sterilely re-prepped and draped. The umbilical area was incised with a #15 scalpel blade and the umbilical stalk was separated from the skin down to the abdominal fascia. The low transverse incision was then incised with a #10 scalpel blade. The abdominal skin flap was raised using electrocautery. The umbilical stalk was carefully maintained. The flap was elevated to the costal margin and xiphoid area. The upper central portion of the flap was thinned slightly, using sharp scissors. Hemostasis was assured. The abdominal fascia was then plicated in the midline using a running #1 Prolene from the xiphoid to the umbilicus. A second Prolene suture was used from the umbilicus to the pubis. A narrowing of the waist was carried out by tightening an ellipse of the fascia, just above the umbilicus bilaterally. A 10-mm Jackson-Pratt drain was placed through a stab incision. The abdominal skin was redraped. Skin excess on the flap was excised, along with some additional excess along the upper lateral hip area. Closure was then carried out using interrupted 2-0 Vicryl to close Scarpa fascia. Interrupted 3-0 Monocryl was used to close the deep dermis. Running 3-0 Monocryl was used to close the transverse incision. The umbilicus was closed using interrupted 3-0 Vicryl for the deep dermis and a running 5-0 chromic suture. Then 10 cc of 0.25% Marcaine was infiltrated along the fascia on either side of the plication sutures. After closure of the abdominal incision, 40 cc of Marcaine was infiltrated into the drain, which was clamped. The wounds were dressed with Steri-Strips and sterile gauze. The patient was placed in foam over the hips with an abdominal binder. She was then awakened, extubated, and discharged from the operating room in stable condition.

SAMPLE TUMESCENT SYRINGE LIPOSUCTION

TITLE OF OPERATION:	Tumescent syringe liposuction of bilateral hips, abdomen, and bilateral thigh area.
PREOPERATIVE DIAGNOSIS:	Adipose excess bilateral hips, abdomen, and bilateral lateral thigh area.
POSTOPERATIVE DIAGNOSIS:	Adipose excess bilateral hips, abdomen, and bilateral lateral thigh area.

INDICATION FOR OPERATION: Patient is a 53-year-old woman who is seen for evaluation of relative adipose excess in the hip, abdomen, and lateral thigh areas. Examination confirmed relative adipose excess in these areas with significant bulging in the hip and lateral thigh and lower abdominal areas. Skin elasticity is judged to be good. Correction of this deformity by tumescent liposuction of these areas was discussed. The nature of the procedure and risks, including bleeding, hematoma, infection, poor wound healing, scarring, tissue loss, asymmetry, skin irregularity, sensory or pigmentary changes and uneven skin contour were all discussed. The patient is noted to have some skin irregularity and cellulite-type changes in the posterior thigh regions. The patient understands these issues and wishes to proceed as outlined.

PROCEDURE IN DETAIL: The patient was prepped in the standing position and then placed supine on the sterile OR table. General laryngeal mask anesthesia was then introduced. The procedure started in the abdominal area with tumescent infiltration of 800 cc of dilute lidocaine/epinephrine and lactated Ringer's. Total volume of 800 cc was infused. Tumescent syringe-type liposuction was then carried out using 3.7-mm cannulas through multiple sites in multiple directions. Cross-tunneling was carried out while maintaining adequate subcutaneous adipose layer. After good contour was achieved, the patient was placed in the left lateral decubitus position. Tumescent fluid was then infiltrated into the right hip and right lateral thigh areas. A total of 600 cc and 800 cc was infiltrated into each area, respectively. Syringe liposuction was then carried out using 3.7-mm cannulas. This was carried out through multiple sites in multiple directions with cross-tunneling and careful maintenance of adequate subcutaneous tissue layer. Suctioning was carried out first in the hip and lateral thigh area. Suctioning was continued until satisfactory contour was achieved. Aspirates were slightly blood tinged at completion. The patient was then placed in the right lateral decubitus position and the left hip and lateral thigh areas were again infiltrated with dilute tumescent fluid 600 cc in the hip and 800 cc in the lateral thigh area. Suctioning was then carried out using 3.7-mm cannulas. The hip was suctioned initially and the lateral thigh was then suctioned. Suctioning was carried out with cross-tunneling through multiple sites. Some additional contouring and smoothing in the posterior left thigh area was also carried out using a 3-mm cannula. This was performed to correct some existing skin irregularity. A total of 1,200 cc was aspirated from the left lateral thigh and 700 cc from the left hip area. On the right hip a total of 675 cc was aspirated from the hip and 950 cc from the lateral thigh area. All incision sites were closed with a single 5-0 nylon. These were dressed with sterile gauze. The patient was placed in foam and a compression garment. She was then awakened, extubated, and discharged to the recovery area in stable condition. Total intraoperative IV fluid was 700 cc. The procedure was well-tolerated.

Common Terms by Procedure

Blepharoplasty Terms
arcus marginalis
blepharoplasty
brow ptosis
carbon dioxide laser (CO_2 laser)
continuous-wave mode
defocusing
Desmarres (pronounced Dah-Mah-Rah)
eyelid
fat pad
globe
laryngeal mask anesthesia
left-hand side
lid dysfunction
lidocaine with epinephrine
moist swab
ocular shield
orbicularis oculi
orbiculopexy
orbital rim
Prolene
pseudoherniation
retro-orbicularis oculi resection
right-hand side
skin markings
Vicryl

Rhinoplasty Terms
aesthetic rhinoplasty
airway difficulties
ala, pl. alae
alar dome
asymmetry
bone biter
bone-biting instrument
broach
cartilage
caudal septum
chevron incision

columella
columellar show
contour
crus, pl. crura
deglove
fibrofatty
footplate
infracture
nasal tip
nasal spine
nasal dorsum
osteotome
palpable nasal structure
PDS suture
plain gut suture
projection
rasp
secondary procedure
shave excision
skin redrape
splint
stab incision
thermoplast
visible nasal structure
Xeroform pack

Septoplasty Terms
airway obstruction
bone-biting instrument
cartilaginous spur
concha, pl. conchae
doughnut
Freer elevator
hemitransfixion incision
mucosal elevation
naris, pl. nares
septal mucosa
septoplasty
septum
straight scissors

submucous resection
swivel knife
transfixion incision
turbinate
turbinated bone
turbinectomy
Xeroform

Osseointegrated Dental Implant Terms

alveolar processes
bilateral incisions
buccal
bur
cover screws
crest of bone
extender
guide-pin
hard palate
implant fixtures
irrigation unit
labial gingiva
lingual gingiva
maxillary frenulum
mucoperiosteal
periosteal elevator
povidone-iodine
root tip
round bur
screw inserter
sublingual gland
submandibular gland
titanium alloy
twist drill
vestibule
wax spatula

Augmentation Mammoplasty Terms

asymmetry
augmentation
B-cup
bacitracin

breast tissue involution
C-cup
capsular contracture
chest wall
deep dermis
deflated
electrocautery
extubated
fascia
fill tube
hematoma
implant valve
implant position
inflated
inframmary incision
left-hand side
mammoplasty
McGhan implant
mid-nipple line
natural-appearing
palpable implant
pectoralis major muscle
pocket
Prolene
right-hand side
scarring
semi-sitting position
Steri-Strips
subcuticular
supportive Ace wrap
symmetry
unfurled
visible implant

Tumescent Liposuction and Abdominoplasty (Tummy Tuck) Terms

abdominal binder
abdominal fascia
abdominoplasty
adipose excess
aspirate
asymmetry
chromic suture

A69

Common Terms by Procedure

costal margin
cross-tunneling
ellipse
foam dressing
hematoma
high-cut bathing suit
Jackson-Pratt drain
lactated Ringer solution
lidocaine
Mercedes-tip cannula
Monocryl
pigmentary changes
plicate
plication suture
Scarpa fascia
secondary procedure
sharp scissors
skin redrape
skin rippling
skin laxity
stab incision
Steri-Strips
stria, pl. striae
tissue loss
tumescent liposuction
umbilical stalk
umbilical loss

umbilicus
Vicryl
xiphoid area

Tumescent Syringe Liposuction Terms

adipose
adipose excess
adiposity
aspirate
blood tinged
blood-tinged aspirate
cannula
cellulite
compression garment
contouring
cross-tunneling
epinephrine
lactated Ringer solution
lidocaine
skin irregularity
skin elasticity
smoothing
subcutaneous tissue
suction, suctioning, suctioned
tumescent syringe liposuction
tumescent fluid

Appendix 4
Common Herbs

Common Name	Latin Name
anise	*Pimpinella anisum*
black cohosh	*Cimicifuga racemosa*
alfalfa	*Medicago sativa*
arnica	*Arnica montana*
balm, lemon	*Melissa officinalis*
barberry	*Berberis vulgaris*
bayberry	*Myrica cerifera, M. pensylvanicum*
bearberry or uva-ursi	*Arctostaphylos uva-ursi*
belladonna	*Atropa belladonna*
bilberry	*Vaccinium myrtillus*
bladderwrack	*Fucus vesiculosus*
blue cohosh	*Caulophyllum thalictroides*
blue flag, iris	*Iris versicolor*
bloodroot	*Sanguinaria canadensis*
burdock	*Arctium lappa*
buckthorn, cascara sagrada	*Rhamnus purshiana*
butcher's broom	*Ruscus aculeatus*
cactus	*Selenicereus grandiflorus*
calendula	*Calendula officinalis*
cayenne	*Capsicum frutescens*
celery	*Apium graveolens*
chamomile	*Matricaria recutita*
chaparral	*Larrea tridentata*
chaste tree berry	*Vitex agnus-castus*
cherry, wild	*Prunus serotina*
cleavers	*Gallium aparine*
clover, red	*Trifolium pratense*
coltsfoot	*Tussilago farfara*
couchgrass	*Agropyron repens*
crampbark	*Viburnum opulus*
comfrey	*Symphytum officinale*
damiana	*Turnera diffusa*
dandelion	*Taraxacum officinale*
devil's claw	*Harpagophytum procumbens*
dong quai	*Angelica sinensis*
eyebright	*Euphrasia officinalis*
elecampane	*Inula helenium*
false unicorn root	*Helonias dioica*
fennel	*Foeniculum vulgare*

Common Herbs

feverfew	*Tanacetum parthenium*
garlic	*Allium sativum*
ginger	*Zingiber officinalis*
feverfew	*Chrysanthemum parthenium*
ginseng, American	*Panax quinquefolius*
ginseng, Asian	*Panax ginseng*
ginseng, Siberian	*Eleutherococcus senticosus*
goldenseal	*Hydrastis canadensis*
juniper berries	*Juniperus communis*
hawthorn berry	*Crataegus laevigata* or *Crataegus oxyacantha*
horse chestnut	*Aesculus hippocastanum*
horsetail	*Equisetum arvense*
kava-kava	*Piper methysticum*
lavender	*Lavandula officinalis*
licorice	*Glycyrrhiza glabra*
licorice, gastrointestinal	*Glcyrrhiza uralensis*
lungwort	*Pulmonaria officinalis*
marsh mallow	*Althaea officinalis*
milk thistle	*Silybum marianum*
nettle	*Urtica dioica*
old man's beard	*Usnea spp.*
onion	*Allium cepa*
osha	*Ligusticum porterii*
pau d'arco	*Tabebuia impetiginosa*
passionflower	*Passiflora incarnata*
peppermint	*Mentha piperita*
pleurisy root	*Asclepias tuberosa*
purple cone flower	*Echinacea angustifolia*
red clover	*Trifolium pratense*
rosemary	*Rosmarinus officinalis*
red raspberry	*Rubus strigosus*
saffron	*Crocus sativus*
saw palmetto	*Serenoa repens*
sarsaparilla	*Smilax officinalis*
senna	*Cassia senna*
St. John's wort	*Hypericum perforatum*
shepherd's purse	*Capsella bursa-pastoris*
skullcap	*Scutellaria lateriflora*
slippery elm	*Ulmus fulva*
squaw vine	*Mitchella repens*
thyme	*Thymus vulgaris*
turmeric	*Curcuma domestica*
yarrow	*Achillea millefolium*
yellow dock or sour dock	*Rumex crispus*